# Evidence-Based Practice in Cardiac Surgery

# Evidence-Based Practice in Cardiac Surgery

Editor: Jessica Clan

AMERICAN
MEDICAL PUBLISHERS
www.americanmedicalpublishers.com

AMERICAN
MEDICAL PUBLISHERS
www.americanmedicalpublishers.com

**Cataloging-in-Publication Data**

Evidence-based practice in cardiac surgery / edited by Jessica Clan.
p. cm.
Includes bibliographical references and index.
ISBN 979-8-88740-116-4
1. Heart--Surgery. 2. Cardiovascular system--Surgery. 3. Hemostasis, Surgical.
4. Surgery, Operative. 5. Heart--Diseases--Treatment. 6. Evidence-based medicine.
7. Cardiology. I. Clan, Jessica.
RD598 .E95 2023
617.412--dc23



American Medical Publishers,
41 Flatbush Avenue,
1st Floor, New York,
NY 11217, USA

ISBN 979-8-88740-116-4 (Hardback)

## Contents

# Preface

This book was inspired by the evolution of our times; to answer the curiosity of inquisitive minds. Many developments have occurred across the globe in the recent past which has transformed the progress in the field.

A surgical process that involves the heart or the blood vessels that carry blood to and from the heart is called cardiovascular surgery or cardiac surgery. This form of surgery is used for treating complex diseases such as ischemic heart disease, congenital heart disease, valvular heart disease, etc. There are various types of cardiac surgeries including open-heart surgery, heart transplant, coronary artery bypass grafting (CABG), and minimally invasive surgery. Advancements in cardiac surgery and cardiopulmonary bypass techniques have remarkably lowered the mortality rates of these procedures. Neurological damage is one of the major concerns associated with cardiac surgery. Another complication related to cardiopulmonary bypass is postperfusion syndrome. Postoperative pulmonary complications such as pneumonia and atelectasis can be reduced by non-pharmacological approaches. Preventive approaches such as preoperative physical therapy and avoidance of smoking can reduce the risk of atrial fibrillation after an operation. This book will be of immense help as a guiding source for students, and surgeons in the sphere of cardiac surgery. Those in search of information to further their knowledge will be greatly assisted by it.

This book was developed from a mere concept to drafts to chapters and finally compiled together as a complete text to benefit the readers across all nations. To ensure the quality of the content we instilled two significant steps in our procedure. The first was to appoint an editorial team that would verify the data and statistics provided in the book and also select the most appropriate and valuable contributions from the plentiful contributions we received from authors worldwide. The next step was to appoint an expert of the topic as the Editor-in-Chief, who would head the project and finally make the necessary amendments and modifications to make the text reader-friendly. I was then commissioned to examine all the material to present the topics in the most comprehensible and productive format.

I would like to take this opportunity to thank all the contributing authors who were supportive enough to contribute their time and knowledge to this project. I also wish to convey my regards to my family who have been extremely supportive during the entire project.

**Editor**

1

# Mitral Valve Surgery in Patients with Rheumatic Heart Disease: Repair vs. Replacement

*Guangguo Fu* [1,2†], *Zhuoming Zhou* [1,2†], *Suiqing Huang* [1,2], *Guangxian Chen* [1,2], *Mengya Liang* [1,2], *Lin Huang* [1,2] *and Zhongkai Wu* [1,2*]

[1] Department of Cardiac Surgery, First Affiliated Hospital of Sun Yat-sen University, Guangzhou, China, [2] NHC Key Laboratory of Assisted Circulation, Sun Yat-sen University, Guangzhou, China

***Correspondence:**
Zhongkai Wu
wuzhk@mail.sysu.edu.cn

† These authors have contributed equally to this work and share first authorship

**Background:** High morbidity and mortality caused by rheumatic heart disease (RHD) are global burdens, especially in low-income and developing countries. Whether mitral valve repair (MVP) benefits RHD patients remains controversial. Thus, we performed a meta-analysis to compare the perioperative and long-term outcomes of MVP and mitral valve replacement (MVR) in RHD patients.

**Methods and Results:** A systematic literature search was conducted in major databases, including Embase, PubMed, and the Cochrane Library, until 17 December 2020. Studies comparing MVP and MVR in RHD patients were retained. Outcomes included early mortality, long-term survival, freedom from reoperation, postoperative infective endocarditis, thromboembolic events, hemorrhagic events, and freedom from valve-related adverse events. Eleven studies that met the inclusion criteria were included. Of a total of 5,654 patients, 1,951 underwent MVP, and 3,703 underwent MVR. Patients who undergo MVP can benefit from a higher long-term survival rate (HR 0.72; 95% CI, 0.55–0.95; $P = 0.020$; $I^2 = 44\%$), a lower risk of early mortality (RR 0.62; 95% CI, 0.38–1.01; $P = 0.060$; $I^2 = 42\%$), and the composite outcomes of valve-related adverse events (HR 0.60; 95% CI, 0.38–0.94; $P = 0.030$; $I^2 = 25\%$). However, a higher risk of reoperation was observed in the MVP group (HR 2.60; 95% CI, 1.89–3.57; $P<0.001$; $I^2 = 4\%$). Patients who underwent concomitant aortic valve replacement (AVR) in the two groups had comparable long-term survival rates, although the trend still favored MVP.

**Conclusions:** For RHD patients, MVP can reduce early mortality, and improve long-term survival and freedom from valve-related adverse events. However, MVP was associated with a higher risk of reoperation.

**Systematic Review Registration**: https://www.crd.york.ac.uk/PROSPERO/display_record.php?RecordID=228307.

**Keywords: mitral valve, repair, replacement, rheumatic heart disease, meta-analysis**

## INTRODUCTION

Currently, more than 30 million patients worldwide suffer from rheumatic heart disease (RHD), which leads to approximately 300,000 deaths and 10 million disabilities every year (1). High morbidity and mortality caused by RHD are global burdens, especially in low-income and developing countries (1–3). As RHD progresses, it can cause severe mitral stenosis (MS) and/or mitral regurgitation (MR) (4) and concomitantly affects more than 30% of patients' aortic valves

(5). Although the current American College of Cardiology/American Heart Association guidelines prioritize the use of percutaneous mitral balloon commissurotomy (PMBC) for the intervention of RHD-related conditions (6), the use of this safe and effective method is restricted by the absence of left atrium thrombus and calcification and the severity of MR (7). Patients require surgical treatment when they reach New York Heart Association functional class III/IV, with surgical indications including severe calcification, concomitant valve/coronary disease, or previous unsuccessful PMBC (6, 7). Mitral valve replacement (MVR) and mitral valve repair (MVP) are the most widely used and effective surgical methods. The standard MVP techniques included commissurotomy, subvalvular debridement, ring annuloplasty, artificial chordae replacement, and release of subvalvular apparatus. Mitral valve repair (MVP) often requires different techniques according to the specific pathological features of the valves in different patients. Because MVP employs a higher-level surgical techniques than MVR and is based on a personalized surgical protocol and a higher level of professional knowledge, the MVP rate is limited by the surgeon's and institutional experience (8). The application of MVP in RHD is technically more difficult than that of MVR since lesions of the valve and subvalvular apparatus in RHD are severer than those in non-RHD disease (9, 10). Although MVP is recommended over MVR for degenerative mitral valve disease (11–13), whether MVP benefits patients with RHD remains controversial, and current guidelines do not provide clear recommendations. Therefore, we conducted a meta-analysis based current studies, with the aim of comparing the perioperative and long-term outcomes of MVP and MVR in patients with RHD.

## MATERIALS AND METHODS

### Search Strategy

This meta-analysis was performed based on the Preferred Reporting Items for Systematic reviews and Meta-Analyses (PRISMA) guidelines and has been registered at the International Prospective Register of Systematic Reviews (PROSPERO), number CRD42021228307. A systematic literature search was conducted in major databases, including Embase, PubMed, and the Cochrane Library, until 17 December 2020. The following key terms were used: [RHD OR rheumatic OR (rheumatic heart disease) OR (rheumatic heart diseases) OR (Bouillaud's disease) OR (Bouillauds disease) OR (Bouillaud disease)] AND [annuloplasty OR annuloplasties OR (annulus repair) OR repair OR replacement] AND [mitral OR (mitral valve) OR (mitral valve surgery) OR (mitral valve reconstruction)]. Reference lists of relevant studies were also browsed to reduce possible omissions.

### Selection Criteria and Quality Assessment

The study inclusion criteria were as follows: (1) studies comparing MVP and MVR for patients with RHD; (2) patients over 15 years old; and (3) reporting of at least one of the following outcomes: early mortality, long-term survival, reoperation, postoperative infective endocarditis (IE), thromboembolic events, hemorrhagic events, and Kaplan-Meier curves of long-term survival or all-cause mortality. The exclusion criteria were as follows: (1) studies not published in English and (2) reviews, case reports, conference abstracts, and letters. When two studies came from the same institution and had overlapping populations, only the latest study was retained. All studies were screened independently by two authors (GF and ZZ), and all differences were resolved through discussion. The quality of each included study was evaluated and scored using the Newcastle-Ottawa Scale (NOS) checklist.

### Definition of Outcomes

The outcomes were defined as follows. Early mortality was defined as 30-day mortality after surgery due to any cause. Long-term survival was used to describe the survival time from discharge to death from any cause. Freedom from reoperation was considered freedom from reoperation involving the mitral valve. Valve-related adverse events included infective endocarditis, thromboembolic events (cerebral infarction, peripheral embolism, valve thrombosis, and transient ischemic attack) and hemorrhagic events (any serious bleeding event that resulted in death, hospitalization, permanent injury, or required blood transfusion).

### Data Extraction

The following data were extracted: lead author, publication year, country, study period, number of participants, follow-up years, study design, age, sex, diabetes mellitus, atrial fibrillation, MR, MS, MR+MS, concomitant aortic valve replacement (AVR), concomitant tricuspid valve repair (TVP), and the outcomes mentioned in the inclusion criteria. All data extraction was completed by two authors (GF and ZZ). Calibration was carried out after extraction, and any disagreements between the two authors were resolved by discussion or by seeking the opinion of another author (SH) until a consensus was reached.

### Statistical Analysis

Statistical analysis was performed by RevMan (version 5.4.1). A random-effects model with Mantel-Haenszel weighting was used to estimate the overall risk ratio (RR) and 95% confidence intervals (CIs) for variables with dichotomous outcomes, including early mortality, IE, thromboembolic events, and hemorrhagic events. For studies that did not directly report adjusted hazard risks (HRs), we obtained data from digitized Kaplan-Meier curves produced by Engauge Digitizer software (version 12.1) and then estimated the HRs according to the method introduced by Tierney et al. (14). Similarly, a random-effects model with Inverse-Variance weighting was used to calculate the overall HR and 95% CIs for long-term survival, freedom from reoperation and freedom from valve-related adverse events. Heterogeneity was investigated by the chi$^2$ test and quantified by the $I^2$ statistic. The heterogeneity and overall RR/HR described above are presented as forest plots. Additionally, we reconstructed the aggregated Kaplan-Meier curves by time, survival rate, and number at risk using the MetaSurv package from R software (version 3.6.3). Publication bias is shown by a funnel plot and was assessed statistically

**TABLE 1** | Main characteristics of the included studies.

| Studies | Patients MVP/MVR (*n*) | Country | Study period | Mean follow-up years | Study design | NOS scores |
|---|---|---|---|---|---|---|
| Brescia 2020 | 80/100 | USA | 1997.9–2018.3 | 5.0 ± 3.9 | Unmatched | 8 |
| Chen 2020 | 467/467 | China (Taiwan) | 2000.1–2013.12 | 5.9 ± 4.2/5.8 ± 4.2 | PSM | 8 |
| Fu 2020 | 529/529 | China | 2011.1–2019.4 | median 4.12 | PSM | 8 |
| Kim 2018 | 188/188 | South Korea | 1997.1–2015.12 | 10.9 ± 2.3 | PSM | 8 |
| Russell 2017 | 119/1078 | Australia | 2001.6–2013.12 | NA | Unmatched | 7 |
| Geldenhuys 2012 | 69/69 | South Africa | 2000.1–2010.12 | 4.4 ± 3.0 | PSM | 9 |
| Wang 2008 | 33/59 | China (Taiwan) | 1997.11–2005.7 | 2.8 ± 2.1/3.1 ± 1.8 | Unmatched | 7 |
| Kuwaki 2007 | 47/81 | Japan | 1981–2003 | 9.1 ± 4.2/9.1 ± 4.6 | Unmatched | 7 |
| Talwar 2007 | 76/293 | India | 1995.1–2005.12 | 5.8 ± 3.4/4.3 ± 3.1 | Unmatched | 8 |
| Ho 2004 | 201/408 | Vietnam | 1992–2001 | 9.0 | Unmatched | 7 |
| Yau 2000 | 142/431 | Canada | 1978.10–1995.6 | 5.7 ± 3.8 | Unmatched | 8 |

*MVP, mitral valve repair; MVR, mitral valve replacement; NA, not available; NOS, Newcastle-Ottawa Scale; PSM, propensity score matching (13, 15–24).*

by Begg's test and Egger's test in Stata (version SE 15.1). Sensitivity analysis was conducted by excluding the studies with the largest proportions or those most likely to be biased and then reanalyzing the data. Subgroup analysis was performed based on different study designs, including propensity score matching (PSM) or unmatched studies, and whether concomitant AVR was performed in all patients.

# RESULTS

## Study Characteristics

Through preliminary searches, a total of 1,159 relevant records were collected, of which 11 studies (13, 15–24) that met the inclusion criteria were included in our meta-analysis (**Supplementary Figure 1**). Among the eleven studies, four were based on PSM analysis, and seven were unmatched (**Table 1**). In addition, three studies focused on patients who had undergone mitral valve surgery with concomitant AVR (**Table 2**). In total, 5,654 patients were included, including 1,951 who underwent MVP and 3,703 who underwent MVR. The baseline characteristics of the included patients are presented in **Table 2**, and the quality assessment scores are presented in **Supplementary Table 2**.

## Early Mortality

Ten studies were included in the analysis of early mortality (6,829 patients, 1,977 underwent MVP and 4,852 underwent MVR). The results indicated a trend in favor of MVP (RR 0.62; 95% CI, 0.38–1.01; $P = 0.060$; $I^2 = 42\%$) (**Figure 1A**), although no significant difference between the two groups was found. Mild heterogeneity was observed.

## Long-Term Survival

A total of eleven studies were included (5,654 patients, 1,951 underwent MVP and 3,703 underwent MVR), of which four directly provided adjusted HRs; for the others, the HR-value and 95% CI were estimated from Kaplan-Meier curves. The analysis of these studies found that the MVP group had a significantly higher long-term survival rate than the MVR group (HR 0.72; 95% CI, 0.55–0.95; $P = 0.020$; $I^2 = 44\%$) (**Figure 1B**). However, a significant difference was not found in PSM studies (HR 0.62; 95% CI, 0.35–1.11; $P = 0.110$; $I^2 = 70\%$) or unmatched studies (HR 0.75; 95% CI, 0.55–1.03; $P = 0.080$; $I^2 = 15\%$). In addition, a significant difference was observed in the non-AVR group (HR 0.71; 95% CI, 0.52–0.98; $P = 0.040$; $I^2 = 51\%$), but not in the AVR group (HR 0.76; 95% CI, 0.39–1.49; $P = 0.42$; $I^2 = 35\%$) (**Figure 2A**). There was moderate heterogeneity in the PSM studies and the non-AVR group and mild heterogeneity in the overall result and the AVR group. Reconstructed Kaplan-Meier curves derived from 10 studies showed that the long-term survival rates at 4, 8, and 12 years were 90.11, 82.95, and 75.73%, respectively, in the MVP group and 88.78, 82.53, and 72.45%, respectively, in the MVR group (**Figure 4A**).

## Freedom From Reoperation

Ten studies were included (4,457 patients, 1,832 underwent MVP and 2,625 underwent MVR), of which four directly provided adjusted HRs or subdistribution hazard ratio (SHRs); in the other six, HRs and 95% CIs were estimated from Kaplan-Meier curves. The analysis of these studies indicated that the MVP group had a significantly higher reoperation rate than the MVR group (HR 2.60; 95% CI, 1.89–3.57; $P < 0.001$; $I^2 = 4\%$) (**Figure 1C**). A higher rate in the MVP group was also observed in the subgroups of PSM studies (HR 2.59; 95% CI, 1.27–5.27; $P = 0.009$; $I^2 = 38\%$), unmatched studies (HR 2.42; 95% CI, 1.69–3.48; $P < 0.001$; $I^2 = 0\%$), the AVR group (HR 2.82; 95% CI, 1.08–7.36; $P = 0.030$; $I^2 = 0\%$), and the non-AVR group (HR 2.60; 95% CI, 1.71–3.97; $P < 0.001$; $I^2 = 23\%$) (**Figure 2B**). There was mild heterogeneity in the PSM studies. Reconstructed Kaplan-Meier curves derived from 10 studies showed that the freedom from reoperation rates at 4, 8, and 12 years were 94.27, 87.87, and 74.45%, respectively, in the MVP group and 96.94, 92.74, and 86.66%, respectively, in the MVR group (**Figure 4B**).

## Freedom From Valve-Related Adverse Events

Five studies were included in the analysis of IE, seven studies were included in the analysis of thromboembolic events, and six studies were included in the analysis of hemorrhagic events.

**TABLE 2** | Baseline characteristics of patients.

| Studies | Patients (*n*) | | Age (years) | | Female (%) | | DM (%) | | MR (%) | | MS (%) | | MR+MS (%) | | AF (%) | | CS AVR (%) | | CS TVP (%) | |
|---|---|---|---|---|---|---|---|---|---|---|---|---|---|---|---|---|---|---|---|---|
| | MVP | MVR | MVP | MVR | MVP | MVR | MVP | MVR | MVP | MVR | MVP | MVR | MVP | MVR | MVP | MVR | MVP | MVR | MVP | MVR |
| Brescia 2020 | 80 | 100 | NA | NA | NA | NA | NA | NA | NA | NA | NA | NA | NA | NA | NA | NA | NA | NA | NA | NA |
| Chen 2020 | 467 | 467 | 56.8 ± 14.2 | 56.7 ± 13.8 | 53.1 | 55.9 | 14.6 | 16.5 | 19.3 | 18.8 | 65.1 | 65.5 | 15.6 | 15.6 | 57.4 | 58.0 | 22.1 | 21.0 | 26.3 | 27.2 |
| Fu 2020 | 529 | 529 | 54.5 ± 10.9 | 54.6 ± 10.0 | 72.2 | 72.2 | 10.0 | 13.0 | 12.7 | 10.2 | 10.4 | 11.9 | 76.9 | 77.9 | 67.9 | 69.6 | 18.9 | 19.8 | 91.1 | 89.2 |
| Kim 2018 | 188 | 188 | 48.8 ± 3.4 | 47.6 ± 2.1 | 71.8 | 75.5 | 11.7 | 13.8 | 50.5 | 47.3 | 30.3 | 33.0 | 19.1 | 19.7 | 64.9 | 63.8 | 23.4 | 20.2 | 38.3 | 35.6 |
| Russell 2017 | 119 | 1078 | 57.3 | 62.0 | 58.0 | 73.1 | 14.3 | 21.1 | 81.5 | 63.9 | 25.2 | 75.3 | NA | NA | 26.1 | 48.9 | NA | NA | NA | NA |
| Geldenhuys 2012 | 69 | 69 | 36.9 ± 14.5 | 40.9 ± 11.7 | 78.3 | 84.1 | NA | NA | 39.0 | 13.0 | 3.0 | 7.0 | 27.0 | 49.0 | 29.0 | 39.0 | NA | NA | 6.0 | 13.0 |
| Wang 2008 | 33 | 59 | 49.7 ± 13.2 | 58.1 ± 11.2 | 63.7 | 66.1 | 12.1 | 6.8 | NA | NA | NA | NA | NA | NA | 93.9 | 96.6 | NA | NA | 45.5 | 61.0 |
| Kuwaki 2007 | 47 | 81 | 48.0 ± 10.0 | 53.0 ± 8.0 | 70.2 | 58.0 | 2.1 | 7.4 | 8.5 | 6.2 | 83.0 | 54.3 | 8.5 | 39.5 | NA | NA | 100 | 100 | 17.0 | 40.7 |
| Talwar 2007 | 76 | 293 | 30.3 ± 10.4 | 32.5 ± 10.7 | 30.3 | 27.8 | NA | NA | 15.8 | 13.2 | 40.8 | 44.4 | 43.4 | 42.4 | 48.7 | 38.3 | 100 | 100 | NA | NA |
| Ho 2004 | 201 | 408 | 32.2 ± 10.4 | 38.7 ± 8.6 | 46.3 | 44.4 | NA | NA | 37.4 | 12.7 | 30.3 | 59.1 | 32.3 | 28.2 | 36.8 | 60.3 | 100 | 100 | 28.9 | 32.4 |
| Yau 2000 | 142 | 431 | 42.0 ± 13.1 | 57.9 | 85.0 | 79.6 | NA | NA | 16.2 | 14.8 | 67.6 | 48.0 | 16.2 | 37.1 | NA | NA | NA | NA | 7.8 | 17.6 |

*MVP, mitral valve repair; MVR, mitral valve replacement; NA, not available; DM, diabetes mellitus; MR, mitral regurgitation; MS, mitral stenosis; AF, atrial fibrillation; CS, concomitant surgery; AVR, aortic valve replacement; TVP, tricuspid valve repair (13, 15–24).*

The risk of thromboembolic events in the MVP group was lower than that in the MVR group (RR 0.61; 95% CI, 0.43–0.85; $P = 0.004$; $I^2 = 42\%$), but the rates of IE (RR 0.98; 95% CI, 0.58–1.64; $P = 0.93$; $I^2 = 0\%$) and hemorrhagic events (RR 0.75; 95% CI, 0.54–1.04; $P = 0.080$; $I^2 = 43\%$) were not significantly different (**Figure 3A**). Four studies that reported the composite outcomes of valve-related adverse events also indicated a lower risk in the MVP group (HR 0.60; 95% CI, 0.38–0.94; $P = 0.030$; $I^2 = 25\%$) (**Figure 3B**). Reconstructed Kaplan-Meier curves derived from four studies showed that the freedom from valve-related adverse event rates at 4, 8, and 12 years were 94.91, 90.91, and 81.59%, respectively, in the MVP group and 93.36, 86.47, and 77.75%, respectively, in the MVR group (**Figure 4C**).

Neither Begg's test nor Egger's test indicated statistically significant publication bias in terms of early mortality, long-term survival, freedom from valve-related adverse events, IE, thromboembolic events, and hemorrhagic events. Funnel plots are provided in the supplemental materials (**Supplementary Figure 2**).

## DISCUSSION

Our meta-analysis demonstrated that in RHD patients, MVP showed significant advantages over MVR in long-term survival rate and valve-related adverse events, especially thromboembolic events. However, the risk of mitral valve reoperation in the MVP group was significantly higher than that in the MVR group. No significant difference was found in IE and hemorrhagic events. However, for RHD patients with concomitant AVR, the long-term survival benefit of MVP was not obvious, and the reoperation rate of MVP was still higher than that of MVR.

Several published previously meta-analyses have compared MVP with MVR in RHD patients. In 2013, Wang et al. (25) included seven studies and reported that MVP provided longer short-term and long-term event-free survival for adult RHD patients. However, for unclear reasons, they included a study that contained young children (26), and the number of studies they included was small. Saurav et al. (27) believed that RHD patients with concomitant AVR were better suited for MVR than for MVP because of the lower rate of reoperation and the absence of a significant difference in long-term survival in their subgroup analysis. However, they did not take time to events into account and used RR rather than HR to assess the long-term outcomes in their analysis. Our meta-analysis included the latest comparative studies, reported time-to-event outcomes, and reconstructed intuitive Kaplan-Meier curves, which provides new evidence for surgical decision-making.

Regarding early mortality, our meta-analysis showed a trend favoring MVP, although it did not show that MVP had a significant reduction effect compared to MVR, which is not consistent with the conclusions of previous studies (25). The 30-day mortality and 1-year mortality after MVP have been shown to be associated with the cardiac surgeon's total annual surgical volume (28, 29). In the study by Chen et al. (15), the multicenter data they collected from the database included fewer than 500 patients with MVP over 14 years. We could estimate that the

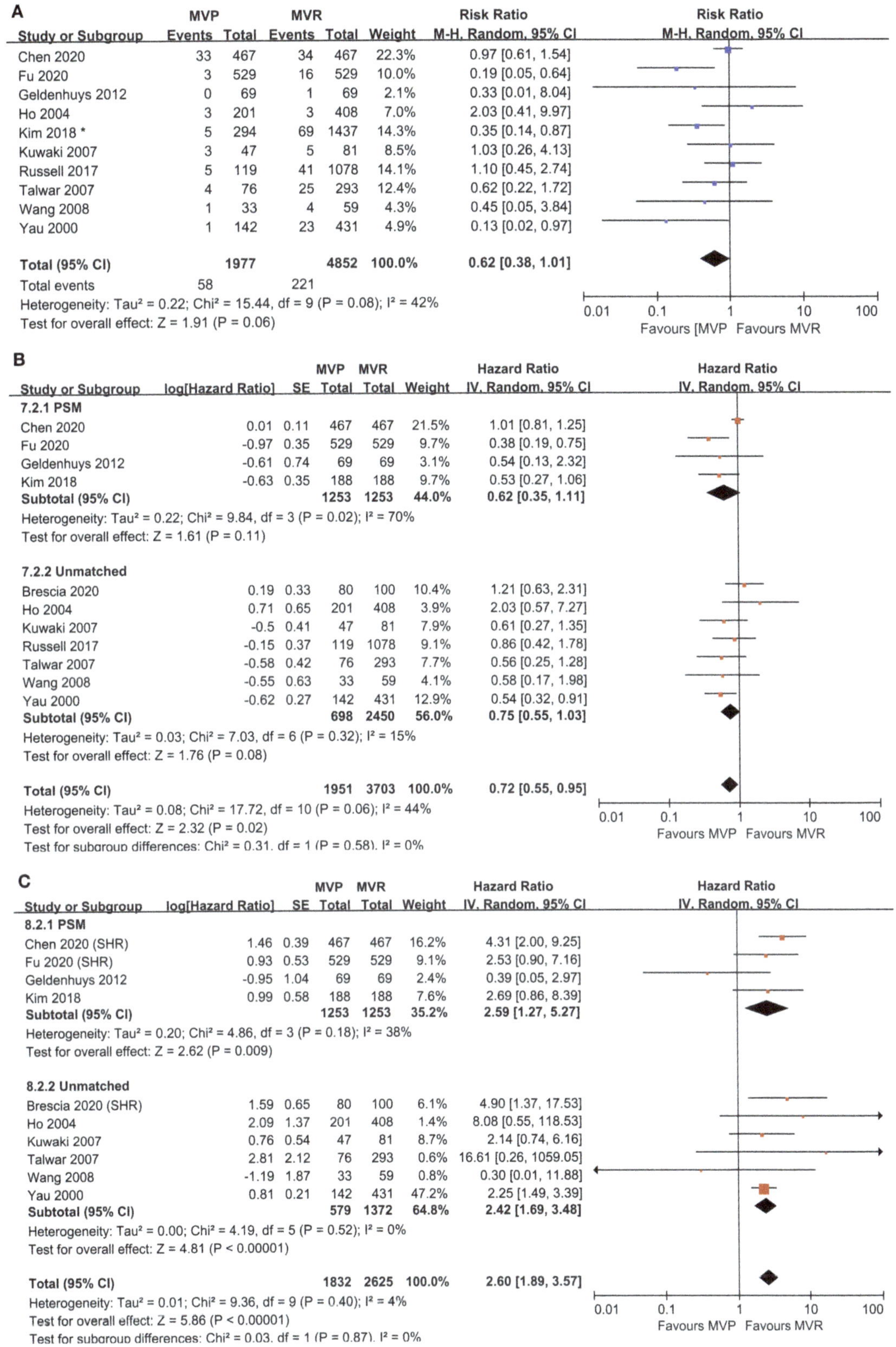


**FIGURE 1 |** Forest plots showing the results of early and late outcomes. **(A)** Early mortality, **(B)** long-term survival, analyzed by study design, and **(C)** freedom from reoperation, analyzed by study design. MVP, mitral valve repair; MVR, mitral valve replacement; M-H, Mantel-Haenszel; CI, confidence interval; SE, standard error; IV, Inverse-Variance; PSM, propensity score matching; SHR, subdistribution hazard ratio; *before matching.

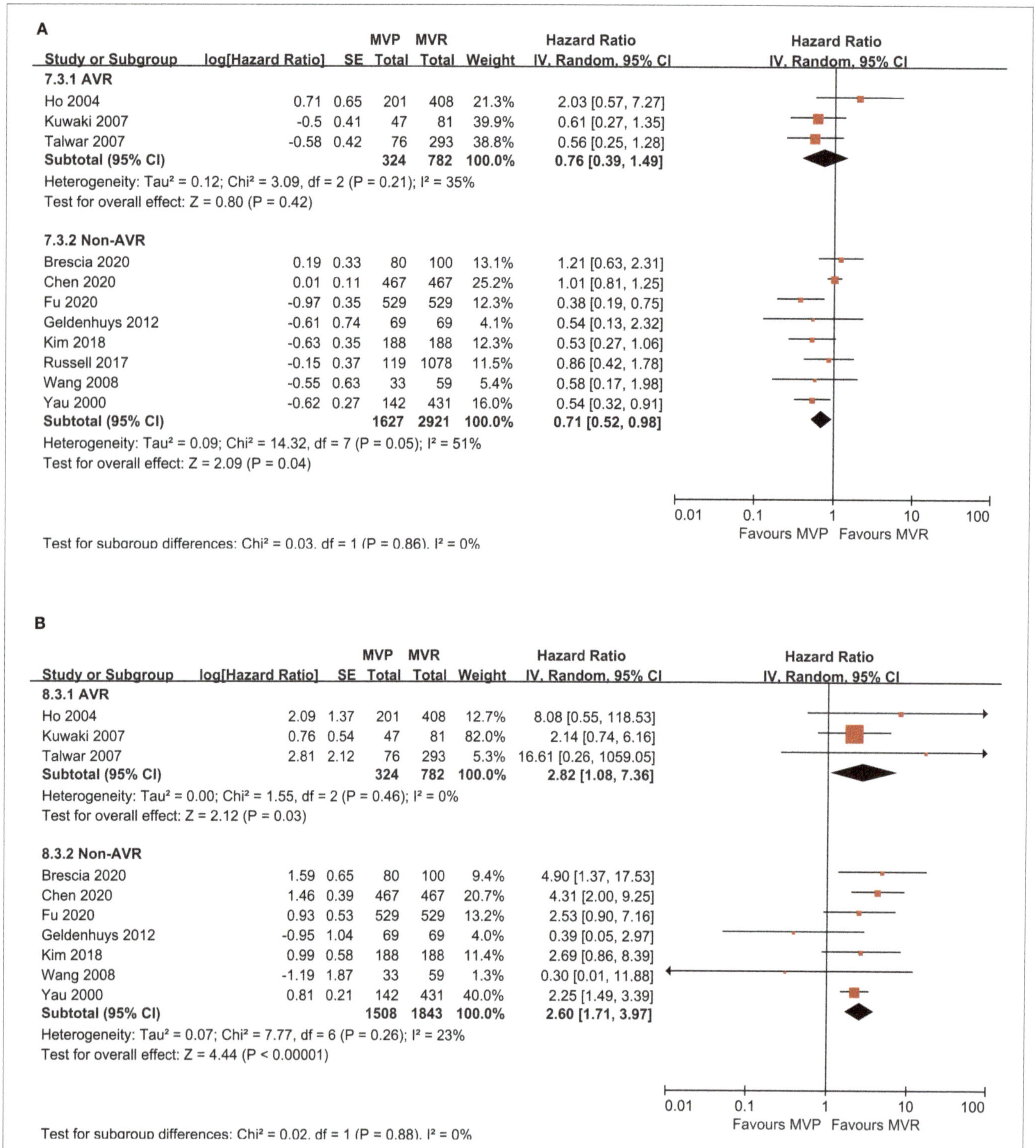


**A**

| Study or Subgroup | log[Hazard Ratio] | SE | MVP Total | MVR Total | Weight | Hazard Ratio IV, Random, 95% CI |
|---|---|---|---|---|---|---|
| **7.3.1 AVR** | | | | | | |
| Ho 2004 | 0.71 | 0.65 | 201 | 408 | 21.3% | 2.03 [0.57, 7.27] |
| Kuwaki 2007 | -0.5 | 0.41 | 47 | 81 | 39.9% | 0.61 [0.27, 1.35] |
| Talwar 2007 | -0.58 | 0.42 | 76 | 293 | 38.8% | 0.56 [0.25, 1.28] |
| **Subtotal (95% CI)** | | | **324** | **782** | **100.0%** | **0.76 [0.39, 1.49]** |
| Heterogeneity: Tau² = 0.12; Chi² = 3.09, df = 2 (P = 0.21); I² = 35% | | | | | | |
| Test for overall effect: Z = 0.80 (P = 0.42) | | | | | | |
| **7.3.2 Non-AVR** | | | | | | |
| Brescia 2020 | 0.19 | 0.33 | 80 | 100 | 13.1% | 1.21 [0.63, 2.31] |
| Chen 2020 | 0.01 | 0.11 | 467 | 467 | 25.2% | 1.01 [0.81, 1.25] |
| Fu 2020 | -0.97 | 0.35 | 529 | 529 | 12.3% | 0.38 [0.19, 0.75] |
| Geldenhuys 2012 | -0.61 | 0.74 | 69 | 69 | 4.1% | 0.54 [0.13, 2.32] |
| Kim 2018 | -0.63 | 0.35 | 188 | 188 | 12.3% | 0.53 [0.27, 1.06] |
| Russell 2017 | -0.15 | 0.37 | 119 | 1078 | 11.5% | 0.86 [0.42, 1.78] |
| Wang 2008 | -0.55 | 0.63 | 33 | 59 | 5.4% | 0.58 [0.17, 1.98] |
| Yau 2000 | -0.62 | 0.27 | 142 | 431 | 16.0% | 0.54 [0.32, 0.91] |
| **Subtotal (95% CI)** | | | **1627** | **2921** | **100.0%** | **0.71 [0.52, 0.98]** |
| Heterogeneity: Tau² = 0.09; Chi² = 14.32, df = 7 (P = 0.05); I² = 51% | | | | | | |
| Test for overall effect: Z = 2.09 (P = 0.04) | | | | | | |

Test for subgroup differences: Chi² = 0.03, df = 1 (P = 0.86), I² = 0%

**B**

| Study or Subgroup | log[Hazard Ratio] | SE | MVP Total | MVR Total | Weight | Hazard Ratio IV, Random, 95% CI |
|---|---|---|---|---|---|---|
| **8.3.1 AVR** | | | | | | |
| Ho 2004 | 2.09 | 1.37 | 201 | 408 | 12.7% | 8.08 [0.55, 118.53] |
| Kuwaki 2007 | 0.76 | 0.54 | 47 | 81 | 82.0% | 2.14 [0.74, 6.16] |
| Talwar 2007 | 2.81 | 2.12 | 76 | 293 | 5.3% | 16.61 [0.26, 1059.05] |
| **Subtotal (95% CI)** | | | **324** | **782** | **100.0%** | **2.82 [1.08, 7.36]** |
| Heterogeneity: Tau² = 0.00; Chi² = 1.55, df = 2 (P = 0.46); I² = 0% | | | | | | |
| Test for overall effect: Z = 2.12 (P = 0.03) | | | | | | |
| **8.3.2 Non-AVR** | | | | | | |
| Brescia 2020 | 1.59 | 0.65 | 80 | 100 | 9.4% | 4.90 [1.37, 17.53] |
| Chen 2020 | 1.46 | 0.39 | 467 | 467 | 20.7% | 4.31 [2.00, 9.25] |
| Fu 2020 | 0.93 | 0.53 | 529 | 529 | 13.2% | 2.53 [0.90, 7.16] |
| Geldenhuys 2012 | -0.95 | 1.04 | 69 | 69 | 4.0% | 0.39 [0.05, 2.97] |
| Kim 2018 | 0.99 | 0.58 | 188 | 188 | 11.4% | 2.69 [0.86, 8.39] |
| Wang 2008 | -1.19 | 1.87 | 33 | 59 | 1.3% | 0.30 [0.01, 11.88] |
| Yau 2000 | 0.81 | 0.21 | 142 | 431 | 40.0% | 2.25 [1.49, 3.39] |
| **Subtotal (95% CI)** | | | **1508** | **1843** | **100.0%** | **2.60 [1.71, 3.97]** |
| Heterogeneity: Tau² = 0.07; Chi² = 7.77, df = 6 (P = 0.26); I² = 23% | | | | | | |
| Test for overall effect: Z = 4.44 (P < 0.00001) | | | | | | |

Test for subgroup differences: Chi² = 0.02, df = 1 (P = 0.88), I² = 0%

**FIGURE 2 |** Forest plots showing the results of subgroup analysis according to whether concomitant AVR was performed. **(A)** Long-term survival and **(B)** freedom from reoperation. MVP, mitral valve repair; MVR, mitral valve replacement; AVR, aortic valve replacement; IV, Inverse-Variance; CI, confidence interval; SE, standard error.

average annual operation volume per center was small. The low volume of annual operations reflected insufficient experience with repair surgery among the cardiac surgeons, which can cause an increase in early mortality. In addition, they did not report the heart function data of the surgical patients; there may have been heterogeneity of cardiac insufficiency, which could present a significant limitation. We conducted a sensitivity analysis and eliminated this study, which accounted for the largest proportion

**A**

| Study or Subgroup | MVP Events | MVP Total | MVR Events | MVR Total | Weight | Risk Ratio M-H, Random, 95% CI |
|---|---|---|---|---|---|---|
| **10.1.1 Infective endocarditis** | | | | | | |
| Chen 2020 | 10 | 467 | 13 | 467 | 40.7% | 0.77 [0.34, 1.74] |
| Ho 2004 | 1 | 201 | 0 | 408 | 2.6% | 6.07 [0.25, 148.45] |
| Kim 2018 * | 5 | 294 | 19 | 1437 | 28.3% | 1.29 [0.48, 3.42] |
| Talwar 2007 | 2 | 76 | 6 | 293 | 10.8% | 1.29 [0.26, 6.24] |
| Yau 2000 | 3 | 142 | 13 | 431 | 17.5% | 0.70 [0.20, 2.42] |
| **Subtotal (95% CI)** | | **1180** | | **3036** | **100.0%** | **0.98 [0.58, 1.64]** |
| Total events | 21 | | 51 | | | |
| Heterogeneity: Tau² = 0.00; Chi² = 2.28, df = 4 (P = 0.68); I² = 0% | | | | | | |
| Test for overall effect: Z = 0.09 (P = 0.93) | | | | | | |
| **10.1.2 Thromboembolic events** | | | | | | |
| Chen 2020 | 59 | 467 | 65 | 467 | 28.2% | 0.91 [0.65, 1.26] |
| Ho 2004 | 1 | 201 | 3 | 408 | 2.1% | 0.68 [0.07, 6.46] |
| Kim 2018 * | 13 | 294 | 118 | 1437 | 18.8% | 0.54 [0.31, 0.94] |
| Kuwaki 2007 | 11 | 47 | 23 | 81 | 16.8% | 0.82 [0.44, 1.54] |
| Talwar 2007 | 8 | 76 | 62 | 293 | 14.8% | 0.50 [0.25, 0.99] |
| Wang 2008 | 1 | 33 | 7 | 59 | 2.6% | 0.26 [0.03, 1.99] |
| Yau 2000 | 10 | 142 | 87 | 431 | 16.7% | 0.35 [0.19, 0.65] |
| **Subtotal (95% CI)** | | **1260** | | **3176** | **100.0%** | **0.61 [0.43, 0.85]** |
| Total events | 103 | | 365 | | | |
| Heterogeneity: Tau² = 0.08; Chi² = 10.36, df = 6 (P = 0.11); I² = 42% | | | | | | |
| Test for overall effect: Z = 2.87 (P = 0.004) | | | | | | |
| **10.1.3 Hemorrhagic events** | | | | | | |
| Chen 2020 | 63 | 467 | 61 | 467 | 31.2% | 1.03 [0.74, 1.43] |
| Ho 2004 | 8 | 201 | 19 | 408 | 11.9% | 0.85 [0.38, 1.92] |
| Kim 2018 * | 5 | 294 | 88 | 1437 | 10.3% | 0.28 [0.11, 0.68] |
| Kuwaki 2007 | 7 | 47 | 16 | 81 | 11.9% | 0.75 [0.33, 1.70] |
| Talwar 2007 | 29 | 76 | 148 | 293 | 32.4% | 0.76 [0.56, 1.03] |
| Wang 2008 | 1 | 33 | 5 | 59 | 2.3% | 0.36 [0.04, 2.93] |
| **Subtotal (95% CI)** | | **1118** | | **2745** | **100.0%** | **0.75 [0.54, 1.04]** |
| Total events | 113 | | 337 | | | |
| Heterogeneity: Tau² = 0.06; Chi² = 8.70, df = 5 (P = 0.12); I² = 43% | | | | | | |
| Test for overall effect: Z = 1.74 (P = 0.08) | | | | | | |

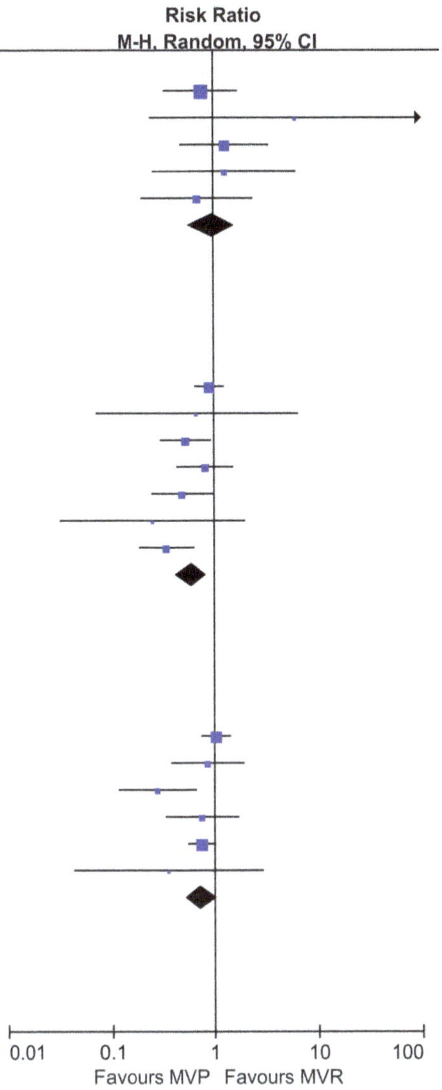


**B**

| Study or Subgroup | log[Hazard Ratio] | SE | MVP Total | MVR Total | Weight | Hazard Ratio IV, Random, 95% CI |
|---|---|---|---|---|---|---|
| Fu 2020 (SHR) | -0.82 | 0.37 | 529 | 529 | 27.5% | 0.44 [0.21, 0.91] |
| Ho 2004 | -0.92 | 0.43 | 201 | 408 | 22.0% | 0.40 [0.17, 0.93] |
| Kuwaki 2007 | 0.39 | 0.66 | 47 | 81 | 10.7% | 1.48 [0.41, 5.38] |
| Yau 2000 | -0.31 | 0.28 | 142 | 431 | 39.8% | 0.73 [0.42, 1.27] |
| **Total (95% CI)** | | | **919** | **1449** | **100.0%** | **0.60 [0.38, 0.94]** |
| Heterogeneity: Tau² = 0.05; Chi² = 3.98, df = 3 (P = 0.26); I² = 25% | | | | | | |
| Test for overall effect: Z = 2.23 (P = 0.03) | | | | | | |

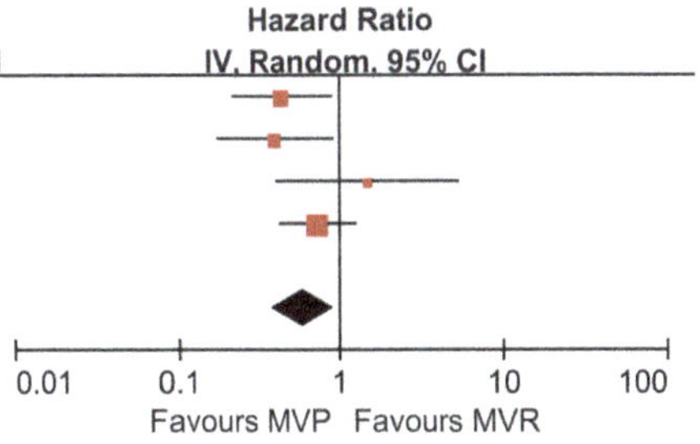


**FIGURE 3 |** Forest plots showing the results for valve-related adverse events. **(A)** Adverse events, including infective endocarditis, thromboembolic events, and hemorrhagic events and **(B)** freedom from valve-related adverse events. MVP, mitral valve repair; MVR, mitral valve replacement; M-H, Mantel-Haenszel; CI, confidence interval; SE, standard error; IV, Inverse-Variance; SHR, subdistribution hazard ratio; *before matching.

and had potential bias. The results of the sensitivity analysis were completely contrary to the original conclusion (RR 0.55; 95% CI, 0.31–0.96; $P = 0.030$; $I^2 = 34\%$). Thus, we tend to consider MVP better for early mortality.

In terms of the long-term survival rate, the analysis of all of the included studies showed that the long-term survival rate of MVP was higher, and this conclusion remained stable (HR 0.65; 95% CI, 0.50–0.86; $P = 0.002$; $I^2 = 15\%$) after the study with the

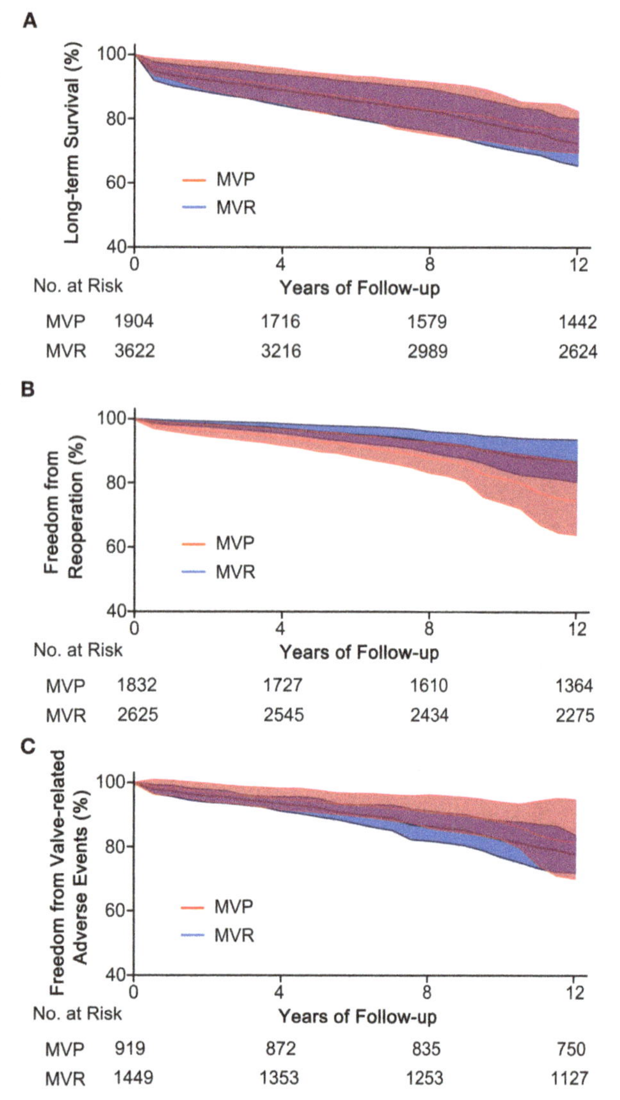


**FIGURE 4 |** Reconstructed Kaplan-Meier curves for MVP and MVR in patients with RHD. **(A)** Reconstructed curves of long-term survival from 10 studies, **(B)** reconstructed curves of freedom from reoperation from 10 studies, and **(C)** reconstructed curves of freedom from valve-related adverse events from four studies. MVP, mitral valve repair; MVR, mitral valve replacement; RHD, rheumatic heart disease.

highest proportion was removed. In the PSM subgroup analysis, the sensitivity analysis indicated that the high heterogeneity was caused by Chen et al. (15), and the conclusion became completely homogeneous and statistically significant once that study was removed (HR 0.46; 95% CI, 0.29–0.73; $P < 0.001$; $I^2 = 0\%$). For patients who have only undergone mitral valve surgery, the benefits of MVP are well-explained. On the one hand, MVP can better preserve the subvalvular apparatus to protect the normal physiological function of the left ventricle (30). Tirone et al. (31) believed that even mild impairment of left ventricle function could adversely affect long-term survival. As a result, deaths associated with left ventricular failure are reduced after MVP. On the other hand, MVP avoids the long-term use of anticoagulants after surgery, which effectively reduces coagulation-related complications (20, 25, 32). From the perspective of MVP development, the survival rate of RHD patients after mitral valve surgery has improved significantly over the past decade in conjunction with a greater understanding of MVP and more reasonable assessments of the feasibility of MVP (13). In addition to long-term mortality, MVP also decreased the total treatment cost during the survival period of over 10 years (33). Patients who underwent MVP did not have to bear the burden of prosthetic valves and ongoing anticoagulant use. This additional benefit of MVP is undoubtedly more cost-effective for developing countries with the ability to implement MVP. However, although the trend was in favor of the AVR+MVP group in the subgroup analysis, RHD patients in this group did not appear to survive longer. Therefore, it can be considered that the long-term survival rate of patients who underwent AVR+MVP or AVR+MVR may not be substantially different. The use of AVR made long-term anticoagulation necessary, thus increasing complications, which may reduce the long-term survival benefits of MVP for patients (21). Currently, few cohort studies have compared these two groups, and conclusions should be drawn with caution. Similarly, AVR+MVP reduced hospitalization costs compared to AVR+MVR (34).

Without exception, the overall and subgroup analysis results for reoperation indicatedthat the MVP group was more likely to undergo mitral valve surgery again. The inevitable residue of diseased valve tissue, the presence of lesions involving the subvalvular apparatus, and younger age may make the reoperation rate significantly higher with MVP than with MVR (27, 35). The continuous natural progression of RHD also inevitably reduces the durability of repair surgery. In degenerative valve disease, a high recurrence of MVP after surgery has also been found by Ciarka et al. (36). However, several studies (35, 37, 38) have demonstrated that valve durability after the repair of RHD was equivalent to that of degenerative valve disease in a long-term follow-up. Previous studies reported that the mortality rate (39, 40), the acute kidney injury rate, and the possibility of longer ICU and hospital stays (41) after the second MVR operation tended to be higher than those rates for MVP. It is known that MVP requires that surgeons have more surgical skills and professional capabilities. In addition to the early mortality mentioned above, repair durability was also related to the annual volume of surgery performed by cardiac surgeons (28). Zhou et al. (42) reported that surgery before atrial fibrillation and left ventricular dysfunction improved the durability of MVP. Therefore, early MVP performed by experienced surgeons was considered to reduce the risk of reoperation.

The incidence of valve-related adverse events, especially thromboembolic events, was lower for patients who underwent MVP in this study. We removed the study with the highest proportions of each item for a sensitivity analysis, and the conclusions remained unchanged. Hemorrhagic events are a common complication with long-term use of anticoagulant drugs. The results indicated that MVP had a favorable effect on hemorrhagic events, although we did not find a significant difference between the two groups. Mitral valve repair (MVP) was associated with a lower risk of thromboembolic events. Long-term oral anticoagulant use after MVR requires a narrow range of international normalized ratios (INRs), and excessively high or low INRs can cause complications (43, 44). Hemorrhagic and thromboembolic events were more likely in the MVR group as a result of decreased long-term drug compliance and the maintenance time of the INR standard range (45, 46). In another study (27), the benefits of MVP in terms of thromboembolic events were demonstrated to extend to RHD patients with concomitant AVR.

It should be pointed out that for children and young unmarried women, MVR is not the optimal surgical method. The degeneration of biologic prostheses is not suitable for growing children. Lifelong anticoagulation of mechanical prostheses has adverse consequences for growth in children and during pregnancy in young women (32). For patients who need MVR because of non-reparable valve structural lesions or unsuccessful repair, a retrospective cohort study showed that compared to biological prostheses, mechanical prostheses reduced the risk of death and reoperation, although it increased the possibility of bleeding (47). This benefit continued until the age of 70 years, while another study suggested that the age threshold should be considered at 65 (48). For people over 70 years old, the risk of hemorrhagic and thromboembolic events caused by biological prostheses was lower, associated with a better survival advantage (47).

## LIMITATION

We must acknowledge that our meta-analysis has some limitations. First, the included studies were mainly retrospective cohort studies, and patients were not randomly divided into MVP and MVR groups. Usually, the surgical treatment of a patient is primarily decided at the surgeon's discretion and inevitably leads to selection bias. Second, these studies came from different centers. There may be heterogeneity due to variations in surgical techniques and patient baseline conditions, such as the proportion of concomitant coronary artery bypass grafting, the NYHA functional class, and the mean left ventricular ejection fraction. Third, the data extracted from the Kaplan-Meier curves before merging was obtained through digital estimation. The digitalization and aggregation of survival curves inevitably reduced the accuracy of the primary data and led to potential deviation. Forth, few included studies have reported the detailed information of subvalvular apparatus. More well-designed studies are warranted to further explore the function of subvalvular apparatus in mitral valves and its clinical implications in mitral valve surgery. Finally, limited by the information provided by the included studies, no further stratification according to the use of biological prostheses vs. mechanical prostheses in MVR or the age of the patient can be performed.

## CONCLUSION

For RHD patients, MVP can reduce early mortality, and improve long-term survival and freedom from valve-related adverse events, although it was associated with a higher risk of reoperation. The results remained generally consistent in patients undergoing concomitant AVR. In summary, MVP is a promising strategy for selective RHD patients, and experienced cardiac centers are encouraged to apply MVP more routinely in clinical practice.

## AUTHOR CONTRIBUTIONS

GC and ML: conception and design. ZW: administrative support. GF, ZZ, and SH: literature search, selection and quality assessment, and data extraction. GF and ZZ: data analysis and interpretation. All authors contributed to the article and approved the submitted version.

## REFERENCES


1. Watkins DA, Johnson CO, Colquhoun SM, Karthikeyan G, Beaton A, Bukhman G, et al. Global, Regional, and National Burden of Rheumatic Heart Disease, 1990–2015. *N Engl J Med.* (2017) 377:713–22. doi: 10.1056/NEJMoa1603693
2. Marijon E, Mirabel M, Celermajer DS, Jouven X. Rheumatic heart disease. *Lancet.* (2012) 379:953–64. doi: 10.1016/S0140-6736(11)61171-9
3. Coffey S, Cairns BJ, Iung B. The modern epidemiology of heart valve disease. *Heart.* (2016) 102:75–85. doi: 10.1136/heartjnl-2014-307020
4. Manjunath CN, Srinivas P, Ravindranath KS, Dhanalakshmi C. Incidence and patterns of valvular heart disease in a tertiary care high-volume cardiac center: a single center experience. *Indian Heart J.* (2014) 66:320–6. doi: 10.1016/j.ihj.2014.03.010
5. Hwang HY, Kim KH, Ahn H. Attitude after a mild aortic valve lesion during rheumatic mitral valve surgery. *J Thorac Cardiovasc Surg.* (2014) 147:1540–6. doi: 10.1016/j.jtcvs.2013.05.040
6. Otto CM, Nishimura RA, Bonow RO, Carabello BA, Erwin JP III, Gentile F, et al. 2020 ACC/AHA guideline for the management of patients with valvular heart disease: executive summary: a report of the American College of Cardiology/American Heart Association Joint Committee on Clinical Practice Guidelines. *Circulation.* (2021) 143:e35–71. doi: 10.1161/CIR.0000000000000932
7. Wunderlich NC, Dalvi B, Ho SY, Küx H, Siegel RJ. Rheumatic mitral valve stenosis: diagnosis and treatment options. *Curr Cardiol Rep.* (2019) 21:14. doi: 10.1007/s11886-019-1099-7
8. LaPar DJ, Ailawadi G, Isbell JM, Crosby IK, Kern JA, Rich JB, et al. Mitral valve repair rates correlate with surgeon and institutional experience. *J Thorac Cardiovasc Surg.* (2014) 148:995–1003; discussion 1003–4. doi: 10.1016/j.jtcvs.2014.06.039
9. Bernal JM, Rabasa JM, Vilchez FG, Cagigas JC, Revuelta JM. Mitral valve repair in rheumatic disease. The flexible solution. *Circulation.* (1993) 88(4 Pt 1):1746–53. doi: 10.1161/01.cir.88.4.1746
10. Piciché M, El Khoury G, D'udekem D'akoz Y, Noirhomme P. Surgical repair for degenerative and rheumatic mitral valve disease. Operative and mid-term results. *J Cardiovasc Surg (Torino).* (2002) 43:327–35.
11. Vassileva CM, McNeely C, Spertus J, Markwell S, Hazelrigg S. Hospital volume, mitral repair rates, and mortality in mitral valve surgery in the elderly: an analysis of US hospitals treating medicare fee-for-service patients. *J Thorac Cardiovasc Surg.* (2015) 149:762.e1–8.e1. doi: 10.1016/j.jtcvs.2014.08.084
12. Badhwar V, Peterson ED, Jacobs JP, He X, Brennan JM, O'Brien SM, et al. Longitudinal outcome of isolated mitral repair in older patients: results from 14,604 procedures performed from 1991 to 2007. *Ann Thorac Surg.* (2012) 94:1870–7; discussion 1877–9. doi: 10.1016/j.athoracsur.2012.05.105
13. Brescia AA, Watt TMF, Murray SL, Rosenbloom LM, Kleeman KC, Allgeyer H, et al. Rheumatic mitral valve repair or replacement in the valve-in-valve era. *J Thorac Cardiovasc Surg.* (2020) 2020:S0022-5223(20)31090-4. doi: 10.1016/j.jtcvs.2020.04.118

14. Tierney JF, Stewart LA, Ghersi D, Burdett S, Sydes MR. Practical methods for incorporating summary time-to-event data into meta-analysis. *Trials.* (2007) 8:16. doi: 10.1186/1745-6215-8-16
15. Chen SW, Chen CY, Chien-Chia Wu V, Chou AH, Cheng YT, Chang SH, et al. Mitral valve repair versus replacement in patients with rheumatic heart disease. *J Thorac Cardiovasc Surg.* (2020) 2020:S0022-5223(20)32459-4. doi: 10.1016/j.jtcvs.2020.07.117
16. Fu J, Li Y, Zhang H, Han J, Jiao Y, Du J, et al. Outcomes of mitral valve repair compared with replacement for patients with rheumatic heart disease. *J Thorac Cardiovasc Surg.* (2020) 2020:S0022-5223(20)30286-5. doi: 10.1016/j.jtcvs.2020.01.053
17. Kim WK, Kim HJ, Kim JB, Jung SH, Choo SJ, Chung CH, et al. Clinical outcomes in 1731 patients undergoing mitral valve surgery for rheumatic valve disease. *Heart.* (2018) 104:841–8. doi: 10.1136/heartjnl-2017-312249
18. Russell EA, Walsh WF, Reid CM, Tran L, Brown A, Bennetts JS, et al. Outcomes after mitral valve surgery for rheumatic heart disease. *Heart Asia.* (2017) 9:e010916. doi: 10.1136/heartasia-2017-010916
19. Geldenhuys A, Koshy JJ, Human PA, Mtwale JF, Brink JG, Zilla P. Rheumatic mitral repair versus replacement in a threshold country: the impact of commissural fusion. *J Heart Valve Dis.* (2012) 21:424–32.
20. Wang YC, Tsai FC, Chu JJ, Lin PJ. Midterm outcomes of rheumatic mitral repair versus replacement. *Int Heart J.* (2008) 49:565–76. doi: 10.1536/ihj.49.565
21. Kuwaki K, Kawaharada N, Morishita K, Koyanagi T, Osawa H, Maeda T, et al. Mitral valve repair versus replacement in simultaneous mitral and aortic valve surgery for rheumatic disease. *Ann Thorac Surg.* (2007) 83:558–63. doi: 10.1016/j.athoracsur.2006.08.015
22. Talwar S, Mathur A, Choudhary SK, Singh R, Kumar AS. Aortic valve replacement with mitral valve repair compared with combined aortic and mitral valve replacement. *Ann Thorac Surg.* (2007) 84:1219–25. doi: 10.1016/j.athoracsur.2007.04.115
23. Ho HQ, Nguyen VP, Phan KP, Pham NV. Mitral valve repair with aortic valve replacement in rheumatic heart disease. *Asian Cardiovasc Thorac Ann.* (2004) 12:341–5. doi: 10.1177/021849230401200413
24. Yau TM, El-Ghoneimi YA, Armstrong S, Ivanov J, David TE. Mitral valve repair and replacement for rheumatic disease. *J Thorac Cardiovasc Surg.* (2000) 119:53–60. doi: 10.1016/s0022-5223(00)70217-0
25. Wang Z, Zhou C, Gu H, Zheng Z, Hu S. Mitral valve repair versus replacement in patients with rheumatic heart disease. *J Heart Valve Dis.* (2013) 22:333–9.
26. Antunes MJ. Mitral valvuloplasty, a better alternative. Comparative study between valve reconstruction and replacement for rheumatic mitral valve disease. *Eur J Cardiothorac Surg.* (1990) 4:257–62; discussion 263–4. doi: 10.1016/1010-7940(90)90249-y
27. Saurav A, Alla VM, Kaushik M, Hunter CC, Mooss AV. Outcomes of mitral valve repair compared with replacement in patients undergoing concomitant aortic valve surgery: a meta-analysis of observational studies. *Eur J Cardiothorac Surg.* (2015) 48:347–53. doi: 10.1093/ejcts/ezu421
28. Chikwe J, Toyoda N, Anyanwu AC, Itagaki S, Egorova NN, Boateng P, et al. Relation of mitral valve surgery volume to repair rate, durability, and survival. *J Am Coll Cardiol.* (2017) 2017:S0735-1097(17)30677-0. doi: 10.1016/j.jacc.2017.02.026
29. Badhwar V, Vemulapalli S, Mack MA, Gillinov AM, Chikwe J, Dearani JA, et al. Volume-outcome association of mitral valve surgery in the United States. *JAMA Cardiol.* (2020) 5:1–10. doi: 10.1001/jamacardio.2020.2221
30. Lee EM, Shapiro LM, Wells FC. Importance of subvalvular preservation and early operation in mitral valve surgery. *Circulation.* (1996) 94:2117–23. doi: 10.1161/01.cir.94.9.2117
31. David TE, David CM, Tsang W, Lafreniere-Roula M, Manlhiot C. Long-term results of mitral valve repair for regurgitation due to leaflet prolapse. *J Am Coll Cardiol.* (2019) 74:1044–53. doi: 10.1016/j.jacc.2019.06.052
32. Fu JT, Popal MS, Zhang HB, Han W, Hu QM, Meng X, et al. A meta-analysis of late outcomes of mitral valve repair in patients with rheumatic heart disease. J Thorac Dis. (2017) 9:4366–75. doi: 10.21037/jtd.2017.10.97
33. Beresniak A, Sabatier B, Achouh P, Menasché P, Fabiani JN. Cost-effectiveness of mitral valve repair versus replacement by biologic or mechanical prosthesis. *Ann Thorac Surg.* (2013) 95:98–104. doi: 10.1016/j.athoracsur.2012.08.005
34. Kilic A, Grimm JC, Magruder JT, Sciortino CM, Whitman GJ, Baumgartner WA, et al. Trends, clinical outcomes, and cost implications of mitral valve repair versus replacement, concomitant with aortic valve replacement. *J Thorac Cardiovasc Surg.* (2015) 149:1614–9. doi: 10.1016/j.jtcvs.2015.02.044
35. Yakub MA, Dillon J, Krishna Moorthy PS, Pau KK, Nordin MN. Is rheumatic aetiology a predictor of poor outcome in the current era of mitral valve repair? Contemporary long-term results of mitral valve repair in rheumatic heart disease. *Eur J Cardiothorac Surg.* (2013) 44:673–81. doi: 10.1093/ejcts/ezt093
36. Ciarka A, Braun J, Delgado V, Versteegh M, Boersma E, Klautz R, et al. Predictors of mitral regurgitation recurrence in patients with heart failure undergoing mitral valve annuloplasty. *Am J Cardiol.* (2010) 106:395–401. doi: 10.1016/j.amjcard.2010.03.042
37. DiBardino DJ, ElBardissi AW, McClure RS, Razo-Vasquez OA, Kelly NE, Cohn LH. Four decades of experience with mitral valve repair: analysis of differential indications, technical evolution, and long-term outcome. *J Thorac Cardiovasc Surg.* (2010) 139:76–83; discussion 83–4. doi: 10.1016/j.jtcvs.2009.08.058
38. Dillon J, Yakub MA, Kong PK, Ramli MF, Jaffar N, Gaffar IF. Comparative long-term results of mitral valve repair in adults with chronic rheumatic disease and degenerative disease: is repair for "burnt-out" rheumatic disease still inferior to repair for degenerative disease in the current era? *J Thorac Cardiovasc Surg.* (2015) 149:771–7; discussion 777–9. doi: 10.1016/j.jtcvs.2014.08.066
39. Albeyoglu SC, Filizcan U, Sargin M, Cakmak M, Goksel O, Bayserke O, et al. Determinants of hospital mortality after repeat mitral valve surgery for rheumatic mitral valve disease. *Thorac Cardiovasc Surg.* (2006) 54:244–9. doi: 10.1055/s-2006-923946
40. Aphram G, De Kerchove L, Mastrobuoni S, Navarra E, Solari S, Tamer S, et al. Re-repair of the failed mitral valve: insights into aetiology and surgical management. *Eur J Cardiothorac Surg.* (2018) 54:774–80. doi: 10.1093/ejcts/ezy111
41. Keenan NM, Newland RF, Baker RA, Rice GD, Bennetts JS. Outcomes of redo valve surgery in indigenous Australians. *Heart Lung Circ.* (2019) 28:1102–11. doi: 10.1016/j.hlc.2018.05.198
42. Zhou T, Li J, Lai H, Zhu K, Sun Y, Ding W, et al. Benefits of early surgery on clinical outcomes after degenerative mitral valve repair. *Ann Thorac Surg.* (2018) 106:1063–70. doi: 10.1016/j.athoracsur.2018.05.011
43. Clarkesmith DE, Pattison HM, Khaing PH, Lane DA. Educational and behavioural interventions for anticoagulant therapy in patients with atrial fibrillation. *Cochrane Database Syst Rev.* (2017) 4:CD008600. doi: 10.1002/14651858.CD008600.pub3
44. Lip GY, Edwards SJ. Stroke prevention with aspirin, warfarin and ximelagatran in patients with non-valvular atrial fibrillation: a systematic review and meta-analysis. *Thromb Res.* (2006) 118:321–33. doi: 10.1016/j.thromres.2005.08.007
45. Toth PP. Direct oral anticoagulants as alternative treatment options for the effective long-term treatment of patients with pulmonary embolism in primary care: a review. *Ann Med.* (2014) 46:341–52. doi: 10.3109/07853890.2014.912833
46. Willey VJ, Bullano MF, Hauch O, Reynolds M, Wygant G, Hoffman L, et al. Management patterns and outcomes of patients with venous thromboembolism in the usual community practice setting. *Clin Ther.* (2004) 26:1149–59. doi: 10.1016/s0149-2918(04)90187-7
47. Goldstone AB, Chiu P, Baiocchi M, Lingala B, Patrick WL, Fischbein MP, et al. Mechanical or biologic prostheses for aortic-valve and mitral-valve replacement. *N Engl J Med.* (2017) 377:1847–57. doi: 10.1056/NEJMoa161379
48. Chen CY, Chan YH, Wu VC, Liu KS, Cheng YT, Chu PH, et al. Bioprosthetic versus mechanical mitral valve replacements in patients with rheumatic heart disease. *J Thorac Cardiovasc Surg.* (2021) 18:S0022-5223(21)00512-2. doi: 10.1016/j.jtcvs.2021.03.033

2

# Exploring the Correlation and Protective Role of Diabetes Mellitus in Aortic Aneurysm Disease

*Divyatha Arun [1†], Wahaj Munir [2†], Lara Victoria Schmitt [2], Rohan Vyas [2], Jeuela Iris Ravindran [2], Mohamad Bashir [3], Ian Michael Williams [4], Bashi Velayudhan [3] and Mohammed Idhrees [3*]*

*[1] Department of Endocrinology, Columbia Asia Referral Hospital, A Unit of Manipal Hospital, Yeshwanthpur, Bengaluru, India, [2] Barts and the London School of Medicine and Dentistry, Queen Mary University of London, London, United Kingdom, [3] Institue of Cardiac and Aortic Disorders, SRM Institutes for Medical Science (SIMS Hospitals), Chennai, India, [4] Vascular Surgery, University Hospital of Wales, Cardiff, United Kingdom*

***Correspondence:**
*Mohammed Idhrees*
*a.m.idhrees@gmail.com*

*These authors share first authorship*

**Introduction:** Diabetes mellitus is recognised as a significant risk factor for cardiovascular and peripheral vascular disease, as the abnormal metabolic state increases the risk for atherosclerosis, occlusive arterial disease and vascular dysfunction. There have been reports of potential association across the literature that illustrates a link between diabetes mellitus and aortic aneurysm, with the former having a protective role on the development of the latter.

**Methods:** A thorough literature search was performed through electronic databases, to provide a comprehensive review of the study's reporting on the association of diabetes mellitus and aortic aneurysm, discussing the mechanisms that have been reported; furthemore, we reviewed the reports of the impact of oral hypoglycameic agents on aortic aneurysms.

**Results:** Various proposed mechanisms are involved in this protective process including endothelial dysfunction, chronic hyperglycemia and insulin resistance. The evidence suggests a negative association between these disease process, with prevelance of diabetes mellitus resulting in lower rates of aortic aneurysm, *via* its protective mechanistic action. The increase in advanced glycation end products, increased arterial stiffness and vascular remodelling seen in diabetes, was found to have a profound impact on aneurysm development, its slow progression and lower rupture rate in these individuals. This review has also highlighted the role of oral hypoglycaemic agents having a protective effect against AA disease.

**Conclusion:** A decrease in development, progression and mortality from aortic aneurysms as well as reduced rates of dissection, have been observed in those with diabetes. This review has provided a comprehensive insight on the effect of diabetes and its physiological processes, and elements of its con-committant treatment, having a protective role against these aortic diseases.

**Keywords: diabetes mellitus, aorta, aneurysm, dissection, hyperglycemia, insulin resistance, protection**

# INTRODUCTION

Diabetes mellitus (DM) is one of today's fastest rising healthcare challenges that we are facing, with almost half a billion adults between the ages of 20 and 79 estimated to currently have the disease. This is equivalent to just under 10% of the global population in this given age range. Predictions concerning the rising diabetic population expect a rapid growth to near 600 and 700 million by 2030 and 2045, respectively. In 2019, deaths associated with DM and the consequent complications of the disease were approximated at 4.2 million (1).

Aortic aneurysms (AA), caused by underlying weakness of the aortic wall which subsequently develops into permanent dilation of the aortic lumen, are most commonly asymptomatic until the catastrophic event of rupture and are associated with a mortality rate of 80%. Whilst AA can occur at any level of the thoracic or abdominal aorta, the most common locations are the infrarenal and proximal thoracic regions. AA show a male preponderance with advancing age, smoking, positive family history, hypertension, hyperlipidaemia and atherosclerosis attributed as the other risk factors (2, 3). Abdominal aortic aneurysms (AAA) are responsible for 1–3% of male deaths between the ages of 65 and 85 in developed regions (2, 4, 5).

Whilst there are many similarities in the mechanism of thoracic aortic aneurysms (TAA) and AAA, distinctive features also contrast the two. The complex pathological process leading to AAA formation involves alteration or depletion of vascular smooth muscle cells (VSMC) linked to inflammatory cell infiltration, re-modelling of the extra-cellular matrix (ECM), intraluminal thrombus development and oxidative stress. Changes in the ECM and the tone of VSMC have significant associations with TAA development, which typically occurs at a younger age, is associated with genetic disorders and frequently leads to aortic dissection (AD).

DM represents a major cardiovascular risk factor but numerous epidemiological reports have shown a negative association between DM and both AAA and TAA, thereby conferring a protective effect on them (6, 7). This review aims to summarise the current available knowledge on the underlying mechanisms of this inverse relationship between these disease processes.

# PATHOLOGY OF ANEURYSM FORMATION

Aneurysm, derived from the Greek term *Aneurysma*, meaning widening, is characterised by permanent irreversible dilatation of a vessel. Conventional diagnosis of AAA requires an aortic diameter of greater than 30 mm, affecting all three layers of the arterial wall (4).

The mechanism of AA formation is complex, with inflammatory cell infiltrate (namely monocytes and macrophages) in the tunica media layer of the aortic wall playing an important role. The macrophage increase results in ECM remodelling which requires a balance between proteases like matrix metalloproteinases (MMPs) and its inhibitors (8). The characteristic dilatation of the aortic wall seen in AA, could partially be due to an imbalanced relation between wall stress and strength. Furthermore, studies have suggested an unmediated association between significant aortic wall stress and AA rupture risk. Aortic wall remodelling is both an expected and vital response to increased wall stress (9–13).

The walls of AAA show widespread inflammation, VSMC depletion and ECM degradation. These changes in the ECM are associated with extensive proteolysis causing the destruction of collagen and elastin. MMPs are a type of proteolytic enzyme whose activity is thought to be augmented in AAA, as evidenced by analysis of human aneurysmal tissue (14, 15). The increase in MMPs and a decrease in tissue inhibitors of MMPs lead to the break down of collagen and elastin in the ECM as well as VSMC depletion, resulting in degradation of the ECM. This leads to thinning and destruction of the normal aortic wall architecture, predisposing the individual to dilational changes and aneurysm development (8, 16–18). Apoptosis of VSMC characterised by inflammatory cell infiltrate, reactive oxygen species (ROS), and endoplasmic reticulum stress with the degeneration of aortic media, are the hallmark of AAA pathology (19).

Data related to the mechanism of TAA represent it as more than just a degenerative process, but rather a multifaceted culmination of both intracellular and extracellular alterations. It is characterised by abnormalities in ECM that compromise the structural integrity of the aorta (19).

# DIABETES MELLITUS IMPACTING AORTIC ANEURYSMS

## The Epidemiological Picture

DM, a chronic metabolic disorder characterised by hyperglycemia, insulin resistance and/or deficiency (relative or absolute), is associated with various microvascular and macrovascular complications contributing to major morbidity and mortality (20). DM is a significant risk factor for cardiovascular disease and reports have shown an inverse relationship between the disease and both AA prevalence and incidence (21, 22).

An ultrasound screening done in a regional veterans health care system as part of the Aneurysm Detection and Management study showed a lower prevalence of AA in the diabetic group. A significant number of other epidemiological studies have also confirmed the negative association of DM and AA, suggesting it to be protective in the formation and expansion of AA (23). A paradoxical inverse relationship was observed between the severity of DM and AA and also a reduced prevalence was seen in an Asian population study (24). Experimental studies in animal models also show attenuation of AA development in the presence of hyperglycemia.

The Viborg Vascular randomised screening trials of Central Denmark showed an inverse relationship between AA growth rate and HbA1c concentration (25). Certain retrospective studies have also observed a realistic association between DM and AA indicating a diabetic subset less likely to have an aneurysmal rupture and death (26). Another epidemiological study investigated the comparison of age at rupture and showed diabetics under the age of 65 had no aneurysmal rupture. Conversely, 15% non-diabetics developed rupture under the age of 65 years (26, 27). Other studies showed the growth rate of smaller AA and associated expansion much slower than in non-diabetics, again suggesting a negative association (28).

Furthermore, the effect DM has on the outcome of AA repair revealed no significant difference in the morbidity and mortality (29, 30), whereas a few other studies showed lower mortality rates in the diabetic population (31). Complications associated with open AAA repair can include myocardial infarction, pancreatitis and infections such as pneumonia; higher rates of these complications were observed in the diabetic population post-operatively (30).

## Impact on TAA

TAA in the vast majority is asymptomatic and diagnosed *via* echocardiography or CT performed for other indications, until a catastrophic event like AD-related complications occur, such as cardiac tamponade, acute aortic regurgitation or stroke (32). A negative correlation between DM and TAA formation and growth rate was also found. Additionally, a case study analysis showed the prevalence of DM in TAA was significantly lower (8). Prakash et al. (33) found an inverse association between DM and hospitalisations due to TAA. Also, those with DM complications had the lowest rate of TAA. Hyperglycemia, which is associated with reduced adventitial neovascularisation and decreased inflammatory cell infiltration in the medial layer of the aorta, probably inhibits progression of TAA by reducing VSMC death and ECM degradation (33). A Spanish study involving Spanish national data revealed a higher indicidence of TAA in the non-diabetic population compared to the diabetic population. Additionally, the mortality associated was significantly lower in the diabetic than the non-diabetic population (34).

## Impact on AAA

AAA have increased in the past two decades adding substantial burden to the healthcare of developed countries. They are often asymptomatic, being detected incidentally *via* routine imaging or as a medical emergency in case of rupture (3, 4). Multiple studies were done to determine the impact of DM on the incidence, growth rate, prevalence, morbidity and mortality of AAA.

De Rango et al. (35) and other prospective studies showed significant decrease in the incidence of new AAA in a diabetic population. Takagi et al. (36) assessed the growth rate in both diabetic and non-diabetic groups and established that DM is associated with a reduced rate of AAA growth. Reduced aneurysmal growth rate and expansion was also confirmed by Vega et al. (27). The life threatening complication of aneurysmal rupture and the associated mortality was also found to be lower in diabetics than non-diabetics (26, 28). The association was also more significant in diabetic males than females (36, 37).

Golledge et al. demonstrated the role of DM and glycation on AAA expansion: DM was associated with slower progression of AAA. The glycated ECM was found to markedly inhibit monocyte MMP production thus explaining the protective role of DM on AAA. There were lower levels of IL-6, MMP-2 and MMP-9 being secreted in the glycated ECM (7). On the contrary, a higher myocardial infarction and wound infection rate in the first 30 days was observed in diabetics with AAA by Treiman et al. Also the long term survival was found to be lower in diabetic patients adding to the increased cardio-vascular burden in a series of studies (35, 38, 39).

A study in the Asian population revealed significant reduction in association of advanced and severe Type 2 DM (T2DM) with AAA without rupture and also a decreased prevalence of AAA in the diabetic population (24). Dua et al. demonstrated an increase in the PAI-1 level with decreased plasmin and thus a low MMP-2 and MMP-9 levels in the DM-AAA induced mice population. This reinforces the protective role of hyperglycemia might have on aneurysm formation and aortic diameter (40). A study by Miyama et al. (41) investigated the role hyperglycemia has on aneurysm progression and found reduced levels of macrophage infiltration, neovessel density and MMP-9 levels, thus conferring protection against aneurysm formation.

Data surveillance from CAESAR, a multicentre randomised trial that compares the efficacy of surveillance vs. endovascular aortic repair in small AAA, by De Rango et al. compared diabetics and non-diabetics. Though the aneurysmal growth rate in the first year was similar in both the groups, later increase was higher in the non-diabetic group. Patients with DM in the surveillance group required lower rates of endovascular aortic repair after 30 months but no significant difference in adverse events between diabetics and non-diabetics was observed (35).

## Impact on AD

Acute Aortic dissection is relatively uncommon and first described over 200 years ago (42). AD involves a tear of the aortic intima, resulting in the formation of a false lumen, with inflow of blood in to the medial layer. The consequential false lumen may propagate distally or even retrogradely making it an aortic emergency (43). The pathology involves acute separation of layers within the aortic wall following an initial intimal tear. Luminal blood enters the intima-media layer creating a life threatening condition requiring immediate assessment and management with 20% patients dying before they reach the hospital and 30% during the hospital admission. Patients with enlarged AA, carry with them a risk of 10% per-year of sudden death as a result of the occurrence of AD. Hypertension, substance abuse, connective tissue disorders, family history of thoracic aortic diseases, vascular inflammation, congenital disorders are all risk factors for the occurrence of AD (43).

Data from inpatient sampling to determine the association between AD and DM established that DM was significantly and negatively associated with TAA and AD; this was found to be independent of multiple clinical characterisitcs and variables, including: type of hospital, the region, age of the patient and income. Hospitalisation due to TAA and AD occurred at a lower rate in diabetics (33). The achieved results in the literature that illustrated this inverse association was seen in both men and women, appearing to be strongest amongst those with diabetic complications. Therefore, the aforementioned suggests that the inverse relation of DM with TAA and AD may further be influenced by the severity and duration of hyperglycemia, as well as the level of susceptibilty a patient has to vascular injury. A nationwide observational study comparing T2DM patient group with a control group, reported a lower short term mortality post-hospitalisation, reaching upto greater results at 2-years with better survival rates for the diabetes group (33). Alteration of aortic tissue through systemic cross linkages contribute to the protective effect of diabetes toward stabilisation of the aorta, preventing dilatation, growth and rupture (44).

A non-western population case control study performed to assess the correlation between AD risk and DM also concluded that DM was significantly associated with a decreased risk of AD. However, it is important to note that the authors reported no significant difference in in-hospital mortality when comparing the DM and non-diabetic patients (45).

## OVERCOMING A CHALLENGE: THE USE OF ANIMAL MODELS

It is challenging to define AA mechanisms in humans, which commonly results in the use of animal models to gain a deeper understanding of the pathophysiology. Although it is difficult to obtain the exact pathophysiology using animals, several probable mechanisms have been studied addressing the deficiencies in animal models (46). Dissecting and non-dissecting AAA models are used, with the non-dissecting AAA created through calcium chloride or porcine pancreatic elastase (PPE) perfusion.

There is evidence of reduced expression of Cell Division AutoAntigen (CDA-1) in the aortic biopsies of human AAA. The CDA-1 which enhances transforming growth factor (TGF)-β signalling is found to be upregulated in diabetes and is also found to play a key role in the protective effect conferred by DM on AA (47). In a study by Jiaze Li et al., DM was induced in male wild-type CDA-1 knockout (KO), Apolipoprotein E (ApoE) KO and CDA-1/ApoE double KO mice. This model was characterised by Angiotensin II (Ag-II) induced aneurysms, and the results demonstrated that CDA-1 lacking mice with diabetes developed aneurysms. On the other hand, with CDA-1 present, the severity of these aneurysms was reduced in diabetic mice and was characterised by reduced fatal aortic rupture and attenuated supra-aortic expansion (47).

The study by Miyama et al. involved hyperglycemic and euglycemic murine (mice) models. Through intra-aortic PPE infusion or by Ag-II subcutaneous infusion, the formation of AA was induced in the mice. To assess the effect of decreasing serum glucose levels, insulin therapy was also instituted in a separate cohort. The study showed hyperglycemia was linked with reduced mural neovascularisation, macrophage infiltration, and medial elastolysis. Also insulin mediated glucose reductions did partially negate the protection rendered by hyperglycemia on AA (41).

Calcium phosphate can contribute to aneurysm formation by causing apoptosis of VSMCs with subsequent macrophage infiltration. The study done by Tanaka et al. was on Type 1 and Type 2 Diabetic mice (murine models) and in them calcium phosphate induced aneurysm formation was found to be significantly suppressed in the presence of hyperglycemia. The mechanism was found to be through suppression of macrophage activation and aneurysmal degeneration through the activation of Nr1h2 (liver X receptor α and β) (48).

## DIABETES, A PROTECTIVE FACTOR? POTENTIAL MECHANISMS LEADING THE WAY

### Wall Stress

In comparison to other arteries, the aortic wall suffers from much greater stress. A typical ageing process is aortic dilation, which occurs in about a quarter of otherwise fit and healthy patients. Although the aortic wall is thicker alongside increasing age, wall stress autoregulation seems to be faulty in males, implying that the aorta is an artery susceptible to damage. Compared to non-diabetics, the AAA expansion rate is at 30%, which is not a substantial difference. An altered remodelling response observed in diabetic patients with AA compared to healthy subjects leads the protective response of AA in DM (49–51).

One of the critical factors in causing and enlarging AAA is aortic wall stress. However, diabetics are known to have a larger matrix volume leading to thicker aortic walls, which reduce aortic wall stress (7, 49, 52). Recent studies show the hyperglycemia associated with DM plays a significant role in stabilising the collagen network through crosslinking of collagen in the aortic wall media (7, 49).

### Matrix Metalloproteinases

MMPs are secreted *via* endothelial cells and macrophages, which exhibit increased activity, through proteolytic action in human aneurysmal tissue and are activated by wall stress. Specifically, through the enzymatic process of disintegrating various proteins such as elastin and collagen within the vessel wall, both MMP-2 (released *via* smooth muscle) and MMP-9 (released *via* macrophages) are involved in destructing the matrix. It has been observed that both MMP-2 and MMP-9 are increased in patients with AAA, whereas mice lacking these enzymes do not develop any dilatation of the aorta (53–57). This may be the potential mechanism through which diabetic patients have a preserved aortic matrix- due to decreased MMP activity. A lower concentration of MMP-1, MMP-2, and MMP-9 has been observed by a study that investigated the differences in MMP activity and presence in both diabetics and non-diabetics (58). Hence, it can be concluded that the potential mechanism for reduced aneurysmal events in diabetics may be through reduced MMP activity primarily, through the effects of high glucose levels (21, 49, 50).

### ECM Remodelling, Glycation, and Advanced Glycation End Products

The vascular ECM contributes to the cellular structure and tissue organisation, which comprises a vast system of components that include: elastin, basement membrane, collagen and proteoglycans (6). The interaction of the ECM and the various cells of the arterial wall play an important role when it comes to vessel remodelling. An example of this cellular remodelling can be seen in diabetic patients, with the advanced glycation of ECM proteins such as collagen, as a result of hyperglycemia. A crucial step involved in the formation and progression of AA is the secretion of MMPs, which result in proteolysis. The crosslinking of collagen and elastin resultant of the advanced glycation of the ECM within the aortic wall of the abdomen, results in the inhibition of MMP secretion and subsequently the aforementioned mechanism (6, 7).

Polysacchiride glycosaminoglycans are a component of the ECM by covalent bonding with the existing proteins forming proteoglycans. There is an abundance of biglycans in the normal aorta, however, it is decreased in the setting of AAA. Biglycans can regulate TGF-beta signalling pathway and *vice-versa*. This implies the presence of regulation *via* a mutual positive feedback mechanism, allowing the ECM's preservation, thereby providing protection against the progression of AA. The direct impact of DM on biglycans is uncertain; there may be the augmented pathway of the TGF-β signalling caused by upregulation of CDA-1 (59, 60). Furthermore, the physiological process of other glycosaminoglycans in the aorta, involving deposition, production and degradation, can be affected by the presence of DM (61).

DM and chronic hyperglycemia lead to advanced glycation end products (AGE), which influence the activation of monocyte-macrophages. This is achieved *via* unique receptors for AGE (RAGE), the engagement of which results in AGEs bringing about non-enzymatic crosslinking between ECM basement membrane components (6, 7). These mechanistic processes add to the pathophysiology of atherosclerosis, and result in numeorus signalling pathways being stimulated. It thus contributes to arterial stiffness, protecting against mechanical structural loss and resists proteolysis. The distinct properties of ECM in diabetic patients confer a protective effect on AAA (6, 7, 14, 62, 63).

## The Role of Inflammation

Inflammatory processes have a vital role in AAA and have a significant influence on many of the factors of remodelling of the wall of the aorta (16). The role inflammation plays in the negative association of DM and AAA is complex (16). The exact mechanism through which DM influences inflammation in AAA might include the stimulation of T-cell insulin receptors, the monocyte-macrophage system or through C-peptide production (41). Patients with T2DM often have increased C-peptide levels.

A study by Cifarelli et al. demonstrated that physiological levels of C-peptide can decrease hyperglycemia induced VSMC proliferation (41, 64). Haidet et al. investigated the effect of C-peptide presence on monocyte cell lines surrounded by a glucose solution. The study demonstrated a decreased expression of multiple pro-inflammatory cytokines through the NF-KB mediated pathway in the presence of C-peptide (65, 66). Studies in mice have shown low levels of IL-6 restricts both TAA and AAA progression. Glycation additionally has the potential to alter monocyte-macrophage function toward an anti-inflammatory phenotype which decreases IL-6 production (7). Additionally, Mendelian randomisation approaches support the involvement of IL-6 receptor pathway in human AAA. Glycation of IL-6 could be another factor contributing to the protective effect of DM on AA (67).

## Aortic Mural Neoangiogenesis

An important element in pathophysiological processes for aneurysms, and potential rupture, is the role played by aortic mural neoangiogenesis. In the event of AAA, there is often the linked formation of a mural thrombus; the thrombus undergoes continuous remodelling as a result of the maintained blood flow throught the abdominal aorta. The thrombus can significantly lower the wall stress, there is the impeding influence of the greater wall thickness. This structural change can subsequently result in the inner aspect of the media to be exposed to hypoxic conditions locally, which consequently leads to inflammatory response and augmented medial neovascularisation (68).

In hyperglycaemic mice, it has been found that the reduced AA diameter is concomittant with lower levels of medial elastolysis, macrophage infiltration, in addition to lower level of this neoangiogenesis. In murine models, hyperglycemia inhibiting neovessel formation by down regulation of activation of vascular endothelial growth factor expression and angiogenic response was observed. Beyond neovascularisation and macrophage infiltration, additional mechanisms include hyperglycaemic influence on the fibrinolytic system, RAGE and progenitor cell function (41).

## Intra-luminal Thrombus

Intra luminal thrombus (ILT) implicated in the pathogenesis of AA, has high concentration of MMP-9 within the thrombus and signs of collagenolytic activity. During the process of thrombus renewal, MMPs that can be found inside the thrombus are released through various processes including fibrinolysis (69–71). Dunn et al. (72) showed the clots in diabetes are denser and lower level of susceptibility to fibrinolysis.

T2DM is often associated with hyperinsulinemia which could also have a protective influence by preventing ILT renewal. Hyperinsulinemia increases PAI-1 levels and inhibits plasmin being converted from plasminogen, which decreases fibrinolysis. This in turn decreases expression of MMP, as plasmin is needed to convert proMMP to its active form (73–75). These fibrinolytic changes and renewal potential reduce clot degradation of ILT in AAA. Stability of the aortic wall can be improved through this along with reducing the rate at which the aneurysm expands (71, 72).

## Vascular Smooth Muscle Cell Homeostasis

Another vital component of the pathophysiological processes involved in the development of an aneurysm are the VSMC. Most VSMC are of contractile phenotype contributing to the vascular tone. These cells play a key role in vascular remodelling due to their ability to differentiate their phenotype, to a synthetic form. Synthetic phenotype switching triggered by oxidative stress, inflammation and injury is characterised by decreased contractile protein expression and increased MMPs. The synthetic phenotype also leads to calcification, in turn leading to risk of aneurysmal progression and rupture. AA is characterised by disrupted vessel wall structure with characteristic histology of VSMC apoptosis. TAA and AAA share a common feature of VSMC depletion and ECM proteolysis (76).

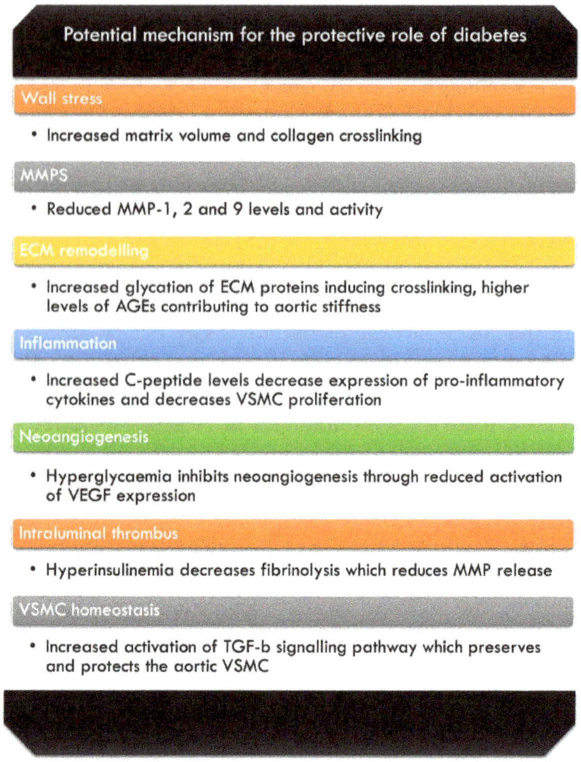


**FIGURE 1 |** Breakdown of some of the potential mechanism for the protective role of diabetes against AA disease (6, 7, 14, 41, 49, 52, 58, 63–66, 69–72).

TGF-β is required for inducing and maintaining the homeostatic and differentiating processes of the VSMC, for the mechanisms discussed. The environment created as a result of DM causes greater stimulation of the TGF-β signalling pathways, which has local and systemic effect on the VSMC of the aorta, hence plays an important protective role (6). Furthermore, as the hyperglycaemic state in the DM patients influences the VSMC, it contributes to the protection against development of aneurysm and AD through its homeostatic actions in the wall of the aorta (6) (**Figure 1**).

## HYPOGLYCAEMIC AGENTS: THE TRUE HEROES?

A number of factors, in DM patients, must be controlled to maintain a tight glycaemic control that is dependent on various medical regimes—these aim to reduce the severe risks associated with DM. Apart from a patient centric approach with life style modification, involving dietary changes and regular exercise regimens, the effective management of diabetes also involves choosing appropriate pharmacological treatment for the blood glucose control. The anti-diabetic medications used include Biguanides, SGLT2-inhibitors, dipeptidyl peptidase (DPP4) inhibitors, thiazolidinediones, glucagon-like-peptide (GLP)-1 receptor agonists, sulfonylureas and insulin therapy (77).

Various studies of different experimental designs have concluded that drugs used to manage DM have a protective role against AA.

### Biguanides—Metformin

Metformin is one of the oldest first line oral hypoglycaemic agent used in DM management. The mechanism of action of Metformin involves a reduction in the hepatic glucose production and also improvement in the tissue sensitivity to insulin. It has pleiotropic anti-inflammatory and vasculoprotective effects through various mechanisms including limiting aortic inflammation, reduction in the ECM remodelling and decreasing the oxidative stress (57, 78).

Studies by Golledge et al. and a nationwide analysis of of Veterans Affairs with DM also showed that Metformin did limit the growth of AAA (79, 80). Mice experiments by Fujimura et al. showed that the administration of Metformin during both aneurysm induction and progression periods reduces the initiation and progression of AAA in non-diabetic mice. The Metformin mediated resistance to AA was associated with reduced inflammation, elastin degradation and VSMC depletion in the histopathologic examination (81).

An improvement in the aortic elasticity was observed in a study by the addition of Metformin to oral contraceptive pills (82). Vasamsetti et al. (83) demonstrated in an Ag-II treated mice that the presence of Metformin reduced the proinflammatory cytokine levels indicating the protective role it has against aneurysm formation.

*In-vitro* studies have shown Metformin additionally reduces MMP-2 and VSMC proliferation in human aortic cells. Additionally, lower incidence of AAA associated events were found in diabetics on Metformin compared to those not on Metformin (14).

### PPAR Gamma Agonists—Thiazolidinediones

Thiazolidenediones include Pioglitazone and Rosiglitazone and these drugs act as PPAR-γ agonists and exhibit their anti-inflammatory effects by lowering tumour necrosis factor (TNF)-α levels.

Motoki et al. studied the effect of PPAR-γ agonists on the aortic wall in patients with AA and found that it may prevent or delay the progression of the aneurysm in patients *via* decreasing the expression of MMP-9 and TNF-α in the wall of the AA (84).

Piranov et al. investigated in ApoE deficient mice, the mechanism of Rosiglitazone in the earlier phases of AAs induced by Ag-II, looking at potential sites at which the drug would act. Rosiglitazone worked by inhibiting c-Jun N-terminal kinase phosphorylation and reduces the regulation of toll-like receptor 4 (TLR4) being expressed at the location at which the lesion is being formed during the initiation stage of experimental AA development. The authors further discussed an additional mechanism *via* which the initiation stages of aneurysm formation is blocked. They explain the relation of the drug with lowered levels of MIP-1α and MCP-1 chemokines, which are pro-inflammatory, as well as declining the level of CD4 antigen (85).

The action of PPAR ligands were studied by Golledje et al. investigating their impact on AA in mouse models. This study reported a significant association of Pioglitazone with lower expansion of the suprarenal aorta. This linkage may potentially be due to down regulation of osteopontin, a chemotactic factor which has an association with AAA in humans (86).

Rosiglitazone could also exert its protective effect on AAA development by reducing serum levels of MMP-9 in individuals with T2DM and thus playing a role in ECM preservation (87). Jones et al. showed that Rosiglitazone led to less inflammation due to the lower amounts of mediators IL-6 and TNF-α. Furthermore, the use of the drug makes the ECM thicker, as a result of its associated amplified production of collagen, thus reducing chances of rupture and death (88).

## Dipeptidyl Peptidase Inhibitors

DPP4 inhibitors like Sitagliptin, Vildagliptin, Teneligliptin and Alogliptin act by inhibiting the proteolytic enzyme DPP4 thus prolonging the action of GLP and delaying gastric emptying, improving glycemic control by increasing meal stimulated insulin secretion and inhibiting glucagon release.

Boa et al. studied the protective effect of DPP-4 inhibitor, Alogliptin. The study investigated on rat AAA models and found that the drug attenuated the formation and expansion of aneurysms in a dose-dependent manner *via* an antioxidative action. Rats on alogliptin showed lower rates of reactive oxygen species (ROS) activity, thus inhibiting aortic wall destruction. A reduction in the MMP-2 and MMP-9 levels were also observed. A significant reduction in aortic dilatation in the DPP-4 inhibitor-treated rats compared to the control group was observed in macroscopic findings (89).

Lu et al. studied the protective effect of Sitagliptin in induced AAA mice models. The incidence of AAA in Sitagliptin treated mice was much lower, around 4–8%. Sitagliptin-treated models showed attenuation of elastin and collagen disruptions with decreased MMP-9 and MMP-2 activity, substantial reduction in macrophage infiltration and reduced apoptosis in the wall of the aorta, thus indicative of a potential protective role of sitagliptin in AA formation (90).

## Sulfonylureas

Sulfonylureas are one of the commonly used potent oral hypoglycaemic agents. A case control analysis done by Hsu et al. with the use of Taiwan's national health insurance research database concluded that diabetic patients on oral hypoglycaemic agents, including sulfonylurea, biguanides and thiazolidinediones were associated with decreased risk of AA development. The exact mechanism by which sulfonylureas exert their protective effect is not known, as no direct clinical or experimental studies are available in this specific area.

The probable mechanism may be through the SUR-2 receptor mainly expressed on the VSMC wall (91). Indirect evidence for the aforementioned was suggested in a study by Hiraki et al. (92) reporting on a patient with AA from a family with Cantu Syndrome, a genetic disorder characterised by ABCC9 mutation affecting both the SUR-2A and SUR-2B.

## GLP-1 Receptor Agonists—Lixisenatide

Yu et al. demonstrated the protective effect of subcutaneous Lixisenatide on development of an aneurysm. The use of Lixisenatide resulted in reduction in ROS and macrophage infiltration; additionally, there is inhibition of the expression of the genes for MMP9, TNF and MMP2 in the walls of the aorta of the experimental rats. These processes instigates the protective action that Lixisenatide has *via* anti-inflammatory and anti-oxidant actions, as well as preserving ECM (93).

In Ag-II infused ApoE KO mice, Liraglutide administration was found to reduce the formation of AAA, as discussed by Lu et al. (90). This was achieved by increasing the circulating active form of GLP-1, reducing the infiltration of macrophages, and decreased expression of MMP-2 and MMP-9, thereby preserving the elastin content (90).

## SGLT2 Inhibitors—Showing Promise?

SGLT2 inhibitors are a more recent hypoglycaemic agent, which inhibit the action of the SGLT2 proteins responsible for the reabsorption of the majority of the glucose that has been filtered. These proteins are situated at the proximal convoluted tubule. The action of these drugs is *via* the blockade of the respective low affinity and high capacity proteins. As a result of this mechanism of action these drugs cause glycosuria, consequently lowering the patients plasma glucose concentration in an insulin and incretin pathway independent manner (94–96). The commonly used drugs of this class are Canagliflozin, Dapagliflozin and Empaglifozin. Apart from the kidneys, the SGLT2 protein is also found to be expressed in other tissues including: adipose tissue, vascular tissue, such as endothelial cells, and the aortic wall (97–99). Therefore, SGLT2 inhibitors have been found to have pleotropic effects, most importantly cardio-protective effect along with their glucose lowering action.

Ortega et al. demonstrated that chronic oral Empagliflozin use reduced the Ag-II induced supra-renal AAA development in ApoE KO mice. The attenuation was a result of reduction in macrophage infiltration within the lesion and down-regulation of pro-inflammatory cytokines that was observed with Empagliflozin administration (100). SGLT2 inhibitors were additonaly seen to have an impact on lowering the levels of MMP-9 and MMP-2, along with reduced atherosclerosis, in ApoE KO mice. The authors also observed a marked reduction in vascular endothelial growth factor levels and neovascularisation in these Empagliflozin co-treated mice. This cotreatment was found to diminish Ag-II induced elastin degradation in immunohistochemistry analysis (100).

*In-vitro* studies in human aortic endothelial cells revealed that Empagliflozin decreased mononuclear-leucocyte endothelial cell interactions and endothelial production of chemokines induced by Ag-II (100). Kaji et al. (101) have also demonstrated *in-vitro* suppression of human endothelial cell proliferation and tubular formation by Canagliflozin. Thus, chronic oral administration of SGLT2 inhibitors show promise as novel glucose lowering agents, displaying pleotrophic effects on AAA. Further research in this field will add greater value to its therapeutic use in DM and beyond.

**TABLE 1** | A brief outline of the mechanism by which various hypoglycaemic agents have a protective impact against AAs.

| Hypoglycaemic agent | Mechanism of aortic aneurysm prevention |
|---|---|
| Biguanides–Metformin (14, 80–82) | • Resistance to AA through: reduced inflammation, elastin degradation and smooth muscle cell depletion |
| | • Combined with oral contraceptive pills, increased aortic elasticity is observed |
| PPAR gamma agonist–Thiazolidinediones (84–86, 88) | • Decreased expression of TNF-a, MMP-9, and IL-6 in AA wall but increased collagen production |
| | • Inhibition of JNK phosphorylation and down-regulation of TLR-4 expression associated with reduced proinflammatory chemokines |
| | • Reduced aortic expansion due to downregulation of osteopontin |
| Dipeptidyl peptidase inhibitors (89, 90) | • Dose dependent suppression of ROS |
| | • Reduced levels of MMP-9 and MMP-2 |
| | • Reduced apoptosis in wall of the aorta and reduced macrophage infiltration |
| Sulfonylureas (91, 92) | • Associated with lower risk of AA development |
| | • Exact protective mechanism is not known |
| | • Proposed mechanism involves action of SUR-2 receptor on VSMC (9) wall. |
| GLP-1 receptor agonists-Lixisenatide (93) | • Reduction in ROS and macrophage infiltration |
| | • Inhibition of TNF-a, MMP-2 and MMP-9 gene expression in the aortic wall |
| SGLT2 inhibitors (94–100) | • Chronic use demonstrated reduced AAA development |
| | • SGLT2 Inhibitors have a pleotropic effect, with cardio-protective effects seen as well as just for DM treatment |
| Insulin therapy (41) | • Insulin therapy negates protective effects of oral hypoglycaemic agents |

*AA, aortic aneurysm; TNF-a, tumour necrosis factor-alpha; MMP, matrix metalloproteinase; IL, interleukin; JNK, C-Jun N-terminal kinase; TLR, toll-like receptor; ROS, reactive oxygen species; VSMC, vascular smooth muscle cell.*

**TABLE 2** | A summary of the key points from the review of the literature discussing the impact of DM on AA disease, and its role as a protective factor.

| Summary table |
|---|
| AA and DM have a well-known significant disease burden |
| DM is a recognised risk factor for cardiovascular disease; however, literature suggests a protective role of DM in AA, thoracic and abdominal, with this association being observed with aortic dissection as well |
| There have been numerous mechanisms proposed for the protective role of AA in DM, these are related to: reduced wall stress, inflammation, neoangiogenesis, lower matrix metalloproteinases, and increased stimulation of transforming growth factor-beta providing protection for the vascular smooth muscle cell |
| Clinical and experimental studies have reported that the drugs used in the management of DM have a protective role against AA |
| Further research, including molecular and genetic studies, into the link between DM and AAs could help with individualising treatment strategies in the future |

*AA, aortic aneurysm; DM, diabetes mellitus.*

## What About Insulin Therapy?

The oral hypoglycaemic agents have shown to confer a protective effect on the incidence and progression of AA. Improvement of hyperglycemia by insulin therapy however, has been found to negate the protective effects (41).

## FUTURE PERSPECTIVES

DM is an established cardiovascular risk factor and accelerates atherosclerosis. Experimental studies and data from epidemiological studies have shown DM to have a protective effect against the development, growth, expansion and rupture of AA. Human and animal studies have shown a spectrum of mechanisms by which DM could exert a protective effect on AA and dissection. Additionally, medications used in the management of hyperglycemia have shown to independently confer a protective effect on the formation and progression of AA.

These observations could help identify high risk groups to help in the primary prevention of AA. Understanding the pathogenesis involved helps in developing future prevention and management strategies both medically and surgically. The evidence of reduced expression of CDA-1 in the human AA walls and the protective effect of CDA-1 seen in experimental mice enables us to plan further involving CDA-1 as a potential therapeutic target in the prevention and management of AA. The downregulation of MMPs observed in animal models, as a potential mechanism involved in the protection observed in diabetes and with oral hypoglycaemic agents, could also act as a potential therapeutic target in future studies.

Further investigations are still needed to establish the mechanism implicated in the beneficial effect of diabetes on AD. Detailed studies into the cellular and molecular mechanisms and other genetic factors contributing to the aneurysm disease process would be required to individualise the treatment strategies in future.

## CONCLUSION

DM has a significant impact on the healthcare of our society and has clearly been shown to be a risk factor for cardiovascular disease. However, our review of the literature has demonstrated the reported protective effects that DM has in the development and progression of AA, as well as with AD.

The literature has reported various mechanisms by which hyperglycemia and presence of DM exerts its protective effects; however, it is important to note that there is yet to be a definitive consensus reached for all the proposed mechanisms. **Figure 1** illustrates these potential mechanisms against AA disease that we have covered in our review of the literature.

Building on the aforementioned, our review has highlighted the impact of oral hypoglycaemic agents themselves playing a role in the protection against AA disease. **Table 1** provides a detailed overview of the classes of drugs that we have discussed, as well as covering the negating action of insulin therapy on the protective effort by the discussed oral hypoglycaemic agents.

There is the need for further research into the association of DM and AA, investigating the molecular and genetic aspects with understanding of the natural history of these diseases. This will allow greater development of decision-making framework for management as we aim toward precision medicine for our patients (**Table 2**).

## AUTHOR CONTRIBUTIONS

DA, WM, LS, RV, JR, MB, IW, BV, and MI have all collectively contributed to the intellectual property of this article, and have been involved in design, structure, data collection and revisions of this article. All authors contributed to the article and approved the submitted version.

## REFERENCES


1. International Diabetes Federation. *IDF Diabetes Atlas.* 9th edn. Brussels: International Diabetes Federation (2019). p. 33
2. Wang L, Zhang X, Song Y. Paradoxical associations of diabetes and obesity with abdominal aortic aneurysm. *North Am J Med Sci.* (2017) 10:83–7.
3. Kuivaniemi H, Elmore JR. Opportunities in abdominal aortic aneurysm research: epidemiology, genetics, and pathophysiology. *Ann Vasc Surg.* (2012) 26:862–70. doi: 10.1016/j.avsg.2012.02.005
4. Sakalihasan N, Limet R, Defawe OD. Abdominal aortic aneurysm. *Lancet.* (2005) 365:1577–89. doi: 10.1016/S0140-6736(05)66459-8
5. Howard D, Banerjee A, Fairhead J, Handa A, Silver L, Rothwell P. Age-specific incidence, risk factors and outcome of acute abdominal aortic aneurysms in a defined population. *Br J Surg.* (2015) 102:907–15. doi: 10.1002/bjs.9838
6. Raffort J, Lareyre F, Clément M, Hassen-Khodja R, Chinetti G, Mallat Z. Diabetes and aortic aneurysm: current state of the art. *Cardiovasc Res.* (2018) 114:1702–13. doi: 10.1093/cvr/cvy174
7. Golledge J, Karan M, Moran C, Muller J, Clancy P, Dear A, et al. Reduced expansion rate of abdominal aortic aneurysms in patients with diabetes may be related to aberrant monocyte-matrix interactions. *Eur Heart J.* (2008) 29:665–72. doi: 10.1093/eurheartj/ehm557
8. Patel K, Zafar M, Ziganshin B, Elefteriades J. Diabetes mellitus: is it protective against aneurysm? *a narrative review. Cardiology.* (2018) 141:107–22. doi: 10.1159/000490373
9. Wassef M, Baxter B, Chisholm R, Dalman R, Fillinger M, Heinecke J, et al. Pathogenesis of abdominal aortic aneurysms: a multidisciplinary research program supported by the National Heart, Lung, and Blood Institute. *J Vasc Surg.* (2001) 34:730–8. doi: 10.1067/mva.2001.116966
10. Cronenwett J, Sargent S, Wall M, Hawkes M, Freeman D, Dain B, et al. Variables that affect the expansion rate and outcome of small abdominal aortic aneurysms. *J Vasc Surg.* (1990) 11:260–9. doi: 10.1016/0741-5214(90)90269-G
11. Hall A, Busse E, McCarville D, Burgess J. Aortic wall tension as a predictive factor for abdominal aortic aneurysm rupture: improving the selection of patients for abdominal aortic aneurysm repair. *Ann Vasc Surg.* (2000) 14:152–7. doi: 10.1007/s100169910027
12. Li Z, Kleinstreuer C. A new wall stress equation for aneurysm-rupture prediction. *Ann Biomed Eng.* (2005) 33:209–13. doi: 10.1007/s10439-005-8979-2
13. Fillinger M, Marra S, Raghavan M, Kennedy F. Prediction of rupture risk in abdominal aortic aneurysm during observation: wall stress versus diameter. *J Vasc Surg.* (2003) 37:724–32. doi: 10.1067/mva.2003.213
14. Shantikumar S, Ajjan R, Porter K, Scott D. Diabetes and the abdominal aortic aneurysm. *Eur J Vasc Endovasc Surg.* (2010) 39:200–7. doi: 10.1016/j.ejvs.2009.10.014
15. Kuivaniemi H, Sakalihasan N, Lederle F, Jones G, Defraigne J, Labropoulos N et al. New insights into aortic diseases. *AORTA.* (2013) 1:23–39. doi: 10.12945/j.aorta.2013.13.006
16. Raffort J, Lareyre F, Clément M, Hassen-Khodja R, Chinetti G, Mallat Z. Monocytes and macrophages in abdominal aortic aneurysm. *Nat Rev Cardiol.* (2017) 14:457–71. doi: 10.1038/nrcardio.2017.52
17. Elefteriades JA. Thoracic aortic aneurysm: reading the enemy's playbook. *Yale J Biol Med.* (2008) 81:175–86. doi: 10.1016/j.cpcardiol.2008.01.004
18. Prasad K, Sarkar A, Zafar M, Shoker A, Moselhi H, Tranquilli M, et al. Advanced glycation end products and its soluble receptors in the pathogenesis of thoracic aortic aneurysm. *AORTA.* (2016) 04:1–10. doi: 10.12945/j.aorta.2016.15.018
19. Quintana RA, Taylor WR. Cellular mechanisms of aortic aneurysm formation. *Circ Res.* (2019) 124:607–18. doi: 10.1161/CIRCRESAHA.118.313187
20. Deshpande AD, Harris-Hayes M, Schootman M. Epidemiology of diabetes and diabetes-related complications. *J Am Phys Ther Assoc.* (2008) 88:1254–64. doi: 10.2522/ptj.20080020
21. Lederle FA, Johnson GR, Wilson SE, Chute EP, Littooy FN, Bandyk N, et al. Prevalence and associations of abdominal aortic aneurysm detected through screening. Aneurysm Detection and Management (ADAM) Veterans Affairs Cooperative Study Group. *Ann Intern Med.* (1997) 126:441–9. doi: 10.7326/0003-4819-126-6-199703150-00004
22. Lederle FA, Johnson GR, Wilson SE, Chute EP, Hye RJ, Makaroun MS, et al. The aneurysm detection and management study screening program: validation cohort and final results. *Aneurysm Detection and Management Veterans Affairs Cooperative Study Investigators Arch Intern Med.* (2000) 160:1425–30. doi: 10.1001/archinte.160.10.1425
23. Climent E, Benaiges D, Chillarón J, Flores-Le Roux J, Pedro-Botet J. La diabetes mellitus como factor protector del aneurisma de aorta abdominal: posibles mecanismos. *Clín Invest Arterioscl.* (2018) 30:181–7. doi: 10.1016/j.arteri.2018.01.002
24. Tsai C, Lin C, Wu Y, Shieh D, Sung F, Kao C. Advanced complicated diabetes mellitus is associated with a reduced risk of thoracic and abdominal aortic aneurysm rupture: a population-based cohort study. *Diabetes Metab Res Rev.* (2015) 31:190–7. doi: 10.1002/dmrr.2585
25. Kristensen K, Dahl M, Rasmussen L, Lindholt J. Glycated hemoglobin is associated with the growth rate of abdominal aortic aneurysms. *Arterioscler Thromb Vasc Biol.* (2017) 37:730–6. doi: 10.1161/ATVBAHA.116.308874
26. Theivacumar N, Stephenson M, Mistry H, Valenti D. Diabetes mellitus and aortic aneurysm rupture. *Vasc Endovascular Surg.* (2013) 48:45–50. doi: 10.1177/1538574413505921
27. Vega M, Gómez R, Estallo L, Rodríguez L, Baquer M, Barba A. Growth rate and associated factors in small abdominal aortic aneurysms. *Eur J Vasc Endovasc Surg.* (2006) 31:231–6. doi: 10.1016/j.ejvs.2005.10.007
28. Takagi H, Umemoto T, ALICE (All-Literature Investigation of Cardiovascular Evidence) Group. Negative association of diabetes

with rupture of abdominal aortic aneurysm. *Diab Vasc Dis Res.* (2016) 13:341–7. doi: 10.1177/1479164116651389
29. Hughes K, Jackson J, Prendergast T, Rose D, Bolorunduro O, Obirieze A, et al. Diabetes mellitus is not associated with major morbidity following open abdominal aortic aneurysm repair. *J Surg Res.* (2013) 184:751–4. doi: 10.1016/j.jss.2013.04.025
30. Weiss JS, Sumpio BE. Review of prevalence and outcome of vascular disease in patients with diabetes mellitus. *Eur J Vasc Endovasc Surg.* (2006) 31:143–50. doi: 10.1016/j.ejvs.2005.08.015
31. Lopez-de-Andrés A, Jiménez-Trujillo I, Jiménez-García R, Hernández-Barrera V, de Miguel-Yanes J, Méndez-Bailón M, et al. National trends in incidence and outcomes of abdominal aortic aneurysm among elderly type 2 diabetic and non-diabetic patients in Spain (2003–2012). *Cardiovasc Diabetol.* (2015) 14:48. doi: 10.1186/s12933-015-0216-1
32. Elefteriades JA, Sang A, Kuzmik G, Hornick M. Guilt by association: paradigm for detecting a silent killer (thoracic aortic aneurysm). *Open Heart.* (2015) 2:e000169. doi: 10.1136/openhrt-2014-000169
33. Prakash SK, Pedroza C, Khalil YA, Milewicz DM. Diabetes and reduced risk for thoracic aortic aneurysms and dissections: a nationwide case-control study. *J Am Heart Assoc.* (2012) 1:e000323. doi: 10.1161/JAHA.111.000323
34. Jiménez-Trujillo I, González-Pascual M, Jiménez-García R, Hernández-Barrera V, de Miguel-Yanes JM, Méndez-Bailón M, et al. Type 2 diabetes mellitus and thoracic aortic aneurysm and dissection: an observational population-based study in spain from 2001 to 2012. *Medicine.* (2016) 95:e3618. doi: 10.1097/MD.0000000000003618
35. De Rango P, Cao P, Cieri E, Parlani G, Lenti M, Simonte G, et al. Effects of diabetes on small aortic aneurysms under surveillance according to a subgroup analysis from a randomized trial. *J Vasc Surg.* (2012) 56:1555–63. doi: 10.1016/j.jvs.2012.05.078
36. Takagi H, Umemoto T, ALICE (All-Literature Investigation of Cardiovascular Evidence) Group. Negative association of diabetes with thoracic aortic dissection and aneurysm. *Angiology.* (2017) 68:216–224. doi: 10.1177/0003319716647626
37. Pafili K, Gouni-Berthold I, Papanas N, Mikhailidis DP. Abdominal aortic aneurysms and diabetes mellitus. *J Diab Comp.* (2015) 29:1330–6. doi: 10.1016/j.jdiacomp.2015.08.011
38. De Rango P, Farchioni L, Fiorucci B, Lenti M. Diabetes and abdominal aortic aneurysms. *Eur J Vasc Endovasc Surg.* (2014) 47:243–61. doi: 10.1016/j.ejvs.2013.12.007
39. Schlösser F, Vaartjes I, Heijden G, Moll F, Verhagen HJM, Muhs BE, et al. Mortality after elective abdominal aortic aneurysm repair. *Ann Surg.* (2010) 251:158–64. doi: 10.1097/SLA.0b013e3181bc9c4d
40. Dua MM, Miyama N, Azuma J, Schultz GM, Sho M, Morser J, et al. Hyperglycemia modulates plasminogen activator inhibitor-1 expression and aortic diameter in experimental aortic aneurysm disease. *Surgery.* (2010) 148:429–35. doi: 10.1016/j.surg.2010.05.014
41. Miyama N, Dua MM, Yeung JJ, Schultz GM, Asagami T, Sho E, et al. Hyperglycemia limits experimental aortic aneurysm progression. *J Vasc Surg.* (2010) 52:975–83. doi: 10.1016/j.jvs.2010.05.086
42. Tsai TT, Trimarchi S, Nienaber CA. Acute aortic dissection: perspectives from the international registry of acute aortic dissection (IRAD). *Eur J Vasc Endovasc Surg.* (2009) 37:149–59. doi: 10.1016/j.ejvs.2008.11.032
43. Karthikesalingam A, Holt PJE, Hinchliffe RJ, Thompson MM, Loftus IM. The diagnosis and management of aortic dissection. *Vasc Endovascular Surg.* (2010) 44:165–9. doi: 10.1177/1538574410362118
44. Avdic T, Franzen S, Zarrouk M, Acosta S, Nilsson P, Gottsäter A, et al. Reduced long-term risk of aortic aneurysm and aortic dissection among individuals with type 2 diabetes mellitus: a nationwide observational study. *J Am Heart Assoc.* (2018) 7:e007618. doi: 10.1161/JAHA.117.007618
45. He X, Liu X, Liu W, Wang B, Liu Y, Li Z, et al. Association between diabetes and risk of aortic dissection: a case-control study in a Chinese population. *PLoS ONE.* (2015) 10:e0142697. doi: 10.1371/journal.pone.0142697
46. Sénémaud J, Caligiuri G, Etienne H, Delbosc S, Michel JB, Coscas R. Translational relevance and recent advances of animal models of abdominal aortic aneurysm. *Arterioscler Thromb Vasc Biol.* (2017) 37:401–10. doi: 10.1161/ATVBAHA.116.308534
47. Li J, Huynh P, Dai A, Wu T, Tu Y, Chow B, et al. Diabetes reduces severity of aortic aneurysms depending on the presence of cell division autoantigen 1 (CDA1). *Diabetes.* (2018) 67:755–68. doi: 10.2337/db17-0134
48. Tanaka T, Takei Y, Yamanouchi D. Hyperglycemia suppresses calcium phosphate-induced aneurysm formation through inhibition of macrophage activation. *J Am Heart Assoc.* (2016) 5:e003062. doi: 10.1161/JAHA.115.003062
49. Astrand H, Ryden-Ahlgren A, Sundkvist G, Sandgren T, Länne T. Reduced aortic wall stress in diabetes mellitus. *Eur J Vasc Endovasc Surg.* (2007) 33:592–8. doi: 10.1016/j.ejvs.2006.11.011
50. Brady AR, Thompson SG, Fowkes GR, Greenhalgh RM, Powell JT, UK. Small aneurysm trial participants. Abdominal aortic aneurysm expansion: risk factors and time intervals for surveillance. *Circulation.* (2004) 110:16–21. doi: 10.1161/01.CIR.0000133279.07468.9F
51. Sonesson B, Länne T, Hansen F, Sandgren T. Infrarenal aortic diameter in the healthy person. *Eur J Vasc Surg.* (1994) 8:89–95. doi: 10.1016/S0950-821X(05)80127-6
52. Mauer SM. Structural-functional correlations of diabetic nephropathy. *Kidney Int.* (1994) 45:612–22. doi: 10.1038/ki.1994.80
53. Death AK, Fisher EJ, McGrath KCY, Yue DK. High glucose alters matrix metalloproteinase expression in two key vascular cells: potential impact on atherosclerosis in diabetes. *Atherosclerosis.* (2003) 168:263–9. doi: 10.1016/S0021-9150(03)00140-0
54. Freestone T, Turner RJ, Coady A, Higman DJ, Greenhalgh RM, Powell JT. Inflammation and matrix metalloproteinases in the enlarging abdominal aortic aneurysm. *Arterioscler Thromb Vasc Biol.* (1995) 15:1145–51. doi: 10.1161/01.ATV.15.8.1145
55. Goodall S, Crowther M, Hemingway DM, Bell PR, Thompson MM. Ubiquitous elevation of matrix metalloproteinase-2 expression in the vasculature of patients with abdominal aneurysms. *Circulation.* (2001) 104:304–9. doi: 10.1161/01.CIR.104.3.304
56. McMillan WD, Tamarina NA, Cipollone M, Johnson DA, Parker MA, Pearce WH. Size matters: the relationship between MMP-9 expression and aortic diameter. *Circulation.* (1997) 96:2228–32. doi: 10.1161/01.CIR.96.7.2228
57. Golledge J, Morris DR, Pinchbeck J, Rowbotham S, Jenkins J, Bourke M, et al. Metformin prescription is associated with a reduction in the combined incidence of surgical repair and rupture related mortality in patients with abdominal aortic aneurysm. *Eur J Vasc Endovasc Surg.* (2019) 57:94–101. doi: 10.1016/j.ejvs.2018.07.035
58. Portik-Dobos V, Anstadt MP, Hutchinson J, Bannan M, Ergul A. Evidence for a matrix metalloproteinase induction/activation system in arterial vasculature and decreased synthesis and activity in diabetes. *Diabetes.* (2002) 51:3063–8. doi: 10.2337/diabetes.51.10.3063
59. Mallat Z, Ait-Oufella H, Tedgui A. The pathogenic transforming growth factor-beta overdrive hypothesis in aortic aneurysms and dissections: a mirage? *Circ Res.* (2017) 120:1718–20. doi: 10.1161/CIRCRESAHA.116.310371
60. Lareyre F, Clement M, Raffort J, Pohlod S, Patel M, Esposito B, et al. TGFbeta (Transforming Growth Factor-beta) blockade induces a human-like disease in a nondissecting mouse model of abdominal aortic aneurysm. *Arterioscler Thromb Vasc Biol.* (2017) 37:2171–81. doi: 10.1161/ATVBAHA.117.309999
61. Ferdous Z, Wei VM, Iozzo R, Höök M, Grande-Allen KJ. Decorin-transforming growth factor- interaction regulates matrix organization and mechanical characteristics of three-dimensional collagen matrices. *J Biol Chem.* (2007) 282:35887–98. doi: 10.1074/jbc.M705180200
62. Goldin A, Beckman JA, Schmidt AM, Creager MA. Advanced glycation end products: sparking the development of diabetic vascular injury. *Circulation.* (2006) 114:597–605. doi: 10.1161/CIRCULATIONAHA.106.621854
63. Norman PE, Davis TM, Le MT, Golledge J. Matrix biology of abdominal aortic aneurysms in diabetes: mechanisms underlying the negative association. *Connect Tissue Res.* (2007) 48:125–31. doi: 10.1080/03008200701331524
64. Viardot A, Grey ST, Mackay F, Chisholm D. Potential antiinflammatory role of insulin via the preferential polarization of effector T cells toward a T helper 2 phenotype. *Endocrinology.* (2007) 148:346–53. doi: 10.1210/en.2006-0686

65. Cifarelli V, Luppi P, Tse HM, He J, Piganelli J, Trucco M. Human proinsulin C-peptide reduces high glucose-induced proliferation and NF-kappaB activation in vascular smooth muscle cells. *Atherosclerosis.* (2008) 201:248–57. doi: 10.1016/j.atherosclerosis.2007.12.060
66. Haidet J, Cifarelli V, Trucco M, Luppi P. C-peptide reduces pro-inflammatory cytokine secretion in LPS-stimulated U937 monocytes in condition of hyperglycemia. *Inflamm Res.* (2012) 61:27–35. doi: 10.1007/s00011-011-0384-8
67. Harrison SC, Smith AJ, Jones GT, Swerdlow DI. Rampuri, R, Bown MJ, et al. Interleukin-6 receptor pathways in abdominal aortic aneurysm. *Eur Heart J.* (2013) 34:3707–16. doi: 10.1093/eurheartj/ehs354
68. Vorp DA, Lee PC, Wang DH, Makaroun MS, Nemoto EM, Ogawa S, et al. Association of intraluminal thrombus in abdominal aortic aneurysm with local hypoxia and wall weakening. *J Vasc Surg.* (2001) 34:291–9. doi: 10.1067/mva.2001.114813
69. Dattani N, Sayers RD, Bown MJ. Diabetes mellitus and abdominal aortic aneurysms: a review of the mechanisms underlying the negative relationship. *Diab Vasc Dis Res.* (2018) 15(5) 367–374. doi: 10.1177/1479164118780799
70. Touat Z, Ollivier V, Dai J, Huisse M, Bezeaud A, Sebbag U, et al. Renewal of mural thrombus releases plasma markers and is involved in aortic abdominal aneurysm evolution. *Am J Pathol.* (2006) 168:1022–30. doi: 10.2353/ajpath.2006.050868
71. Houard X, Rouzet F, Touat Z, Philippe M, Dominguez M, Fontaine V, et al. Topology of the fibrinolytic system within the mural thrombus of human abdominal aortic aneurysms. *J Pathol.* (2007) 212:20–8. doi: 10.1002/path.2148
72. Dunn EJ, Ariëns RA, Grant PJ. The influence of type 2 diabetes on fibrin structure and function. *Diabetologia.* (2005) 48:1198–206. doi: 10.1007/s00125-005-1742-2
73. Festa A, Williams K, Tracy RP, Wagenknecht LE, Haffner SM. Progression of plasminogen activator inhibitor-1 and fibrinogen levels in relation to incident type 2 diabetes. *Circulation.* (2006) 113:1753–9. doi: 10.1161/CIRCULATIONAHA.106.616177
74. Murphy G, Atkinson S, Ward R, Gavrilovic J, Reynolds JJ. The role of plasminogen activators in the regulation of connective tissue metalloproteinases. *Ann N Y Acad Sci.* (1992) 667:1–12. doi: 10.1111/j.1749-6632.1992.tb51590.x
75. Festa A, D'Agostino Jr R, Mykkänen L, Tracy RP, Zaccaro DJ, Hales CN, et al. Relative contribution of insulin and its precursors to fibrinogen and PAI-1 in a large population with different states of glucose tolerance. The Insulin Resistance Atherosclerosis Study (IRAS). *Arterioscler Thromb Vasc Biol.* (1999) 19:562–8. doi: 10.1161/01.ATV.19.3.562
76. Petsophonsakul P, Furmanik M, Forsythe R, Dweck M, Schurink GW, Natour E, et al. Role of vascular smooth muscle cell phenotypic switching and calcification in aortic aneurysm formation. Involvement of vitamin k-dependent processes. *Arterioscler Thromb Vasc Bio.* (2019) 39:1351–68. doi: 10.1161/ATVBAHA.119.312787
77. American Diabetes Association. Pharmacologic approaches to glycemic treatment: standards of medical care in diabetes 2020. *Diab Care.* (2020) 43(Suppl 1): S98–110. doi: 10.2337/dc20-S009
78. Isoda K, Young JL, Zirlik A, MacFarlane LA, Tsuboi N, Gerdes N, et al. Metformin inhibits proinflammatory responses and nuclear factor-kappaB in human vascular wall cells. *Arterioscler Thromb Vasc Biol.* (2006) 26:611–7. doi: 10.1161/01.ATV.0000201938.78044.75
79. Golledge J, Moxon J, Pinchbeck J, Anderson G, Rowbotham S, Jenkins J, et al. Association between metformin prescription and growth rates of abdominal aortic aneurysms. *Br J Surg.* (2017) 104:1486–93. doi: 10.1002/bjs.10587
80. Itoga NK, Rothenberg KA, Suarez P, Ho TV, Mell MW, Xu B, et al. Metformin prescription status and abdominal aortic aneurysm disease progression in the U. S. veteran population. *J Vasc Surg.* (2019) 69:710–6. doi: 10.1016/j.jvs.2018.06.194
81. Fujimura N, Xiong J, Kettler EB, Xuan H, Glover KJ, Mell MW, et al. Metformin treatment status and abdominal aortic aneurysm disease progression. *J Vasc Surg.* (2016) 64:46–54. doi: 10.1016/j.jvs.2016.02.020
82. Kaya MG, Calapkorur B, Karaca Z, Yildirim S, Celik A, Akpek M, et al. The effects of treatment with drospirenone/ethinyl oestradiol alone or in combination with metformin on elastic properties of aorta in women with polycystic ovary syndrome. *Clin Endocrinol.* (2012) 77:885–92. doi: 10.1111/j.1365-2265.2012.04436.x
83. Vasamsetti SB, Karnewar S, Kanugula AK, Thatipalli AR, Kumar JM, Kotamraju S. Metformin inhibits monocyte-to-macrophage differentiation *via* AMPK-mediated inhibition of STAT3 activation: potential role in atherosclerosis. *Diabetes.* (2015) 64:2028–41. doi: 10.2337/db14-1225
84. Motoki T, Kurobe H, Hirata Y, Nakayama T, Kinoshita H, Rocco KA, et al. PPAR-γ agonist attenuates inflammation in aortic aneurysm patients. *Gen Thorac Cardiovasc Surg.* (2015) 63:565–71. doi: 10.1007/s11748-015-0576-1
85. Pirianov G, Torsney E, Howe F, Cokerill GW. Rosiglitazone negatively regulates c-Jun N-terminal kinase and toll-like receptor 4 proinflammatory signalling during initiation of experimental aortic aneurysms. *Atherosclerosis.* (2012) 225:69–75. doi: 10.1016/j.atherosclerosis.2012.07.034
86. Golledge J, Cullen B, Rush C, Moran CS, Secomb E, Wood F, et al. Peroxisome proliferator-activated receptor ligands reduce aortic dilatation in a mouse model of aortic aneurysm. *Atherosclerosis.* (2010) 210:51–6. doi: 10.1016/j.atherosclerosis.2009.10.027
87. Haffner SM, Greenberg AS, Weston WM, Chen H, Williams K, Freed MI. Effect of rosiglitazone treatment on nontraditional markers of cardiovascular disease in patients with type 2 diabetes mellitus. *Circulation.* (2002) 106:679–84. doi: 10.1161/01.CIR.0000025403.20953.23
88. Jones A, Deb R, Torsney E, Howe F, Dunkley M, Gnaneswaran Y, et al. Rosiglitazone reduces the development and rupture of experimental aortic aneurysms. *Circulation.* (2009) 119:3125–32. doi: 10.1161/CIRCULATIONAHA.109.852467
89. Bao W, Morimoto K, Hasegawa T, Sasaki N, Yamashita T, Hirata K, et al. Orally administered dipeptidyl peptidase-4 inhibitor (alogliptin) prevents abdominal aortic aneurysm formation through an antioxidant effect in rats. *J Vasc Surg.* (2014) 59:1098–108. doi: 10.1016/j.jvs.2013.04.048
90. Lu HY, Huang CY, Shih CM, Chang WH, Tsai CS, Lin FY, et al. Dipeptidyl peptidase-4 inhibitor decreases abdominal aortic aneurysm formation through GLP-1-dependent monocytic activity in mice. *PLoS ONE.* (2015) 10:e0121077. doi: 10.1371/journal.pone.0121077
91. Hsu CY, Su YW, Chen YT, Tsai SH, Chang CC Li SY, et al. Association between use of oral-antidiabetic drugs and the risk of aortic aneurysm: a nested case-control analysis. *Cardiovasc Diabetol.* (2016) 15:125. doi: 10.1186/s12933-016-0447-9
92. Hiraki Y, Miyatake S, Hayashidani M, Nishimura Y, Matsuura H, Kamada M, et al. Aortic aneurysm and craniosynostosis in a family with Cantu syndrome. *Am J Med Genet A.* (2014). 164A:231–6. doi: 10.1002/ajmg.a.36228
93. Yu J, Morimoto K, Bao W, Yu Z, Okita Y, Okada K. Glucagon-like peptide-1 prevented abdominal aortic aneurysm development in rats. *Surg Today.* (2016) 46:1099–107. doi: 10.1007/s00595-015-1287-z
94. Hummel CS, Lu C, DDF. Loo, Hirayama BA, Voss AA, Wright EM. Glucose transport by human renal Na+/D-glucose cotransporters SGLT1 and SGLT2. *Am J Physiol Cell Physiol.* (2011) 300:C14–21. doi: 10.1152/ajpcell.00388.2010
95. Kalra S. Sodium glucose co-transporter-2 (SGLT2) inhibitors: a review of their basic and clinical pharmacology. *Diabetes Ther.* (2014) 5:355–66. doi: 10.1007/s13300-014-0089-4
96. Joshi SS, Singh T, Newby DE, Singh J. Sodium-glucose co-transporter 2 inhibitor therapy: mechanisms of action in heart failure. *Heart.* (2021) 107:1032–8. doi: 10.1136/heartjnl-2020-318060
97. El-Daly M, Venu VKP, Saifeddine M, Mihara K, Kang S, Fedak PWM, et al. Hyperglycaemic impairment of PAR2-mediated vasodilation: prevention by inhibition of aortic endothelial sodium-glucose-co-transporter-2 and minimizing oxidative stress. *Vascul Pharmacol.* (2018) 109:56–71. doi: 10.1016/j.vph.2018.06.006
98. Díaz-Rodríguez E, Agra RM, Fernández ÁL, Adrio B, Garcia-Caballero T, Gonzalez-Juanatey JR, et al. Effects of dapagliflozin on human epicardial adipose tissue: modulation of insulin resistance, inflammatory chemokine production, and differentiation ability. *Cardiovasc Res.* (2018) 114:336–46. doi: 10.1093/cvr/cvx186
99. Mancini SJ, Boyd D, Katwan OJ, Strembitska A, Almabrouk TA, Kennedy S, et al. Canagliflozin inhibits interleukin-1β-stimulated cytokine and chemokine secretion in vascular endothelial cells by AMP-activated protein kinase-dependent and -independent mechanisms. *Sci Rep.* (2018) 8:5276. doi: 10.1038/s41598-018-23420-4

100. Ortega R, Collado A, Selles F, Gonzalez-Navarro H, Sanz MJ, Real JT, et al. SGLT-2 (sodium-glucose cotransporter 2) inhibition reduces Ang II (Angiotensin II)–induced dissecting abdominal aortic aneurysm in ApoE (apolipoprotein E) knockout mice. *Arterioscl. Thromb. Vasc. Biol.* (2019) 39:1614–28. doi: 10.1161/ATVBAHA.119.312659

101. Kaji K, Nishimura N, Seki K, Sato S, Saikawa S, Nakanishi K, et al. Sodium glucose cotransporter 2 inhibitor canagliflozin attenuates liver cancer cell growth and angiogenic activity by inhibiting glucose uptake. *Int J Cancer.* (2018) 142:1712–22. doi: 10.1002/ijc.31193

3

# One-Stop Hybrid Coronary Revascularization Versus Off-Pump Coronary Artery Bypass Grafting in Patients with Multivessel Coronary Artery Disease

*Dongjie Li*[1]*, Yulin Guo*[1]*, Yingdi Gao*[1]*, Xiangguang An*[1]*, Yan Liu*[1]*, Song Gu*[1]*, Xitao Zhang*[1]*, Jiuchang Zhong*[2]*, Jie Gao*[1*] *and Pixiong Su*[1*]

[1] Department of Cardiac Surgery, Heart Center and Beijing Key Laboratory of Hypertension, Beijing Chaoyang Hospital, Capital Medical University, Beijing, China, [2] Heart Center and Beijing Key Laboratory of Hypertension, Beijing Chaoyang Hospital, Capital Medical University, Beijing, China

***Correspondence:**
Jie Gao
gaojie19750824@163.com
Pixiong Su
supixiong1130@163.com

**Background:** Data on one-stop hybrid coronary revascularization (HCR) are limited. This study aimed to compare the early and midterm outcomes of one-stop HCR with off-pump coronary artery bypass grafting (OPCAB) in patients with multivessel coronary artery disease.

**Methods:** From April 2018 to May 2021, 752 patients with multivessel coronary artery disease who underwent isolated one-stop HCR or OPCAB were retrospectively included in this analysis. After exclusion and propensity score matching, 151 patients who underwent HCR were matched with 151 patients who underwent OPCAB. The primary endpoints were midterm major adverse cardiovascular and cerebrovascular events (MACCE) after the procedure. The secondary endpoints were in-hospital complications and outcomes.

**Results:** The preprocedural characteristics were well balanced between the two groups after matching. The HCR group was associated with a lower rate of perioperative transfusion (23.8 vs. 53.0%, $p < 0.001$) and new-onset atrial fibrillation (AF) (5.3 vs. 15.2%, $p = 0.004$), shorter time of mechanical ventilation (h) [15 (16, 17) vs. 17 (16, 20), $p < 0.001$], and shorter length of stay (LOS) in the hospital (days) [19 (16, 24) vs. 22 (18, 27), $p = 0.001$]. Cumulated MACCE rates were similar between the two groups (15.9 vs. 14.0%, $p = 0.59$) during a median follow-up of 20 months.

**Conclusions:** One-stop HCR is safe and efficacious with less invasiveness and faster postoperative recovery in selected patients with multivessel coronary artery disease. Randomized controlled trials with larger sample sizes and long-term follow-up are warranted to confirm these findings.

**Keywords: hybrid coronary revascularization (HCR), off-pump coronary artery bypass graft (OPCAB), percutaneous coronary intervention (PCI), minimally invasive direct coronary artery bypass (MIDCAB), major adverse cardiovascular and cerebrovascular events (MACCE)**

## INTRODUCTION

Coronary artery bypass grafting (CABG) remains the gold standard for the treatment of multivessel coronary artery disease (1–3). The left internal mammary artery (LIMA) to left anterior descending (LAD) graft provides most of the survival benefit of CABG due to its long-term patency rate, which can reach 90% at 10 years. However, the 10-year patency for saphenous vein graft (SVG) was only 60%, and conventional CABG is a relatively invasive and high-risk procedure via sternotomy (4–6). In-stent restenosis was <6% in patients undergoing percutaneous coronary intervention (PCI) with drug eluting stents (DESs) (7). However, the long-term outcomes of PCI were not superior to those of CABG in patients with intermediate or high SYNTAX scores (>22) (8, 9).

Hybrid coronary revascularization (HCR) was first introduced by Angelini in 1996 and consisted of LIMA-LAD anastomosis using a minimally invasive left thoracotomy approach and PCI procedure for non-LAD lesions (10). HCR combines the advantages of CABG and PCI, avoids their relative deficiencies, and achieves complete revascularization. The HYBRID trial and several observational studies have shown similar short and long-term outcomes compared with off-pump or on-pump CABG (11–14). Nevertheless, data comparing HCR and off-pump CABG (OPCAB) are still limited, and the safety and efficacy of HCR in multivessel coronary artery disease have not been completely indicated, especially for one-stop HCR patients, due to the majority composition of staged HCR in these studies. Considering the potentially different strengths and disadvantages between one-stop and staged HCR, the results of one-stop HCR need to be separately evaluated.

Therefore, we sought to investigate the early and midterm outcomes of one-stop HCR compared with OPCAB in patients with multivessel coronary artery disease to evaluate the safety and effectiveness of this procedure.

## METHODS

### Study Population

This was a retrospective single-center observational study conducted at Beijing Chaoyang Hospital, Capital Medical University. From April 2018 to May 2021, data from a total of 752 patients with multivessel coronary artery disease who underwent isolated one-stop HCR or OPCAB were collected. Patients with ST-segment elevation myocardial infarction within 30 days before the procedure, ejection fraction <30%, hemodynamic instability, and creatinine clearance <30 ml/min were excluded. Finally, 151 patients underwent one-stop HCR (HCR group), and 531 patients who received OPCAB (OPCAB group) were enrolled in this study. **Figure 1** shows the detailed flow of this study.

For the choice of revascularization strategies, all patients were reviewed and discussed preoperatively by the heart team of our center, which consisted of cardiac surgeons, interventional cardiologists, and anesthesiologists, to make the most appropriate decision regarding PCI, CABG, or HCR. The selection criteria of patients who underwent one-stop HCR were as follows: patients with multivessel disease in whom the LAD lesion was not suitable for PCI but was suitable for surgical revascularization and in whom the non-LAD lesions were amenable to PCI; and patients who were not good candidates for traditional CABG, such as poor right coronary or circumflex arteries for bypass, relative contraindication for sternotomy, porcelain aorta, lack of acceptable conduits, and patient desire for minimally invasive procedures.

### Data Collection

Preoperative risk profile and demographic features, including age, sex, body mass index (BMI), hypertension, hyperlipoidemia, diabetes mellitus (DM), and smoking status, were retrospectively extracted for all patients from the database of Chaoyang Hospital. Intraoperative and postoperative variables were also collected. The SYNTAX score and EuroSCORE II were calculated based on the anatomy of the lesions and preoperative risk factors. The study was conducted in accordance with the Declaration of Helsinki (as revised in 2013). The study was approved by the local research ethics board of Chaoyang Hospital (No.: 2021-D-5), and individual consent for this retrospective analysis was waived.

### Surgical Technique and Intervention

For the HCR group, all patients underwent one-stop HCR in the hybrid operating room. Surgical procedures were performed by minimally invasive direct coronary artery bypass (MIDCAB) or endoscopic assisted coronary artery bypass. LIMA was harvested as a pedicle directly through a small anterior thoracotomy (5–7 cm) at the fourth to fifth intercostal space using special retractors or via an endoscope to avoid chest wall retraction and rib spreading. Then, LIMA was hand sewn to the LAD territory via direct vision. All surgical procedures were performed by one experienced surgeon (Pixiong Su). A partial dose of protamine was administrated to neutralize heparin after LIMA-LAD anastomosis. Then, a loading dose of clopidogrel was administrated before closure of the thorax. The PCI procedures were performed according to practice guidelines and standard techniques (15). PCI for non-LAD lesions was performed through the femoral artery, and the femoral arterial sheath was placed before heparinization to avoid potential access site hematomas. The guidewire and stent selection were performed according to the interventionist's discretion. LIMA-LAD graft patency was immediately confirmed by angiography after chest closure. Then, DESs or drug-coated balloons (DCBs) were used to treat the non-LAD lesions.

For the OPCAB group, standard procedures described previously were followed (16). Aspirin was administered 100 mg daily after HCR and OPCAB procedures and then continued for life, while clopidogrel was administered at a dose of 75 mg/day for 12 months.

### Follow-Up

All patients needed to return to the outpatient department for a postoperative review at 1 and 6 months after discharge from the hospital and then once a year after surgery. Patients who did not return for review visits were contacted via telephone during the study period by the research staff using standard procedures and forms.

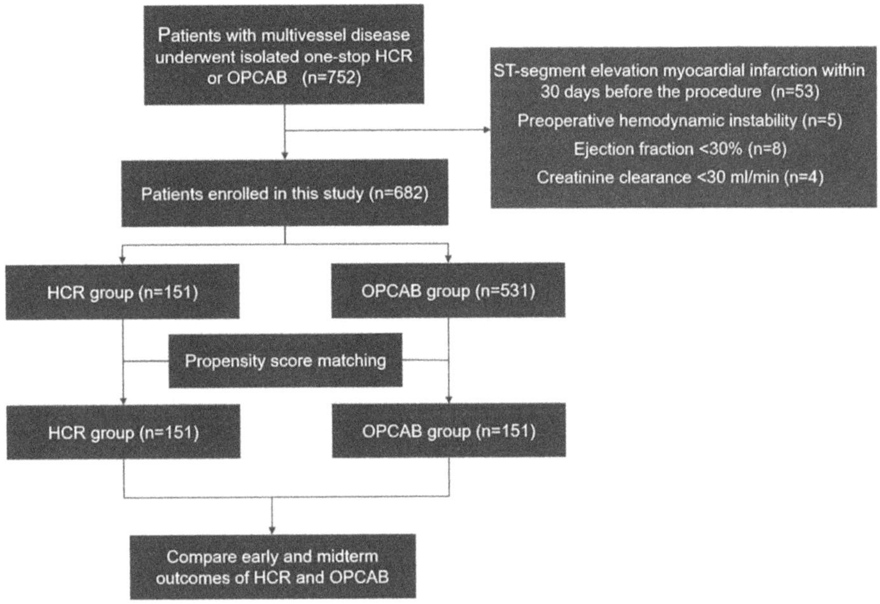


**FIGURE 1** | Flow chart of the study. HCR, hybrid coronary revascularization; OPCAB, off-pump coronary artery bypass graft.

The primary endpoints of this study were midterm major adverse cardiovascular and cerebrovascular events (MACCE) after the procedure, including death, myocardial infarction (MI), stroke, and repeat revascularization (defined as any revascularization after the HCR procedure or isolated OPCAB procedure). The secondary endpoints were in-hospital complications and outcomes, defined as in-hospital death, MI, stroke, repeat revascularization, reoperation for bleeding, time of mechanical ventilation, mechanical ventilation (PMV), perioperative transfusion, renal failure requiring dialysis, new onset atrial fibrillation (AF), incision infection, intensive care unit (ICU) stay, and length of stay (LOS) in hospital (days).

## Statistical Analysis

To reduce the impact of selection bias and potential confounding factors in this observational study, propensity score matching was performed using a logistic regression model. We chose nearest-neighbor caliper matching without a replacement, and the matching ratio was 1:1. Key variables and risk factors were involved in the matching. The standardized differences (SD) were calculated to assess the balance for the baseline characteristics before and after matching. SD values <10% indicated good matching. All matching procedures were performed by R (version 4.0.3).

Continuous variables were expressed as the means ± standard deviation or medians (the 25th percentile and the 75th percentile), and categorical data were summarized as a proportion. Comparisons of baseline characteristics and outcomes between the HCR group and OPCAB group were assessed by *t test* or Mann–Whitney *U* test for continuous variables and chi-square test or Fisher exact test for categorical variables before and after matching. Kaplan–Meier curves and log-rank tests were performed to compare cumulative events and MACCE rates between the two groups after matching. All statistical data analyses were performed by SPSS (IBM Corp. Released 2013. IBM SPSS Statistics for Windows, Version 22.0. Armonk, NY: IBM Corp). $P < 0.05$ was considered statistically significant.

# RESULTS

## Baseline Characteristics

Before propensity score matching, there were significant differences in demographics and comorbidities between the two groups. The HCR group had a higher BMI, a higher proportion of hyperlipidemia patients, administration of statins, and better heart function. Additionally, there were significantly lower EuroSCORE II scores, a lower proportion of diabetes mellitus patients, previous MI, and preoperative intra-aortic balloon pump (IABP) insertion compared with the OPCAB group. Variables of the unmatched population are shown in **Table 1**.

There were 151 patients in each group after 1:1 propensity score matching, and the baseline characteristics were similar between the two groups (**Table 2**). In the HCR group, no patients required conversion to sternotomy or cardiopulmonary bypass (CPB), and the mean number of DESs or DCBs used in each patient was 2.3 ± 1.5. The LIMA-LAD anastomosis, mean graft flow (MGF), and pulsatility index (PI) were comparable between the two groups (**Table 3**).

## In-Hospital Outcomes

The in-hospital outcomes are illustrated in **Table 4**. The incidences of in-hospital death, MI, stroke, and repeat

**TABLE 1 |** Preoperative characteristics of unmatched patients who underwent hybrid coronary revascularization (HCR) and off-pump coronary artery bypass (OPCAB).

| Preoperative characteristics | HCR group, N = 151 | OPCAB group, N = 531 | SD | P |
|---|---|---|---|---|
| Age (years) | 64.6 ± 9.4 | 63.6 ± 8.8 | 0.051 | 0.58 |
| Male | 75.5 | 77.0 | 0.036 | 0.70 |
| BMI (kg/m2) | 26.0 ± 3.3 | 25.3 ± 3.2 | 0.189 | 0.04 |
| Hypertension | 72.8 | 68.9 | 0.085 | 0.35 |
| Hyperlipidemia | 64.9 | 54.0 | 0.218 | 0.02 |
| Diabetes mellitus | 37.1 | 46.1 | 0.187 | 0.048 |
| Smoker | 55 | 50.1 | 0.098 | 0.29 |
| COPD | 1.3 | 2.3 | 0.063 | 0.75 |
| Peripheral vascular disease | 9.9 | 6.6 | 0.135 | 0.16 |
| Preoperative arrhythmia | 7.9 | 9.2 | 0.044 | 0.63 |
| Previous stroke | 19.9 | 21.7 | 0.043 | 0.64 |
| Previous MI | 16.6 | 45.6 | 0.583 | < 0.001 |
| Previous PCI | 21.9 | 19.8 | 0.052 | 0.57 |
| Acute coronary syndrome | 98.7 | 96.2 | 0.128 | 0.19 |
| Left main disease | 41.7 | 36.9 | 0.100 | 0.28 |
| LVEF (%) | 63.6 ± 9.0 | 60.7 ± 11.0 | 0.265 | 0.001 |
| LVEDD (mm) | 48.0 ± 4.6 | 49.4 ± 5.8 | 0.235 | 0.003 |
| Preoperative IABP | 2.0 | 7.3 | 0.205 | 0.02 |
| SYNTAX Score | 30.1 ± 9.4 | 31.7 ± 8.0 | 0.195 | 0.07 |
| EuroSCORE II | 1.97 ± 1.67 | 2.93 ± 2.27 | 0.424 | < 0.001 |
| β blocker | 64.9 | 70.1 | 0.113 | 0.23 |
| ACEI/ARB | 40.4 | 35.2 | 0.109 | 0.24 |
| Statin | 96.0 | 86.8 | 0.272 | 0.002 |

*Values are presented as mean ± SD or %.*
*HCR, hybrid coronary revascularization; OPCAB, off pump coronary artery bypass grafting; SD, standardized difference; BMI, body mass index; COPD, chronic obstructive pulmonary disease; MI, myocardial infarction; PCI, percutaneous coronary intervention; LVEF, left ventricular ejection fraction; LVEDD, left ventricular end-diastolic dimension; IABP, intra-aortic balloon pump; ACEI, angiotensin converting enzyme inhibitor; ARB, angiotensin receptor blockers.*

revascularization were comparable between the two matched groups. Meanwhile, differences in the rate of reoperation for bleeding, PMV (≥48 h), renal failure requiring dialysis, incision infection, and length of ICU stay (h) were not statistically significant. The HCR group had a lower rate of perioperative transfusion (23.8 vs. 53.0%, $p < 0.001$) and new-onset AF (5.3 vs. 15.2%, $p = 0.004$), shorter time of mechanical ventilation (h) [15 (16, 17) vs. 17 (16, 20), $p < 0.001$], and shorter LOS in the hospital (days) [19 (16, 24) vs. 22 (18, 27), $p = 0.001$]. No patient developed vascular access complications under anticoagulation therapy. One patient developed postoperative stroke caused by atherosclerotic plaques detached from the left subclavian artery in selective LIMA angiography. For in-hospital death, one patient died of cardiogenic shock caused by postoperative MI, the other patient died of severe lung infection in the HCR group, and one patient died of stroke in the OPCAB group.

**TABLE 2 |** Preoperative characteristics of matched patients who underwent HCR and OPCAB.

| Preoperative characteristics | HCR group, N = 151 | OPCAB group, N = 151 | SD | P |
|---|---|---|---|---|
| Age (years) | 64.6 ± 9.4 | 64.4 ± 8.6 | 0.011 | 0.92 |
| Male | 75.5 | 77.5 | 0.047 | 0.68 |
| BMI (kg/m$^2$) | 26.0 ± 3.3 | 25.3 ± 3.3 | 0.193 | 0.10 |
| Hypertension | 72.8 | 72.8 | 0.000 | 1.00 |
| Hyperlipidemia | 64.9 | 61.6 | 0.066 | 0.55 |
| Diabetes mellitus | 37.1 | 33.8 | 0.066 | 0.55 |
| Smoker | 55.0 | 51.7 | 0.066 | 0.56 |
| COPD | 1.3 | 2.0 | 0.045 | 1.00 |
| Peripheral vascular disease | 9.9 | 9.3 | 0.027 | 0.85 |
| Preoperative arrhythmia | 7.9 | 7.3 | 0.023 | 0.83 |
| Previous stroke | 19.9 | 19.9 | 0.000 | 1.00 |
| Previous MI | 16.6 | 16.6 | 0.000 | 1.00 |
| Previous PCI | 21.9 | 19.2 | 0.067 | 0.57 |
| Acute coronary syndrome | 98.7 | 98.7 | 0.000 | 1.00 |
| Left main disease | 41.7 | 43.7 | 0.041 | 0.73 |
| LVEF (%) | 63.6 ± 9.0 | 63.3 ± 9.2 | 0.021 | 0.83 |
| LVEDD (mm) | 48.0 ± 4.6 | 48.2 ± 5.4 | 0.028 | 0.78 |
| Preoperative IABP | 2.0 | 0.0 | 0.076 | 0.25 |
| SYNTAX Score | 30.1 ± 9.4 | 31.2 ± 7.4 | 0.081 | 0.51 |
| EuroSCORE II | 1.97 ± 1.67 | 2.36 ± 2.40 | 0.155 | 0.15 |
| β blocker | 64.9 | 65.6 | 0.015 | 0.90 |
| ACEI/ARB | 40.4 | 39.7 | 0.014 | 0.91 |
| Statin | 96.0 | 98.0 | 0.059 | 0.50 |

*Values are presented as mean ± SD or %.*
*HCR, hybrid coronary revascularization; OPCAB, off pump coronary artery bypass grafting; SD, standardized difference; BMI, body mass index; COPD, chronic obstructive pulmonary disease; MI, myocardial infarction; PCI, percutaneous coronary intervention; LVEF, left ventricular ejection fraction; LVEDD, left ventricular end-diastolic dimension; IABP, intra-aortic balloon pump; ACEI, angiotensin converting enzyme inhibitor; ARB, angiotensin receptor blockers.*

## Midterm Outcomes

At a median follow-up time of 20 months (interquartile range: 10–30 months), the cumulative mortality in the HCR and OPCAB groups was 5.1 and 7.1%, respectively (log rank $p = 0.91$) (**Table 5**, **Figure 2**). Significant differences in the estimated rates of MI (4.3 vs. 4.3%, $p = 0.56$), stroke (4.0 vs. 4.5%, $p = 0.66$), repeat revascularization (4.7 vs. 5.0%, $p = 0.61$), and MACCE (15.9 vs. 14.0%, $p = 0.59$) were not observed for the HCR and CABG groups (**Table 5**, **Figure 3**).

# DISCUSSION

Minimally invasive techniques for surgical myocardial revascularization have received much attention in recent years, especially the HCR technique (17). Compared with staged HCR, one-stop HCR can achieve complete revascularization in a single procedure, which avoids ischemic events during the

**TABLE 3 |** Intraoperative characteristics of matched patients who underwent HCR and OPCAB.

| Intraoperative characteristics | HCR group, $N = 151$ | OPCAB group, $N = 151$ | $P$ |
|---|---|---|---|
| Conversion to sternotomy | 0 | NA | NA |
| LIMA-LAD | 98.7 | 95.4 | 0.17 |
| MGF (ml/min) | 23.5 ± 13.9 | 26.6 ± 19.7 | 0.11 |
| PI | 2.5 ± 1.4 | 2.4 ± 1.6 | 0.23 |
| Number of DES/DCB | 2.3 ± 1.5 | NA | NA |

*Values are presented as mean ± SD or %.*
*HCR, hybrid coronary revascularization; OPCAB, off pump coronary artery bypass grafting; LIMA, left internal mammary artery; LAD, left anterior descending artery; MGF, mean graft flow; PI, pulsatility index; DES, drug-eluting stents; DCB, drug-coated balloon.*

**TABLE 4 |** In-hospital outcomes of matched patients who underwent HCR and OPCAB.

| Variables | HCR group, $N = 151$ | OPCAB group, $N = 151$ | $P$ |
|---|---|---|---|
| In-hospital death | 2 (1.3) | 1 (0.7) | 1.00 |
| MI | 3 (2.0) | 4 (2.6) | 1.00 |
| Stroke | 3 (2.0) | 2 (1.3) | 1.00 |
| Repeat revascularization | 0 (0.0) | 1 (0.7) | 1.00 |
| Reoperation for bleeding | 6 (4.0) | 1 (0.7) | 0.12 |
| Time of mechanic ventilation (h)* | 15 (16, 17) | 17 (16,20) | < 0.001 |
| PMV (≥ 48 h) | 17 (11.3) | 19 (12.6) | 0.72 |
| Perioperative transfusion | 36 (23.8) | 80 (53.0) | < 0.001 |
| Renal failure needs dialysis | 2 (1.3) | 1 (0.7) | 1.00 |
| New onset AF | 8 (5.3) | 23 (15.2) | 0.004 |
| Incision infection | 2 (1.3) | 2 (1.3) | 1.00 |
| ICU stay (h)* | 77 (66, 124) | 95 (69, 140) | 0.17 |
| LOS in hospital (day)* | 19 (16, 24) | 22 (18, 27) | 0.001 |

**Non-normal variables are presented as median (P25, P75).*
*Categorical values are presented as n (%).*
*HCR, hybrid coronary revascularization; OPCAB, off pump coronary artery bypass grafting; MI, myocardial infarction; PMV, prolonged mechanic ventilation; AF, atrial fibrillation; ICU, intensive care unit; LOS, length of stay.*

**TABLE 5 |** Midterm outcomes of matched patients who underwent HCR and OPCAB.

| Variables | HCR group, $N = 151$ | OPCAB group, $N = 151$ | HR (95% CI) | $P$ |
|---|---|---|---|---|
| Death | 6 (5.1) | 6 (7.1) | 1.07 (0.34–3.30) | 0.91 |
| MI | 4 (4.3) | 6 (4.3) | 0.69 (0.20–2.38) | 0.56 |
| Stroke | 5 (4.0) | 4 (4.5) | 1.34 (0.36–4.95) | 0.66 |
| Repeat revascularization | 4 (4.7) | 6 (5.0) | 0.72 (0.21 2.49) | 0.61 |
| MACCE | 17 (15.9) | 15 (14.0) | 1.21 (0.60–2.41) | 0.59 |

*Events are presented as n (cumulative incidence rate%) after procedure.*
*HCR, hybrid coronary revascularization; OPCAB, off pump coronary artery bypass grafting; HR, hazard ratio; CI, confidence interval; MI, myocardial infarction; MACCE, major adverse cardiac and cerebrovascular events.*

waiting period caused by incomplete revascularization in staged HCR. Furthermore, LIMA-LAD anastomosis can be evaluated by angiography immediately before PCI, and grafts can be revised if there are any major issues (18). Additionally, high-risk non-LAD PCI is performed with a protected LAD territory, and surgical bailout can be performed for any possible complication or unsuccessful PCI with a surgical team in a hybrid suite. Finally, this single-step procedure reduces hospital stay and readmission, provides convenience for patients, and improves patient satisfaction (19).

On the other hand, the simultaneous procedure requires a costly hybrid room featuring advanced surgical and interventional equipment. In addition, adopting an appropriate antiplatelet therapy strategy to balance the risk of bleeding and stent thrombosis is a major challenge (20).

To date, a series of published data comparing HCR with conventional CABG and OPCAB from different centers with variable surgical techniques and study methodologies have demonstrated limited conclusions (11, 12, 21, 22). Most of the patients involved in these studies underwent staged HCR, and the one-stop HCR approach accounted for only 15% of all HCR procedures in the United States (23). Outcomes of one-stop HCR should be proven, particularly due to their different natural attributes.

The present study compared early and midterm results between one-stop HCR and standard OPCAB, which revealed similar excellent in-hospital and midterm outcomes. In addition, the HCR group was associated with a lower rate of perioperative transfusion (23.8 vs. 53.0%), new-onset AF (5.3 vs. 15.2%), shorter time of mechanical ventilation, and LOS in the hospital. Consistent with our results, Reynolds et al. (24) evaluated a total of 4,260 patients (1,350 of whom underwent HCR) in a meta-analysis. They confirmed that HCR had a significantly lower rate of blood transfusion than CABG (22.8 vs. 46.1%) and a shorter time of mechanical ventilation and LOS in the hospital, but no significant differences were found in ICU stay, postoperative atrial fibrillation, renal failure, perioperative myocardial infarction, or death. Similar conclusions were also investigated by Sardar et al. (25). These findings indicated the advantages of minimally invasive and rapid recovery of HCR.

Another particular potential benefit of HCR procedures is completely avoiding manipulation of the aorta, which could theoretically reduce the risk of neurological events. However, in our study, the incidence of in-hospital stroke was low and was comparable between the two groups. Three (HCR group) and two (OPCAB group) patients developed stroke. Among the stroke patients in the HCR group, two patients had a history of cerebral infarction, and one stroke patient was caused by atherosclerotic plaques detached from the left subclavian artery in selective LIMA angiography. Meanwhile, in the OPCAB group, using proximal anastomosis devices (Heartstring or Enclose) was a routine procedure in our center. This surgical approach reduced aortic manipulation and was associated with a lower risk of perioperative stroke (26). Nevertheless, HCR is still an optimal strategy for patients with severe aortic atherosclerosis.

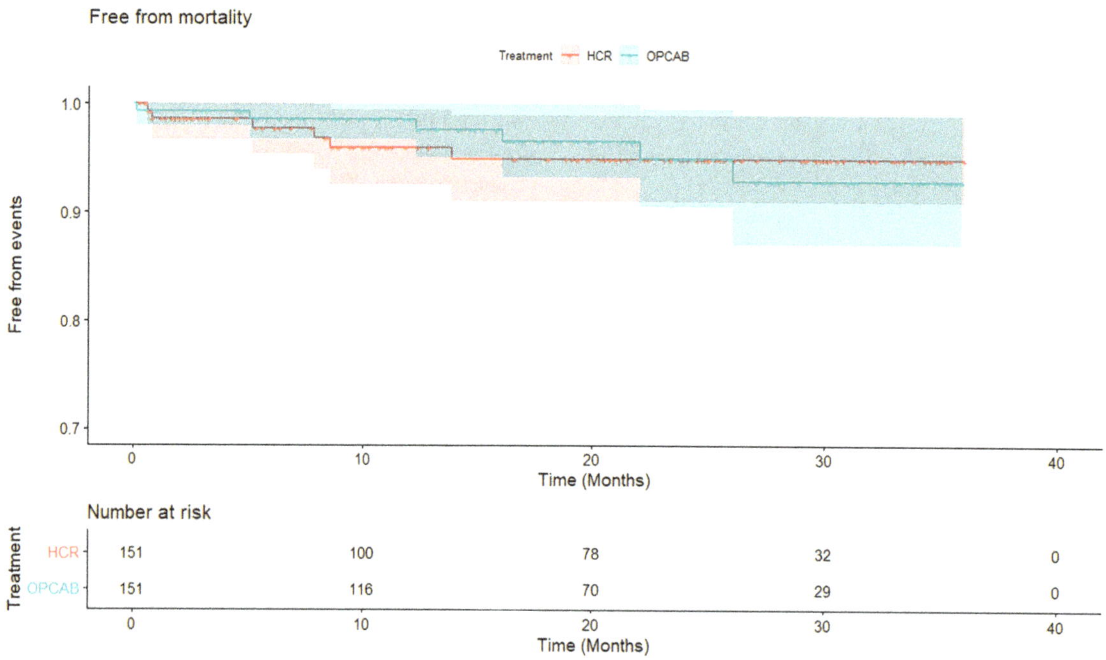


**FIGURE 2 |** Cumulative survival rate in hybrid coronary revascularization (HCR) and off-pump coronary artery bypass (OPCAB) group. Kaplan–Meier curve estimates similar cumulated survival rate in HCR and OPCAB groups (94.9 vs. 92.9%, $p = 0.91$) during the follow-up. HCR, hybrid coronary revascularization; OPCAB, off-pump coronary artery bypass graft.

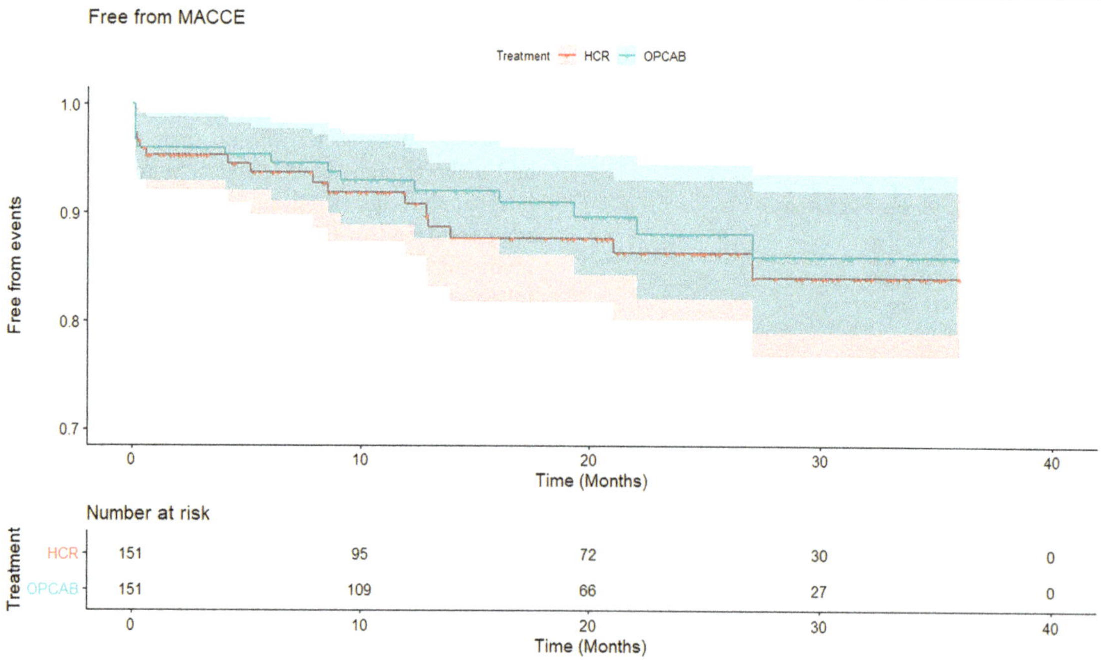


**FIGURE 3 |** Cumulative free from major adverse cardiovascular and cerebrovascular events (MACCE) rate in HCR and OPCAB group. Kaplan–Meier curve estimates similar cumulated free from MACCE rate in HCR and OPCAB groups (84.1 vs. 86%, $p = 0.59$) during the follow-up. MACCE, major adverse cardiovascular and cerebrovascular events; HCR, hybrid coronary revascularization; OPCAB, off-pump coronary artery bypass grafting.

Appropriate antiplatelet therapy to preserve stent patency and minimize the risk of postoperative bleeding is challenging in one-stop HCR procedures. Exposure to potent antiplatelet drugs may increase the risk of postoperative bleeding events. Coincidentally, in the present study, the reoperation rate for bleeding was higher in the HCR group (4.0 vs.0.7%), although the difference was not significant ($p = 0.12$), which is consistent with the rate of 3 to 6.8% reported by Zhao et al. and Harskamp et al. (18). Most of the reoperation cases occurred early after introducing one-stop HCR into our center, and the LIMA pedicle was harvested through direct vison at that time. Then, endoscopy was used in LIMA harvesting, which could reduce the trauma of the LIMA bed. We strengthened surgical hemostasis, such as by using the "LIMA bed closure" technique. As a consequence, few patients now develop major bleeding events requiring reoperation.

During midterm follow-up, we revealed no differences between the two groups in cumulative survival (94.9 vs. 92.9%, $p = 0.91$) or free from MACCE (84.1 vs. 86%, $p = 0.59$) after the procedure. These findings are consistent with recently published data. The HYBRID (POL-MIDES) trial (11), the largest prospective randomized study comparing HCR with conventional CABG, involved 98 HCR patients and 102 conventional CABG patients. The 5-year survival rates were 93.6% in the HCR group and 90.8% in the CABG group ($p = 0.69$), and the rates of freedom from MACCE were 45.2 and 53.4%, respectively ($p = 0.39$). No differences were found between the two groups. There were also no differences in the rates of MI, stroke, or repeat revascularization. Shen et al. (27) compared one-stop HCR, CABG, and PCI in an observational study. At the 3-year follow-up, actuarial survival was 99.3% in the HCR group and 97.2% in the CABG group, and the cumulative rate of freedom from MACCE was 93.6% after HCR and 86.5% after CABG ($p = 0.14$). In Shen's study, surgical revascularization was completed through a lower partial ministernotomy, which is different from the widely used technique through a small anterior thoracotomy.

In the present study, the rate of any repeat revascularization was comparable between the HCR and OPCAB groups (4.7 vs. 5.0%; OR.72; 95% CI.21–2.49; $p = 0.61$) during the follow-up. Hage et al. (12) compared HCR ($n = 147$, robotic-assisted minimally invasive direct CABG) and OPCAB ($n = 216$) using inverse-probability weighting. The HCR was associated with a higher in-hospital reintervention rate (HCR 3.4% vs. CABG 0%, $p = 0.03$). For long-term follow-up, freedom from any form of revascularization was similar between the two groups (91 vs. 92%; $p = 0.80$), which is consistent with our results. In contrast, a meta-analysis from Nolan et al. (28) found that HCR was also associated with a higher risk of long-term repeat target vessel revascularization (TVR) than CABG.

Several limitations need to be addressed. First, this study was a single-center retrospective study, and the risk of selection bias was inevitable despite the benefits of propensity score matching. Second, the sample size was limited. Finally, the follow-up time was short, and long-term follow-up to verify the effectiveness of one-stop HCR is warranted.

## CONCLUSIONS

One-stop HCR is safe and efficacious with less invasiveness and faster postoperative recovery in selected patients with multivessel coronary artery disease. Compared with OPCAB, one-stop HCR is associated with a lower rate of perioperative transfusion and new-onset AF, shorter time of mechanical ventilation and LOS in the hospital, and excellent similar midterm outcomes. Randomized controlled trials with larger sample sizes and long-term follow-up are warranted to confirm these findings.

## ETHICS STATEMENT

The studies involving human participants were reviewed and approved by Research Ethics Board of Chaoyang Hospital. Written informed consent for participation was not required for this study in accordance with the national legislation and the institutional requirements.

## AUTHOR CONTRIBUTIONS

DL, PS, and JG: conception and design. YL, JZ, and PS: administrative support. DL, JG, YGu, XA, and XZ: provision of study materials or patients. DL and YGa: collection and assembly of data. DL, JG, and SG: data analysis and interpretation. DL: manuscript writing. All authors read and approved the final manuscript.

## REFERENCES

1. Serruys P, Morice M, Kappetein A, Colombo A, Holmes D, Mack M, et al. Percutaneous coronary intervention versus coronary-artery bypass grafting for severe coronary artery disease. *N Engl J Med.* (2009) 360:961–72. doi: 10.1056/NEJMoa0804626
2. Park S, Ahn J, Kim Y, Park D, Yun S, Lee J, et al. Trial of everolimus-eluting stents or bypass surgery for coronary disease. *N Engl J Med.* (2015) 372:1204–12. doi: 10.1056/NEJMoa1415447
3. Bangalore S, Guo Y, Samadashvili Z, Blecker S, Xu J, Hannan E. Everolimus-eluting stents or bypass surgery for multivessel coronary disease. *N Engl J Med.* (2015) 372:1213–22. doi: 10.1056/NEJMoa1412168
4. Loop F, Lytle B, Cosgrove D, Stewart R, Goormastic M, Williams G, et al. Influence of the internal-mammary-artery graft on 10-year survival and other cardiac events. *N Engl J Med.* (1986) 314:1–6. doi: 10.1056/NEJM198601023140101
5. Zacharias A, Schwann T, Riordan C, Durham S, Shah A, Habib R. Late results of conventional versus all-arterial revascularization based on internal thoracic and radial artery grafting. *Ann Thorac Surg.* (2009) 87:19–26.e2. doi: 10.1016/j.athoracsur.2008.09.050
6. Goldman S, Zadina K, Moritz T, Ovitt T, Sethi G, Copeland JG, et al. Long-term patency of saphenous vein and left internal mammary artery grafts after coronary artery bypass surgery: results from a Department of Veterans Affairs Cooperative Study. *J Am Coll Cardiol.* (2004) 44:2149–56. doi: 10.1016/j.jacc.2004.08.064
7. Dangas G, Claessen B, Caixeta A, Sanidas E, Mintz G, Mehran R. In-stent restenosis in the drug-eluting stent era. *J Am Coll Cardiol.* (2010) 56:1897–907. doi: 10.1016/j.jacc.2010.07.028
8. Head S, Milojevic M, Daemen J, Ahn J, Boersma E, Christiansen E, et al. Mortality after coronary artery bypass grafting versus percutaneous coronary intervention with stenting for coronary artery disease: a pooled

analysis of individual patient data. *Lancet (London, England).* (2018) 391:939–48. doi: 10.1016/S0140-6736(18)30423-9

9. Neumann FJ, Sousa-Uva M, Ahlsson A, Alfonso F, Banning AP, Benedetto U, et al. 2018 ESC/EACTS Guidelines on myocardial revascularization. *Eur Heart J.* (2019) 40:87–165. doi: 10.1093/eurheartj/ehy855
10. Lloyd CT, Calafiore AM, Wilde P, Ascione R, Paloscia L, Monk CR, et al. Integrated left small thoracotomy and angioplasty for multivessel coronary artery revascularisation. *Lancet (London, England).* (1996) 347:757–8. doi: 10.1016/S0140-6736(96)90107-5
11. Tajstra M, Hrapkowicz T, Hawranek M, Filipiak K, Gierlotka M, Zembala M, et al. Hybrid coronary revascularization in selected patients with multivessel disease: 5-Year clinical outcomes of the prospective randomized pilot study. *JACC Cardiovasc Interv.* (2018) 11:847–52. doi: 10.1016/j.jcin.2018.01.271
12. Hage A, Giambruno V, Jones P, Chu MW, Fox S, Teefy P, et al. Hybrid coronary revascularization versus off-pump coronary artery bypass grafting: comparative effectiveness analysis with long-term follow-up. *J Am Heart Assoc.* (2019) 8:e014204. doi: 10.1161/JAHA.119.014204
13. Hannan EL, Wu Y, Cozzens K, Sundt TM. 3rd, Girardi L, Chikwe J, et al. Hybrid coronary revascularization versus conventional coronary artery bypass surgery: utilization and comparative outcomes. *Circ Cardiovasc Interv.* (2020) 13:e009386. doi: 10.1161/CIRCINTERVENTIONS.120.009386
14. Giambruno V, Jones P, Khaliel F, Chu MW, Teefy P, Sridhar K, et al. Hybrid coronary revascularization versus on-pump coronary artery bypass grafting. *Ann Thorac Surg.* (2018) 105:1330–5. doi: 10.1016/j.athoracsur.2017.11.019
15. Patel MR, Calhoon JH, Dehmer GJ, Grantham JA, Maddox TM, Maron DJ, et al. ACC/AATS/AHA/ASE/ASNC/SCAI/SCCT/STS 2017 appropriate use criteria for coronary revascularization in patients with stable ischemic heart disease: a report of the american college of cardiology appropriate use criteria task force, american association for thoracic surgery, american heart association, american society of echocardiography, american society of nuclear cardiology, society for cardiovascular angiography and interventions, society of cardiovascular computed tomography, and society of thoracic surgeons. *J Am Coll Cardiol.* (2017) 69:2212–41. doi: 10.1007/s12350-017-0917-9
16. Li D, Gu S, Liu Y, Zhang X, An X, Yan J, et al. Outcomes of left internal mammary artery with saphenous vein composite graft to bypass the left anterior descending artery: a propensity-matched study. *J Thorac Dis.* (2020) 12:6629–39. doi: 10.21037/jtd-20-2358
17. Gaudino M, Bakaeen F, Davierwala P, Di Franco A, Fremes SE, Patel N, et al. New strategies for surgical myocardial revascularization. *Circulation.* (2018) 138:2160–8. doi: 10.1161/CIRCULATIONAHA.118.035956
18. Zhao DX, Leacche M, Balaguer JM, Boudoulas KD, Damp JA, Greelish JP, et al. Routine intraoperative completion angiography after coronary artery bypass grafting and 1-stop hybrid revascularization results from a fully integrated hybrid catheterization laboratory/operating room. *J Am Coll Cardiol.* (2009) 53:232–41. doi: 10.1016/j.jacc.2008.10.011
19. Kon ZN, Brown EN, Tran R, Joshi A, Reicher B, Grant MC, et al. Simultaneous hybrid coronary revascularization reduces postoperative morbidity compared with results from conventional off-pump coronary artery bypass. *J Thorac Cardiovasc Surg.* (2008) 135:367–75. doi: 10.1016/j.jtcvs.2007.09.025
20. Moreno PR, Stone GW, Gonzalez-Lengua CA, Puskas JD. The hybrid coronary approach for optimal revascularization: JACC review topic of the week. *J Am Coll Cardiol.* (2020) 76:321–33. doi: 10.1016/j.jacc.2020.04.078
21. McKiernan M, Halkos ME. Hybrid coronary revascularization. *Current Opinion in Cardiology.* (2020) Publish Ahead of Print. doi: 10.1097/HCO.0000000000000784
22. Patel NC, Hemli JM, Kim MC, Seetharam K, Pirelli L, Brinster DR, et al. Short- and intermediate-term outcomes of hybrid coronary revascularization for double-vessel disease. *J Thorac Cardiovasc Surg.* (2018) 156:1799–807 e3. doi: 10.1016/j.jtcvs.2018.04.078
23. Harskamp RE, Brennan JM, Xian Y, Halkos ME, Puskas JD, Thourani VH, et al. Practice patterns and clinical outcomes after hybrid coronary revascularization in the United States: an analysis from the society of thoracic surgeons adult cardiac database. *Circulation.* (2014) 130:872–9. doi: 10.1161/CIRCULATIONAHA.114.009479
24. Reynolds AC, King N. Hybrid coronary revascularization versus conventional coronary artery bypass grafting: Systematic review and meta-analysis. *Medicine (Baltimore).* (2018) 97:e11941. doi: 10.1097/MD.0000000000011941
25. Sardar P, Kundu A, Bischoff M, Chatterjee S, Owan T, Nairooz R, et al. Hybrid coronary revascularization versus coronary artery bypass grafting in patients with multivessel coronary artery disease: A meta-analysis. *Catheter Cardiovasc Interv.* (2018) 91:203–12. doi: 10.1002/ccd.27098
26. Borgermann J, Hakim K, Renner A, Parsa A, Aboud A, Becker T, et al. Clampless off-pump versus conventional coronary artery revascularization: a propensity score analysis of 788 patients. *Circulation.* (2012) 126:S176–82. doi: 10.1161/CIRCULATIONAHA.111.084285
27. Shen L, Hu S, Wang H, Xiong H, Zheng Z, Li L, et al. One-stop hybrid coronary revascularization versus coronary artery bypass grafting and percutaneous coronary intervention for the treatment of multivessel coronary artery disease: 3-year follow-up results from a single institution. *J Am Coll Cardiol.* (2013) 61:2525–33. doi: 10.1016/j.jacc.2013.04.007
28. Nolan S, Filion K, Atallah R, Moss E, Reynier P, Eisenberg M. Hybrid coronary revascularization vs complete coronary artery bypass grafting for multivessel coronary artery disease: a systematic review and meta-analysis. *J Invasive Cardiol.* (2018) 30(12):E131–E49.

# 4

# The Relationship Between Body Mass Index and In-Hospital Mortality in Patients Following Coronary Artery Bypass Grafting Surgery

*Gabby Elbaz-Greener[1,2*†], Guy Rozen[3,4,5†], Shemy Carasso[6,7], Fabio Kusniec[6,7], Merav Yarkoni[1,2], Ibrahim Marai[6,7], Bradley Strauss[8], Harindra C. Wijeysundera[8], Frank W. Smart[9], Eldad Erez[10], Ronny Alcalai[1,2], David Planer[1,2] and Offer Amir[1,2,6,7]*

*[1] Department of Cardiology, Hadassah Medical Center, Jerusalem, Israel, [2] Faculty of Medicine, Hebrew University of Jerusalem, Jerusalem, Israel, [3] Cardiology Division, Hillel Yaffe Medical Center, Hadera, Israel, [4] The Ruth and Bruce Rappaport Faculty of Medicine, Technion, Haifa, Israel, [5] Cardiology Division, Harvard Medical School, Massachusetts General Hospital, Boston, MA, United States, [6] Division of Cardiovascular Medicine, Baruch Padeh Medical Center, Poriya, Israel, [7] The Azrieli Faculty of Medicine in the Galilee, Bar-Ilan University, Safed, Israel, [8] Division of Cardiology, Schulich Heart Centre, Sunnybrook Health Sciences Centre, University of Toronto, Toronto, ON, Canada, [9] Louisiana State University School of Medicine, New Orleans, LA, United States, [10] Department of Cardio Surgery, Hadassah Medical Center, Hebrew University of Jerusalem, Jerusalem, Israel*

***Correspondence:***
*Gabby Elbaz-Greener*
*Gabby@hadassah.org.il*

*† These authors have contributed equally to this work*

**Background:** The association between Body Mass Index (BMI) and clinical outcomes following coronary artery bypass grafting (CABG) remains controversial. Our objective was to investigate the real-world relationship between BMI and in-hospital clinical course and mortality, in patients who underwent CABG.

**Methods:** A sampled cohort of patients who underwent CABG between October 2015 and December 2016 was identified in the National Inpatient Sample (NIS) database. Outcomes of interest included in-hospital mortality, peri-procedural complications and length of stay. Patients were divided into 6 BMI (kg/m$^2$) subgroups; (1) under-weight $\leq$19, (2) normal-weight 20–25, (3) over-weight 26–30, (4) obese I 31–35, (5) obese II 36–39, and (6) extremely obese $\geq$40. Multivariable logistic regression model was used to identify predictors of in-hospital mortality. Linear regression model was used to identify predictors of length of stay (LOS).

**Results:** An estimated total of 48,710 hospitalizations for CABG across the U.S. were analyzed. The crude data showed a U-shaped relationship between BMI and study population outcomes with higher mortality and longer LOS in patients with BMI $\leq$ 19 kg/m$^2$ and in patients with BMI $\geq$ 40 kg/m$^2$ compared to patients with BMI 20–39 kg/m$^2$. In the multivariable regression model, BMI subgroups of $\leq$19 kg/m$^2$ and $\geq$40 kg/m$^2$ were found to be independent predictors of mortality.

**Conclusions:** A complex, U-shaped relationship between BMI and mortality was documented, confirming the "obesity paradox" in the real-world setting, in patients hospitalized for CABG.

**Keywords: body mass index (BMI), coronary artery bypass grafting surgery (CABG), ischemic heart, outcome, mortality**

## INTRODUCTION

Body mass index (BMI) is widely used for routine characterization of weight status in epidemiological and clinical research, however with some limitations, for instance not distinguishing fat from muscle mass (1). The World Health Organization (WHO) classifies a patient body weight by six categorical subgroups, (1) under-weight, BMI $\leq$ 18.5 kg/m$^2$; (2) normal-weight, BMI 18.5–24.9 kg/m$^2$; (3) over-weight, BMI 25–29.9 kg/m$^2$; (4) obese class I, BMI 30–34.9 kg/m$^2$; (5) obese class II, BMI 35–39.9 kg/m$^2$; and (6) extremely obese BMI $\geq$ 40 Kg/m$^2$ (1, 2). In population-based studies, higher BMI was associated with increased incidence of major cardiovascular risk factors (1, 3). BMI has been proven an independent risk factor for various cardiovascular conditions such as acute coronary syndrome, congestive heart failure, sudden cardiac death, atrial and ventricular arrhythmia and stroke (3, 4).

Several studies investigated the effect of different BMI arrays on short- and long-term mortality rates post cardiac surgery with contradictory conclusions. Some studies suggested that obesity was an independent negative predictor of morbidity and mortality (5–8) while others showed more favorable outcomes after cardiac surgery in obese patients (9–13). This phenomenon has been referred to as the obesity paradox (9–13). One explanation for this paradox is that patients with higher BMI may have a lower postoperative bleeding volume and transfusion rate; thus, such patients may save blood products during on-pump CABG factor that contributes to higher survival rates (14). On the other hand, sternal wound infections are more prevalent in obese patients and prior studies have shown increased morbidity and mortality rates in obese patients (15–17).

In the current study, we aimed to describe the BMI distribution and in-hospital outcomes among different BMI subgroups post-CABG, during the index hospitalization.

## METHODS

### Data Source

The data were drawn from the National Inpatient Sample (NIS), the Healthcare Cost and Utilization Project (HCUP), and Agency for Healthcare Research and Quality (AHRQ) (18, 19). The NIS database only includes de-identified data; therefore, this study was considered exempt from institutional review by the Human Research Committee.

The NIS is the largest collection of data on all-payer hospitalizations in the United States (U.S.), and represents an approximate 20% stratified sample of all inpatient discharges from U.S. hospitals (20). This includes information at the hospital-level, such as hospital region, teaching status, bed size and cost of hospitalization, and other data at the patient-level, including demographic characteristics, primary and secondary diagnoses and procedures, comorbidities and length of stay (LOS). National estimates can be calculated using the patient-level and hospital-level sampling weights that are provided by the HCUP.

For the purpose of this study, we obtained data for the years 2015 and 2016. The International Classification of Diseases, 10th Revision, Clinical Modification (ICD-10-CM) was used from the last quarter of 2015 and thereafter for reporting diagnoses and procedures in the NIS database during the study period. For each index hospitalization, the database provides a principal discharge diagnosis and a maximum of 14 or 24 additional diagnoses, in addition to a maximum of 15 procedures. We restricted our cohort to the period during which data was coded with ICD-10 codes, because the ICD-10 system includes individual codes for BMI values and ranges.

### Study Population and Variables

We identified patients 18 years of age or older with a primary diagnosis of CABG procedure based on ICD-10-CM code starting with I10.PR1 with 0210-0213xxx codes, who have one of the Z68.x codes as I10-Dx1 to I10-Dx30. These codes represent the six subgroups in our study; Z68, Z68.20–25, Z68.26–30, Z68.31–35, Z68.36–39, and Z68.4 (BMI $\leq$ 19 under-weight group; BMI 20–25 normal-weight group; BMI 26–30 over-weight group; BMI 31–35 obese I group, BMI 36–39 obese II group and BMI equal or $\geq$40 extremely obese group, respectively).

The following patient demographics were collected from the database: age, sex, and race. Prior comorbidities were identified by measures from the AHRQ. For the purpose of calculating Deyo-Charlson Comorbidity Index (Deyo-CCI), additional comorbidities were identified from the database using ICD-10-CM codes. Deyo-CCI is a modification of the Charlson Comorbidity Index, containing 17 comorbid conditions of differential weights, with a total score ranging from 0 to 33 (detailed information on Deyo-CCI is provided in the **Appendix Table 1**). Higher Deyo-CCI scores indicate a greater burden of comorbid diseases and is associated with mortality 1-year after admission (21). The index has been used extensively in studies from administrative databases, with proved validity in predicting short- and long-term outcomes (22, 23).

Our primary outcome in this study was in-hospital mortality. The secondary outcomes included in-hospital periprocedural complications and length of stay in the hospital. In-hospital complications were defined as previously reported (24–26) and included known cardiac surgery related complications as follows: (1) Pericardial complications as tamponade, hemopericardium, pericarditis and pericardiocentesis; (2) Cardiac complications (during or resulting from procedure), defined as cardiac block, myocardial infarction, cardiac arrest, congestive heart failure, cardiogenic shock and others; (3) Pulmonary complications, defined as pneumothorax/hemothorax, diaphragm paralysis, post-operative respiratory failure, and other iatrogenic respiratory complications; (4) Vascular complications, defined as accidental puncture or laceration during a procedure, injury to blood vessels, arteriovenous fistula, injury to retroperitoneum, vascular complication requiring surgical repair, re-open, and other vascular complications; (5) Infection, defined as fever, septicemia, and post-procedural aspiration pneumonia; (6) Neurological, defined as nervous system complication, unspecified, central nervous system complication, iatrogenic cerebrovascular infarction or hemorrhage cerebrovascular effect, and transient ischemic attack; (7) Acute renal failure; (8) Cardiogenic shock; (9) Diaphragmatic paralysis; (10) Re-open

**TABLE 1** | Frequency distribution of baseline characteristics by BMI group in CABG patients.

| BMI groups (Kg/m²) | ≤19 Under-weight | 20–25 Normal-weight | 26–30 Over-weight | 31–35 Obese I group | 36–39 Obese II group | ≥40 Extremely obese | Total | *P*-value |
|---|---|---|---|---|---|---|---|---|
| Unweighted[a] | 137 | 263 | 1,570 | 3,544 | 1,952 | 2,276 | 9,742 | |
| Weighted[b] | 685 | 1,315 | 7,850 | 17,720 | 9,760 | 11,380 | 48,710 | |
| Age group, %, years | | | | | | | | <0.001 |
| 18-44 | 1.5 | 0.8 | 1.8 | 3.0 | 4.8 | 5.2 | 3.6 | |
| 45-59 | 20.4 | 22.8 | 24.7 | 29.7 | 31.2 | 34.0 | 29.9 | |
| 60-74 | 50.4 | 48.7 | 54.5 | 53.8 | 54.0 | 53.1 | 53.6 | |
| ≥ 75 | 27.7 | 27.8 | 19.0 | 13.5 | 10.0 | 7.6 | 12.9 | |
| Gender, % | | | | | | | | <0.001 |
| Male | 67.2 | 71.1 | 72.9 | 74.6 | 68.6 | 62.5 | 70.1 | |
| Female | 32.8 | 28.9 | 27.1 | 25.3 | 31.3 | 37.5 | 29.9 | |
| Race, % | | | | | | | | <0.001 |
| White | 70.1 | 71.9 | 73.6 | 76.6 | 75.4 | 78.1 | 76.0 | |
| Non-white | 25.5 | 17.9 | 19.7 | 15.9 | 16.3 | 15.4 | 16.7 | |
| Comorbidity, % | | | | | | | | |
| Hypertension | 48.9 | 58.6 | 66.2 | 67.3 | 67.9 | 65.4 | 66.3 | <0.001 |
| Congestive heart failure | 21.9 | 15.2 | 13.9 | 11.8 | 13.8 | 17.2 | 14.1 | <0.001 |
| Diabetes mellitus | 16.8 | 34.2 | 36.9 | 41.4 | 44.9 | 50.1 | 42.9 | <0.001 |
| Chronic renal disease | 28.5 | 24.7 | 20.8 | 20.3 | 21.8 | 24.3 | 21.9 | <0.001 |
| Chronic obstructive pulmonary disease | 47.4 | 23.6 | 22.7 | 21.9 | 24.4 | 27.0 | 24.1 | <0.001 |
| Peripheral vascular disease | 30.7 | 20.5 | 17.8 | 14.3 | 13.1 | 12.0 | 14.5 | <0.001 |
| Atrial Fibrillation/Flutter | 40.9 | 31.9 | 33.0 | 31.8 | 33.5 | 35.6 | 33.3 | <0.001 |
| Prior MI | 20.4 | 22.1 | 19.3 | 19.7 | 18.9 | 18.9 | 19.3 | 0.085 |
| Deyo-CCI, % | | | | | | | | <0.001 |
| 1 | 9.5 | 18.3 | 20.0 | 19.9 | 20.6 | 17.6 | 19.3 | |
| 2 or higher | 87.6 | 74.5 | 70.3 | 69.2 | 70.7 | 75.8 | 71.6 | |

*MI, Myocardial Infraction; Deyo-CCI, Deyo-Charlson Comorbidity Index.*
*[a]Represents the number of observations in the NIS database.*
*[b]Represents total national estimates after applying sampling weights.*

surgery; (11) Permanent pacemaker implantation (PPM); (12) New onset atrial fibrillation; (13) Wound infection.

Detailed information on all ICD-10-CM codes used to identify in-hospital complications, is summarized in the **Appendix Table 2**.

## Statistical Analysis

The chi-square ($\chi^2$) and Wilcoxon Rank Sum tests were used to compare categorical variables and continuous variables, respectively. The NIS provides discharge sample weights that are calculated within each sampling level as the ratio of discharges in the universe to discharges in the sample (25). We generated a weighted logistic regression model to identify independent predictors of in-hospital mortality. Candidate variables included patient-level characteristics, Deyo-CCI and hospital-level factors. We included all candidate variables that were associated with our primary and secondary outcome in our final multivariable regression model. A linear regression model was used to identify predictors of LOS.

For all analyses, we used SAS® software version 9.4 (SAS Institute Inc., Cary, NC.) A $p < 0.05$ was considered statistically significant.

# RESULTS

## Study Cohort

A total sample of 9,742 CABG hospitalizations across the U.S. during 2015 (last quarter) and 2016 were included in the analysis. After implementing the weighting method, these represented an estimated total of 48,710 hospitalizations for CABG, in patients who had BMI information during the index hospitalization. The majority of patients (70.1%) were male, and the mean age of the cohort was 63.4 ± 22.1 years. A smaller proportion of CABG patients were underweight with a BMI ≤ 19 kg/m² (**Table 1**).

## Patient Characteristics, Presentation of Acute Myocardial Infraction, and Treatment Approach by BMI Group

Study population baseline and clinical characteristics are presented in detail in **Tables 1, 2**. Male predominance and higher prevalence of comorbidities such as chronic obstructive pulmonary disease, chronic renal disease, atrial fibrillation/flutter and higher Deyo-CCI scores were observed in both under-weight (BMI ≤ 19 kg/m²⁾ and extremely obese groups (BMI ≥ 40 kg/m²; **Table 1**). Forty-five percent of the patients underwent coronary

**TABLE 2 |** Frequency distribution of clinical course and outcomes by BMI group.

| | ≤19 Under-weight | 20–25 Normal-weight | 26–30 Over-weight | 31–35 Obese I group | 36–39 Obese II group | ≥40 Extremely obese | Total | *P*-value |
|---|---|---|---|---|---|---|---|---|
| NSTEMI, % | 38.7 | 33.5 | 29.4 | 27.9 | 28.1 | 29.7 | 28.9 | <0.0001 |
| STEMI, % | 10.2 | 7.2 | 5.6 | 5.4 | 4.6 | 4.1 | 5.1 | <0.0001 |
| Coronary angiography, % | 44.5 | 47.5 | 46.9 | 45.5 | 42.0 | 44.4 | 44.8 | <0.0001 |
| Percutaneous coronary intervention, % | 1.5 | 1.9 | 2.2 | 2.7 | 2.2 | 2.5 | 2.4 | 0.048 |
| Concomitant valve surgery, % | 3.6 | 3.8 | 2.9 | 2.5 | 3.1 | 3 | 2.9 | 0.005 |
| Mortality, % | 4.4 | 1.5 | 1.3 | 1.0 | 1.0 | 2.2 | 1.4 | <0.0001 |
| LOS (days), Mean ± SEM | 14.89 ± 0.77 | 10.54 ± 0.55 | 9.18 ± 0.16 | 8.83 ± 0.10 | 9.00 ± 0.13 | 10.69 ± 0.18 | 9.51 ± 0.09 | <0.0001 |

*LOS, Length of Stay; NSTEMI, Non-ST Segment Elevation Myocardial Infraction; STEMI, ST segment Myocardial Infraction.*

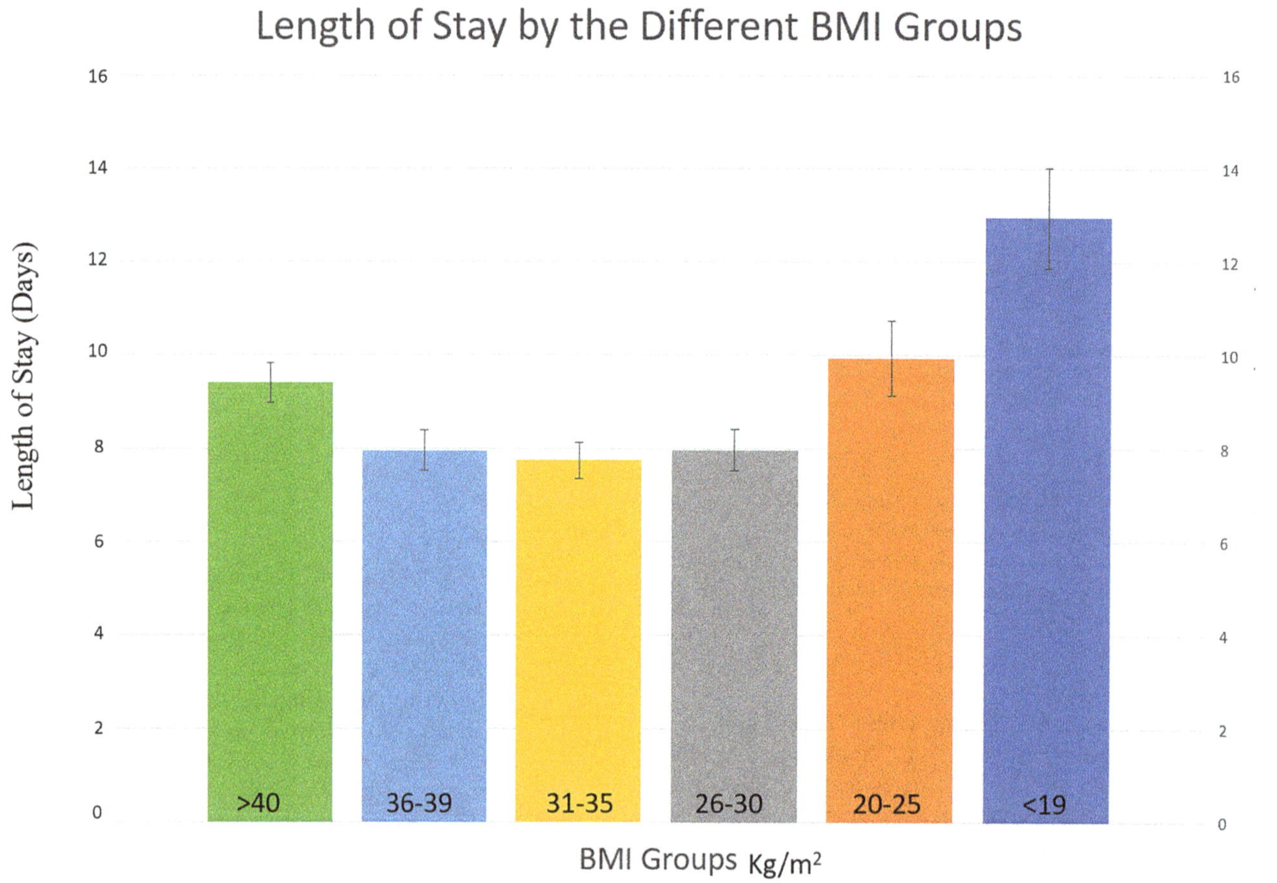


**FIGURE 1 |** Length of Stay per BMI groups.

angiogram and CABG in the same index hospitalization. These patients presented more frequently with NSTEMI compared to STEMI. A very small portion (3%) underwent CABG concomitant with valve surgery.

## Peri-Procedural Complications

Peri-procedural complications in the study population are reported in **Appendix Table 3**. A U-shaped relation between the BMI and several periprocedural complications was noted

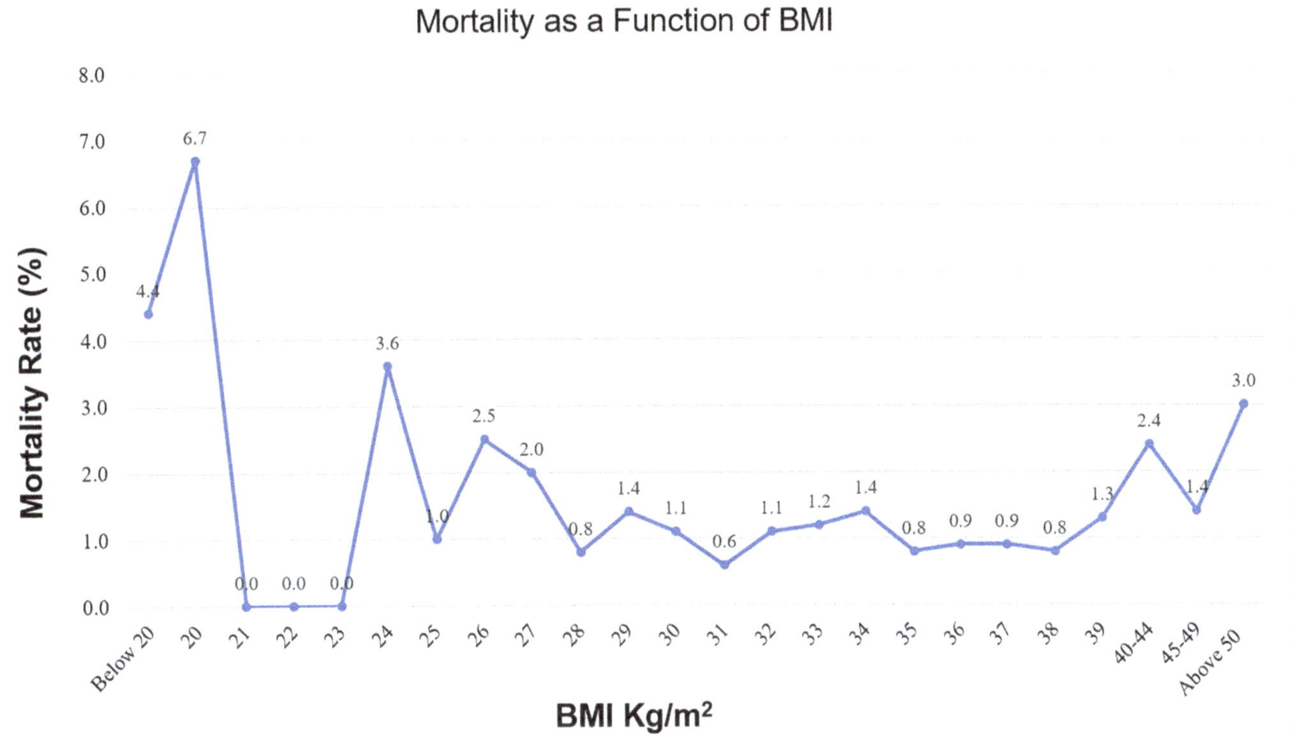


**FIGURE 2** | Mortality as a function of BMI.

including in acute renal failure, infectious, pulmonary, and vascular complications. In most instances, the underweight population had the highest prevalence of complications including acute renal failure, new atrial fibrillation, cardiac complications, cardiogenic shock, need for a pacemaker, and pulmonary complications (**Appendix Table 3**).

## Length of Stay and Mortality by BMI Groups

We observed a complex U-shaped relationship between the BMI and the study outcomes. Both the extremely obese (BMI $\geq$ 40 kg/m$^2$) and underweight patients (BMI $\leq$ 19 kg/m$^2$) had a higher crude mortality and longer LOS (**Figure 1**). The relationship between mortality and BMI as continuous variable is presented in **Figure 2**. The overall rate of total mortality during the study period was 1.4% with a significantly higher mortality rate in under-weight (4.4%) and in extremely obese (2.2%) patient population groups ($p$ < 0.001; **Figure 1**). The mean LOS in the total cohort was 9.51 $\pm$ 0.09 days. Longer LOS was documented in the under-weight (14.9 $\pm$ 0.77 days) and in the extremely obese subgroup (10.7 $\pm$ 0.18 days; **Figure 2**).

## Predictors of In-hospital Mortality

In the univariate analysis, we found that baseline characteristics as older age, increasing Deyo-CCI score, chronic renal failure, atrial fibrillation/flutter, congestive heart failure, peripheral vascular disease, female sex, chronic obstructive pulmonary disease and prior sternotomy all increased the odds of in-hospital mortality ($p$ < 0.001; **Table 3**).

The U-shaped relationship between BMI and outcomes were again seen in the multivariable analyses. BMI $\leq$ 19 kg/m$^2$ and BMI $\geq$ 40 kg/m$^2$ remained independent predictors of in-hospital mortality after adjusting for potential confounders, with a higher risk of mortality in the underweight patients compared to extremely obese patients (OR 2.64; [95% CI: 1.48–4.71], $p$ < 0.001 vs. OR 1.71; [95% CI: 1.07–2.72], $p$ = 0.025, respectively; **Table 4**).

## Predictors of LOS

Linear regression models for LOS are represented in the **Appendix Tables 4**, **5**. BMI $\leq$ 19 kg/m$^2$ was found to be an independent predictor of longer hospitalization [OR = 12.95; (95% CI: 11.88–14.03), $p$ < 0.001]. Other predictors for longer LOS were older age, Deyo-CCI score $\pm$2, atrial fibrillation, congestive heart failure, and chronic renal failure. Additionally, were patients who presented with acute coronary syndrome and who underwent percutaneous coronary intervention or concomitant valve surgery in the same index hospitalization (**Appendix Tables 4**, **5**).

## DISCUSSION

Utilizing data from the NIS, the largest all-payer inpatient database in the U.S., we identified a weighted total of 48,710

**TABLE 3** | Univariate analysis for predictors of in-hospital mortality, 2015–2016.

| Predictor | Odds ratio (95% CI) | *P*-value |
|---|---|---|
| BMI kg/m$^2$ group | | <0.001 |
| ≤19 | 2.97 (1.67–5.27) | <0.001 |
| 20–25 | 1.00 (reference) | N/A |
| 26–30 | 0.88 (0.54–1.42) | 0.596 |
| 31–35 | 0.66 (0.42–1.06) | 0.085 |
| 36–39 | 0.64 (0.39–1.03) | 0.068 |
| ≥40 | 1.45 (0.92–2.30) | <0.001 |
| Age group, years | | <0.001 |
| 18–44 | 1.00 (reference) | N/A |
| 45–59 | 1.70 (0.89–3.23) | 0.106 |
| 60–74 | 2.41 (1.28–4.53) | 0.006 |
| ≥75 | 5.02 (2.65–9.51) | <0.001 |
| Deyo-CCI | | <0.001 |
| 0 | 0.43 (0.22–0.84) | 0.01 |
| 1 | 1.00 (reference) | N/A |
| 2 or higher | 3.39 (2.54–4.52) | <0.001 |
| Gender | | <0.001 |
| Male | 1.00 (reference) | N/A |
| Female | 1.66 (1.42–1.93) | <0.001 |
| Race | | 0.42 |
| Non-white | 1.00 (reference) | N/A |
| White | 0.92 (0.75–1.13) | 0.42 |
| **Comorbidities** | | <0.001 |
| Atrial fibrillation/flutter | | |
| No | 1.00 (reference) | N/A |
| Yes | 2.08 (1.79–2.42) | <0.001 |
| Chronic obstructive pulmonary disease | | 0.02 |
| No | 1.00 (reference) | N/A |
| Yes | 1.22 (1.03–1.45) | 0.02 |
| Congestive heart failure | | <0.001 |
| No | 1.00 (reference) | N/A |
| Yes | 1.90 (1.59–2.28) | <0.001 |
| Diabetes mellitus | | 0.009 |
| No | 1.00 (reference) | N/A |
| Yes | 1.22 (1.05–1.42) | 0.009 |
| Hypertension | | <0.001 |
| No | 1.00 (reference) | N/A |
| Yes | 0.42 (0.36–0.49) | <0.001 |
| Peripheral vascular disease | | <0.001 |
| No | 1.00 (reference) | N/A |
| Yes | 2.78 (2.36–3.28) | <0.001 |
| Chronic renal failure | | <0.001 |
| No | 1.00 (reference) | N/A |
| Yes | 2.54 (2.18–2.97) | <0.001 |
| **Clinical Course** | | |
| NSTEMI | | <0.001 |
| No | 1.00 (reference) | N/A |
| Yes | 2.09 (1.79–2.43) | <0.001 |
| STEMI | | <0.001 |
| No | 1.00 (reference) | N/A |
| Yes | 3.12 (2.50–3.88) | <0.001 |
| Percutaneous coronary intervention | | <0.001 |
| No | 1.00 (reference) | N/A |
| Yes | 2.58 (1.87–3.57) | <0.001 |
| Prior sternotomy | | 0.021 |
| No | 1.00 (reference) | N/A |
| Yes | 1.23 (1.03–1.48) | 0.02 |
| Concomitant valve surgery | | <0.001 |
| No | 1.00 (reference) | N/A |
| Yes | 4.05 (3.14–5.21) | <0.001 |
| VF/VT | | <0.001 |
| No | 1.00 (reference) | N/A |
| Yes | 9.17 (7.79–10.81) | <0.001 |

*BMI, Body Mass Index; Deyo-CCI, Deyo-Charlson Comorbidity Index; NSTEMI, Non-ST Segment Elevation Myocardial Infraction; STEMI, ST segment Myocardial Infraction; VF/VT, Ventricular Flutter/Ventricular Fibrillation.*

patients to investigate the relationship between BMI and in-hospital outcomes among patients undergoing CABG. To our knowledge, this is the single largest study analyzing the relationship between BMI and CABG in-hospital outcomes. This nationwide data analysis revealed a U-shaped relationship between the BMI and in-hospital mortality during hospitalization for CABG in the U.S. during the study period. BMI $\leq$ 19 kg/m$^2$ and BMI $\geq$ 40 kg/m$^2$ were both independent predictors of higher mortality and longer length of stay in patients post CABG in the U.S. during the study period.

Several studies investigated the effect of different BMI arrays on short- and long-term mortality with contradictory results. Some studies suggested that obesity was an independent negative predictor of morbidity and mortality (5–8) while other showed more favorable outcomes after cardiac surgery in obese patients (9–13). This could partially be explained by the poor association between obese and non-obese groups in comparing morbidity and mortality; many of the studies lacked the "under-weight" and "severe obesity" patient populations in their statistical comparisons of different BMI groups.

Obesity is a rising global epidemic affecting 10–20% of the world's adult population (24), and is further known to complicate anesthesia (27) and surgery with fatal and non-fatal events. Prior studies showed higher rates of surgical site infections in obese patients, venous thromboembolism, more significant blood loss and the need of blood transfusions, as well as longer surgical times (28, 29). Other studies showed increased rates of urine and respiratory infections and post-surgery myocardial infarction events in obese patients (29). Specifically, after CABG surgery, obesity is a strong risk factor for deep sternal wound infections and as such serves an indicator of higher morbidity rates (30).

**TABLE 4** | Multivariable analysis for predictors of in-hospital mortality, 2015–2016.

| Predictor | Odds ratio (95% CI) | *P*-value |
|---|---|---|
| BMI kg/m² group | | <0.001 |
| 20–25 | 1.00 (reference) | N/A |
| ≤19 | 2.64 (1.48–4.71) | <0.001 |
| 26–30 | 0.86 (0.52–1.40) | 0.541 |
| 31–35 | 0.70 (0.43–1.12) | 0.140 |
| 36–39 | 0.76 (0.47–1.25) | 0.288 |
| ≥40 | 1.71 (1.07–2.73) | 0.025 |
| Age group, years | | <0.001 |
| 18–44 years | 1.00 (reference) | N/A |
| 45–59 years | 1.68 (0.88–3.21) | 0.116 |
| 60–74 years | 2.32 (1.23–4.38) | 0.009 |
| 75 years or older | 4.53 (2.37–8.66) | <0.001 |
| Deyo-CCI | | <0.001 |
| 1 | 1.00 (reference) | N/A |
| 2 or higher | 3.46 (2.50–4.77) | <0.001 |
| Gender | | <0.001 |
| Male | 1.00 (reference) | N/A |
| Female | 1.42 (1.21–1.68) | <0.001 |
| Race | | 0.470 |
| Non-white | 1.00 (reference) | N/A |
| White | 0.93 (0.75–1.14) | 0.470 |
| **Comorbidities** | | <0.001 |
| Atrial fibrillation/flutter | | |
| No | 1.00 (reference) | N/A |
| Yes | 1.80 (1.53–2.12) | <0.001 |
| COPD | | 0.208 |
| No | 1.00 (reference) | N/A |
| Yes | 0.89 (0.74–1.07) | 0.208 |
| Congestive heart failure | | 0.002 |
| No | 1.00 (reference) | N/A |
| Yes | 1.36 (1.13–1.65) | 0.002 |
| Diabetes mellitus | | 0.718 |
| No | 1.00 (reference) | N/A |
| Yes | 0.97 (0.82–1.14) | 0.718 |
| Hypertension | | <0.001 |
| No | 1.00 (reference) | N/A |
| Yes | 0.56 (0.47–0.66) | <0.001 |
| Peripheral vascular disease | | <0.001 |
| No | 1.00 (reference) | N/A |
| Yes | 2.25 (1.89–2.68) | <0.001 |
| Chronic renal failure | | <0.001 |
| No | 1.00 (reference) | N/A |
| Yes | 1.72 (1.45–2.03) | <0.001 |
| **Clinical course** | | <0.001 |
| NSTEMI | | |
| No | 1.00 (reference) | N/A |
| Yes | 1.62 (1.38–1.90) | <0.001 |
| STEMI | | <0.001 |
| No | 1.00 (reference) | N/A |
| Yes | 2.99 (2.36–3.77) | <0.001 |
| Percutaneous coronary intervention | | <0.001 |
| No | 1.00 (reference) | N/A |
| Yes | 2.22 (1.56–3.16) | <0.001 |
| Prior sternotomy | | 0.224 |
| No | 1.00 (reference) | N/A |
| Yes | 1.13 (0.93–1.36) | 0.224 |
| Concomitant valve surgery | | <0.001 |
| No | 1.00 (reference) | N/A |
| Yes | 3.12 (2.36–4.12) | <0.001 |
| VF/VT | | <0.001 |
| No | 1.00 (reference) | N/A |
| Yes | 8.02 (6.72–9.57) | <0.001 |

*(Continued)*

**TABLE 4** | Continued

*BMI, Body Mass Index; Deyo-CCI, Deyo-Charlson Comorbidity Index; NSTEMI, Non-ST Segment Elevation Myocardial Infraction; STEMI, ST segment Myocardial Infraction; VF/VT, Ventricular Flutter/Ventricular Fibrillation.*

Currently, there is a lack of publications studying cachexia and survival rates in post CABG patients.

On the contrary to the abovementioned studies, others showed that higher weight individuals conferred better survival after surgery. One possible explanation is that high BMI may be beneficial by providing nutritional and caloric reserves in severely and critically ill patients. This is supported by previous studies in additional chronic, debilitating cardiovascular and non-cardiovascular conditions, in which both under-weight and normal weight BMI was associated with increased mortality rates, compared to higher-BMI groups (3, 31–33). Further studies supported that severe cardiovascular disease, such as heart failure, results in tissue hypoperfusion and cardiac cachexia. The hypothesis is that this state resulting from a heightened metabolic or increased catabolic state is associated with worse prognosis (34, 35). On the other hand, elevated BMI might indicate a better metabolic reserve and tolerance to metabolic stress and consequently to a better prognosis (36).

Our study results improve the available literature on the negative association of extremely obese BMI subgroups and early mortality following CABG. Of note, the Society of Thoracic Surgeons (STS) uses statistical models to create risk-adjusted performance metrics for Adult Cardiac Surgery Database (ACSD) participants. BSA and BMI were both independently associated with mortality, and O'Brien et al. (26) found that inclusion of both variables was needed to capture variation in the residuals. In line with our findings, they also demonstrated a U-shape relationship between BMI and mortality (26), reflected in the STS score. In contrast, BMI has not been directly included in the current European (EuroSCORE II) score (37). We believe that this important correlation between BMI and mortality should be reflected in all surgical risk scores.

Contrary to many previous clinical studies, we included the "real world" BMI spectrum including the underweight, normal weight and extremely obese patients for a complete representation. Our results showed that underweight patients undergoing CABG (BMI $\leq$ 19 kg/m$^2$) have the highest risk of mortality compared to the other BMI groups.

This study population represents the entire, nationwide population of patients who underwent CABG in the U.S between October 2015 and December 2016, hence eliminating the "selection bias" in some of the prior studies regarding CABG patients.

The current study should be interpreted in the contexts of several limitations. First, the NIS database is a retrospective administrative database that contains discharge-level records and as such is susceptible to coding errors. The NIS database does not include detailed information about the patients' clinical characteristics, medication, blood tests such as level of cholesterol and markers of inflammation, all of which have been independently linked with adverse cardiovascular events, therefore we cannot rule out residual confounding of the associations we observed. Unfortunately, no data about the number/type of diseased vessels (SYNTAX score etc.), the number of coronary bypass and the techniques preferred (venous vs. arteriosus graft, off-pump BH, etc.) have been included in our study, despite of increasing interest. In addition, the lack of patient identifiers in the NIS precluded us from using other outcome variables and mortality measures such as at 30-days, we could only capture events that occurred in the same index hospitalization. These limitations are counterbalanced by the real world, nationwide nature of the data, as well as mitigation of reporting bias introduced by selective publication of results from specialized centers.

In conclusion, a U-shaped relationship between BMI and mortality was documented in patients hospitalized for CABG in the recent years. Accordingly, BMI should be addressed and considered as part of the risk assessment for in-hospital mortality in patients who are planned for CABG.

## ETHICS STATEMENT

Ethical review and approval was not required for the study on human participants in accordance with the local legislation and institutional requirements. Written informed consent for participation was not required for this study in accordance with the national legislation and the institutional requirements.

## AUTHOR CONTRIBUTIONS

All authors listed have made a substantial, direct, and intellectual contribution to the work, and approved it for publication.

## ACKNOWLEDGMENTS

The GE-G affirms that she has listed everyone who contributed significantly to the work, had access to all the study data, takes responsibility for the accuracy of the analysis, and had authority over the manuscript preparation and the decision to submit the manuscript for publication, and confirms that all authors read and approved the manuscript.

## REFERENCES

1. Khan SS, Ning H, Wilkins JT, Allen N, Carnethon M, Berry JD, et al. Association of body mass index with lifetime risk of cardiovascular disease and compression of morbidity. *JAMA Cardiol.* (2018) 3:280–7. doi: 10.1001/jamacardio.2018.0022
2. Available online at: http://www.euro.who.int/en/health-topics/disease-prevention/nutrition/a-healthy-lifestyle/body-mass-index-bmi (accessed July 7, 2020).
3. Lavie CJ, Milani RV, Ventura HO. Obesity and cardiovascular disease: risk factor, paradox, and impact of weight loss. *J Am Coll Cardiol.* (2009) 53:1925–32. doi: 10.1016/j.jacc.2008.12.068
4. Muller MJ, Braun W, Enderle J, Bosy-Westphal A. Beyond BMI: conceptual issues related to overweight and obese patients. *Obes Facts.* (2016) 9:193–205. doi: 10.1159/000445380
5. Sun Y, Jiang D, Zhang B, Yu H, Gao Y, Li Y, Qi G. Impact of obesity on the outcome of Chinese patients with ST-segment myocardial infarction undergoing urgent percutaneous coronary intervention. *Acta Cardiol.* (2012) 67:541–8. doi: 10.1080/AC.67.5.2174128
6. Montazerghaem H, Safaie N, Samiei Nezhad V. Body mass index or serum albumin levels: which is further prognostic following cardiac surgery? *J Cardiovasc Thorac Res.* (2014) 6:123–6. doi: 10.5681/jcvtr.2014.026
7. Zittermann A, Becker T, Gummert JF, Borgermann J. Body mass index, cardiac surgery and clinical outcome. A single-center experience with 9125 patients. *Nutr Metab Cardiovasc Dis.* (2014) 24:168–75. doi: 10.1016/j.numecd.2013.06.013
8. Caliskan E, Gusewell S, Seifert B, Theusinger OM, Starck CT, Pavicevic J, et al. Does body mass index impact the early outcome of surgical revascularization? A comparison between off-pump and on-pump coronary artery bypass grafting. *Interact Cardiovasc Thorac Surg.* (2014) 19:749–55. doi: 10.1093/icvts/ivu246
9. Reeves BC, Ascione R, Chamberlain MH, Angelini GD. Effect of body mass index on early outcomes in patients undergoing coronary artery bypass surgery. *J Am Coll Cardiol.* (2003) 42:668–76. doi: 10.1016/S0735-1097(03)00777-0
10. Wiedemann D, Schachner T, Bonaros N, Weidinger F, Kolbitsch C, Friedrich G, et al. Does obesity affect operative times and perioperative outcome of patients undergoing totally endoscopic coronary artery bypass surgery? *Interact Cardiovasc Thorac Surg.* (2009) 9:214–7. doi: 10.1510/icvts.2009.203059
11. Le-Bert G, Santana O, Pineda AM, Zamora C, Lamas GA, Lamelas J. The obesity paradox in elderly obese patients undergoing coronary artery bypass surgery. *Interact Cardiovasc Thorac Surg.* (2011) 13:124–7. doi: 10.1510/icvts.2010.256677
12. Wang TK, Ramanathan T, Stewart R, Gamble G, White H. Lack of relationship between obesity and mortality or morbidity after coronary artery bypass grafting. *N Z Med J.* (2013) 126:56–65.
13. Zhang Y, Zheng Q, Dai X, Xu X, Ma L. Overweight is associated with better one-year survival in elderly patients after cardiac surgery: a retrospective analysis of the MIMIC-III database. *J Thorac Dis.* (2021) 13:562–74. doi: 10.21037/jtd-20-2824
14. Wang M, Chen M, Ao H, Chen S, Wang Z. The effects of different BMI on blood loss and transfusions in Chinese patients undergoing coronary artery bypass grafting. *Ann Thorac Cardiovasc Surg.* (2017) 23:83–90. doi: 10.5761/atcs.oa.16-00219
15. Brunet A, N'Guyen Y, Lefebvre A, Poncet A, Robbins A, Bajolet O, et al. Obesity and preoperative anaemia as independent risk factors for sternal wound infection after coronary artery bypass graft surgery with pedicled (non-skeletonized) internal mammary arteries: the role of thoracic wall ischemia? *Vasc Health Risk Manag.* (2020) 16:553–9. doi: 10.2147/VHRM.S264415
16. Atik FA, Pegado HM, de Brito LMR, Macedo MT, Franca EP Jr, Dias AKA, et al. Does the anthropometric profile influence infection morbidity

after coronary artery bypass grafting? *J Card Surg.* (2021) 36:1194–200. doi: 10.1111/jocs.15334

17. Buschmann K, Wrobel J, Chaban R, Rosch R, Ghazy A, Hanf A, et al. Body mass index (BMI) and its influence on the cardiovascular and operative risk profile in coronary artery bypass grafting patients: impact of inflammation and leptin. *Oxid Med Cell Longev.* (2020) 2020:5724024. doi: 10.1155/2020/5724024
18. Healthcare Cost Utilization Project (HCUP). *Agency for Healthcare Research Quality R* (2000–2011). Available online at: www.hcup-us.ahrq.gov/nisoverview.jsp (accessed July 7, 2020).
19. HCUP National Inpatient Sample (NIS). *Healthcare Cost Utilization Project (HCUP).* Agency for Healthcare Research Quality R, MD (2012–2013). Available online at: www.hcup-us.ahrq.gov/nisoverview.jsp (accessed July 07, 2020).
20. Steiner C, Elixhauser A, Schnaier J. The healthcare cost and utilization project: an overview. *Eff Clin Pract.* (2002) 5:143–51.
21. Deyo RA, Cherkin DC, Ciol MA. Adapting a clinical comorbidity index for use with ICD-9-CM administrative databases. *J Clin Epidemiol.* (1992) 45:613–9. doi: 10.1016/0895-4356(92)90133-8
22. Chu YT, Ng YY, Wu SC. Comparison of different comorbidity measures for use with administrative data in predicting short- and long-term mortality. *BMC Health Serv Res.* (2010) 10:140. doi: 10.1186/1472-6963-10-140
23. Radovanovic D, Seifert B, Urban P, Eberli FR, Rickli H, Bertel O, et al. Validity of Charlson Comorbidity Index in patients hospitalised with acute coronary syndrome. Insights from the nationwide AMIS Plus registry 2002-2012. *Heart.* (2014) 100:288–94. doi: 10.1136/heartjnl-2013-304588
24. Kappetein AP, Head SJ, Genereux P. Updated standardized endpoint definitions for transcatheter aortic valve implantation: the Valve Academic Research Consortium-2 consensus document (VARC-2). *Eur J Cardiothorac Surg.* (2012) 42:45–60. doi: 10.1093/ejcts/ezs533
25. Hosseini SM, Moazzami K, Rozen G, Vaid J, Saleh A, Heist KE, et al. Utilization and in-hospital complications of cardiac resynchronization therapy: trends in the United States from 2003 to 2013. *Eur Heart J.* (2017) 38:2122–28. doi: 10.1093/eurheartj/ehx100
26. O'Brien SM, Liqi F, He X, Xian Y, Jacobs JP, Badhwar V, et al. The STS 2018 adult cardiac surgery risk models: part 2 - statistical methods & results. *Ann Thorac Surg.* (2018) 105:1419–28. doi: 10.1016/j.athoracsur.2018.03.00
27. Lotia S, Bellamy MC. Anaesthesia and morbid obesity. Continuing education in anaesthesia. *Crit Care Pain.* (2008) 8:151–6. doi: 10.1093/bjaceaccp/mkn030
28. Jiang J, Teng Y, Fan Z, Khan S, Xia Y. Does obesity affect the surgical outcome and complication rates of spinal surgery? A meta-analysis. *Clin Orthop Relat Res.* (2014) 472:968–75. doi: 10.1007/s11999-013-3346-3
29. Bamgbade OA, Rutter TW, Nafiu OO, Dorje P. Postoperative complications in obese and nonobese patients. *World J Surg.* (2007) 31:556–60; discussion 561. doi: 10.1007/s00268-006-0305-0
30. Hollenbeak CS, Murphy DM, Koenig S, Woodward RS, Dunagan WC, Fraser VJ. The clinical and economic impact of deep chest surgical site infections following coronary artery bypass graft surgery. *Chest.* (2000) 118:397–402. doi: 10.1378/chest.118.2.397
31. Oliveros H, Villamor E. Obesity and mortality in critically ill adults: a systematic review and meta-analysis. *Obesity (Silver Spring).* (2008) 16:515–21. doi: 10.1038/oby.2007.102
32. Kalantar-Zadeh K, Horwich TB, Oreopoulos A, Kovesdy CP, Younessi H, Anker SD, et al. Risk factor paradox in wasting diseases. *Curr Opin Clin Nutr Metab Care.* (2007) 10:433–42. doi: 10.1097/MCO.0b013e3281a30594
33. Habbu A, Lakkis NM, Dokainish H. The obesity paradox: fact or fiction? *Am J Cardiol.* (2006) 98:944–8. doi: 10.1016/j.amjcard.2006.04.039
34. Kenchaiah S, Pocock SJ, Wang D, Finn PV, Zornoff LAM, Skali H, et al. Body mass index and prognosis in patients with chronic heart failure insights from the candesartan in heart failure: assessment of reduction in mortality and morbidity (CHARM) program. *Circulation.* (2007) 116:627–36. doi: 10.1161/CIRCULATIONAHA.106.679779
35. Berry C, Clark AL. Catabolism in chronic heart failure. *Eur Heart J.* (2000) 21:521–32. doi: 10.1053/euhj.1999.1882
36. Coats A, Anker SD, Roecker EB, Schultz MK, Staiger C, Amann-Zalan I, et al. Prevention and reversal of cardiac cachexia in patients with severe heart failure by carvedilol: results of the COPERNICUS study. *Circulation.* (2001) 10:4II–437.
37. *EuroSCORE Models.* Available online at: http://www.euroscore.org/calcold.html (accessed July 7, 2020).

5

# Application of Homograft Valved Conduit in Cardiac Surgery

*Yige Huyan, Yuan Chang and Jiangping Song**

*The Cardiomyopathy Research Group at Fuwai Hospital, State Key Laboratory of Cardiovascular Disease, Chinese Academy of Medical Sciences and Peking Union Medical College, Beijing, China*

***Correspondence:***
*Jiangping Song*
*fwsongjiangping@126.com*

Valved conduits often correct the blood flow of congenital heart disease by connecting the right ventricle to the pulmonary artery (RV-PA). The homograft valved conduit was invented in the 1960s, but its wide application is limited due to the lack of effective sterilization and preservation methods. Modern cryopreservation prolongs the preservation time of homograft valved conduit, which makes it become the most important treatment at present, and is widely used in Ross and other operations. However, homograft valved conduit has limited biocompatibility and durability and lacks any additional growth capacity. Therefore, decellularized valved conduit has been proposed as an effective improved method, which can reduce immune response and calcification, and has potential growth ability. In addition, as a possible substitute, commercial xenograft valved conduit has certain advantages in clinical application, and tissue engineering artificial valved conduit needs to be further studied.

**Keywords: homograft valved conduit, cardiac surgery, xenograft valved conduit, decellularized valved conduit, tissue engineered substitutes**

## INTRODUCTION

In tetralogy of Fallot combined with pulmonary atresia or other types of severe cardiac malformations, the use of valved conduits to reconstruct the ventricular outflow tract is required to restore normal hemodynamics. From the 1960s, when valved conduits were first used, improvements in preservation methods have greatly expanded the use of homograft valved conduits in clinical practice. This technology has been rapidly developed at present. The basic research, clinical trials, and follow-up reports on valved conduits have been published continuously, opening up new avenues for the treatment of complex precordial and vascular disease. This article reviews the advances in homograft valved conduit and its clinical applications and provides an outlook on this field.

## METHODS

An electronic search in PubMed was performed from inception until 31 April 2021. The search strategy consisted of free and controlled terms for homograft valved conduit. The search was limited to publications in English. Reference lists of previous reviews of the subject as well as the included articles were hand-searched to identify additional eligible studies. Following retrieval of the search results, the title and abstract of the remaining records were screened. Relevant articles and articles of which eligibility could not be assessed properly were selected for full-text assessment. Then select relevant articles to be included in this review.

## THE HISTORY OF HOMOGRAFT VALVED CONDUIT

In 1966, Ross et al. used homograft valved conduit to connect right ventricular outflow tract and pulmonary artery for the first time. They used valved homograft aorta and pulmonary artery to treat pulmonary atresia, and then gradually expanded to tetralogy of Fallot, double outlet of right ventricle, transposition of great arteries, single ventricle, permanent truncus arteriosus, and many other complex congenital heart diseases. In the 1960s, five cases of pulmonary atresia variant transposition of aorta with occlusion of left ventricular outflow tract were reported, all of which were repaired with valved homograft aorta at the site of pulmonary artery (1, 2). At the Mayo Clinic, there is relatively large early experience in radiation cryopreservation of homograft valved conduit. However, the graft was found to have calcification and rapid degeneration 1–3 years after operation, resulting in severe stenosis (3). Subsequently, several international centers disinfected the homograft valved conduit with antibiotics and preserved them in a tissue medium at 4°C (4, 5). In the experience of a limited number of centers, these conduits performed well in the location of the pulmonary artery. However, the shelf life of this kind of conduits is very short, so it is difficult to become a widely used homograft technology.

The development of homograft valved conduit preservation methods can be broadly divided into four phases: the first stage (mid-1960s) was the *in situ* operation method, in which fresh homograft valved conduit was obtained under sterile conditions and perform surgical treatment within a few hours. In the second stage (mid-1960s to mid-1970s), chemical reagents or radiation sterilization were used, followed by cryopreservation at −79°C (6). Because sterilization also leads to loss of biological activity of the homograft valve, the valve is prone to degeneration, calcification after surgery, and poor long-term results. In the third stage (mid-1970s to mid-1980s), isolated homograft valved conduit were sterilized in antibiotic solution for 24 h and then stored at a low temperature of 4°C in a nutrient solution containing low concentrations of antibiotics, which maintained their biological activity and short and long-term clinical outcomes, but the maximum storage time was only 6 weeks, which was still unsatisfactory (7). The fourth stage (after the mid-1980s) used antibiotic sterilization, controlled rate cooling, and liquid nitrogen deep cryopreservation (8). This is currently the most widely used and studied method internationally. The main process is to sterilize isolated homograft valved conduit with antibiotic solution at 37°C for 24 h, then put into RPMI1640 medium containing dimethyl sulfoxide (DMSO) and cool down to −80°C at a rate of −1°C/min, and then transfer to liquid nitrogen for deep cryopreservation for long-term storage. **Figure 1** illustrates the development of valved conduits, including milestones of homograft valved conduits and some xenograft valved conduit.

## PRESERVATION METHODS FOR HOMOGRAFT VALVED CONDUIT

The biological activity of homograft valved conduit and the integrity of its tissue structure are the keys to preserve its function. The biological activity of homograft valved conduit refers to the number of living cells it contains and its functional state, while the integrity of tissue structure refers to the composition and structural integrity of the extracellular matrix. Fibroblasts can synthesize extracellular matrix and play an important role in maintaining the stability of valved conduit (9). The increased possibility of thrombosis caused by the loss of endothelial cells will also accelerate the failure of homograft (10). Current research advances in homograft valved conduit preservation methods focus on donor conditions, warm ischemia time, sterilization methods, freezing methods, and rewarming methods (11).

The health status of the donor itself determines the biological activity and the structural integrity of the tissue of the homograft valved conduit. In clinical applications, Sadowski et al. found that valves removed from elderly donors were prone to complications such as degeneration and incomplete closure (12). Verghese et al. noted that homograft valved conduit from individuals after organ or tissue transplantation readily induces an immune response in the recipient and should not be used as a donor (13). Gall et al. quantitatively evaluated the initial activity of homograft valved conduit in normal and cardiac arrest donors by thin-layer radiographic autoradiography, and the initial activity of homograft valved conduit in normal donors was significantly higher (92 ± 2)% than that in cardiac arrest donors (66 ± 3)%, suggesting that the biological activity of homograft valved conduit is significantly reduced after cardiac arrest due to the lack of oxygen and nutrient supply (14). Therefore, to maximize preservation of homograft valved conduit activity prior to operation, it should be removed as soon as possible after donor cardiac arrest, or if the corpse is cryopreserved it can still be collected within 24 h. Donors currently used in clinical practice are generally selected from brain dead or autopsied patients under 45 years of age (6) who have no major vascular disease, valve disease, infectious disease or autoimmune disease in their lifetime. Homograft valved conduit are removed under strict aseptic conditions, placed in saline or Hank's solution containing antibiotics, packed in double-layer sterile bags, and shipped as soon as possible at 4°C for trimming and subsequent processing.

Warm ischemia time is a period of time between when homograft valved conduit loses blood supply after cardiac arrest and when it is taken out and stored at 0–4°C. Mohan et al. found that when warm ischemia time >24 h, homograft valved conduit endothelial cells basically die and fall off, and the synthesis of prostacyclin stops. The collagen fibers in the artery wall are destroyed, and the structural integrity is also destroyed (14). Suh et al. studied the activity of porcine aortic valve fibroblasts under different conditions. Fibroblast activity was (92.25 ± 2.7)% at 2 h of heat ischemia and (57.0 ± 10)% at 24 h of heat ischemia ($P < 0.05$), suggesting a significant decrease in fibroblast activity with increasing warm ischemia time. Suh et al. studied

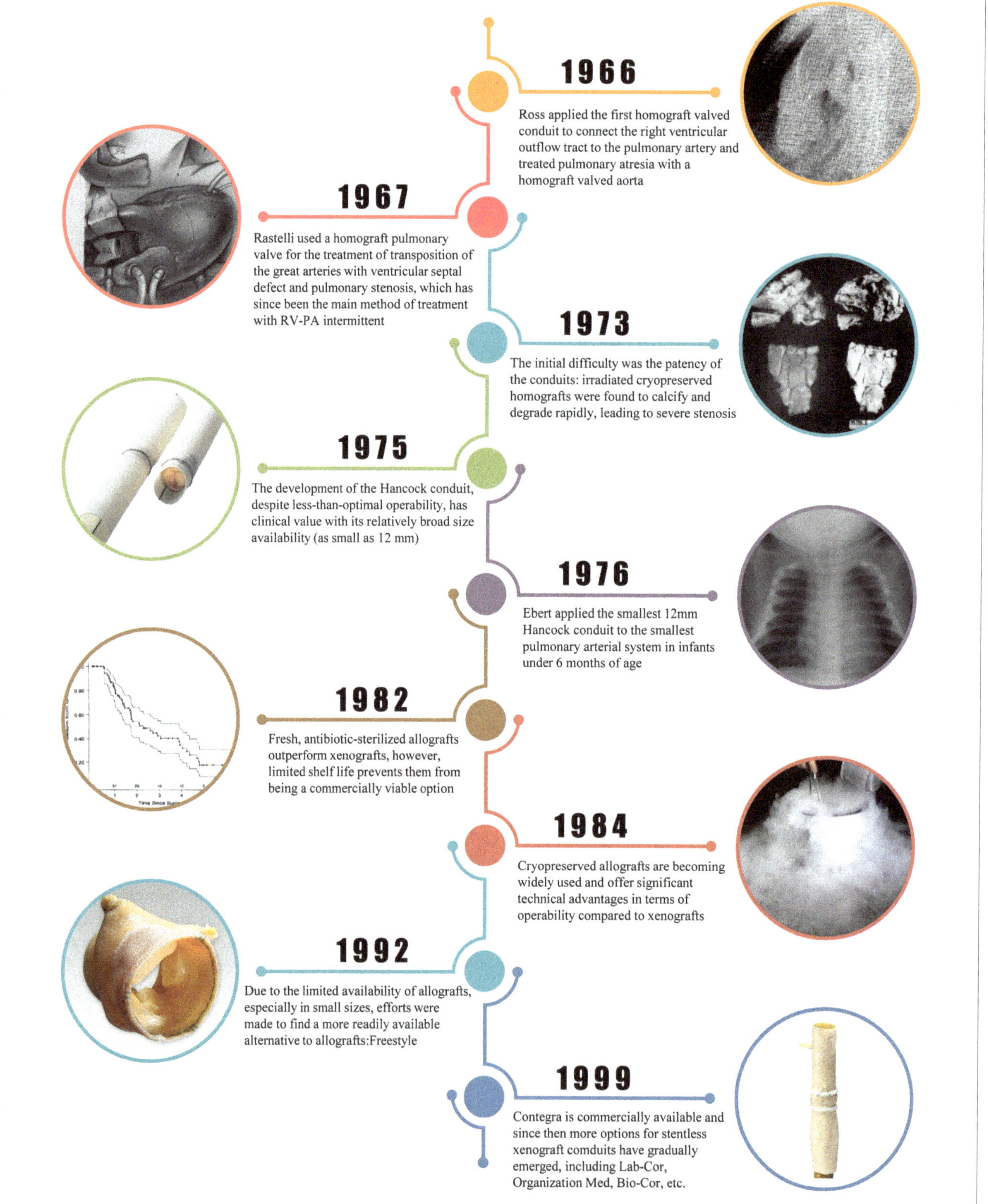


**FIGURE 1 |** Historical progression since 1966 when Ross first applied homograft valved conduit.

the activity of porcine aortic valve fibroblasts under different conditions. Fibroblast activity was (92.25 ± 2.7)% at 2 h of warm ischemia and (57.0 ± 10)% at 24 h of warm ischemia ($P < 0.05$), suggesting a significant decrease in fibroblast activity with increasing warm ischemia time (15). Burkert et al. applied scanning electron microscopy to observe the effects of different warm ischemia time on human aortic valves. When the valve was left at room temperature for 12 h, the continuity between valve endothelial cells was disrupted, some endothelial cells were shed into the lumen, and endothelial cell loss occurred. When warm ischemia time reached 48 h, the vascular endothelial cells were completely shed, while the vessel wall structure was destroyed. By comparing the degree of damage to the homograft valved conduit by different warm ischemia time, it is recommended that warm ischemia time should be controlled within 24 h as much as possible (16). Stemper et al. found that vascular tissue mechanics were significantly reduced after more than 24 h compared to fresh vessels, even after storage at 4°C (17). The above studies provide an objective experimental basis for clinical control of homograft valved conduit with a warm ischemia time of <24 h.

The classic antibiotic solution formulation is penicillin 50 U/ml, streptomycin 50 μg/ml, and amphotericin B 10 μg/ml. However, Strickett et al. found that amphotericin B and streptomycin are highly cytotoxic and can significantly reduce the activity of valvular fibroblasts (17). Yu Haibin et al. used cefoxitin 240 mg/L, polymyxin B 100 mg/L, lincomycin 120 mg/L, and vancomycin 50 mg/L for sterilization treatment, which ensured sterilization and avoided the effect of streptomycin and amphotericin B on cell activity. Jashari et al. found that the removal of cefoxitin and the use of lower concentrations of lincomycin, polymyxin B, and vancomycin had no significant effect on cell survival and the sterilization effect was reliable (18). Since antibiotics are sterilized primarily during the bacterial multiplication phase, antibiotic sterilization activity is greatest at 37°C. However, the normal metabolic rate of valve tissue at 37°C inevitably leads to inactivation of valve tissue cells due to hypoxia and nutrient deficiency. The 4°C incubation sterilization protocol was first proposed by Kinklin et al. found that valve sterilization at 4°C for 20 h resulted in a slower metabolic rate and increased tolerance to lack of oxygen and nutrients, but a positive sterilization effect (19).

Currently, the main clinical methods used are incubation sterilization with antibiotic solution, controlled rate cooling, and liquid nitrogen freezing, as proposed by O'Brien. The main mechanism is that the deep cryogenic environment can interfere with cell metabolism and inhibit the biochemical activities of the organism. Brockbank et al. compared the protein synthesis function of homograft valved conduit fibroblasts preserved by different methods. After 2 years of preservation by liquid nitrogen freezing, the fibroblasts still had protein synthesis function, and the protein synthesis function of freeze-dried fibroblasts gradually decreased with time. The protein synthesis function of fibroblasts preserved at 4°C for 2 weeks was only 15% of that of the liquid nitrogen preservation group (20). Liquid nitrogen freezing is effective in preserving tissues and organs, but cryoinjury still exists. Dimethyl sulfoxide is currently the most commonly used homograft valved conduit liquid nitrogen cryoprotectant. It can rapidly penetrate cell membranes, lower the freezing point, slow down the cryopreservation process, increase the intracellular ion concentration, and reduce intracellular ice crystal formation, thereby reducing cellular damage. However, high concentrations of DMSO are inherently cytotoxic and can cause osmotic damage. The optimal concentration of DMSO in cryopreservation solution is currently considered to be 15% (21). Wosteman et al. found that replacing sodium salts with vitamin B complexes in cryopreservation solutions prevented DMSO from exerting its toxic effects (22). Mazur et al. found that during rapid freezing, water molecules in the intracellular fluid do not have time to penetrate outside the cell and form ice crystals inside the cell, which disrupt the ultrastructure of the cell and lead to cell death. During slow freezing, cells are exposed to hyperosmotic extracellular fluid and toxic antifreeze for too long, which may also lead to cell death (23). Therefore, the cooling rate is very important to maintain the biological activity of cells. The use of a program-controlled hypothermia instrument to control homograft valved conduit cooling at a relatively stable and reasonable rate can minimize cryo-damage. −1°C/min was found by Vander et al. to be the best cooling rate to maximize fibroblast activity (24). In recent years, the concept of phase change point has received increasing attention in the process of programmed cooling. The phase change point is the temperature point at which the sample transforms from liquid to solid during the freezing process, and a large amount of melt heat is released during the morphological transformation, causing the local sample to condense, and then increase in temperature and melt, and then condense again. During this process, the cells are susceptible to repeated damage by ice crystals, which affects the preservation effect of homograft valved conduit. To overcome the phase transition heat, increasing the cooling rate near the phase transition point to prevent the temperature increase during the phase transition and decreasing the cooling rate after complete phase transition to continue cooling at −1°C/min can reduce the damage to the homograft valved conduit from the phase transition. The phase transition point of human homograft aortic valved conduits is −4 to −6°C. During this period, increasing the cooling rate to −4°C/min instead of −1°C/min can effectively reduce cell damage.

Liquid nitrogen cryopreserved homograft valved conduit needs to be thawed and resuscitated before it can be used in the clinic. Rapid rewarming in a 42°C water bath is now commonly accepted in clinical practice. Rapid rewarming is particularly important for frozen cells. For cells containing ice crystals, rapid rewarming can limit the phenomenon of migratory recrystallization within the cells and reduce the damage caused by repeated crystallization, thus improving cell survival for cytoprotection. Since DMSO is toxic to cells at room temperature, when homograft valved conduit is rewarmed and melted, it should be quickly removed and replaced by "graded series rinsing" to reduce its damage to cells. This preservation method not only retains the biological activity of the valved conduit, but also retains a certain degree of antigenicity. Most patients implanted with valved conduit have humoral immunity against human leukocyte antigen (HLA) (25). It has been found that donor-derived dendritic cells and endothelial cells expressing HLA-II molecules in valved conduits can directly present antigens and activate receptor immunity (26, 27). Other studies have shown that there are mild to moderate mononuclear inflammatory cell infiltration composed of T cells and macrophages in valvular tissue (28). **Figure 2** summarizes the processing flow of homograft valved conduit preservation method (29).

## CLINICAL APPLICATION OF HOMOGRAFT VALVED CONDUIT

One of the tasks frequently faced by congenital heart surgeons is the reconstruction of the right ventricular outflow tract, i.e., the creation of a channel between the right ventricle and the pulmonary artery. Depending on the etiology of the pathological changes of the pulmonary outflow tract, it can be classified as tetralogy of Fallot combined with pulmonary atresia, congenital arterial trunk right ventricular outflow tract or pulmonary artery agenesis, transposition of the great arteries with ventricular septal defect and pulmonary stenosis, corrected transposition of the great arteries with pulmonary stenosis, complex right ventricular double outlet, and Ross procedure of medical origin (30).

The Ross procedure, using the autograft pulmonary valve to replace the diseased aortic valve and a non-autograft valved conduit to replace the pulmonary valve, has become the procedure of choice for young people with irreparable aortic root disease. There are two main techniques for Ross procedure: the subcoronary and root replacement techniques. The subcoronary technique can be technically challenging because the aortic and pulmonary roots often have different dimensions and commissural distribution. Therefore, many surgeons use the full root replacement technique for Ross procedures (31, 32). The Ross procedure is reserved for patients with non-repairable, non-spareable aortic valves. Otherwise, isolated aortic valve repair or valve-sparing root replacement should be chosen. Ideal candidates for the Ross procedure are young or middle-aged (<50 years old). Patients presenting with mechanical or bioprosthetic aortic valve dysfunction and patients with active endocarditis also appear to be appropriate candidates for

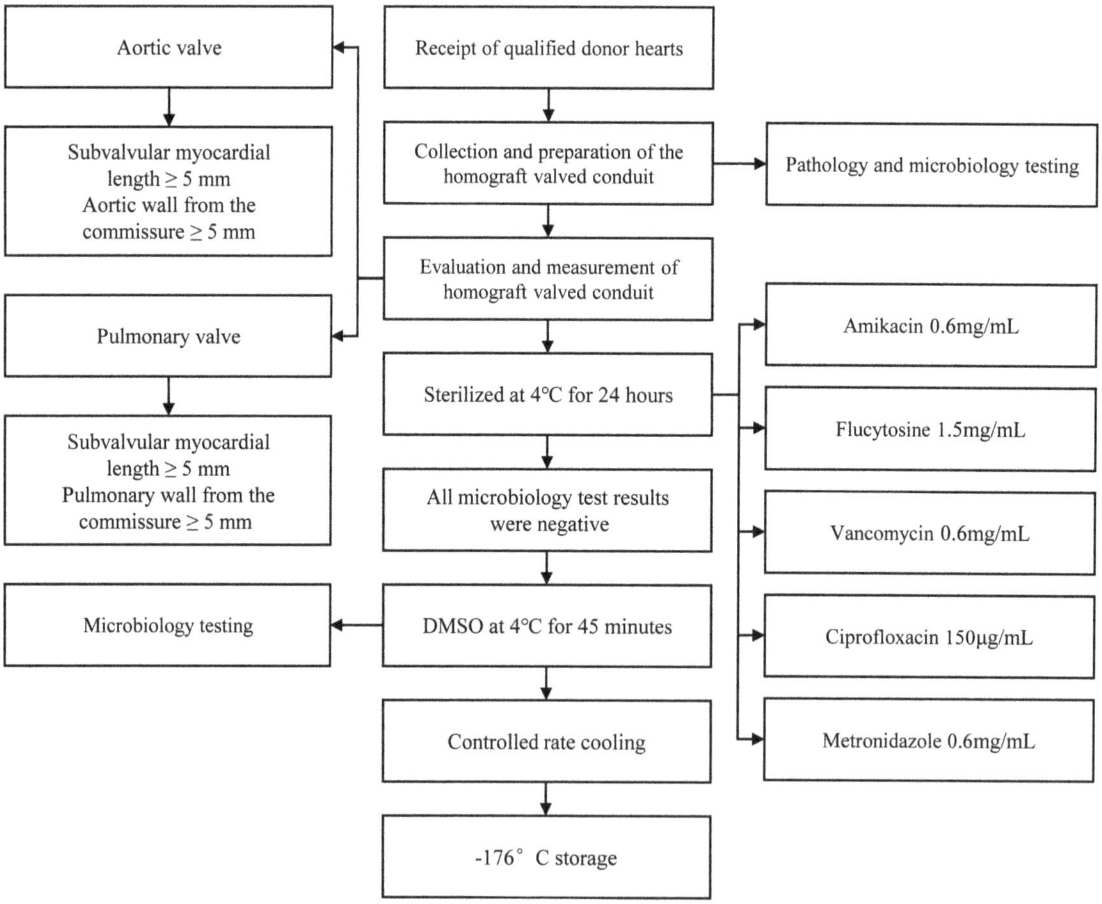


**FIGURE 2 |** Specific handling of homograft valved conduit from donor acquisition to deep cryogenic storage. It is important to note that (1) extra care must be taken throughout the processing and repeated microbiological tests must be performed to ensure complete sterile processing and storage, as any contamination could be catastrophic to the recipient; (2) the sterilization recipe in the figure is the protocol of Berlin, Germany, and different sterilization protocols may exist in other institutions, and there is no uniform protocol yet, sterilization to meet microbiological testing standards is a feasible solution.

surgery. Athletes are also suitable because of the absence of anticoagulation and extreme physiological and hemodynamic consequences (33). Chronic complications after the Ross surgery including aortic valve insufficiency, right ventricular outflow tract obstruction, autograft aortic valve dilatation, and homograft pulmonary valve stenosis. Potential long-term failure of both valves (aortic and pulmonary) has been considered the Achilles' heel of the Ross procedure (34). Reece et al. (35) reported a three-fold increase in mortality with the Ross procedure compared with conventional AVR. However, the Ross procedure is more complex than standard AVR. Some of the steps required in the Ross procedure—but not in conventional AVR—include dissection of the aortic root, mobilization of the coronary arteries, harvesting of the pulmonary autograft, proximal autograft anastomosis, coronary artery reimplantation, and pulmonary homograft implantation. Each of these steps increases the risk of the procedure (36). Importantly, the increase in mortality was mainly observed in low-volume centers. Therefore, for the complex surgery, these suboptimal outcomes are not surprising (37). In contrast, several experienced high-volume centers have demonstrated that the mortality rate for performing Ross surgery is similar to that of conventional AVR (31). This emphasizes the importance of the surgeon expertise and adequate surgical volume to achieve excellent outcomes in Ross surgery.

There are some findings in echocardiograms at follow-up after right ventricular outflow tract reconstruction. Pulmonary autograft dilatation is common in adults after Ross surgery, which may be the reason for reoperation. This dilatation develops over time and is usually accompanied by a dilatation of the native aorta. In a study of 71 patients with a median follow-up of 8.9 years (38), the proportion of patients with enlarged autografts and proximal ascending aorta was 13 and 16%, increasing to 33 and 44%, respectively. A retrospective multicenter international cohort study monitored the peak transvalvular gradients and regurgitation grade. Female sex, tricuspid natural aortic valve, and higher preoperative gradients were significantly associated with higher autograft gradients. Female sex was significantly associated with lower gradients of homografts, but also increased the likelihood of significant regurgitation. In contrast, the use of homografts rather than bioprosthesis and older donor age was associated with a lower likelihood of significant regurgitation (39). Another study showed that age and homograft diameter at the time of operation was also associated with valve function (40).

Homograft pulmonary artery is the best option for reconstructing RVOT, has good durability, and is not necessary for adults to undergo valve replacement again. Alexander et al. (41) evaluated 741 adult patients who underwent the Ross procedure. Right ventricular outflow tract reconstruction included 175 (23.6%) homograft pulmonary arteries, 561 (75.7%) porcine or bovine grafts, and 5 (0.7%) polytetrafluoroethylene duct reconstructions. The mean follow-up time was 5.8 ± 2.2 years. The 10-year survival rate was 90.7%, comparable to the age- and sex-matched general population. The 5- and 10-year graft reoperation rates were 94.1 and 88.3%, respectively. The probability of not reoperation at 10 years for allografts, pericardial xenografts treated with bicycloxide or glutaraldehyde, and porcine aortic root grafts was 100, 94.4, 82.7, and 80.6%, respectively. Jamie et al. (40) reported the implantation of 701 homograft pulmonary valved conduits in 604 patients. At 25 years of follow-up, the survival rate was 84 ± 4% and the valve replacement rate was 56 ± 6%. The probability of not requiring valve replacement after 15 years was 28 ± 14% in patients younger than 1 year, 59 ± 8% in patients 1–18 years, and 82 ± 5% in patients older than 18 years. Patients reported lower levels of physical strength and general health compared with the sex- and age-matched Dutch population, but significantly less physical pain. Pieter et al. (42) reported a total of 133 homograft valved conduits implanted in 126 patients with tetralogy of Fallot, including 126 pulmonary valved conduits and 7 aortic valved conduits. At long-term follow-up, the homograft conduits functioned satisfactorily in the pulmonary artery location. Clinical study data from Parth et al. (43) showed good mid-term durability of the homograft pulmonary valved conduits when used for right ventricular outflow tract reconstruction for the Ross procedure. At present, the main clinical application is pulmonary valved conduit, while aortic valved conduit is less. The reason may be that atherosclerosis and calcification are easy to involve the aorta, so the source of this kind of valved conduit is relatively limited. Anatomical, histological and biomechanical tests *in vitro* show that both conduits can meet the needs of clinical application (44, 45), but there is a lack of randomized controlled trials to compare the two conduits. The results of retrospective clinical studies are controversial. Some studies do not show significant differences (46, 47), while other studies have shown that the survival rate of pulmonary valved conduit is higher than that of aortic valved conduit (48, 49).

Homograft pulmonary arteries perform well in adult cardiac surgery, but have no significant clinical advantage in pediatric cardiac surgery due to limited sources and size. John et al. (50) reported 40 cases of Rastelli's procedure. There were 32 cases of right ventricular outflow tract obstruction and eight cases of atresia. Follow-up was obtained in all but one case with a mean of (8.6 ± 5.6) years. The right ventricular outflow tract was reconstructed using homograft conduits (25 cases), bovine jugular vein (BJV) (eight cases), valveless polyester conduits (five cases), and porcine valved conduits (two cases). The conduit-free replacement rates at 5, 10, 15, and 20 years were 86, 74, 63, and 59%, respectively. Multifactorial analysis showed that younger intraoperative age was a risk factor for conduit replacement ($p < 0.001$). Early performance of small BJVs may be more favorable than homografts. Andrew et al. (51) compared the results of initial placement of smaller diameter BJVs (12–14 mm) and homograft pulmonary valved conduits (10–15 mm) in children younger than 2.84 years (mean age 8.4 ± 8.5 months). Eighty-four children received BJV ($n = 51$) or homograft pulmonary artery ($n = 32$) conduit placement. Early and late mortality rates were similar (BJV 80%; pulmonary artery 88%; $P = 0.55$). None of the deaths were graft-related. The degree of functional recovery was significantly better in the BJV group at 5 and 10 years after surgery (85 and 90% in the bovine jugular group; 71 and 24% in the pulmonary artery group, respectively; $P < 0.05$). In the pulmonary valved conduit cohort, the probability of conduit failure at 5 and 10 years was higher (85 and 67% in the BJV group; 75 and 45% in the pulmonary artery group, respectively; $P = 0.06$). The probability of avoiding reoperation was significantly better in patients with implanted BJV conduits than in the pulmonary artery group (85 and 47%, respectively; $P < 0.001$). Although the early performance of BJVs may be superior to that of homografts, the incidence of infective endocarditis after right ventricle-pulmonary artery conduit implantation suggests that conduits of bovine origin are more susceptible to endocarditis (52, 53), which may be associated with suboptimal hemodynamics (54) and thrombus apposition at the basis of conduit valve sinus (55). Meanwhile, Mercer et al. (56) demonstrated that polytetrafluoroethylene conduits with mitral valves are ideal for right ventricular outflow tract reconstruction in children under 2 years of age. Their availability, low cost, and lack of potential sensitization make them an attractive alternative to homograft conduits. Based on the above problems, we can consider using bicuspidalized to reduce the size of valved conduit in infants (57, 58). A retrospective study analyzed 93 conduits which are <20 mm implanted for more than 23 years, including 40 standard pulmonary conduits, 12 standard aortic conduits, 17 bicuspidalized conduits and 24 xenografts (59). The average follow-up time was 7.6 ± 5.9 years. The percentage of patients without structural valve degeneration for 10 years was 47 ± 6%, including 68 ± 8% of pulmonary conduits, 42 ± 16% of bicuspidalized conduits, 31 ± 15% of aortic conduits, and 20 ± 9% of xenografts (log rank $P < 0.001$). Therefore, the appropriate size of pulmonary valved conduit is still the most durable choice for right ventricular outflow tract in children. However, when there is no available size, the mid-term follow-up results show that bicuspidalization can provide an effective alternative compared to xenograft. Other studies have also shown that bicuspidalized valved conduit seems to be a feasible option to solve the problem of limited supply of small size allografts, with acceptable survival rate and reoperation rate (60–62).

Homograft valved femoral veins with both smaller size and less risk of infection have shown good potential in pediatric cardiac surgery. The Yasui procedure is indicated for ventricular septal defects with interrupted aortic arch and associated subaortic stenosis. Manan et al. (63) described a modified Yasui procedure in which aortic reconstruction is simplified using a valveless homograft femoral vein connecting the pulmonary artery to the descending aorta. The homograft femoral vein is laterally anastomosed to the ascending aorta to complete the new aortic reconstruction. The anomalous opening from the left ventricle to the pulmonary artery is repaired with a patch, followed by restoration of continuity of the right ventricular outflow tract using a valved homograft femoral vein. This eponymous repair technique for aortic arch disruption and severe left ventricular outflow tract obstruction using a homograft valved femoral vein was first described in a case report by Yasui. According to Kumar et al. (64), the homograft femoral vein is safe as a conduit from the right ventricle to the pulmonary artery (RV-PA) in the Norwood procedure, and echocardiography shows good pulmonary artery growth and preserved ventricular function. Ofer et al. (65) reported that homograft valved femoral veins have similar short- and medium-term performance to homograft aorta or pulmonary artery in reconstructing the right ventricular outflow tract and are an attractive alternative to the smaller conduits used in neonates and infants. Histopathological evaluation showed that the valve maintained most of its function, and venous wall remodeling included only mild inflammation and calcification (66). A summary of clinical trials of homograft valved conduits over the past decade is shown in **Table 1**.

Homograft valved conduit has good biological properties and clinical results, but its durability is not very satisfactory (67). Age ≤9 years old is one of the main factors affecting durability (68, 69). Small size congduits (<19 mm) are also associated with decreased graft survival (70, 71). The type of conduits is considered to be one of the most important factors in long-term durability, for example, the survival rate of pulmonary conduit is higher than that of aortic conduit (70, 72). Baltivala et al. found that the graft survival rate of patients with a history of transplantation was worse than that of other patients (73). The relationship between bioactivity and durability of homograft valved conduit is still controversial. Fibroblasts living in the graft can reshape and reconstruct collagen structure and extracellular matrix, thus enhancing durability (74). However, these unevenly distributed fibroblasts may have phenotypic change and abnormal biological behavior due to immune response or environmental changes. Valve distortion or loss of elasticity caused by punctate or extensive hypertrophy, resulting in easy to rupture (75). The existence of endothelial cells reduces the possibility of thrombosis, but at the same time increases the antigenicity of the graft. The immune response is related to the early degeneration and dysfunction of the graft (76). Other factors related to the preservation process, including donor conditions, WIT, etc. will also affect the durability of valved conduits.

## XENOGRAFT VALVED CONDUITS AND OTHER POSSIBLE ALTERNATIVES

Xenograft valved conduit can prolong the time of freedom from operation and has a good long-term survival rate (77). The Medtronic Freestyle (Minneapolis, MN) is a glutaraldehyde fixed stentless porcine aortic valved conduit. Because of its standard availability from 19 to 29 mm in diameter and potential for longer valve function compared to homograft, several authors have published a series of studies on the Freestyle implantation, primarily for phase II RVOT reconstruction (78, 79). Early results performed satisfactorily with minimal pressure gradients and little or no valvular regurgitation. In the published reports, the follow-up time was <3 years. Long-term data for this conduit have not been published. Although the Freestyle performs well *in situ*, in most adult patients, the Freestyle is usually not long enough to reach the pulmonary artery from the free wall of the right ventricle, which can be addressed by anastomosing the Freestyle graft to the pulmonary artery and then connecting the Freestyle proximally to the right ventricle with an expanded large-bore polytetrafluoroethylene or braided polyester conduit. Ezelsoy et al. (80) reported 77 patients with ascending aortic aneurysm combined with aortic valve insufficiency who underwent total root replacement using Freestyle. The median follow-up was 11.2 years. The probability of freedom from aortic

**TABLE 1** | Clinical trial data of homograft valved conduits in the last decade.

| Period | Number of patients | Number of patients receiving homograft valved conduit | Mean age (years) | Mean follow-up time (years) | Surgical procedure | Avoiding of valve replacement rates | Conference |
|---|---|---|---|---|---|---|---|
| 1998–2014 | 741 | 175 | 47.4 | 5.8 | Ross | 10 years: 100% | (41) |
| 1986–2017 | 604 | 604 | 19.5 | 11.4 | RVOT reconstruction | 25 years: 76% | (40) |
| 1987–2009 | 126 | 126 | 27.8 | 8.1 | TOF | 10years: 83% | (42) |
| 1998–2016 | 30 | 15 | 3.3 | 6.8 | Ross | 5 years: 87% | (43) |
| 1988–2008 | 40 | 25 | 4 | 8.6 | Rastelli | 10 years: 74% | (50) |
| 1998–2009 | 84 | 32 | 0.7 | 5.9 | RVOT reconstruction | 10 years: 55% | (51) |
| 2004–2014 | 54 | 26 | 0.35 | 2.7 | RVOT reconstruction | End of follow-up: 48% | (56) |

valve reoperation at 5 and 10 years was 97.4 ± 1.2 and 93.4 ± 4.9%, respectively. Freestyle demonstrated favorable clinical outcomes in terms of survival and structural degeneration of the valve. Freestyle is a viable option for patients who are undergoing bioprosthetic aortic valve replacement and expect long-term durability. Mehdiani et al. found that the mid-term clinical and hemodynamic results of BioIntegral composite biological and stentless Freestyle conduits in patients undergoing full aortic root replacement are similar, but the simplified implantation technique of BioIntegral shortens the time of cardiopulmonary bypass and operation (81). The RVOT Elan conduit consists of a stentless valve (Vascutek Elan porcine stentless heart valve) sewn into a vascular graft (Vascutek Biblex Valsalva), showed good hemodynamic performance during an one-year short-term follow-up (82). Another type of diepoxy-treated porcine aortic conduit showed a higher risk of calcification during follow-up (83).

Despite satisfactory early outcome data for porcine-derived valved conduits, manufacturers are now focusing on another xenograft conduit for pediatric RVOT reconstruction, the valved BJV. Originally developed by VenPro (Irvine, CA) and currently owned and marketed by Medtronic, ConIntegra is a glutaraldehyde-fixed BJV conduit for RVOT reconstruction conduit option. Although several centers have reported that this conduit is more clinically beneficial than homograft (84, 85). However, these data are rather preliminary due to the published mean follow-up period of 12 months or less. At the same time, TakashiKido et al. have shown that early conduit dysfunction can still be caused by more than mild pulmonary hypertension and lower body weight during surgery of <3.0 kg (86). In addition, one center reported significant early fibrous epidermis formation at the distal anastomosis, as well as significant dilation and regurgitation of the conduit in the case of pulmonary hypertension or distal obstruction of the aforementioned distal anastomosis (87). Some studies have shown that BJV conduits have good medium-term durability, but have not been compared with the homograft or other types of conduits (88, 89). Therefore, this conduit will require further observation at longer follow-up times to clarify the differences in performance compared to equivalent sized cryopreserved homograft (43). Alessandro et al. (90) suggests that the 12 mm ConIntegra is an effective alternative to small homogaft valved conduit in the neonatal patient population.

In addition to xenograft valved conduits, synthetic material conduits or conduits containing part of synthetic materials are also gradually being developed for clinical use. The mid-term results of a multicenter clinical trial of simplified tricuspid polytetrafluoroethylene valved conduit show that it has an acceptable functional outcome and service life, freedom from conduit dysfunction was 58.5% at 5 years (91). KONECT RESILIA aortic valved conduit (Edwards Lifesciences, Irvine, Calif) is a noval type of bovine pericardial valved conduit, preassembled with the PERIMOUNT Magna Ease valve and RESILIA tissue with stent. This kind of conduit improves the anti-calcification performance and has dry storage capacity. *In vitro* experiments show that the simulation of sinuses of valsalva structure improves the hemodynamic performance (92).

Porcine small intestinal submucosa extracellular matrix (CorMatrix; CorMatrix Cardiovascular, Rosewell, GA) is a relatively novel tissue substitute. Preclinical experiments applied to pig models show that this biodegradable conduit cannot be reconstructed in a structured and anatomical in the arterial environment. Fibrosis, scarring, and calcification begin at 4 months, and chronic inflammation persists (93). There are also no satisfactory results in the sheep models (94). PTFE valved conduits show excellent hemodynamic performance in preclinical *in vitro* and *in vivo* experiments (95–97). The results of mid-term clinical trials showed less need for further intervention and severe valvular dysfunction (98, 99), especially in valvular regurgitation (100). And the failure incidence of this conduit is lower than that of autologous pericardial valved conduit operation (101). A clinical study involving 502 patients also showed satisfactory long-term results, freedom from conduit explantation was 89.0% at 10 years (102). Histopathological analysis showed that protein infiltration into the valve was thought to be the cause of future calcification and subsequent stenosis failure. Modification of polytetrafluoroethylene to prevent protein infiltration may help to improve the durability of the pipeline (103).

## ADVANTAGES AND DISADVANTAGES OF HOMOGRAFT AND XENOGRAFT VALVED CONDUIT

Although homograft valved conduit was used as early as the 1960s, its widespread use was limited by the lack of effective sterilization and preservation methods (1). Early methods of dealing with homograft valved conduit led to early calcification and progressive stenosis. Current storage methods, deep cryopreservation, delay the onset of these problems, but they still occur in the medium to long term (104). Despite this, compared with other types of valved conduits, homograft valved conduits still have the advantages of biological activity and tissue structural integrity, ease of use, good hemodynamics, intact valve function, long valve life, and no need for anticoagulation. The patency of the conduit after operation is excellent and basically conforms to the anatomical structure of the ventricular outflow tract, corrects cardiac malformations anatomically and hemodynamically, facilitates the recovery of cardiac function, and is less prone to heart failure. The homograft valved conduit has good resistance to infection, and complications caused by implantation such as bacterial endocarditis and hemolysis are rare, but its access is limited.

The BJV graft was introduced in 1999 as an option, which contains a trilobular venous valve (105). Preservation with glutaraldehyde solution under vacuum conditions preserves the flexibility of the valve (106). Because a variety of sizes are readily available, these tubes are more commonly used in clinical practice. The good valvular performance of BJV may be associated with an enlarged leaflet alignment area and reduced sensitivity to deformation of surrounding structures, including the right ventricle, aorta, and chest wall. BJV is associated with distal anastomotic stenosis and a higher incidence of endocarditis compared with homograft (107–112). The Hancock, a stented polyester conduit with porcine valve (113), can also be used in adult cardiac surgery. However, in pediatric applications, calcification as well as poor intraoperative properties due to the polyester conduit, make the Hancock not a common choice.

Current homograft and xenograft conduits lack any capacity for additional growth. As children grow, the fixed size of the conduit means that there is a progressive size mismatch between the patient and the conduit, which necessitates future reoperation. Typically, a new conduit is required approximately 4–5 years after the initial conduit placement in an infant or young child (110). Critically, studies reporting the time of reoperation often combine patients with very different anatomic features, thereby confounding the analysis of outcomes. For example, placement of an RV-PA conduit in pulmonary atresia involves a non-*in situ* and tortuous pathway that allows blood to flow anteriorly from the right ventricle, across the surface of the heart, and then backward to the pulmonary artery. In contrast, placement of the RV-PA conduit in Ross procedure is essentially *in situ* placement of the implant. This may have less turbulence and energy loss than in patients with pulmonary artery atresia, factors that may affect the durability of the conduit.

In addition to body growth, a variety of other problems can lead to conduit failure. These include distal anastomotic stenosis, sternal compression, aneurysm formation at the proximal anastomotic enlargement site, valve stenosis (114), and donor-specific and non-specific immune responses. A study has shown that both homograft and xenograft can trigger an immune response in the recipient, leading to calcification, endothelial thickening or vascular membrane formation, stenosis, and deterioration of valve function (115).

## POSSIBLE FUTURE DIRECTIONS FOR IMPROVEMENT

Cryopreserved homograft valved conduit has low clotting activity, good hemodynamic properties, and high resistance to infection, but cannot grow and develop in the recipient. Because cryopreserved homograft valved conduits carry donor cells that express relevant antigens, these cells can cause adverse host immune responses and lead to calcification, which in turn may require reoperation in young patients who receive a homograft valved conduit. Therefore, removal of the cellular component of the homograft valved conduit prior to implantation may reduce the immune response and calcification (116). In addition, removal of donor cells may encourage the proliferation of the cells with the ability to repair and remodel in receptor, thereby overcoming the limitations of degeneration of the homograft valved conduit over time and creating a valve with growth potential in younger patients, thus eliminating the need for reoperation. Decellularized valved conduits demonstrate almost complete removal of cells and cellular components by histological and immunocytochemical analysis without corresponding changes in biomechanics *in vitro* (117). Previous studies have shown that the decellularization process does not affect the *in vivo* performance of homograft valved conduit, and good clinical performance in the short to medium term has been reported for decellularized pulmonary valves, with similar (118–122) or better (123–125) outcomes than conventional deep cryopreserved homograft in adults and children at a mean follow-up of 4 years. However, longer-term data are needed to determine whether they can reduce or eliminate the need for reoperation (126).

SynerGraft (CryoLife Inc., Kennesaw, GA) decellularized pulmonary allograft (SGDPA) is an alternative to standard cryopreserved allograft (SCA) Ross aortic valve replacement. John et al. (127) reported 29 patients underwent SGDPA and 34 underwent SCA during Ross aortic valve replacement. Early clinical and hemodynamic outcomes were favorable but not significantly different from SCA. There were no early or late deaths or major pathologic events during a mean follow-up of 4.9 $\pm$ 2.7 years. None of the patients required reoperation. No deterioration in conduit or valve function was seen in the SGDPA group. Several patients with SCA developed mild regurgitation, and one patient developed moderate regurgitation. Thus, the SynerGraft technique may provide a more durable option for patients requiring right ventricular outflow tract reconstruction. Mark et al. (124) also suggests that the medium-term performance of decellularized cryopreserved homograft may be superior to that of standard cryopreserved homograft. Decellularized aortic homograft can withstand the stresses of the body circulation, provide a good effective orifice area, and may be an alternative graft for aortic valve replacement in younger patients. Enlarged aortic root replacement using decellularized aortic homograft is a further option for aortic valve disease associated with dilatation of the ascending aorta, as it avoids the use of any prosthetic material. Igor et al. (128) reported the replacement of the dilated ascending aorta with decellularized aortic homograft in 18 patients with enlarged aortic root replacement. None of the grafts had any degree of dilatation observed during the relatively short follow-up period (mean 2.0 ± 1.8 years, maximum 7.6 years). Intraoperative and postoperative histological analysis of the grafts showed no calcification and revealed extensive recellularization and no inflammation.

Reconstruction of the right ventricular outflow tract in children with decellularized homograft has a low incidence of structural deterioration of the valve and conduit failure. Francisco et al. (129) reported 59 patients who underwent decellularized allograft RVOT reconstruction. The most common procedure was the Ross procedure (34%) and the mean follow-up was 5.4 years. Structural valve deterioration occurred in 13 patients, including five with stenosis and eight with valvular insufficiency. The incidence of no structural valve deterioration from any cause 8 years after surgery was 64.9%. During the follow-up period, CT scans showed no or minimal calcification of the conduit. Grauss et al. (130) believes that decellularization techniques cause much less damage to the valve than recipient's immune response. *In vitro* removal of live cells from cryopreserved homograft may reduce the probability of graft failure. Implantation of autologous or major histocompatibility complex-matched donor endothelial cells would be necessary to reduce damage due to lack of blood-tissue barrier. Willem et al. (131) found that encapsulation of decellularized homograft with FN/SDF-1α prevented cryopreserved heart valve-mediated immune responses, conduit calcification and vascular scar formation, and stimulated reendothelialization.

Decellularization as a promising improvement method not only improves the performance of homografts, but decellularized xenografts also perform well in clinical practice. Decellularized porcine pulmonary artery valved conduits have excellent potential as a substitute for right ventricular outflow tract reconstruction. Ji Luo et al. (132) developed a method for decellularization of porcine pulmonary arterial with minimal effects on biomechanical, hydrodynamic, and leaflet dynamics properties, and immunohistochemical labeling and antibody uptake assays confirmed the lack of α-gal epitopes in decellularized porcine pulmonary artery valve and conduit. *In vitro* biocompatibility studies demonstrated no cytotoxicity in decellularized pulmonary artery valve and conduit. Decellularized bovine pericardial valves also exhibited potent anti-calcification effects in a sheep circulating model (133). However, study by Higuita et al. has shown that the commonly used SDS acellular method may change or eliminate ECM protein, and will lead to the destruction of valve function, while the use of antigen removal tissue treatment can retain the subtle ECM structure and composition of natural tissue, thus preserving the function of natural valve (134). Therefore, the best acellular method needs to be further explored in the field of tissue engineering. **Table 2** compares in detail the advantages and disadvantages of different types of valved conduit.

## PROSPECT

Tissue engineering is an emerging technology with the potential to create implants that can provide structural and mechanical support and are biologically functional. Ideally, grafts with good biocompatibility, the ability to grow in proportion to host tissue growth, and minimal clinical complications will be produced, thus eliminating the need for further surgery. Considering the specific and highly variable cardiac anatomy of patients with congenital heart disease, significant research challenges remain in the design and fabrication of well-durable valved conduits.

Artificial conduit biomaterials need to mimic the mechanical properties of natural arteries and their biomechanical behavior such as hemodynamics while possessing good biocompatibility to avoid clinical complications. In addition, the human arterial structure consists of cytoskeletal proteins such as collagen and elastin deposited in a directional manner, which ensures that natural vessels exhibit complex anisotropic mechanical behavior (135). For example, arterial walls exhibit non-linear elastic properties under stress and hysteresis behavior in response to changes in circulating pressure (136). The key point is that none of the currently available tissue engineering valved conduits has the same material properties as natural tissues, especially anisotropic properties. Computational fluid dynamics can be used to optimize the geometric design of valved conduits and tissue engineering materials. Therefore, fluid mechanics and structural calculation models will continue to play an important role in optimizing the design and manufacturing of patient-specific conduit.

With the development of manufacturing technology, the use of tissue engineering technology to construct artificial valved conduits is under continuous exploration. Traditional 3D porous biodegradable scaffolds planted with cells usually lack the ability of cell differentiation and function, and cannot fully reconstruct the characteristics of natural tissues (137). The advent of technologies such as electrospinning and 3D bioprinting has led to the creation of more complex designs that mimic valved conduit (138). Poly(lactic acid-caprolactone) [P(LA-CL)]-reinforced electrospinning polyglycolic acid (PGA) mesh has been used as a promising composite scaffold and were able to survive in patients, but some developed conduit stenosis, which may be related to the acidic environment caused by the degradation product lactic acid (139). Electrospinning nanofiber grafts are made from composite materials such as polyethylene

**TABLE 2 |** Advantages and disadvantages of the three types of valved conduits in current clinical application.

| Type of valved conduit | Advantages | Disadvantages |
|---|---|---|
| Homograft valved conduit | Good hemodynamic and valvular performance, better medium- to long-term clinical outcomes than xenograft valved conduits, relatively low reoperate rates | Restricted source especially in small sizes, presence of some antigenicity that may lead to rejection and early calcification of the conduit especially in pediatric patients, no potential for *in vivo* growth |
| Xenograft valved conduit | The 12–22 mm size with unlimited sources provides a wide range of applications in pediatric patients | Risk of thrombosis, higher risk of postoperative infection than homograft valved conduit, no potential for *in vivo* growth |
| SynerGraft decellularized pulmonary allograft | Minimizing rejection and calcification and improving long-term durability, *in vivo* growth potential, current clinical results show that the function and longevity of the conduit is no less than homograft valved conduit and with more significant advantages in pediatric patients | The available evidence is not sufficient to demonstrate the advantages of the long-term effects of decellularized valved conduit and further long-term follow-up is needed |

glycol dimethacrylate, PLA, PCL, and polyvinyl alcohol to mimic the structural and mechanical properties of natural valves, but electrospinning scaffolds are less efficient to fabricate and have limited ability to create complex 3D structures (140). The Xeltis graft is a pulmonary artery valved conduit made from a range of synthetic materials, including a wall made of polycaprolactone and a valve made of polycarbonate, with modifiable mechanical properties and biodegradability, and has demonstrated good and durable hemodynamic performance in preclinical studies with no stenosis or obstruction or severe regurgitation 2 years after implantation (141). Compared with the histology of Hancock conduit, significant calcification was rarely observed in Xeltis, while Hancock formed more neointimal thickness with the calcification of aortic root (142). 3D bioprinted trilobular valved conduits based on hyaluronic acid methacrylate and gelatin methacrylate have been successfully implanted in mouse models and have shown high cell survival and remodeling potential (143). But 3D printing geometrically complex structures with similar biological behavior to natural tissues remains a great challenge, and ideal scaffold materials and conduit fabrication methods remain an area for continued effort and innovation. Current research advances in tissue engineering scaffolds are mostly limited to preclinical trials (144).

The clinical use of homograft valved conduits is widespread with good long-term outcomes. Although there are still some limitations, with the development of cardiac surgery and other disciplines, research is continuously exploring the best ways to improve the efficacy of homograft valved conduit operation by improving preservation methods, using low-dose immunosuppressive agents, and matching ABO and HLA antigens to mitigate post-transplant immune reactions to extend the life of homograft valved conduits. The development of genetic engineering technology is expected to induce immune tolerance and mitigate immune response through molecular biology techniques. It is also expected that the construction of recipient cellularized tissue-engineered conduit by implanting recipient-derived endothelial cells on decellularized valved conduits or degradable synthetic materials will be an ideal biologic valved conduits substitution for heart disease treatment.

## AUTHOR CONTRIBUTIONS

YH wrote the text, performed the literature search, and review under guidance from YC. JS reviewed the text. YC and JS revising the manuscript. All authors contributed to the article and approved the submitted version.

## REFERENCES

1. Ross DN, Somerville J. Correction of pulmonary atresia with a homograft aortic valve. *Lancet.* (1966) 2:1446–7. doi: 10.1016/s0140-6736(66)90600-3
2. Rastelli GC, McGoon DC, Wallace RB. Anatomic correction of transposition of the great arteries with ventricular septal defect and subpulmonary stenosis. *J Thorac Cardiovasc Surg.* (1969) 58:545–52.
3. Merin G, McGoon DC. Reoperation after insertion of aortic homograft as a right ventricular outflow tract. *Ann Thorac Surg.* (1973) 16:122–6. doi: 10.1016/s0003-4975(10)65826-2
4. Alexiou C, Keeton BR, Salmon AP, Monro JL. Repair of truncus arteriosus in early infancy with antibiotic sterilized aortic homografts. *Ann Thorac Surg.* (2001) 71(5 Suppl):S371–4. doi: 10.1016/s0003-4975(01)02547-4
5. Shabbo FP, Wain WH, Ross DN. Right ventricular outflow reconstruction with aortic homograft conduit: analysis of the long-term results. *Thorac Cardiovasc Surg.* (1980) 28:21–5. doi: 10.1055/s-2007-1022045
6. Ross D, Yacoub MH. Homograft replacement of the aortic valve. A critical review. *Prog Cardiovasc Dis.* (1969) 11:275–93. doi: 10.1016/0033-0620(69)90054-1
7. Barratt-Boyes BG, Roche AH, Whitlock RM. Six year review of the results of freehand aortic valve replacement using an antibiotic sterilized homograft valve. *Circulation.* (1977) 55:353–61. doi: 10.1161/01.cir.55.2.353
8. O'Brien MF, Stafford G, Gardner M, Pohlner P, McGiffin D, Johnston N, et al. The viable cryopreserved allograft aortic valve. *J Card Surg.* (1987) 2(1 Suppl):153–67. doi: 10.1111/jocs.1987.2.1s.153
9. Kneebone JM, Lupinetti FM. Procollagen synthesis by fresh and cryopreserved rat pulmonary valve grafts. *J Thorac Cardiovasc Surg.* (2000) 120:596–603. doi: 10.1067/mtc.2000.107681
10. Lupinetti FM, Tsai TT, Kneebone JM, Bove EL. Effect of cryopreservation on the presence of endothelial cells on human valve allografts. *J Thorac Cardiovasc Surg.* (1993) 106:912–7. doi: 10.1016/S0022-5223(19)34047-4
11. Rendal Vázquez ME, Román TD, Cuesta MG, Botta CZ, Ibáñez JS, Díaz SP, et al. Viability and histologic structure of

porcine valves after cryopreservation. *Ann Thorac Surg.* (2004) 77:186–90. doi: 10.1016/s0003-4975(03)01491-7
12. Sadowski J, Kapelak B, Bartus K, Podolec P, Rudzinski P, Myrdko T, et al. Reoperation after fresh homograft replacement: 23 years' experience with 655 patients. *Eur J Cardiothorac Surg.* (2003) 23:996–1000; discussion 1000-1. doi: 10.1016/s1010-7940(03)00109-x
13. Verghese S, Padmaja P, Sindhu B, Elizabeth SJ, Lesley N, Cherian KM. Homograft valve bank: our experience in valve banking. *Indian Heart J.* (2004) 56:299–306.
14. Gall KL, Smith SE, Willmette CA, O'Brien MF. Allograft heart valve viability and valve-processing variables. *Ann Thorac Surg.* (1998) 65:1032-8. doi: 10.1016/s0003-4975(98)00085-x
15. Suh H, Lee JE, Park JC, Han DW, Yoon CS, Park YH, et al. Viability and enzymatic activity of cryopreserved porcine heart valve. *Yonsei Med J.* (1999) 40:184–90. doi: 10.3349/ymj.1999.40.2.184
16. Burkert J, Krs O, Vojácek J, Mokrácek A, Slízová D, Hlubocký J, et al. Cryopreserved semilunar heart valve allografts: leaflet surface damage in scanning electron microscopy. *Zentralbl Chir.* (2008) 133:367-73. doi: 10.1055/s-2008-1076872
17. Stemper BD, Yoganandan N, Stineman MR, Gennarelli TA, Baisden JL, Pintar FA. Mechanics of fresh, refrigerated, and frozen arterial tissue. *J Surg Res.* (2007) 139:236–42. doi: 10.1016/j.jss.2006.09.001
18. Jashari R, Tabaku M, Van Hoeck B, Cochéz C, Callant M, Vanderkelen A. Decontamination of heart valve and arterial allografts in the European Homograft Bank (EHB): comparison of two different antibiotic cocktails in low temperature conditions. *Cell Tissue Bank.* (2007) 8:247–55. doi: 10.1007/s10561-007-9040-5
19. Fan YD, Van Hoeck B, Holovska V, Jashari R. Evaluation of decontamination process of heart valve and artery tissues in European Homograft Bank (EHB): a retrospective study of 1,055 cases. *Cell Tissue Bank.* (2012) 13:297-304. doi: 10.1007/s10561-011-9255-3
20. Brockbank KG, Carpenter JF, Dawson PE. Effects of storage temperature on viable bioprosthetic heart valves. *Cryobiology.* (1992) 29:537–42. doi: 10.1016/0011-2240(92)90058-a
21. Xu Y, Hua TC, Sun DW, Zhou GY, Xu F. Effects of freezing rates and dimethyl sulfoxide concentrations on thermal expansion of rabbit aorta during freezing phase change as measured by thermo mechanical analysis. *J Biomech.* (2007) 40:3201–6. doi: 10.1016/j.jbiomech.2007.04.010
22. Wusteman M, Rauen U, Simmonds J, Hunds N, Pegg DE. Reduction of cryoprotectant toxicity in cells in suspension by use of a sodium-free vehicle solution. *Cryobiology.* (2008) 56:72–9. doi: 10.1016/j.cryobiol.2007.10.178
23. Mazur P, Leibo SP, Chu EH. A two-factor hypothesis of freezing injury. Evidence from Chinese hamster tissue-culture cells. *Exp Cell Res.* (1972) 71:345–55. doi: 10.1016/0014-4827(72)90303-5
24. van der Kamp AW, Visser WJ, van Dongen JM, Nauta J, Galjaard H. Preservation of aortic heart valves with maintenance of cell viability. *J Surg Res.* (1981) 30:47–56. doi: 10.1016/0022-4804(81)90069-x
25. Lisy M, Kalender G, Schenke-Layland K, Brockbank KG, Biermann A, Stock UA. Allograft heart valves: current aspects and future applications. *Biopreserv Biobank.* (2017) 15:148–57. doi: 10.1089/bio.2016.0070
26. Austyn JM, Larsen CP. Migration patterns of dendritic leukocytes. Implications for transplantation. *Transplantation.* (1990) 49:1–7. doi: 10.1097/00007890-199001000-00001
27. Oei FB, Stegmann AP, van der Ham F, Zondervan PE, Vaessen LM, Baan CC, et al. The presence of immune stimulatory cells in fresh and cryopreserved donor aortic and pulmonary valve allografts. *J Heart Valve Dis.* (2002) 11:315–24; discussion 25.
28. Mitchell RN, Jonas RA, Schoen FJ. Structure-function correlations in cryopreserved allograft cardiac valves. *Ann Thorac Surg.* (1995) 60(2 Suppl):S108–12; discussion S13. doi: 10.1016/0003-4975(95)00258-m
29. Delmo Walter EM, de By TMMH, Meyer R, Hetzer R. The future of heart valve banking and of homografts: perspective from the Deutsches Herzzentrum Berlin. *HSR Proc Intensive Care Cardiovasc Anesth.* (2012) 4:97–108.
30. Forbess JM. Conduit selection for right ventricular outflow tract reconstruction: contemporary options and outcomes. *Semin Thorac Cardiovasc Surg Pediatr Card Surg Annu.* (2004) 7:115–24. doi: 10.1053/j.pcsu.2004.02.004
31. Sievers HH, Stierle U, Charitos EI, Takkenberg JJ, Horer J, Lange R, et al. A multicentre evaluation of the autograft procedure for young patients undergoing aortic valve replacement: update on the German Ross Registrydagger. *Eur J Cardiothorac Surg.* (2016) 49:212-8. doi: 10.1093/ejcts/ezv001
32. Berdajs DA, Muradbegovic M, Haselbach D, Kofmehl R, Steurer J, Ferrari E, et al. Ross procedure: is the root replacement technique superior to the sub-coronary implantation technique? Long-term results. *Eur J Cardiothorac Surg.* (2014) 46:944–51. doi: 10.1093/ejcts/ezu176
33. Oury JH. Clinical aspects of the Ross procedure: indications and contraindications. *Semin Thorac Cardiovasc Surg.* (1996) 8:328–35.
34. Klieverik LM, Takkenberg JJ, Bekkers JA, Roos-Hesselink JW, Witsenburg M, Bogers AJ. The Ross operation: a Trojan horse? *Eur Heart J.* (2007) 28:1993–2000. doi: 10.1093/eurheartj/ehl550
35. Reece TB, Welke KF, O'Brien S, Grau-Sepulveda MV, Grover FL, Gammie JS. Rethinking the Ross procedure in adults. *Ann Thorac Surg.* (2014) 97:175–81. doi: 10.1016/j.athoracsur.2013.07.036
36. Mazine A, El-Hamamsy I, Verma S, Peterson MD, Bonow RO, Yacoub MH, et al. Ross procedure in adults for cardiologists and cardiac surgeons: JACC state-of-the-art review. *J Am Coll Cardiol.* (2018) 72:2761-77. doi: 10.1016/j.jacc.2018.08.2200
37. Hughes GC, Zhao Y, Rankin JS, Scarborough JE, O'Brien S, Bavaria JE, et al. Effects of institutional volumes on operative outcomes for aortic root replacement in North America. *J Thorac Cardiovasc Surg.* (2013) 145:166-70. doi: 10.1016/j.jtcvs.2011.10.094
38. Aljassim O, Svensson G, Perrotta S, Jeppsson A, Bech-Hanssen O. Dilatation of the pulmonary autograft and native aorta after the Ross procedure: a comprehensive echocardiographic study. *J Thorac Cardiovasc Surg.* (2011) 142:634.e1–40.e1. doi: 10.1016/j.jtcvs.2010.11.025
39. Romeo JLR, Papageorgiou G, da Costa FFD, Sievers HH, Bogers A, El-Hamamsy I, et al. Long-term clinical and echocardiographic outcomes in young and middle-aged adults undergoing the Ross procedure. *JAMA Cardiol.* (2021) 6:539–48. doi: 10.1001/jamacardio.2020.7434
40. Romeo JLR, Mokhles MM, van de Woestijne P, de Jong P, van den Bosch A, van Beynum IM, et al. Long-term clinical outcome and echocardiographic function of homografts in the right ventricular outflow tractdagger. *Eur J Card Thorac Surg.* (2019) 55:518–26. doi: 10.1093/ejcts/ezy265
41. Karaskov A, Sharifulin R, Zheleznev S, Demin I, Lenko E, Bogachev-Prokophiev A. Results of the Ross procedure in adults: a single-centre experience of 741 operations. *Eur J Card Thorac Surg.* (2016) 49:e97-104. doi: 10.1093/ejcts/ezw047
42. van de Woestijne PC, Mokhles MM, de Jong PL, Witsenburg M, Takkenberg JJM, Bogers AJJC. Right ventricular outflow tract reconstruction with an allograft conduit in patients after tetralogy of Fallot correction: long-term follow-up. *Ann Thorac Surg.* (2011) 92:161–6. doi: 10.1016/j.athoracsur.2011.02.036
43. Patel PM, Herrmann JL, Rodefeld MD, Turrentine MW, Brown JW. Bovine jugular vein conduit versus pulmonary homograft in the Ross operation. *Cardiol Young.* (2020) 30:323–7. doi: 10.1017/S1047951119003007
44. Gorczynski A, Trenkner M, Anisimowicz L, Gutkowski R, Drapella A, Kwiatkowska E, et al. Biomechanics of the pulmonary autograft valve in the aortic position. *Thorax.* (1982) 37:535–9. doi: 10.1136/thx.37.7.535
45. Vesely I, Casarotto DC, Gerosa G. Mechanics of cryopreserved aortic and pulmonary homografts. *J Heart Valve Dis.* (2000) 9:27–37.
46. Junnil P, Cheanvechai C, Namchaisiri J, Saprungruang A, Thitivaraporn P, Chomvilailuk M, et al. Long-term course after pediatric right ventricular outflow tract reconstruction. *Asian Cardiovasc Thorac Ann.* (2021) 29:483-9. doi: 10.1177/0218492320983449
47. Nasirov T, Maeda K, Reinhartz O. Aortic or pulmonary valved homograft right ventricle to pulmonary artery conduit in the Norwood procedure. *World J Pediatr Congenit Heart Surg.* (2019) 10:499–501. doi: 10.1177/2150135119842865
48. Kalfa D, Feier H, Loundou A, Fraisse A, Mace L, Metras D, et al. Cryopreserved homograft in the Ross procedure: outcomes and prognostic factors. *J Heart Valve Dis.* (2011) 20:571–81.
49. Mokhles MM, van de Woestijne PC, de Jong PL, Witsenburg M, Roos-Hesselink JW, Takkenberg JJ, et al. Clinical outcome and health-related quality of life after right-ventricular-outflow-tract reconstruction

with an allograft conduit. *Eur J Card Thorac Surg.* (2011) 40:571–8. doi: 10.1016/j.ejcts.2010.10.023
50. Brown JW, Ruzmetov M, Huynh D, Rodefeld MD, Turrentine MW, Fiore AC. Rastelli operation for transposition of the great arteries with ventricular septal defect and pulmonary stenosis. *Ann Thorac Surg.* (2011) 91:188–93; discussion 93–4. doi: 10.1016/j.athoracsur.2010.07.057
51. Fiore AC, Ruzmetov M, Huynh D, Hanley S, Rodefeld MD, Turrentine MW, et al. Comparison of bovine jugular vein with pulmonary homograft conduits in children less than 2 years of age. *Eur J Card Thorac Surg.* (2010) 38:318–25. doi: 10.1016/j.ejcts.2010.01.063
52. Gröning M, Tahri NB, Søndergaard L, Helvind M, Ersbøll MK, Ørbæk Andersen H. Infective endocarditis in right ventricular outflow tract conduits: a register-based comparison of homografts, contegra grafts and melody transcatheter valves. *Eur J Card Thorac Surg.* (2019) 56:87–93. doi: 10.1093/ejcts/ezy478
53. Beckerman Z, De Leon LE, Zea-Vera R, Mery CM, Fraser CD, Jr. High incidence of late infective endocarditis in bovine jugular vein valved conduits. *J Thorac Cardiovasc Surg.* (2018) 156:728e2–34.e2. doi: 10.1016/j.jtcvs.2018.03.156
54. Chen H, Shi G, Qiu L, Wang S, Chen H, Xu Z. Outcomes of prosthetic valved conduits for right ventricular outflow tract reconstruction. *Pediatr Cardiol.* (2019) 40:848–56. doi: 10.1007/s00246-019-02081-8
55. Jewgenow P, Schneider H, Bokenkamp R, Horer J, Cleuziou J, Foth R, et al. Subclinical thrombus formation in bioprosthetic pulmonary valve conduits. *Int J Cardiol.* (2019) 281:113–8. doi: 10.1016/j.ijcard.2019.01.095
56. Mercer CW, West SC, Sharma MS, Yoshida M, Morell VO. Polytetrafluoroethylene conduits versus homografts for right ventricular outflow tract reconstruction in infants and young children: an institutional experience. *J Thorac Cardiovasc Surg.* (2018) 155:2082.e1–91.e1. doi: 10.1016/j.jtcvs.2017.11.107
57. Michler RE, Chen JM, Quaegebeur JM. Novel technique for extending the use of allografts in cardiac operations. *Ann Thorac Surg.* (1994) 57:83–7. doi: 10.1016/0003-4975(94)90369-7
58. Santini F, Mazzucco A. Bicuspid homograft reconstruction of the right ventricular outflow tract in infants. *Ann Thorac Surg.* (1995) 60(6 Suppl):S624–5. doi: 10.1016/0003-4975(96)81282-3
59. Francois K, De Groote K, Vandekerckhove K, De Wilde H, De Wolf D, Bove T. Small-sized conduits in the right ventricular outflow tract in young children: bicuspidalized homografts are a good alternative to standard conduits. *Eur J Card Thorac Surg.* (2018) 53:409–15. doi: 10.1093/ejcts/ezx354
60. Bramer S, Mokhles MM, Takkenberg JJ, Bogers AJ. Long-term outcome of right ventricular outflow tract reconstruction with bicuspidalized homografts. *Eur J Card Thorac Surg.* (2011) 40:1392–5. doi: 10.1016/j.ejcts.2011.02.066
61. Romeo JLR, Papageorgiou G, van de Woestijne PC, Takkenberg JJM, Westenberg LEH, van Beynum I, et al. Downsized cryopreserved and standard-sized allografts for right ventricular outflow tract reconstruction in children: long-term single-institutional experience. *Interact Cardiovasc Thorac Surg.* (2018) 27:257–63. doi: 10.1093/icvts/ivy057
62. Perri G, Polito A, Gandolfo F, Albanese SB, Carotti A. Outcome of standard and bicuspidalized cryopreserved homografts for primary right ventricular outflow tract reconstruction. *J Heart Valve Dis.* (2015) 24:83–8.
63. Desai MH, Sinha P, Jonas RA, Ramakrishnan K. Modified Yasui operation using cryopreserved femoral vein homograft. *Ann Thorac Surg.* (2020) 110:e147–9. doi: 10.1016/j.athoracsur.2020.02.031
64. Kumar TKS, Zurakowski D, Briceno-Medina M, Shah A, Sathanandam S, Allen J, et al. Experience of a single institution with femoral vein homograft as right ventricle to pulmonary artery conduit in stage 1 Norwood operation. *J Thorac Cardiovasc Surg.* (2019) 158:853.e1–62.e1. doi: 10.1016/j.jtcvs.2019.03.123
65. Schiller O, Sinha P, Zurakowski D, Jonas RA. Reconstruction of right ventricular outflow tract in neonates and infants using valved cryopreserved femoral vein homografts. *J Thorac Cardiovasc Surg.* (2014) 147:874–9. doi: 10.1016/j.jtcvs.2013.11.006
66. Carreon CK, Benini A, Baird C, Hoganson D, Borisuk M, Emani S, et al. Pathology of valved venous homografts used as right ventricle-to-pulmonary artery conduits in congenital heart disease surgery. *J Thorac Cardiovasc Surg.* (2019) 157:342.e3–50.e3. doi: 10.1016/j.jtcvs.2018.08.102
67. Heidary Rouchi A, Radmehr H, Tavakoli SA, Jafarzadeh Kashi TS, Mahdavi-Mazdeh M. Iranian homograft heart valves: assessment of durability and late outcome. *Cell Tissue Bank.* (2016) 17:603–10. doi: 10.1007/s10561-016-9573-6
68. Etnel JR, Elmont LC, Ertekin E, Mokhles MM, Heuvelman HJ, Roos-Hesselink JW, et al. Outcome after aortic valve replacement in children: a systematic review and meta-analysis. *J Thorac Cardiovasc Surg.* (2016) 151:143–52.e1–3. doi: 10.1016/j.jtcvs.2015.09.083
69. Fukushima S, Tesar PJ, Pearse B, Jalali H, Sparks L, Fraser JF, et al. Long-term clinical outcomes after aortic valve replacement using cryopreserved aortic allograft. *J Thorac Cardiovasc Surg.* (2014) 148:65.e2–72.e2. doi: 10.1016/j.jtcvs.2013.07.038
70. Poynter JA, Eghtesady P, McCrindle BW, Walters HL III, Kirshbom PM, Blackstone EH, et al. Association of pulmonary conduit type and size with durability in infants and young children. *Ann Thorac Surg.* (2013) 96:1695–701; discussion 701–2. doi: 10.1016/j.athoracsur.2013.05.074
71. Buber J, Assenza GE, Huang A, Valente AM, Emani SM, Gauvreau K, et al. Durability of large diameter right ventricular outflow tract conduits in adults with congenital heart disease. *Int J Cardiol.* (2014) 175:455–63. doi: 10.1016/j.ijcard.2014.06.023
72. David TE, David C, Woo A, Manlhiot C. The Ross procedure: outcomes at 20 years. *J Thorac Cardiovasc Surg.* (2014) 147:85–93. doi: 10.1016/j.jtcvs.2013.08.007
73. Batlivala SP, Emani S, Mayer JE, McElhinney DB. Pulmonary valve replacement function in adolescents: a comparison of bioprosthetic valves and homograft conduits. *Ann Thorac Surg.* (2012) 93:2007–16. doi: 10.1016/j.athoracsur.2012.02.039
74. McNally RT, Brockbank KG. Issues surrounding the preservation of viable allograft heart valves. *J Med Eng Technol.* (1992) 16:34–8. doi: 10.3109/03091909209021955
75. Armiger LC. Postimplantation leaflet cellularity of valve allografts: are donor cells beneficial or detrimental? *Ann Thorac Surg.* (1998) 66(6 Suppl):S233–5. doi: 10.1016/s0003-4975(98)00984-9
76. Yankah AC, Alexi-Meskhishvili V, Weng Y, Schorn K, Lange PE, Hetzer R. Accelerated degeneration of allografts in the first two years of life. *Ann Thorac Surg.* (1995) 60(2 Suppl):S71–6; discussion 576–7. doi: 10.1016/0003-4975(95)00289-w
77. Alfieris GM, Swartz MF, Lehoux J, Bove EL. Long-term survival and freedom from reoperation after placement of a pulmonary xenograft valved conduit. *Ann Thorac Surg.* (2016) 102:602–7. doi: 10.1016/j.athoracsur.2016.02.045
78. Kanter KR, Fyfe DA, Mahle WT, Forbess JM, Kirshbom PM. Results with the freestyle porcine aortic root for right ventricular outflow tract reconstruction in children. *Ann Thorac Surg.* (2003) 76:1889–94; discussion 94–5. doi: 10.1016/s0003-4975(03)01304-3
79. Hartz RS, Deleon SY, Lane J, Dorotan J, Joyce J, Urbina E, et al. Medtronic freestyle valves in right ventricular outflow tract reconstruction. *Ann Thorac Surg.* (2003) 76:1896–900. doi: 10.1016/s0003-4975(03)01301-8
80. Ezelsoy M, Oral K, Saracoglu KT, Saracoglu A, Bayramoglu Z, Akpinar B. Long term outcomes of freestyle stentless aortic bioprosthesis: a single center experience. *Heart Surg Forum.* (2020) 23:E034–E8. doi: 10.1532/hsf.2661
81. Mehdiani A, Sorokin VA, Sule J, Smiris K, Stadnik D, Lichtenberg A, et al. Mid-term single-center outcomes of BioIntegral compared to freestyle aortic conduit implantation. *J Cardiovasc Surg (Torino).* (2020) 61:512–9. doi: 10.23736/S0021-9509.19.11098-1
82. Liebrich M, Hemmer W, Uhlemann F, Merz C, Voth W, Scheid M, et al. A novel designed valved conduit for RVOT reconstruction in grown-up congenital heart patients: a glimpse down the road. *Thorac Cardiovasc Surg.* (2016) 64:36–43. doi: 10.1055/s-0035-1564930
83. Nichay NR, Zhuravleva IY, Kulyabin YY, Timchenko TP, Voitov AV, Kuznetsova EV, et al. In search of the best xenogeneic material for a paediatric conduit: an analysis of clinical data. *Interact Cardiovasc Thorac Surg.* (2018) 27:34–41. doi: 10.1093/icvts/ivy029
84. Breymann T, Thies WR, Boethig D, Goerg R, Blanz U, Koerfer R. Bovine valved venous xenografts for RVOT reconstruction: results after 71 implantations. *Eur J Card Thorac Surg.* (2002) 21:703–10; discussion 710. doi: 10.1016/s1010-7940(02)00049-0

85. Bové T, Demanet H, Wauthy P, Goldstein JP, Dessy H, Viart P, et al. Early results of valved bovine jugular vein conduit versus bicuspid homograft for right ventricular outflow tract reconstruction. *Ann Thorac Surg.* (2002) 74:536–41; discussion 541. doi: 10.1016/s0003-4975(02)03728-1
86. Kido T, Hoashi T, Kagisaki K, Fujiyoshi T, Kitano M, Kurosaki K, et al. Early clinical outcomes of right ventricular outflow tract reconstruction with small caliber bovine jugular vein conduit (Contegra((R))) in small children. *J Artif Organs.* (2016) 19:364–71. doi: 10.1007/s10047-016-0908-7
87. Boudjemline Y, Bonnet D, Massih TA, Agnoletti G, Iserin F, Jaubert F, et al. Use of bovine jugular vein to reconstruct the right ventricular outflow tract: early results. *J Thorac Cardiovasc Surg.* (2003) 126:490–7. doi: 10.1016/s0022-5223(03)00232-0
88. Patel PM, Tan C, Srivastava N, Herrmann JL, Rodefeld MD, Turrentine MW, et al. Bovine jugular vein conduit: a mid- to long-term institutional review. *World J Pediatr Congenit Heart Surg.* (2018) 9:489–95. doi: 10.1177/2150135118779356
89. Erek E, Temur B, Suzan D, Aydin S, Yildiz O, Kirat B, et al. Outcomes of truncus arteriosus repair with bovine jugular vein conduit. *Turk Gogus Kalp Damar Cerrahisi Derg.* (2018) 26:365–9. doi: 10.5606/tgkdc.dergisi.2018.14841
90. Falchetti A, Demanet H, Dessy H, Melot C, Pierrakos C, Wauthy P. Contegra versus pulmonary homograft for right ventricular outflow tract reconstruction in newborns. *Cardiol Young.* (2019) 29:505–10. doi: 10.1017/S1047951119000143
91. Choi KH, Sung SC, Kim H, Lee HD, Kim G, Ko H, et al. Simplified tricuspid polytetrafluoroethylene valved conduit: midterm results of multicenter study. *Ann Thorac Surg.* (2019) 108:1228–33. doi: 10.1016/j.athoracsur.2019.04.018
92. Sadri V, Madukauwa-David ID, Yoganathan AP. *In vitro* evaluation of a new aortic valved conduit. *J Thorac Cardiovasc Surg.* (2021) 161(2):581.e6–590.e6. doi: 10.1016/j.jtcvs.2019.09.181
93. Mosala Nezhad Z, Poncelet A, de Kerchove L, Fervaille C, Banse X, Bollen X, et al. CorMatrix valved conduit in a porcine model: long-term remodelling and biomechanical characterization. *Interact Cardiovasc Thorac Surg.* (2017) 24:90–8. doi: 10.1093/icvts/ivw314
94. van Rijswijk JW, Talacua H, Mulder K, van Hout GPJ, Bouten CVC, Grundeman PF, et al. Failure of decellularized porcine small intestinal submucosa as a heart valved conduit. *J Thorac Cardiovasc Surg.* (2020) 160:e201–e15. doi: 10.1016/j.jtcvs.2019.09.164
95. Chang TI, Hsu KH, Luo CW, Yen JH, Lu PC, Chang CI. *In vitro* study of trileaflet polytetrafluoroethylene conduit and its valve-in-valve transformation. *Interact Cardiovasc Thorac Surg.* (2020) 30:408–16. doi: 10.1093/icvts/ivz274
96. Chen WL, Kan CD. *In vitro* hemodynamic evaluation of right ventricle-pulmonary artery continuity reconstruction through a trileaflet expanded polytetrafluoroethylene valved conduit. *Annu Int Conf IEEE Eng Med Biol Soc.* (2018) 2018:4548–51. doi: 10.1109/EMBC.2018.8513179
97. Kan CD, Wang JN, Chen WL, Lu PJ, Chan MY, Lin CH, et al. Applicability of handmade expanded polytetrafluoroethylene trileaflet-valved conduits for pulmonary valve reconstruction: an *ex vivo* and *in vivo* study. *J Thorac Cardiovasc Surg.* (2018) 155:765.e3–74.e3. doi: 10.1016/j.jtcvs.2017.09.049
98. Ootaki Y, Welch AS, Walsh MJ, Quartermain MD, Williams DA, Ungerleider RM. Medium-term outcomes after implantation of expanded polytetrafluoroethylene valved conduit. *Ann Thorac Surg.* (2018) 105:843–50. doi: 10.1016/j.athoracsur.2017.07.013
99. Sharifulin R, Bogachev-Prokophiev A, Demin I, Zheleznev S, Pivkin A, Afanasyev A, et al. Right ventricular outflow tract reconstruction using a polytetrafluoroethylene conduit in Ross patients. *Eur J Card Thorac Surg.* (2018) 54:427–33. doi: 10.1093/ejcts/ezy128
100. Kobayashi K, Shinkawa T, Yamagishi M, Saito S, Nakayama Y, Hoki R, et al. Right ventricle to pulmonary artery conduit with tricuspid expanded polytetrafluoroethylene valves. *Ann Thorac Surg.* (2020). doi: 10.1016/j.athoracsur.2020.06.119
101. Zhang H, Ye M, Chen G. Jia B. 0.1 mm ePTFE versus autologous pericardium for hand-sewn trileaflet valved conduit: a comparative study. *J Artif Organs.* (2019) 22:207–13. doi: 10.1007/s10047-019-01107-5
102. Fujita S, Yamagishi M, Miyazaki T, Maeda Y, Itatani K, Yamamoto Y, et al. Long-term results of large-calibre expanded polytetrafluoroethylene-valved conduits with bulging sinuses. *Eur J Card Thorac Surg.* (2020) 58:1274–80. doi: 10.1093/ejcts/ezaa240
103. Yamamoto Y, Yamagishi M, Maeda Y, Asada S, Hongu H, Fujita S, et al. Histopathologic analysis of explanted polytetrafluoroethylene-valved pulmonary conduits. *Semin Thorac Cardiovasc Surg.* (2020) 32:990–9. doi: 10.1053/j.semtcvs.2019.10.001
104. Niemantsverdriet MBA, Ottenkamp J, Gauvreau K, Del Nido PJ, Hazenkamp MG, Jenkins KJ. Determinants of right ventricular outflow tract conduit longevity: a multinational analysis. *Congenit Heart Dis.* (2008) 3:176–84. doi: 10.1111/j.1747-0803.2008.00190.x
105. Iyer KS. The Contegra bovine jugular valved conduit: living up to expectations? *Ann Pediatr Cardiol.* (2012) 5:34–5.
106. Kirklin JW, Blackstone EH, Maehara T, Pacifico AD, Kirklin JK, Pollock S, et al. Intermediate-term fate of cryopreserved allograft and xenograft valved conduits. *Ann Thorac Surg.* (1987) 44:598–606. doi: 10.1016/s0003-4975(10)62142-x
107. Boethig D, Thies WR, Hecker H, Breymann T. Mid term course after pediatric right ventricular outflow tract reconstruction: a comparison of homografts, porcine xenografts and Contegras. *Eur J Card Thorac Surg.* (2005) 27:58–66. doi: 10.1016/j.ejcts.2004.09.009
108. Brown JW, Ruzmetov M, Rodefeld MD, Vijay P, Darragh RK. Valved bovine jugular vein conduits for right ventricular outflow tract reconstruction in children: AN attractive alternative to pulmonary homograft. *Ann Thorac Surg.* (2006) 82:909–16. doi: 10.1016/j.athoracsur.2006.03.008
109. Christenson JT, Sierra J, Manzano NEC, Jolou J, Beghetti M, Kalangos A. Homografts and xenografts for right ventricular outflow tract reconstruction: long-term results. *Ann Thorac Surg.* (2010) 90:1287–94. doi: 10.1016/j.athoracsur.2010.06.078
110. Mery CM, Guzman-Pruncda FA, De Leon LE, Zhang W, Terwelp MD, Bocchini CE, et al. Risk factors for development of endocarditis and reintervention in patients undergoing right ventricle to pulmonary artery valved conduit placement. *J Thorac Cardiovasc Surg.* (2016) 151: 432–9, 441.e1–2. doi: 10.1016/j.jtcvs.2015.10.069
111. Rastan AJ, Walther T, Daehnert I, Hambsch J, Mohr FW, Janousek J, et al. Bovine jugular vein conduit for right ventricular outflow tract reconstruction: evaluation of risk factors for mid-term outcome. *Ann Thorac Surg.* (2006) 82:1308–15. doi: 10.1016/j.athoracsur.2006.04.071
112. Sekarski N, van Meir H, Rijlaarsdam MEB, Schoof PH, Koolbergen DR, Hruda J, et al. Right ventricular outflow tract reconstruction with the bovine jugular vein graft: 5 years' experience with 133 patients. *Ann Thorac Surg.* (2007) 84:599–605. doi: 10.1016/j.athoracsur.2007.04.026
113. Belli E, Salihoglu E, Leobon B, Roubertie F, Ly M, Roussin R, et al. The performance of hancock porcine-valved dacron conduit for right ventricular outflow tract reconstruction. *Ann Thorac Surg.* (2010) 89:152–8. doi: 10.1016/j.athoracsur.2009.09.046
114. Wells WJ, Arroyo H, Bremner RM, Wood J, Starnes VA. Homograft conduit failure in infants is not due to somatic outgrowth. *J Thorac Cardiovasc Surg.* (2002) 124:88–96. doi: 10.1067/mtc.2002.121158
115. Shinkawa T, Chipman C, Bozzay T, Tang X, Gossett JM, Imamura M. Outcome of right ventricle to pulmonary artery conduit for biventricular repair. *Ann Thorac Surg.* (2015) 99:1357–64. doi: 10.1016/j.athoracsur.2014.07.095
116. Wan J, Zhong X, Xu Z, Gong D, Li D, Xin Z, et al. A decellularized porcine pulmonary valved conduit embedded with gelatin. *Artif Organs.* (2021) 45:1068–82. doi: 10.1111/aor.13955
117. Elkins RC, Dawson PE, Goldstein S, Walsh SP, Black KS. Decellularized human valve allografts. *Ann Thorac Surg.* (2001) 71(5 Suppl):S428–32. doi: 10.1016/s0003-4975(01)02503-6
118. Bechtel JFM, Gellissen J, Erasmi AW, Petersen M, Hiob A, Stierle U, et al. Mid-term findings on echocardiography and computed tomography after RVOT-reconstruction: comparison of decellularized (SynerGraft) and conventional allografts. *Eur J Card Thorac Surg.* (2005) 27:410–5. doi: 10.1016/j.ejcts.2004.12.017
119. Bechtel JEM, Stierle U, Sievers H-H. Fifty-two months' mean follow up of decellularized SynerGraft (TM)-treated pulmonary valve allografts. *J Heart Valve Dis.* (2008) 17:98–104.
120. Brown JW, Elkins RC, Clarke DR, Tweddell JS, Huddleston CB, Doty JR, et al. Performance of the CryoValve* SG human decellularized pulmonary

valve in 342 patients relative to the conventional CryoValve at a mean follow-up of four years. *J Thorac Cardiovasc Surg.* (2010) 139:339–48. doi: 10.1016/j.jtcvs.2009.04.065
121. Burch PT, Kaza AK, Lambert LM, Holubkov R, Shaddy RE, Hawkins JA. Clinical performance of decellularized cryopreserved valved allografts compared with standard allografts in the right ventricular outflow tract. *Ann Thorac Surg.* (2010) 90:1301–5. doi: 10.1016/j.athoracsur.2010.05.024
122. Hawkins JA, Hillman ND, Lambert LM, Jones J, Di Russo GB, Profaizer T, et al. Immunogenicity of decellularized cryopreserved allografts in pediatric cardiac surgery: comparison with standard cryopreserved allografts. *J Thorac Cardiovasc Surg.* (2003) 126:247–53. doi: 10.1016/s0022-5223(03)00116-8
123. Konuma T, Devaney EJ, Bove EL, Gelehrter S, Hirsch JC, Tavakkol Z, et al. Performance of CryoValve SG decellularized pulmonary allografts compared with standard cryopreserved allografts. *Ann Thorac Surg.* (2009) 88:849–55. doi: 10.1016/j.athoracsur.2009.06.003
124. Ruzmetov M, Shah JJ, Geiss DM, Fortuna RS. Decellularized versus standard cryopreserved valve allografts for right ventricular outflow tract reconstruction: a single-institution comparison. *J Thorac Cardiovasc Surg.* (2012) 143:543–9. doi: 10.1016/j.jtcvs.2011.12.032
125. Tavakkol Z, Gelehrter S, Goldberg CS, Bove EL, Devaney EJ, Ohye RG. Superior durability of synergraft pulmonary allografts compared with standard cryopreserved allografts. *Ann Thorac Surg.* (2005) 80:1610–4. doi: 10.1016/j.athoracsur.2005.04.017
126. Vafaee T, Thomas D, Desai A, Jennings LM, Berry H, Rooney P, et al. Decellularization of human donor aortic and pulmonary valved conduits using low concentration sodium dodecyl sulfate. *J Tissue Eng Regen Med.* (2018) 12:e841–e53. doi: 10.1002/term.2391
127. Brown JW, Ruzmetov M, Eltayeb O, Rodefeld MD, Turrentine MW. Performance of SynerGraft decellularized pulmonary homograft in patients undergoing a Ross procedure. *Ann Thorac Surg.* (2011) 91:416–22; discussion 422–3. doi: 10.1016/j.athoracsur.2010.10.069
128. Tudorache I, Horke A, Cebotari S, Sarikouch S, Boethig D, Breymann T, et al. Decellularized aortic homografts for aortic valve and aorta ascendens replacement. *Eur J Card Thorac Surg.* (2016) 50:89–97. doi: 10.1093/ejcts/ezw013
129. da Costa FDA, Etnel JRG, Torres R, Balbi Filho EM, Torres R, Calixto A, et al. Decellularized allografts for right ventricular outflow tract reconstruction in children. *World J Pediatr Congenit Heart Surg.* (2017) 8:605–12. doi: 10.1177/2150135117723916
130. Grauss RW, Hazekamp MG, van Vliet S. Gittenberger-de Groot AC, DeRuiter MC. Decellularization of rat aortic valve allografts reduces leaflet destruction and extracellular matrix remodeling. *J Thorac Cardiovasc Surg.* (2003) 126:2003–10. doi: 10.1016/s0022-5223(03)00956-5
131. Flameng W, De Visscher G, Mesure L, Hermans H, Jashari R, Meuris B. Coating with fibronectin and stromal cell-derived factor-1α of decellularized homografts used for right ventricular outflow tract reconstruction eliminates immune response-related degeneration. *J Thorac Cardiovasc Surg.* (2014) 147:139.e28–404.e2. doi: 10.1016/j.jtcvs.2013.06.022
132. Luo J, Korossis SA, Wilshaw S-P, Jennings LM, Fisher J, Ingham E. Development and characterization of acellular porcine pulmonary valve scaffolds for tissue engineering. *Tissue Eng A.* (2014) 20:2963–74. doi: 10.1089/ten.TEA.2013.0573
133. Collatusso C, Roderjan JG, Vieira ED, Myague NI, de Noronha L, da Costa FDA. Decellularization as an anticalcification method in stentless bovine pericardium valve prosthesis: a study in sheep. *Rev Bras Cir Cardiovasc.* (2011) 26:419–26. doi: 10.5935/1678-9741.20110017
134. Lopera Higuita M, Griffiths LG. Antigen removal process preserves function of small diameter venous valved conduits, whereas SDS-decellularization results in significant valvular insufficiency. *Acta Biomater.* (2020) 107:115–28. doi: 10.1016/j.actbio.2020.03.003
135. Fung YC, Fronek K, Patitucci P. Pseudoelasticity of arteries and the choice of its mathematical expression. *Am J Physiol.* (1979) 237:H620–H31. doi: 10.1152/ajpheart.1979.237.5.H620
136. Ogden RW. Nonlinear elasticity, anisotropy, material stability and residual stresses in soft tissue. In: Holzapfel GA, Ogden RW, editors. *Biomechanics of Soft Tissue in Cardiovascular Systems. International Centre for Mechanical Sciences (Courses and Lectures). Vol 441.* Vienna: Springer (2003). p. 65–108.
137. Norotte C, Marga FS, Niklason LE, Forgacs G. Scaffold-free vascular tissue engineering using bioprinting. *Biomaterials.* (2009) 30:5910–7. doi: 10.1016/j.biomaterials.2009.06.034
138. Paulsen MJ, Kasinpila P, Imbrie-Moore AM, Wang H, Hironaka CE, Koyano TK, et al. Modeling conduit choice for valve-sparing aortic root replacement on biomechanics with a 3-dimensional-printed heart simulator. *J Thorac Cardiovasc Surg.* (2019) 158:392–403. doi: 10.1016/j.jtcvs.2018.10.145
139. Shinoka T. What is the best material for extracardiac Fontan operation? *J Thorac Cardiovasc Surg.* (2017) 153:1551–2. doi: 10.1016/j.jtcvs.2017.02.023
140. Sankaran KK, Krishnan UM, Sethuraman S. Axially aligned 3D nanofibrous grafts of PLA-PCL for small diameter cardiovascular applications. *J Biomater Sci Polym Ed.* (2014) 25:1791–812. doi: 10.1080/09205063.2014.950505
141. Soliman OI, Miyazaki Y, Abdelghani M, Brugmans M, Witsenburg M, Onuma Y, et al. Midterm performance of a novel restorative pulmonary valved conduit: preclinical results. *EuroIntervention.* (2017) 13:e1418–27. doi: 10.4244/EIJ-D-17-00553
142. Bennink G, Torii S, Brugmans M, Cox M, Svanidze O, Ladich E, et al. A novel restorative pulmonary valved conduit in a chronic sheep model: mid-term hemodynamic function and histologic assessment. *J Thorac Cardiovasc Surg.* (2018) 155:2591.e3–601.e3. doi: 10.1016/j.jtcvs.2017.12.046
143. Wise SG, Byrom MJ, Waterhouse A, Bannon PG, Weiss AS, Ng MK, et al. multilayered synthetic human elastin/polycaprolactone hybrid vascular graft with tailored mechanical properties. *Acta Biomater.* (2011) 7:295–303. doi: 10.1016/j.actbio.2010.07.022
144. Manavitehrani I, Ebrahimi P, Yang I, Daly S, Schindeler A, Saxena A, et al. Current challenges and emergent technologies for manufacturing artificial right ventricle to pulmonary artery (RV-PA) cardiac conduits. *Cardiovasc Eng Technol.* (2019) 10:205–15. doi: 10.1007/s13239-019-00406-5

# 6

# Clinical and Surgical Evaluations of Reoperation After Mechanical Mitral Valve Replacement Due to Different Etiologies

*Jiehui Li, Shuiyun Wang*, Hansong Sun, Jianping Xu, Chao Dong, Min Song and Qibin Yu*

*State Key Laboratory of Cardiovascular Disease, Department of Cardiac Surgery, National Center for Cardiovascular Diseases, Peking Union Medical College, Fuwai Hospital, Chinese Academy of Medical Sciences, Beijing, China*

***Correspondence:**
*Shuiyun Wang*
*wangshuiyun@fuwaihospital.org*

**Background:** This study aimed to evaluate the clinical and surgical characteristics of patients who required reoperation after mechanical mitral valve replacement (MVR).

**Methods:** We retrospectively identified 204 consecutive patients who underwent reoperation after mechanical MVR between 2009 and 2018. Patients were categorized according the reason for reoperation (perivalvular leakage, thrombus formation, or pannus formation). The patients' medical and surgical records were studied carefully and the rates of in-hospital complications were calculated.

**Results:** The mean age was 51±12 years and 44% of the patients were male. The reasons for reoperation were perivalvular leakage (117 patients), thrombus formation (35 patients), and pannus formation (52 patients). The most common positions for perivalvular leakage were at the 6–10 o'clock positions (proportions of ≥25% for each hour position). Most patients had an interval of >10 years between the original MVR and reoperation. The most common reoperation procedure was re-do MVR (157 patients), and 155 of these patients underwent concomitant cardiac procedures. There were 10 in-hospital deaths and 32 patients experienced complications. The 10-year survival rate was 82.2 ± 3.9% in general, and the group of lowest rate was patients with PVL (77.5 ± 5.2%). The independent risk factors were "male" (4.62, 95% CI 1.57–13.58, $P = 0.005$) and "Hb<9g/dL before redo MV operation" (3.45, 95% CI 1.13–10.49, $P = 0.029$).

**Conclusion:** Perivalvular leakage was the most common reason for reoperation after mechanical MVR, with a low survival rate in long term follow-up relatively.

**Keywords: prosthesis malfunction, mitral valve replacement, perivalvular leakage, thrombus, pannus**

## INTRODUCTION

Mechanical prosthesis replacement is a valuable treatment option for mitral valve lesions. It offers a much longer life expectancy than a biological prosthesis. However, a few patients require secondary operation after mechanical mitral valve replacement (MVR). In such cases, the most common pathogeneses include perivalvular leakage (PVL), thrombus, or pannus formation. Although coupled with low prevalence (6.5% for 10 years follow-up, or 1,000–2,000 cases per year in Japan or the US), (1–4) the redo operation remains a significant challenge to clinicians and patients.

Several studies and reviews have examined the therapies and prognosis of redo operations after mechanical MVR, especially for patients with PVL (5–7). However, cases of thrombus or pannus were insufficient. In contrast, it was also worth comprehensively analyzing the operative techniques and their impacts on patients by different etiologies. Therefore, the current study aims to report the clinical features, operative techniques, and complications in-hospital of redo operations after mechanical MVR in our medical center.

# MATERIALS AND METHODS

## Patients Selection

More than 2,000 mitral valve surgeries have been completed in recent years in our hospital; (8) however, only a few of these patients underwent secondary operations. This retrospective study evaluated patients undergoing reoperation after mechanical MVR from January 2009 to December 2018. Medical records, including echocardiographic, clinical, operative, and in-hospital outcomes, were collected. For inclusion, patients were also required to have undergone transthoracic Doppler echocardiography and preoperative coronary angiography if older than 45. The cause of redo MVR was attributed to perivalvular leakage, thrombogenesis, and pannus formation. Patients were categorized into groups correspondingly. For patients of PVL, because of the variances of mitral annular, a novel item, "summed points of PVL," was used to evaluate the severity of perivalvular leakage, representing the overall points of a lesion by clock position. The medical records were reviewed carefully to confirm the cause of the operation. The details of lesions were affirmed by the surgery records in cases of inconsistencies with echocardiography or other imaging.

The primary endpoint was defined as the death in the follow-up. The secondary endpoint was defined as the complications in-hospital, including mortality in hospital, bleeding reoperation, continuous renal replacement therapy (CRRT), Intra-Aortic Balloon Pump (IABP), tracheotomy, stroke, ventilator usage ≥96 h, and ICU Stay ≥7 days.

## Statistical Analysis

Continuous variables were expressed as mean ± standard deviation, and categoric variables were represented as percentages. Comparisons were performed by the $\chi^2$ test or Fisher's exact test for categorical variables and Student's *t*-test

**TABLE 1** | Preoperative characteristics of the study patients.

| | PVL* (*n* = 117) | Thrombus (*n* = 35) | Pannus (*n* = 52) | Overall (*n* = 204) | *P*-value† |
|---|---|---|---|---|---|
| Age (y) | 51 ± 13 | 47 ± 13 | 52 ± 10 | 51 ± 12 | 0.10 |
| Male (%) | 69 (59%) | 9 (26%) | 11 (21%) | 89 (44%) | < 0.01 |
| BSA (m$^2$) | 1.5 ± 0.4 | 1.2 ± 0.4 | 1.1 ± 0.3 | 1.3 ± 0.4 | < 0.01 |
| BMI§ (kg/m$^2$) | 22 ± 3 | 23 ± 3 | 23 ± 4 | 22 ± 3 | 0.02 |
| **Risk factors, *n* (%)** | | | | | |
| Atrial fibrillation** | 69 (59%) | 21 (60%) | 36 (69%) | 126 (62%) | 0.44 |
| Tricuspid regurgitation | 74 (63%) | 16 (46%) | 32 (62%) | 122 (60%) | 0.17 |
| Pulmonary hypertension | 45 (39%) | 20 (57%) | 25 (48%) | 90 (44%) | 0.12 |
| Hypertension | 17 (15%) | 4 (11%) | 3 (6%) | 24 (12%) | 0.26 |
| Diabetes mellitus | 6 (5%) | 3 (9%) | 3 (6%) | 12 (6%) | 0.75 |
| History of stroke | 6 (5%) | 1 (3%) | 10 (19%) | 17 (8%) | < 0.01 |
| NYHA III/IV | 69 (59%) | 22 (63%) | 29 (56%) | 120 (59%) | 0.80 |
| History of AVR | 42 (36%) | 9 (28%) | 12 (23%) | 63 (31%) | 0.19 |
| **Echocardiology** | | | | | |
| LVEF, (%)†† | 60 ± 12 | 52 ± 22 | 56 ± 15 | 57 ± 15 | 0.07 |
| < 50%, n (%) | 5 (4%) | 1 (3%) | 6 (12%) | 12 (6%) | 0.13 |
| LVEDD | 56 ± 13 | 40 ± 17 | 45 ± 11 | 53 ± 10 | < 0.01 |
| ≥55mm, *n* (%) | 74 (63%) | 8 (23%) | 11 (21%) | 93 (46%) | < 0.01 |
| MVPG§§ | 9 ± 5 | 14 ± 9 | 11 ± 6 | 10 ± 6 | < 0.01 |
| Hemoglobin (g/dL) | 118 ± 23 | 128 ± 21 | 120 ± 22 | 120 ± 23 | 0.08 |
| Intervals of operations (y) | 11 ± 8 | 9 ± 7 | 15 ± 8 | 12 ± 8 | < 0.01 |
| ≥10y, *n* (%) | 61 (52%) | 19 (54%) | 40 (77%) | 120 (59%) | 0.01 |

**PVL, Perivalvular Leakage.*
*†Comparisons among PVL, thrombus or pannus.*
*BSA, Body Surface Area.*
*§BMI, Body Mass Index.*
***Atrial fibrillation, Atrial fibrillation before redo MV operation.*
*††LVEF, Left Ventricular Ejection Fraction.*
*LVEDD, Left Ventricular End Diastolic Diameter.*
*§§MVPG, Mitral Valve Pressure Gradient.*
*P value < 0.05, with significant difference in statistics.*

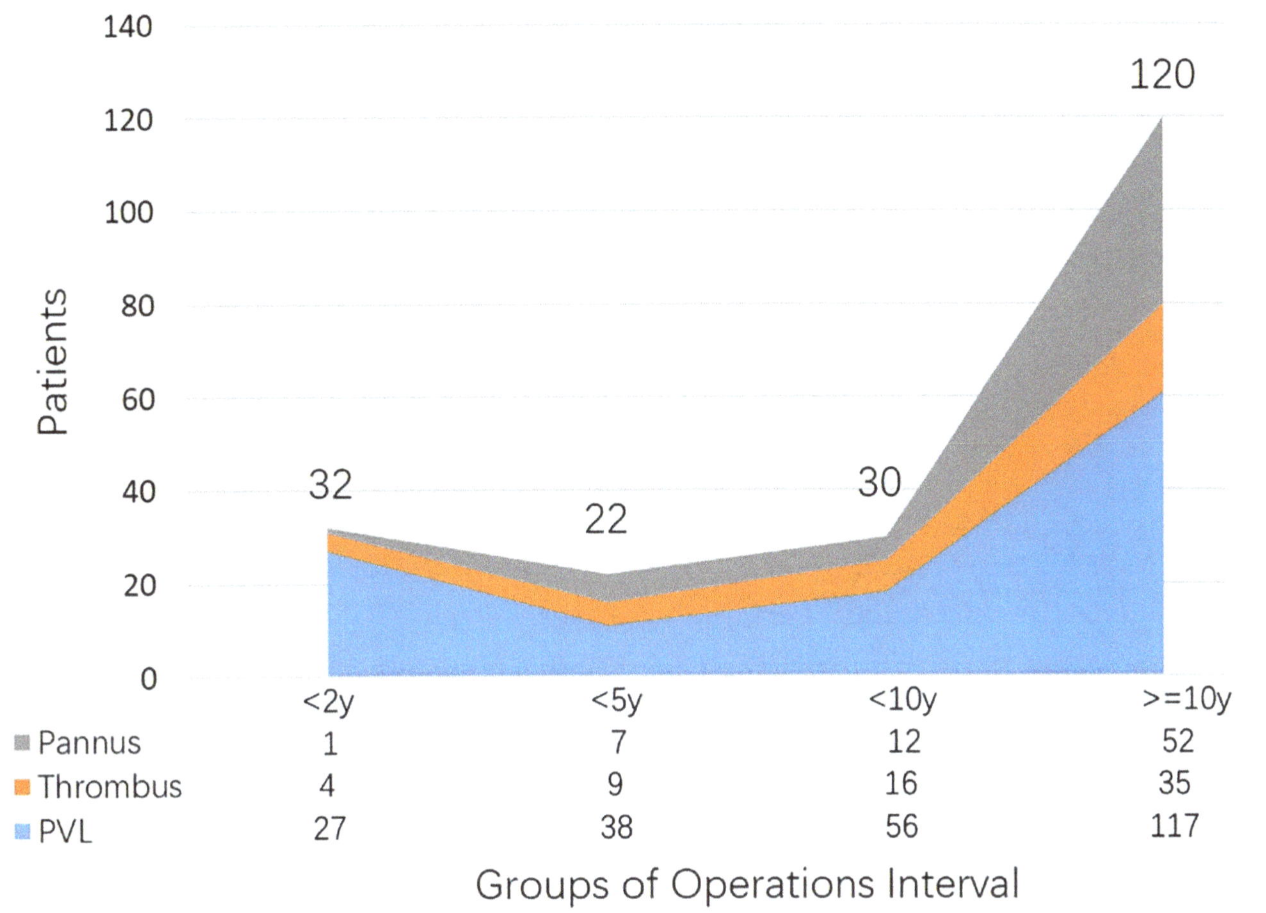


**FIGURE 1** | Patient distributions of etiologies categorized by operations interval.

for continuous variables. Multiple logistic regression models were used to assess associations with the in-hospital outcomes. As appropriate, survival rates were compared between groups, using the log-rank test or Breslow's test. Predictors or risk factors were analyzed by Cox regression. All variables were included in the univariate analysis. Those with a probability value of <0.1 were included in the multivariate regression. In terms of the Cox multivariate model, missing values were replaced by multiple imputation, and predictor selection using backward stepwise regression with Akaike information criterion (AIC) was performed on all imputed datasets. All statistical tests were two-sided, and a probability value of <0.05 was considered statistically significant. Statistical analysis was performed using IBM SPSS software (version 19.0; IBM Corp., Armonk, NY, USA).

## RESULTS

### Characteristics of Patients With Redo Operations After Mechanical MVR

Two hundred and four patients underwent redo operation after mechanical MVR. Their average height was 1.64 ± 0.1 m, and average weight was 61 ± 11 kg, average age was 51 ± 12 years old, and 50 patients (24.5%) were older than 60. Groups were categorized by etiologies: perivalvular leakage ($n$ = 117), thrombus ($n$ = 35), and pannus ($n$ = 52). The baseline and clinical data of patients enrolled are summarized in **Table 1**.

Most baseline characteristics among the patients showed no difference in statistical terms. Patients with perivalvular leakage had more proportion of males ($n$ = 69, 59%), with the highest BSA (1.5 ± 0.4 $m^2$) and the lowest BMI (22 ± 3 kg/$m^2$). The pannus group had the longest interval of operations (15 ± 8 years, $p = 0.001$). Group PVL had the largest left ventricular end-diastolic diameter (LVEDD, 56 ± 13 mm, $p < 0.001$), and group thrombus had the greatest mitral valve pressure gradient (MVPG, 14 ± 9 mmHg, $p = 0.004$).

As displayed in **Figure 1**, more than half of the patients had more than 10 years gap between operations. Especially for patients with pannus, the average interval was 15 ± 8 years, and few of them underwent redo operations <10 years after primary surgery. The majority of PVL patients were in the group "< 2 years" ($n$ = 27, 84.4%). Moreover, among patients with thrombus, the morbidity of redo surgery appeared to be similar in the entire cohort.

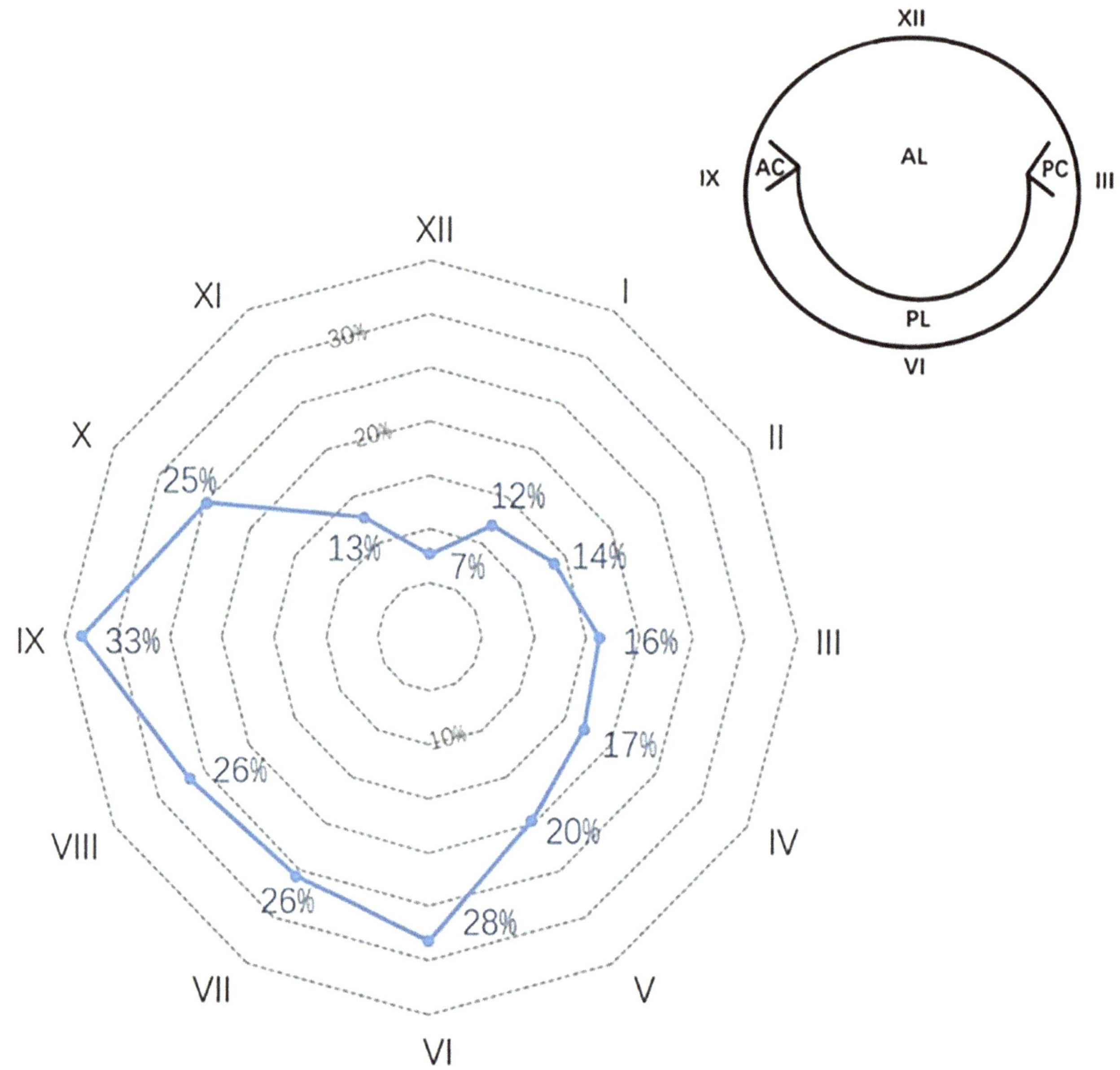


**FIGURE 2 |** Perivalvular leakage of mechanical mitral prosthesis in the native valve anatomy. The percentages show the prevalence in each clock position. The most frequent positions were from 6 to 10 o'clock.

Detailed documentation of perivalvular leakage was available for 109 (93% of PVL group). **Figure 2** illustrates the distribution of perivalvular leakage illustrated by the clock position on a radar chart. Eighty-one patients (74% of PVL records) had more than one point of lesion. The most susceptible regions appeared from six to ten o'clock, with a prevalence of no <25%.

We used a novel item, "summed points of PVL," to evaluate the severity of perivalvular leakage, representing the lesion's overall points by clock position. Generally, patients were found to have 2.6 ± 1.4 points (**Figure 3**), and it had no relationship with the interval of operations ($r = 0.06$, $p = 0.56$). Furthermore, we analyzed the PVL patients combined with AVR simultaneously and found no relationship between "summed points of PVL" and "aortic valve replacement" (eight of one point, eight of two summed points, and seven of more than two points, $p = 0.797$).

## Characteristics of Redo Operations After Mechanical MVR

One hundred and fifty-seven patients underwent repeat MVR, with 147 mechanical prostheses (94% of re-MVR) implanted. Forty patients of perivalvular leakage (34% of PVL group) underwent PVL repair, and seven patients (14% of pannus group) underwent pannus clearance only.

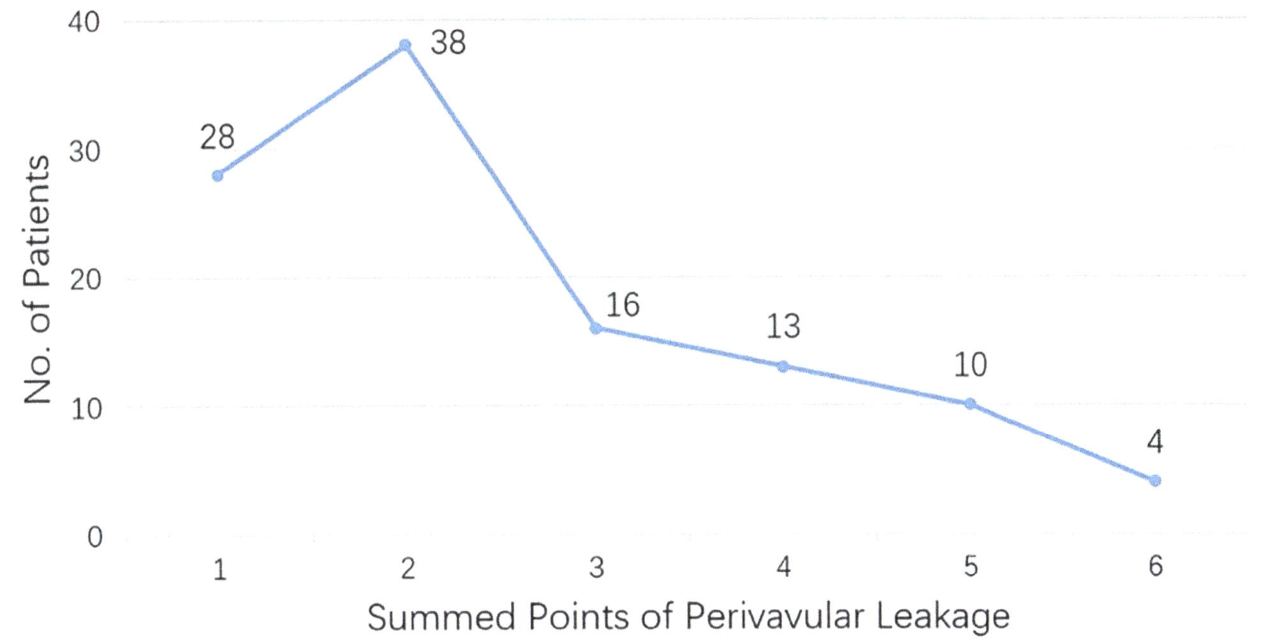


**FIGURE 3** | Patients number for each subgroup with summed points of perivalvular leakage.

One hundred and fifty-five patients underwent concomitant heart procedures, including 131 tricuspid valve repairs and 54 aortic valve replacements (AVR) (**Table 2**). The operation time was 327 ± 104 min, and the aortic cross-clamping (ACC) time was 103 ± 48 min. Operations in the PVL group had a shorter ACC time than non-PVL groups (min: 96 ± 46: 112 ± 50, $p$ = 0.01). We had recorded 10 deaths (mortality of 4.9%) in the hospital. And as shown in **Table 3**, there was no difference among the three groups in terms of complications in general or in detail.

## Follow-Up of Redo Operations After Mechanical MVR

The overall survival rate at 10 years was 82.2 ± 3.9%. As shown in **Figure 4**, there was no difference among the three groups in terms of etiologies (log-rank test, $P = 0.18$). However, differences could be observed after categorizing patients into the PVL group and Others group (non-PVL group) (log-rank test, $P = 0.06$). Univariate and multivariate Cox regression analyses (**Table 4**) revealed that "Male" (4.62, 95% CI 1.57–13.58, $P = 0.005$) and "Hb<9g/dL before secondary MV operation" (3.45, 95% CI 1.13–10.49, $P = 0.029$) were the independent risk factors in patients undergoing redo operations after mechanical MVR. Additionally, LVEF might influence the late outcomes of patients after the redo MV operation (1.07, 95% CI 1–1.14, $P = 0.061$).

# DISCUSSION

## Patients by Different Etiologies of Redo Operations After Mechanical MVR

In the present study, perivalvular leakage was the most important pathogenesis leading to a secondary operation after mechanical MVR. Patients with perivalvular leakage had a longer diameter of left ventricular end-diastole, and the percentage of left ventricular dilation (LVEDD ≥55 mm) was up to 63%. This could be attributed to the fact that the pathophysiology was similar to mitral regurgitation, which also led to a shorter interval between operations than patients with pannus or thrombus (years: 11 ± 8: 13 ± 8, $p = 0.058$). These findings were in line with Botta et al. report (mean: 130 months) (9). Most studies proposed that patients require intervention only with the moderate-severe PVL or coupled with symptoms; mild PVL without symptoms usually had a benign course and could be managed in follow-up carefully (10). However, the surgeries peaked slightly in PVL patients during the first 2 years. This spike in the extremely short interval might be attributed to the surgical techniques being used. Meanwhile, patient numbers in other groups increased gradually with time in 10 years, after former mechanical MVR from our study.

In the current investigation, the perivalvular leakage in the mitral position was predominantly at six to ten o'clock position (≥25% in each point), which was mirror-symmetric to Bouhout et al. study (from two to six o'clock, ≥35% for each point) (6). Meanwhile, another important assessment was the severity of PVL. Because of the different sizes of mitral prostheses, it might be unreasonable to compare them by length or width directly. We analyzed the item, "summed points of PVL" (2.6 ± 1.4 points), which represented the overall leakage points by clock position. These data could benefit further analysis.

Patients with pannus had the greatest MVPG in the cohort (14 ± 9 mmHg, $p = 0.004$). This was in line with previous studies and reports on pannus and thrombus (11, 12). The current consensus showed that pannus always formed as circular mass curved along the ring, and thrombus tended to infest into the prosthesis,

**TABLE 2** | Blood transfusion and operative characteristics of the study patients.

| | PVL*** ($n$ = 117) | Thrombus ($n$ = 35) | Pannus ($n$ = 52) | Overall ($n$ = 204) | $P$-value††† |
|---|---|---|---|---|---|
| **Operative techniques** | | | | | |
| PVL-repairing | 40 (34%) | - | - | 40 (20%) | - |
| Pannus clearance | - | - | 7 (14%) | 7 (3%) | - |
| Mitral valve replacement | 77 (66%) | 35 (100%) | 45 (87%) | 157 (77%) | <0.01 |
| Mechanical prosthesis§§§ | 76 | 30 | 41 | 147 | 0.02 |
| Size of prosthesis (mm) | 27 ± 2 | 26 ± 1 | 26 ± 1 | 26 ± 2 | <0.01 |
| Concomitant procedure, n**** | 87 (74%) | 24 (69%) | 44 (85%) | 155 (76%) | 0.19 |
| Aortic valve replacement | 26 (22%) | 7 (20%) | 21 (40%) | 54 (27%) | 0.03 |
| Tricuspid valve repairing | 76 (65%) | 20 (57%) | 35 (67%) | 131 (64%) | 0.61 |
| Operation time (mins) | 330 ± 107 | 321 ± 114 | 325 ± 98 | 327 ± 104 | 0.93 |
| CPB time†††† | 149 ± 72 | 157 ± 71 | 161 ± 65 | 153 ± 70 | 0.56 |
| ACC time | 96 ± 46 | 105 ± 45 | 117 ± 53 | 103 ± 48 | 0.02 |
| P-ACC time§§§§ | 30 ± 22 | 33 ± 30 | 40 ± 52 | 33 ± 34 | 0.89 |
| P-ACC: ACC | 0.36 ± 0.27 | 0.34 ± 0.29 | 0.36 ± 0.38 | 0.35 ± 0.30 | 0.33 |
| Length of hospital stay (d) | 26 ± 18 | 15 ± 7 | 18 ± 10 | 22 ± 15 | <0.01 |
| Postoperative stay (d) | 13 ± 11 | 11 ± 6 | 10 ± 6 | 12 ± 9 | 0.08 |
| ICU stay (h) | 101 ± 147 | 94 ± 116 | 83 ± 99 | 95 ± 131 | 0.76 |
| Ventilator usage (h) | 48 ± 87 | 46 ± 76 | 37 ± 39 | 45 ± 75 | 0.38 |
| **Blood Transfusion** | | | | | |
| Red blood cell (u) | 8 ± 7 | 9 ± 14 | 6 ± 5 | 8 ± 8 | 0.49 |
| Plasma (ml) | 917 ± 780 | 1,216 ± 2,229 | 741 ± 572 | 939 ± 1163 | 0.63 |
| Platelet (u) | 1.6 ± 1.5 | 1.5 ± 0.8 | 1.5 ± 1.6 | 2.0 ± 3.5 | 0.89 |

*** *PVL, Perivalvular Leakage.*
††† *Comparisons among PVL, thrombus or pannus.*
*Values are n (%), or median (interquartile range).*
§§§ *Comparisons (PVL, Thrombus, & Pannus) in patients received redo MV replacement.*
**** *No. of patients received concomitant procedures.*
†††† *CPB, Cardio-Pulmonary Bypass.*
*ACC, Aortic Cross Clamping.*
§§§§ *P-ACC, CPB time of Post ACC.*
*P value < 0.05, with significant difference in statistics.*

which further restricted leaflet motion and caused a malfunction. Moreover, patients with pannus had the most prolonged interval of operations (15 ± 8 years, $p$ = 0.001). The development of pannus that can affect the hemodynamics of artificial prostheses requires a significant amount of time (13). In contrast, thrombi always give rise to acute symptoms, leading to shorter intervals (9 ± 7 years), similar to our study. These findings were consistent with Separham et al. report (14).

## Techniques and Details of Redo Operations

Thirty-three percent of PVL patients underwent perivalvular leakage repair, with shorter aortic cross-clamping time than redo MVR in the same group (min: 78 ± 45: 105 ± 44, $p$ = 0.002). However, this procedure did not cut down the operation time and Cardio-Pulmonary Bypass (CPB) time in general. Moreover, CPB time after ACC was not significantly different between the three etiology groups. Thus, it could be recognized that the operative techniques would not impact the difficulty of surgery.

The most common type of operative technique was the repeated replacement of mitral prosthesis (re-MVR), received by 66% of patients of PVL in our cohort. However, Bouhout et al. study showed that 76% of patients underwent PVL repair, who also reported the opposite distribution of PVL points mentioned above (6). PVL patients also had a larger prosthesis size than patients with thrombus or pannus in our hospital. All re-MVRs implanted artifacts had a size similar to the previous operation. The mechanical prosthesis was the mainstream choice for surgeons, even for patients aged more than 65 years. There were 11 cases of 14 implantations (three bioprosthetic valves). For these cases, there were four with small aortic annulus (size 19 or 21), two with endocarditis, one with Behcet's disease, and one with patient preference. These results might differ from Fukunaga et al. findings, which suggested that 75% of patients aged 50–69 years had received biological prostheses (15). However, the composition of their cohort was significantly different from ours, as there were only 6.8% cases of PVL in the mechanical MVR group.

Among patients undergoing concomitant operations, 22% (54 patients) had AVR, of which 31 patients underwent secondary replacement. The most common lesion of the aortic prosthesis was pannus formation ($n$ = 16), and there were eight patients with a mean aortic valve pressure gradient >30 mmHg at rest. In our cohort, secondary AVR was more common among patients with a history of AVR [OR 3.54, 95%CI (1.84, 6.81), $p$ < 0.01].

Meanwhile, in the present study, there were seven patients who underwent pannus removal through the transaortic route.

**TABLE 3 |** Complications of redo operations after mechanical MVR*.

| | PVL† (*n* = 117) | Thrombus (*n* = 35) | Pannus (*n* = 52) | Overall (*n* = 204) | *P*-value |
|---|---|---|---|---|---|
| Complications, n (%)§ | 19 (16%) | 6 (17%) | 7 (13%) | 32 (16%) | 0.87 |
| ICU stay ≥ 7d | 12 (10%) | 3 (9%) | 2 (4%) | 17 (8%) | 0.38 |
| Ventilator usage ≥ 96 h | 7 (6%) | 3 (9%) | 4 (8%) | 14 (7%) | 0.84 |
| Mortality in hospital | 4 (3%) | 3 (9%) | 3 (6%) | 10 (5%) | 0.44 |
| CRRT** | 8 (7%) | 3 (9%) | 1 (2%) | 12 (6%) | 0.35 |
| Tracheotomy | 5 (4%) | 1 (3%) | 1 (2%) | 7 (3%) | 0.73 |
| Bleeding reoperation | 5 (4%) | 2 (6%) | 4 (8%) | 11 (5%) | 0.66 |

*Complications: mortality in hospital, bleeding reoperation, CRRT, IABP, tracheotomy, stroke, ventilator usage ≥ 96 h, ICU Stay ≥ 7 d;*
*† PVL, Perivalvular Leakage.*
*Comparisons among PVL, thrombus or pannus.*
*§ No. of patients with complications after redo MV operation.*
*** CRRT, Continuous Renal Replacement Therapy.*

**TABLE 4 |** Univariate/multivariate cox regression of redo operations after mechanical MVR.

| Variables | Univariate regression HR (95% CI) | *P*-value | Multivariate regression HR (95% CI) | *P*-value |
|---|---|---|---|---|
| Age | 1.02 (0.98, 1.06) | 0.256 | | |
| Male | 4.62 (1.69, 12.63) | 0.003 | 4.62 (1.57, 13.58) | 0.005 |
| BMI[xxii] | 1.02 (0.90, 1.16) | 0.728 | | |
| Etiologies[xxiii] | 0.54 (0.26, 1.11) | 0.093 | 0.84 (0.41, 1.76) | 0.649 |
| NYHA III/IV | 1.41 (0.57, 3.50) | 0.457 | | |
| PH[xxiv] | 0.91 (0.38, 2.20) | 0.839 | | |
| Atrial fibrillation[xxv] | 1.19 (0.48, 2.94) | 0.712 | | |
| Hb<9g/dL | 3.67 (1.22, 11.06) | 0.021 | 3.45 (1.13, 10.49) | 0.029 |
| MVR[xxvi] | 0.60 (0.24, 1.49) | 0.269 | | |
| Multi-Operation[xxvii] | 3.12 (0.73, 13.38) | 0.126 | | |
| LVEDD[xxviii] | 1.01 (0.97, 1.05) | 0.770 | | |
| LVEF[xxix] | 1.06 (1, 1.13) | 0.063 | 1.07 (1, 1.14) | 0.061 |

*[xxii] BMI, Body Mass Index.*
*[xxiii] Etiologies, PVL, thrombus, pannus.*
*[xxiv] PH, Pulmonary Hypertension.*
*[xxv] Atrial fibrillation, Atrial fibrillation before redo MV operation.*
*[xxvi] MVR, Patients receiving MVR finally during the redo MV operation.*
*[xxvii] Multi-Operation, Multi-cardiac operations performed simultaneously during the redo MV operation.*
*[xxviii] LVEDD, Left Ventricular End Diastolic Diameter.*
*[xxix] LVEF, Left Ventricular Ejection Fraction.*

Their MVPG was 5 ± 1 mmHg, compared to 11 ± 7 mmHg ($p = 0.001$). Park et al. (16) found that patients with MVPG <5 mmHg could not benefit from the pannus clearance. Our findings were in line with their report.

## Endpoints After Redo Operations

Complications during the perioperative period have already been outlined in the Results section. The in-hospital mortality in our cohort was relatively low in our study compared to previous reports (2, 7, 17). The prevalence of dialysis and postoperative stroke (one case) was at an extremely low level, (18, 19) and the morbidity of bleeding during reoperation in our study was similar to a previous study (20). However, the ICU stay time and length of hospital stay after the operation was longer in our study than that reported earlier (19).

The overall survival rate at 10 years for our study participants was 82.2 ± 3.9%, similar to that reported by Fukunaga et al. (survival rate: 79.2%) (21). In our study cohorts, the PVL group had an outcome of 77.5 ± 5.2% after a 10-year follow-up which was the worst among the three groups. This might be due to the larger LVEDD than other groups (percentage of LVEDD>65 mm; PVL: Thrombus: Pannus; 63: 23: 21%). Patients with PVL always had worse outcomes than those patients with thrombus or pannus (1, 7, 14, 21). However, the survival rate of PVL patients in our study was still higher than in some studies, such as Bouhout et al. (57 ± 6%) (6). This may be attributed to the inclusion of relatively older adults in their group and a higher proportion of patients with NYHA III/IV. Furthermore, Botta et al. reported a survival rate at 5 years similar to our study (88.8: 84.0%) (9). However, these studies had different outcomes after

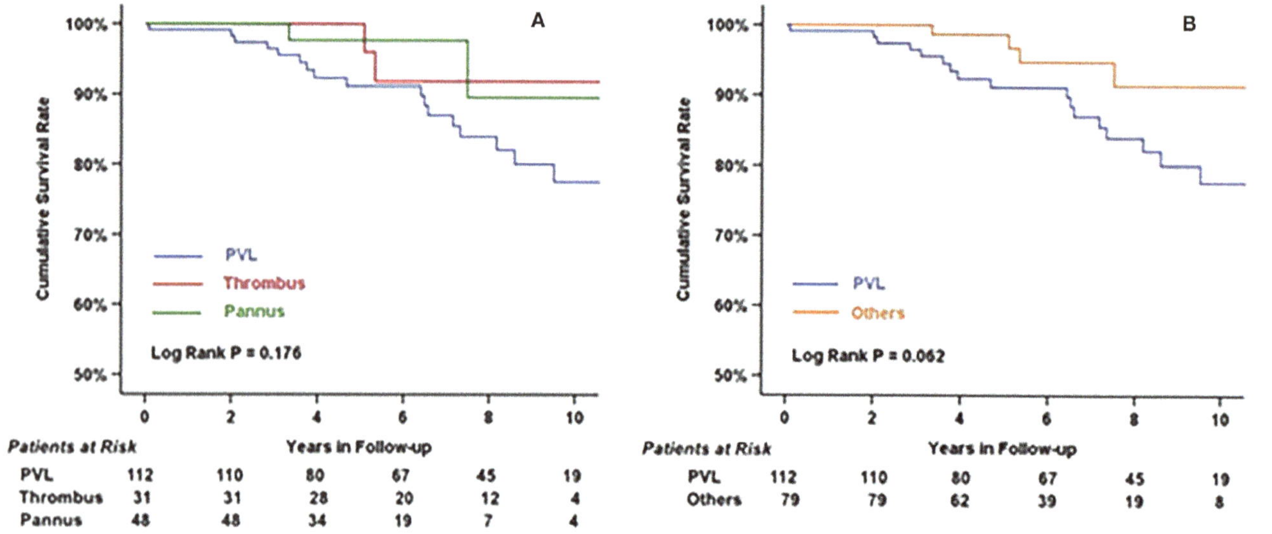


**FIGURE 4** | Cumulative survival rate of patients categorized by etiologies **(A)** and by PVL/Others **(B)**. There was no statistical difference among three groups (log rank $P = 0.176$), but had significant difference between patients with or without perivalvular leakage before redo MV operation (log rank = 0.062).

Cox regression analysis. Our research had found that "male" and "Hb <9g/dL before secondary MV operation" were independent risk factors affecting long-term prognosis.

Patients with thrombus in our study had a 10 years survival rate of 91.8 ± 5.5%, which was mildly lower than that reported by Raman et al. (97.4 ± 1.2%) (22). Furthermore, those with pannus had a moderate survival rate (89.5%) compared with the thrombus group and PVL group, similar to findings reported by Park et al. (87.6%) (23). This suggests that patients with mechanical mitral valve dysfunction would have a good prognosis if they underwent a proper redo procedure.

## Limitations of the Study

There were some limitations to our study. First, due to insufficient or missing clinical data, the insights drawn based on the surgical and patient history might not be fully valid and acceptable. Many patients did not undergo echocardiography in recent 2–3 years, making it further challenging to analyze th functioning of mechanical prostheses.

## CONCLUSION

Despite the low prevalence, reoperation after mechanical mitral valve replacement remains a key challenge. In our study, perivalvular leakage might be the possible cause of operation, which might lead to a low survival rate in the long-term follow-up relatively. Male patients with low hemoglobin (Hb <9g/dL) before the redo MV operation might have a worse outcome during the long-term follow-up compared to other patient subgroups.

## ETHICS STATEMENT

The studies involving human participants were reviewed and approved by the Ethics Committee of Fuwai Hospital, National Center for Cardiovascular Disease. The Ethics Committee waived the requirement of written informed consent for participation.

## AUTHOR CONTRIBUTIONS

SW, HS, JX, and CD: main surgeons of operations. JL, MS, and QY: statistics. JL and SW: writing. SW: general responsibility. All authors contributed to the article and approved the submitted version.

## REFERENCES

1. Nishida T, Sonoda H, Oishi Y, Tanoue Y, Nakashima A, Shiokawa Y, et al. Single-institution, 22-year follow-up of 786 carbomedics mechanical valves used for both primary surgery and reoperation. *J Thorac Cardiovasc Surg.* (2014) 147:1493–8. doi: 10.1016/j.jtcvs.2013.05.017
2. Furukawa H, Tanemoto K. Redo valve surgery–current status and future perspectives. *Ann Thorac Cardiovasc Surg.* (2014) 20:267–75. doi: 10.5761/atcs.ra.13-00380
3. Tanemoto K, Furukawa H. Repeated valve replacement surgery: technical tips and pitfalls. *Gen Thorac Cardiovasc Surg.* (2014) 62:639–44. doi: 10.1007/s11748-014-0473-z
4. Kilic A, Acker MA, Gleason TG, Sultan I, Vemulapalli S, Thibault D, et al. Clinical outcomes of mitral valve reoperations in the United States: an analysis of the society of thoracic surgeons national database. *Ann Thorac Surg.* (2019) 107:754–9. doi: 10.1016/j.athoracsur.2018.08.083
5. Rodríguez Muñoz D, Lázaro Rivera C, Zamorano Gómez JL. Guidance of treatment of perivalvular prosthetic leaks. *Curr Cardiol Rep.* (2014) 16:430. doi: 10.1007/s11886-013-0430-y
6. Bouhout I, Mazine A, Ghoneim A, Millàn X, El-Hamamsy I, Pellerin M, et al. Long-term results after surgical treatment of paravalvular leak in the aortic and mitral position. *J Thorac Cardiovasc Surg.* (2016) 151:1260–6.e1. doi: 10.1016/j.jtcvs.2015.11.046
7. Taramasso M, Maisano F, Denti P, Guidotti A, Sticchi A, Pozzoli A, et al. Surgical treatment of paravalvular leak: long-term results in a single-center

experience (up to 14 years). *J Thorac Cardiovasc Surg.* (2015) 149:1270–5. doi: 10.1016/j.jtcvs.2014.12.041

8. https://www.fuwaihospital.org/News/Columns/List/810
9. Botta L, De Chiara B, Quattrocchi S, Casadei F, Borgia F, Giannattasio C, et al. Mitral periprosthetic leakage: contemporary results of surgical correction at a single centre. *Interact Cardiovasc Thorac Surg.* (2017) 25:185–90. doi: 10.1093/icvts/ivx101
10. Giblett JP, Rana BS, Shapiro LM, Calvert PA. Percutaneous management of paravalvular leaks. *Nat Rev Cardiol.* (2019) 16:275–85. doi: 10.1038/s41569-018-0147-0
11. Gürsoy MO, Kalçik M, Karakoyun S, Özkan M. The current status of fluoroscopy and echocardiography in the diagnosis of prosthetic valve thrombosis-a review article. *Echocardiography.* (2015) 32:156–64. doi: 10.1111/echo.12721
12. Tanis W, Habets J, van den Brink RB, Symersky P, Budde RP, Chamuleau SA. Differentiation of thrombus from pannus as the cause of acquired mechanical prosthetic heart valve obstruction by non-invasive imaging: a review of the literature. *Eur Heart J Cardiovasc Imaging.* (2014) 15:119–29. doi: 10.1093/ehjci/jet127
13. Dangas GD, Weitz JI, Giustino G, Makkar R, Mehran R. Prosthetic heart valve thrombosis. *J Am Coll Cardiol.* (2016) 68:2670–89. doi: 10.1016/j.jacc.2016.09.958
14. Separham A, Ghaffari S, Aslanabadi N, Sohrabi B, Ghojazadeh M, Anamzadeh E, et al. Prosthetic valve thrombosis. *J Card Surg.* (2015) 30:246–50. doi: 10.1111/jocs.12510
15. Fukunaga N, Miyakoshi C, Sakata R, Koyama T. Impact of valve type on outcomes after redo mitral valve replacement in patients aged 50 to 69 years. *Interact Cardiovasc Thorac Surg.* (2018) 27:322–7. doi: 10.1093/icvts/ivy109
16. Park B, Sung K, Park PW. Clinical implication of transaortic mitral pannus removal during repeat cardiac surgery for patients with mechanical mitral valve. *Circ J.* (2018) 82:396–402. doi: 10.1253/circj.CJ-17-0463
17. Huang G, Schaff HV, Sundt TM, Rahimtoola SH. Treatment of obstructive thrombosed prosthetic heart valve. *J Am Coll Cardiol.* (2013) 62:1731–6. doi: 10.1016/j.jacc.2013.07.075
18. Said SM, Schaff HV, Greason KL, Pochettino A, Daly RC, Dearani JA. Reoperation for mitral paravalvular leak: a single-centre experience with 200 patients. *Interact Cardiovasc Thorac Surg.* (2017) 25:806–12. doi: 10.1093/icvts/ivx222
19. Mehaffey HJ, Hawkins RB, Schubert S, FonnerC, Yarboro LT, Quader M, et al. Contemporary outcomes in reoperative mitral valve surgery. *Heart.* (2018) 104:652–6. doi: 10.1136/heartjnl-2017-312047
20. Hwang HY, Choi JW, Kim HK, Kim KH, Kim KB, Ahn H. Paravalvular leak after mitral valve replacement: 20-year follow-up. *Ann Thorac Surg.* (2015) 100:1347–52. doi: 10.1016/j.athoracsur.2015.03.104
21. Fukunaga N, Sakata R, Koyama T. Short- and long-term outcomes following redo valvular surgery. *J Card Surg.* (2018) 33:56–63. doi: 10.1111/jocs.13534
22. Raman K, Mohanraj A, Palanisamy V, Ganesh J, Rawal S, Kurian VM, et al. Thrombolysis and surgery for mitral prosthetic valve thrombosis: 11-year outcomes. *Asian Cardiovasc Thorac Ann.* (2019) 27:633–40. doi: 10.1177/0218492319878015
23. Park PW, Park B, Jeong DS, Sung K, Kim WS, Lee YT, et al. Clinical outcomes of repeat aortic valve replacement for subaortic pannus in mechanical aortic valve. *Circ J.* (2018) 82:2535–41. doi: 10.1253/circj.CJ-18-0352

# 7

# Effects of Transapical Transcatheter Mitral Valve Implantation

*Ming-Chon Hsiung*[1], *Wei-Hsian Yin*[1,2], *Yung-Tsai Lee*[1,3], *Tien-Ping Tsao*[1,4], *Kuo-Chen Lee*[1,4], *Kuan-Chih Huang*[1], *Pei-En Chen*[5,6], *Wei-Hsuan Chiang*[1], *Tao-Hsin Tung*[7] *and Jeng Wei*[1,4*]

[1] *Heart Center, Cheng Hsin General Hospital, Taipei, Taiwan,* [2] *Faculty of Medicine, National Yang Ming University, Taipei, Taiwan,* [3] *School of Medicine, Institute of Microbiology and Immunology, National Yang Ming University, Taipei, Taiwan,* [4] *Faculty of Medicine, National Defense Medical Center, Taipei, Taiwan,* [5] *Institute of Health Policy and Management, National Taiwan University, Taipei, Taiwan,* [6] *Taiwan Association of Health Industry Management and Development, Taipei, Taiwan,* [7] *Department of Medical Research and Education, Cheng Hsin General Hospital, Taipei, Taiwan*

***Correspondence:***
*Jeng Wei*
*jengwei@mac.com*

**Purpose:** In this study, transapical transcatheter mitral valve-in-valve implantation (TAMVI) was compared with surgical redo mitral valve replacement (SRMVR) in terms of clinical outcomes.

**Methods:** We retrospectively identified patients with degenerated mitral bioprosthesis or failed annuloplasty rings who underwent redo SRMVR or TAMVI at our medical center. Clinical outcomes were based on echocardiography results.

**Results:** We retrospectively identified patients with symptomatic mitral bioprosthetic valve dysfunction ($n = 58$) and failed annuloplasty rings ($n = 14$) who underwent redo SRMVR ($n = 36$) or TAMVI ($n = 36$). The Society of Thoracic Surgeons Predicted Risk of Mortality scores were higher in the TAMVI group (median: 9.52) than in the SRMVR group (median: 5.59) ($p$-value = 0.02). TAMVI patients were more severe in New York Heart Association ($p$-value = 0.04). The total procedure time (skin to skin) and length of stay after procedures were significantly shorter in the TAMVI group, and no significant difference in mortality was noted after adjustment for confounding factors ($p$-value = 0.11). The overall mean mitral valve pressure gradient was lower in the TAMVI group than in the SRMVR group at 24 months ($p < 0.01$). Both groups presented a decrease in the severity of mitral and tricuspid regurgitation at 3–24 months.

**Conclusions:** In conclusion, the statistical analysis is still not robust enough to make a claim that TAMVI is an appropriate alternative. The outcome of the patient appears only to be related to the patient's pre-operative STS score. Additional multi-center, longitudinal studies are warranted to adequately assess the effect of TAMVI.

**Keywords: mitral valve implantation, surgical redo mitral valve replacement, cardiac surgery, heart surgery, cardiovascular**

## INTRODUCTION

Over the past two decades, transcatheter aortic valve implantation (TAVI) has been established as a viable alternative treatment to deal with severe aortic stenosis in patients at risk of open-heart surgery. This procedure has also been extended to patients facing low-to-intermediate operative risk. This shift has been prompted by recent studies suggesting that TAVI provides survival benefits for high-risk and intermediate-risk patients (1). Mitral valve disease is the most common valvular disease in developed countries. There has been a notable shift away from mechanical valves toward bioprosthesis valves, despite their finite longevity. Recurrent mitral regurgitation (MR) is frequently encountered after mitral valve repair, particularly in cases of ischemic MR (2). However, reoperation imposes high risks among the aged and those with multiple comorbidities. Transapical transcatheter mitral valve-in-valve implantation (TAMVI) is now regarded as a promising alternative treatment for patients with degenerated bioprosthesis or failed annuloplasty (3). Most cases of TAMVI were reported in large registry and were done in some referral centers. The surgery was only reported with limited cases in Asian patients (4, 5). There have been a relatively small number of reports pertaining to the clinical outcomes and echocardiographic findings following TAMVI or surgical redo mitral valve replacement (SRMVR) for degenerated bioprosthetic valve or failed annuloplasty rings. In this study, we sought to determine whether TAMVI could achieve outcomes on par with those of SRMVR at 3, 6, 12, and 24 months after the procedure in terms of mortality rates and echocardiographic findings.

# METHODS AND MATERIALS

## Study Subjects and Data Collections

We retrospectively identified patients who underwent SRMVR or TAMVI for degenerated mitral bioprosthesis or failed annuloplasty rings at our medical center between 1998 and July 2018. Note that the TAMVI procedure was not performed until 2014 (**Figure 1**). In the SRMVR group, myocardial protection was achieved via aortic clamping and antegrade cardioplegia. The left atrium was approached via Waterson's groove or trans-septal (in cases where tricuspid intervention was required). Following replacement, the left atrium was closed and warmed cardioplegia was delivered prior to removal of the aortic cross clamp. Once the heart started beating and all vital signs were satisfactory, cardio pulmonary bypass (CPB) was weaned off and the sternum was closed. In the TAMVI group, all procedures were conducted using the transapical approach. All procedures were performed using general anesthesia under 2D and 3D trans-esophageal echocardiography guidance (TEE). The left ventricle apex was guided via Transthoracic Echo and agitated normal saline (2 cc) was injected into the left ventricle using a fine needle, whereupon a left anterior thoracotomy was performed through the fifth or sixth intercostal space. A guidewire was advanced through two 3-0 polypropylene purse string surfaces reinforced with Teflon pledget, across the malfunctioning bioprosthesis into the pulmonary vein. This procedure was performed solely under 2D or 3D TEE with no iodinated contrast. A stiffer guidewire (Amplatz Extra stiff; Cook Inc., Bloomington, IN) was then introduced using a Judkins catheter for protection. An Edwards Sapien, Sapien XT, Sapien S3 (Edwards Lifesciences, Irvine, CA), or Lotus (Boston Scientific) was delivered using the standard delivery system (Ascendra, Ascendra +, Commander; Edwards Life sciences) during rapid ventricular pacing 130–180 BPM.

All of the patients included in this study had degenerated mitral bioprosthesis or failed annuloplasty rings. The treatment method was determined by a multi-disciplinary heart team in accordance with the anticipated risk and anatomical specifics of each patient. Echocardiographic parameters were reported in accordance with the guidelines defined by the American Society of Echocardiography and the Mitral Valve Academic Research Consortium (MVARC) consensus document (6–8). All transcatheter procedures were performed using a balloon-expandable transcatheter heart valve (Edward Sapien 3, XT) or heart valve (Lotus, Boston Scientific), which was manually implanted via transapical access, as previous described (9–11). The access route and valve size were based on procedural echocardiographic findings and multidetector computed tomography (MDCT). The exclusion criteria included active endocarditis, cases requiring concomitant procedures for aortic disease or coronary artery disease. We also excluded the patients with a measured new-left ventricular outflow tract area (new-LVOT) $<150$ cm$^2$ at end-systolic phase and aortic-mitral angle $<135^\circ$ (12).

Sample data included detailed clinical information on 72 patients, 36 of whom underwent TAMVI (50%) and 36 of whom underwent SRMVR with cardiopulmonary bypass (50%). Valve type was determined prior to the procedure, whereas valve size was determined during the procedure by calculation with proprietary valve size. None of the patients who needed concomitant aortic valve replacement or had prosthetic valves developed mitral valve endocarditis (in the time period).

In this study, all patient information, outcomes, and complications were derived from electronic medical records. This study was approved by the Regional Ethical Review Board and all patients provided written informed consent.

## Statistical Analysis

Continuous variables were reported as mean ± SD or median (range) and tested using a two-sample independent $t$-test or Mann-Whitney $U$ test, respectively. Categorical variables were examined using the chi-square test or fisher's exact test. A repeated measures analysis of variance and McNemar's test were performed to clarify the results of the echocardiographic findings between the SRMVR and TAMVI groups. Survival curves were analyzed using the Kaplan-Meier method and compared using the log-rank test. A two-sided $p$-value of $<0.05$ was considered statistically significant. All statistical analysis was performed using IBM SPSS statistics, version 20 (IBM, Armonk, NY).

In addition, the estimates of screening for important variables using univariable cox regression and including the significant variables is not the ideal way to approach model construction. Because subjects in the TAMVI and SRMVR groups likely differ for confounding factors and differences in outcomes could reflect differences in baseline conditions rather than a real treatment

**Abbreviations:** TAMVI, transapical transcatheter mitral valve-in-valve implantation; SRMVR, surgical redo mitral valve replacement; NYHA, New York Heart Association; MR, mitral regurgitation; CPB, cardio pulmonary bypass; TEE, trans-esophageal echocardiography; MVARC, Mitral Valve Academic Research Consortium; MDCT, multidetector computed tomography; IPTW, inverse probability of treatment weighting; LVOT, left ventricular outflow tract; TMVIR, the mitral valve in ring; MVARC, Mitral Valve Academic Research Consortium.

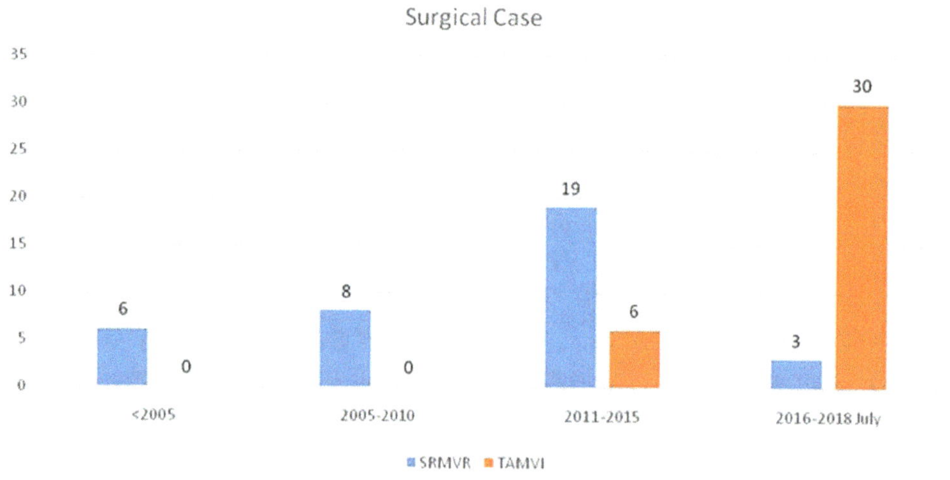


**FIGURE 1** | Change of the number of TAMVI compared with SRMVR in the study hospital ($n$ = 72).

effects, inverse probability of treatment weighting (IPTW) was used to compare the two treatments (13).

## RESULTS

In this study, a total of 72 redo mitral valve replacement patients (TAMVI: $n = 36$; SRMVR: $n = 36$) met the inclusion criteria, including patient characteristics and operative data. Study-patients TAMVI (30/36 = 83.3%) exhibited a more-pronounced proportion after 2016 than SRMVR (3/36 = 8.3%) (**Figure 1**). **Table 1** lists the baseline characteristics of the study population. The age difference is not statistically significant between patients who underwent TAMVI implantation and underwent SRMVR (65.28 ± 13.89 vs. 59.61 ± 15.92, $p = 0.11$). In addition to higher median STS Predicted Risk of Mortality scores (9.52 [range: 1.16–78.41] vs. 5.59 [range: 1.12–44.15], $p = 0.02$ for Mann-Whitney $U$ test), TAMVI patients are also more likely to have liver disease, CAD, and severe heart failure. Indications for reoperation included recurrent severe mitral regurgitation in 16 patients (22.2%), isolated mitral stenosis in 44 (61.1%), and mixed mitral regurgitation and stenosis in 12 (16.7%).

Procedural details for surgical intervention are summarized in the **Table 2**. The main proportion of replacing valve type were ST-JUDE (44.4%) and Edwards Sapien XT (63.9%) in the SRMVR and TAMVI groups, respectively. **Table 3** further indicates the comparisons of in-hospital outcomes between SRMVR and TAMVI groups. To compare the TAMVI groups, SRMVR groups had longer total procedure time (520.97 ± 85.56 min vs. 177.50 ± 115.86 min, $p < 0.001$) and longer length of stay after procedures (28.47 ± 12.15 min vs. 21.89 ± 8.60 min, $p = 0.01$). There was one case of stroke after SRMVR but no cases of stroke after TAMVI. There were no indications of left ventricular outflow tract (LVOT) obstruction in either group. There were no significant differences between the two groups in terms of bleeding or arrhythmia. In addition, the mean cardiopulmonary bypass duration was 181.97 ± 63.20 min, whereas the aortic clamp duration was 153.39 ± 66.96 min. Tricuspid valve repair was performed as a concomitant procedure in six cases and ablation for atrial fibrillation in five cases, based on the judgment of the operating surgeon.

**Table 4** indicates the no statistical significantly for the comparisons of in-hospital outcomes between the two TAVI products. As **Table 5** shows, only borderline significant was found in total ICU stay between failed annuloplasty ring and non-failed annuloplasty (12.33 ± 13.65 vs. 3.76 ± 4.43 days, $p = 0.05$ for Mann-Whitney U test). In addition, in the mitral valve in ring (TMVIR) groups, we did three patients, all patients under TAMVI implantation with two Edwards Sapien XT and one Boston Scientific Lotus valve. As shown in **Table 6**, two of these patients were event-free; however, one of the patients expired 21-day post-operation due to multiple organ failure (STS score = 73.665).

As shown in **Figures 2A–D**, hemodynamic results were deemed satisfactory based on a significant reduction in the mean pressure gradient, transmitral prosthesis gradient, and right ventricular systolic pressure for both SRMVR and TAMVI groups. The significant lower were found of these three hemodynamic results in the SRMVR groups than TAMVI groups (p-value for the repeated ANOVA < 0.001). **Figure 2E** shows that TAMVI groups had lower right ventricular ejection fraction than SRMVR groups during 24-month follow-up ($p = 0.005$).

**Figure 3** shows that the degrees of mitral regurgitation significantly regress to mild or none only after 3 months in both SRMVR (3A) ($p = 0.02$) and TAMVI (3B) ($p = 0.02$) groups. No significant changes were found based on the multiple comparisons. The disparity of tricuspis regurgitation was found between SRMVR (3C) and TAMVI (3D) groups.

As **Figure 4** shows, in the SRMVR patients, the 3-, 6-, 12-, and 24-month cumulative mortality were 2.8%. In TAMVI patients, the 3-, 6-, 12-, and 24-month cumulative mortality

**TABLE 1** | Baseline clinical characteristics between SRMVR and TAMVI groups ($n = 72$).

| | SRMVR ($n = 36$) | TAMVI ($n = 36$) | *P*-value |
|---|---|---|---|
| | Mean ± SD or *n* (%) | Mean ± SD or *n* (%) | |
| Age (years) | 59.61 ± 15.92 | 65.28 ± 13.89 | 0.11 |
| BSA ($m^2$) | 1.58 ± 0.20 | 1.57 ± 0.18 | 0.91 |
| STS score | Median: 5.59; range (1.12–44.15) | Median: 9.52; range (1.16–78.41) | 0.02 |
| Male | 13 (36.1) | 16 (44.4) | 0.63 |
| Diabetes | 7 (19.4) | 8 (22.2) | 1.00 |
| Dyslipidemia | 18 (50.0) | 15 (41.7) | 0.64 |
| AKD | 0 (0.0) | 2 (5.6) | – |
| CKD | 11 (30.6) | 8 (22.2) | 0.59 |
| H/D | 2 (5.6) | 4 (11.1) | 0.67 |
| Lung disease | 7 (19.4) | 10 (27.8) | 0.58 |
| Liver disease | 1 (2.8) | 6 (16.7) | 0.11 |
| CVA | 2 (5.6) | 6 (16.7) | 0.26 |
| CAD | 6 (16.7) | 16 (44.4) | 0.02 |
| PVD | 1 (2.8) | 2 (5.6) | 1.00 |
| Endocarditis history | 7 (19.4) | 4 (11.1) | 0.51 |
| Old MI | 1 (2.8) | 0 (0.0) | – |
| PCI | 2 (5.6) | 6 (16.7) | 0.26 |
| CABG | 3 (8.3) | 8 (22.2) | 0.19 |
| AF | 17 (47.2) | 20 (55.6) | 0.64 |
| PPM | 3 (8.3) | 5 (13.9) | 0.71 |
| LA thrombus | 4 (11.1) | 2 (5.6) | 0.67 |
| Arrhythmia | 9 (25.0) | 4 (11.1) | 1.00 |
| AKD + H/D | 1 (2.8) | 1 (2.8) | 1.00 |
| Indications | | | 0.17 |
| Mitral regurgitation | 6 (16.7) | 10 (27.8) | |
| Isolated mitral stenosis | 26 (72.2) | 18 (50.0) | |
| Mixed mitral regurgitation and stenosis | 4 (11.1) | 8 (22.2) | |
| NYHA | | | 0.04 |
| 2 | 12 (33.3) | 6 (16.7) | |
| 3 | 19 (52.8) | 16 (44.4) | |
| 4 | 5 (13.9) | 14 (38.9) | |
| Previous MV replacement | 25 (69.4) | 33 (91.7) | 0.04 |
| Previous MV repair | 11 (30.6) | 3 (8.3) | 0.04 |
| Previous AV replacement | 5 (13.9) | 10 (28.6) | 0.16 |
| Previous TV repair | 14 (38.9) | 17 (48.6) | 0.48 |

*BSA, body surface area; STS, society of thoracic surgeons; AKD, acute kidney disease; CKD, chronic kidney disease; H/D, hemodialysis; CVA, cerebrovascular accident; CAD, coronary artery disease; PVD, peripheral artery disease; MI, myocardial infarction; PCI, percutaneous coronary intervention; CABG, coronary artery bypass graft; AF, atrial fibrillation; PPM, permanent pacemaker; LA, left atrium; NYHA, New York Heart Association; MV, mitral valve; AV, aortic valve; TV, tricuspid valve.*

were 5.6, 5.6, 9.8, and 21.9%, respectively. The statistical significance ($p = 0.038$) of procedure difference was found for cumulative survival.

**TABLE 2** | Procedure details in SRMVR or TAMVI approaches.

| SRMVR | *n* (%) |
|---|---|
| **APPROACH** | |
| Median sternotomy | 36 (100.0) |
| **REPLACING VALVE TYPE** | |
| Edwards Sapien | 10 (27.8) |
| ST-JUDE | 16 (44.4) |
| ON-X | 5 (13.9) |
| Medtronic-Hancock | 2 (5.6) |
| SORIN BICARBON | 1 (2.8) |
| C-E perimount magna mitral ease | 1 (2.8) |
| Mosaic tissue valve | 1 (2.8) |
| **CONCOMITANT SURGICAL PROCEDURES** | |
| Tricuspid valve repair | 6 (16.7) |
| Ablation for atrial fibrillation | 5 (13.9) |
| **TAMVI** | ***n* (%)** |
| **APPROACH** | |
| Transapical | 36 (100.0) |
| **REPLACING VALVE TYPE** | |
| Edwards Sapien | 6 (16.7) |
| Edwards Sapien XT | 23 (63.9) |
| Boston Scientific Lotus | 7 (19.4) |

The effect of independently associated risk factors upon all-cause mortality among patients after SRMVR or TAMVI surgery was examined using the multiple Cox regression models. As is depicted in **Table 7**, subsequent to adjustment for confounding factors and IPTW, STS score (Hazard ratio = 1.05, 95%CI: 1.01–1.09) appeared to be statistically significantly related to all-cause mortality.

# DISCUSSION

## Clinical Implications

Surgical valve replacement is the gold standard for patients with mitral valve disease or bioprosthesis failure. Nonetheless, recurrent MR is frequently encountered after mitral valve repair, particularly in the setting of functional MR (3). For most individuals, intervention provides functional improvement and increased survival exceeding that of clinical treatment (2, 14). However, many patients (particularly those with comorbidities) require reoperation, which brings with it an elevated risk of surgery-related complications (15–17). Since its introduction in 2009, transcatheter mitral valve-in-valve implantation has been increasingly adopted for the treatment of patients with malfunctioning bioprosthesis (18). Currently, there is a lack of data pertaining to TAMVI, and no direct comparison of TAMVI and SRMVR has been published in Asia. One study reported on 62 patients who underwent TAMVI and 59 patients who underwent SRMVR in three medical centers. They reported no difference between the two groups in terms of mortality at 12-month (19). Our results suggest that TAMVI could achieve results comparable to those of SRMVR in terms of 24-month all

**TABLE 3** | The comparisons of in-hospital outcomes between SRMVR and TAMVI groups ($n = 72$).

| | SRMVR ($n = 36$) | TAMVI ($n = 36$) | *P*-value |
|---|---|---|---|
| | Mean ± SD or *n* (%) | Mean ± SD or *n* (%) | |
| Replacing valve inner diameter (mm) | 28.17 ± 1.88 | 27.92 ± 1.52 | 0.54 |
| Urgent procedure | 7 (19.4) | 2 (5.6) | 0.08 |
| Total procedure time (min) | 520.97 ± 85.56 | 177.50 ± 115.86 | <0.001 |
| CPB time (min) | 181.97 ± 63.20 | – | – |
| Cross-clamp time (min) | 153.39 ± 66.96 | – | – |
| Fluoroscopy time (min) | – | 10.00 ± 2.00 | – |
| Amount of contrast (ml) | – | 0.00 | – |
| IABP utilization (intra-/post-procedure) | 3 (8.3) | 0 (0.0) | 1.00 |
| Total ICU stay (days) | 6.56 ± 5.47 | 4.47 ± 5.86 | 0.12 |
| Length of stay after procedures (days) | 28.47 ± 12.15 | 21.89 ± 8.60 | 0.01 |
| Delayed LV apical pseudoaneurysm | 0 (0.0) | 1 (2.8) | 1.00 |
| **CLINICAL OUTCOMES** | | | |
| Post-PPM | 2 (5.6) | 1 (2.8) | 0.23 |
| In-hospital death | 1 (2.8) | 0 (0.0) | 1.00 |
| Minor complication | 2 (5.6) | 0 (0.0) | 1.00 |
| Bleeding complication | 3 (8.3) | 1 (2.8) | 0.30 |
| Stroke | 1 (2.8) | 0 (0.0) | – |
| Arrhythmia | 9 (25.0) | 4 (11.1) | 0.13 |
| LVOT obstruction | 0 (0.0) | 0 (0.0) | – |

*PPM, permanent pacemaker.*

**TABLE 4** | The comparisons of in-hospital outcomes between the two TAVI products ($n = 36$).

| | Boston Scientific Lotus ($n = 7$) | Edward Sapien ($n = 29$) | *P*-value |
|---|---|---|---|
| | Mean ± SD or *n* (%) | Mean ± SD or *n* (%) | |
| Replacing valve inner diameter (mm) | 27.29 ± 0.76 | 34.97 ± 37.35 | 0.17 |
| Total procedure time (min) | 155.71 ± 52.08 | 182.76 ± 126.69 | 0.70 |
| Total ICU stay (days) | 2.57 ± 2.37 | 4.93 ± 6.38 | 0.14 |
| Length of stay after procedures (days) | 25.71 ± 6.60 | 20.97 ± 8.86 | 0.06 |
| **CLINICAL OUTCOMES** | | | |
| Post-PPM | 0 (0) | 5 (17.2) | – |
| Bleeding complication | 0 (0) | 1 (3.4) | – |
| Arrhythmia | 0 (0) | 4 (13.8) | – |

*PPM, permanent pacemaker.*

**TABLE 5** | The results for value in ring compare to valve in prosthesis ($n = 36$).

| | Failed annuloplasty ring ($n = 3$) | Non-failed annuloplasty ($n = 33$) | *P*-value |
|---|---|---|---|
| | Mean ± SD or *n* (%) | Mean ± SD or *n* (%) | |
| Replacing valve inner diameter (mm) | 27.00 ± 1.73 | 34.06 ± 35.03 | 0.27 |
| Total procedure time (min) | 148.33 ± 42.53 | 180.15 ± 120.34 | 0.91 |
| Total ICU stay (days) | 12.33 ± 13.65 | 3.76 ± 4.43 | 0.05 |
| Length of stay after procedures (days) | 24.67 ± 8.51 | 21.64 ± 8.69 | 0.51 |
| **CLINICAL OUTCOMES** | | | |
| Post-PPM | 0 (0.0) | 5 (15.2) | – |
| Bleeding complication | 1 (33.3) | 0 (0.0) | – |
| Arrhythmia | 0 (0.0) | 4 (12.1) | – |

*PPM, permanent pacemaker.*

causes mortality due to this procedure introduces less surgical trauma and is less invasive (20, 21). Patients with poor left ventricular function were usually precluded SRMVR. Patients received SRMVR have higher risks of post-operative bleeding, longer ventilator usage time, and longer hospital stay (22, 23).

We acknowledge that our findings will have to be confirmed in subsequent research with a larger study population over a longer follow-up period. Note that our findings are also limited by the fact that the mean age in TAMVI group was not higher than in SRMVR group ($p = 0.11$), but the STS Predicted Risk of Mortality scores were higher. Note also that the SRMVR cohort included patients over a far longer period of time (from 1998 to July 2018). Since its introduction, the TAMVI technique has evolved in terms of planning (valve apps, MDCT and 2D, 3D echocardiography) and approach (from transapical), such that the procedure has become more effective, less invasive, and safer. Thus, our overall results may be influenced by difficulties experienced shortly after adoption; however, we were unable to excise the early cases due to the small number of patients in our sample.

Previous evidence-based studies reported mean gradient after TAMVI were 11.3 ± 5.2 to 5.5 ± 3.6 mmHg, 14.0 ± 6.5 to 4.7 ± 3.1 mmHg, and 6.3 ± 2.9 (immediate) to 7.3 ± 2.5 mmHg after 70, 130 days, and 1 year, respectively. The findings were consistent with our TAMVI results at 3 months from 11.64 ± 5.98 to 6.29 ± 1.80 mmHg at 3-month, 6.43 ± 1.91 mmHg at 24-month. This noted that the mean gradient after SRMVR includes mechanical and bioprosthetic valves (24–28). In addition, our results suggest that an elevated post-procedural mean gradient can still be a limitation after a transcatheter valve-in-valve procedure in both the aortic and mitral positions, but new techniques, such as transcatheter bioprosthetic valve fracture during TAMVI maybe a solution for patients with a small bioprosthetic valve (29–31).

**TABLE 6 |** The details of patients with failed annuloplasty rings ($n = 3$).

| No | Age | Valve type | Baseline STS score | Baseline NYHA class | No. of prior thoracotomies | Comorbidities | Clinical outcomes |
|---|---|---|---|---|---|---|---|
| 1 | 72 | Boston Scientific Lotus | 14.24 | IV | 1 | History of mitral valve repaired, HTN, dyslipidemia, CKD, CAD, PCI, AF | Alive |
| 2 | 81 | Edwards Sapien XT | 73.67 | IV | 1 | History of mitral valve repaired, CKD, H/D, lung disease, CAD, PCI, CABG, PPM, bleeding complication | Expired (21days) |
| 3 | 64 | Edwards Sapien XT | 5.25 | III | 1 | History of Mitral Valve Repaired, HTN, CAD, AF | Alive |

*HYN, hypertension; CKD, chronic kidney disease; CAD, coronary artery disease; PCI, percutaneous coronary intervention; AF, atrial fibrillation; H/D, hemodialysis; CABG, coronary artery bypass graft; PPM, permanent pacemaker; STS, society of thoracic surgeons; NYHA, New York Heart Association.*

There is always a risk of left ventricular outflow tract obstruction after TAMVI or SRMVR, due to interference from the surgical implant/TAMVI frame or paradoxical septal motion in patients with right ventricular volume overload following surgery. None of the patients in the current study presented LVOT obstruction after TAMVI (0%), most likely due to pre-procedural planning using 2D and 3D TEE and MDCT (32, 33).

The original idea for valve-in-ring procedures was proposed by Wilbring et al. (34). The most recent series was published by Urena et al. in which 30 Edward Sapien XT and Sapien 3 valves were implanted (35). Post-operative echocardiography results revealed hemodynamic outcomes. Note that valve sizing (and particularly determining the inner diameter) is essential to the success of valve-in-ring procedures; however, it remains the most challenging aspect of the procedure. We used the ring area provided by the manufacturer to estimate the internal diameter, under the assumption that the ring area and circumference would remain constant even after TAMVI implantation. Unfortunately, annuloplasty rings are semi-rigid, and a TAMVI is not capable of reshaping after implantation. Surprisingly, these gaps appear not to have any effect in implantations in terms of paravalvular leakage. We assume that surrounding valvular tissue or pannus formation seal these gaps. All valve-in-ring procedures in our series produced excellent hemodynamic results with good prosthesis function.

Concomitant surgical tricuspid repair is recommended for patients with more than mild tricuspid regurgitation at the time of mitral valve surgery, due to the fact that it does not increase the risk of operative mortality (36–38). Nonetheless, its effect on clinical long-term outcome remains an issue of controversy, despite acute echocardiographic improvement (39–41). Interestingly, in this study, for all SRMVR and TAMVI patients who did not undergo any tricuspid procedures (22 vs. 19), reductions of TR were similar (**Figure 4**) in 12-month mortality.

There are only limited cases in valve-in-ring, and mostly done by complete ring. The sizing guidance is according to the mitral VIV app developed by Bapat et al. incorporation with the technology company UBQO (42). We also performed the bench test according to the sizing chart of the app. Usually, oversizing 20% of the correspondent valve area by overfilling the balloon was done. All these valve-in-ring cases received surgical complete ring (case1: Edwards classic ring; case 2: Edwards Physio I ring; case 3: Sorin Memo 3D). In our bench test, the Edwards classic and Physio ring could be fitted by oversizing the implanted valve. However, Sorin Memo 3D remained some paravalvular space and resulted in paravalvular leakage.

Yoon et al. Reported in the TMVR registry only 80–90% success with relative lower success in the valve in ring group than our results (2). There are several important issues to success in our series. First, patients received pre-operative 4-D MSCT. The neo-LVOT, especially in mitral-valve-ring, was analyzed before surgery. If the neo-LVOT is <30% of original LVOT, we suggested patients should receive redo-surgery. Second, we performed all procedures from transapical access. We belief transapical access providing better coaxiality than trans-septal access. Besides, there are several cases received mitral procedure from trans-septal approach and bi-atrial approaches during first open heart surgery. It makes mitral valve-in-valve and valve-in-ring procedures from trans-septal approach more difficult. Currently, the procedure time of transapical mitral valve-in-valve and valve-in-ring procedures was <3 h. And there was only one case with apical pseudoaneurysm formation. Third, all patients received general anesthesia and transesophageal echocardiography. We belief additional TEE image providing neo-LVOT size and gradient. And also TEE monitoring the depth of the devices and prevent left atrial or left ventricle embolization.

We had a 58-year-old male patient who underwent TAMVI with a 26 mm Sapien 3 valve. After discharge, he remained symptom-free for a period of 3 weeks, at which point he began complaining of shortness of breath. Echocardiographic analysis revealed a large pseudoaneurysm in the left ventricular apex region. The patient subsequently underwent transcatheter closure of the pseudoaneurysm using an 18 mm Amplatzer atrial septal defect occluder (St. Jude Medical). As results indicated in previous mitral transcatheter studies, prescribing warfarin may prevent early valve thrombosis; however, there is no clear evidence to prevent the pseudoaneurysm in patients (25, 33). The Coumadin was routinely prescript in valve-in-valve,

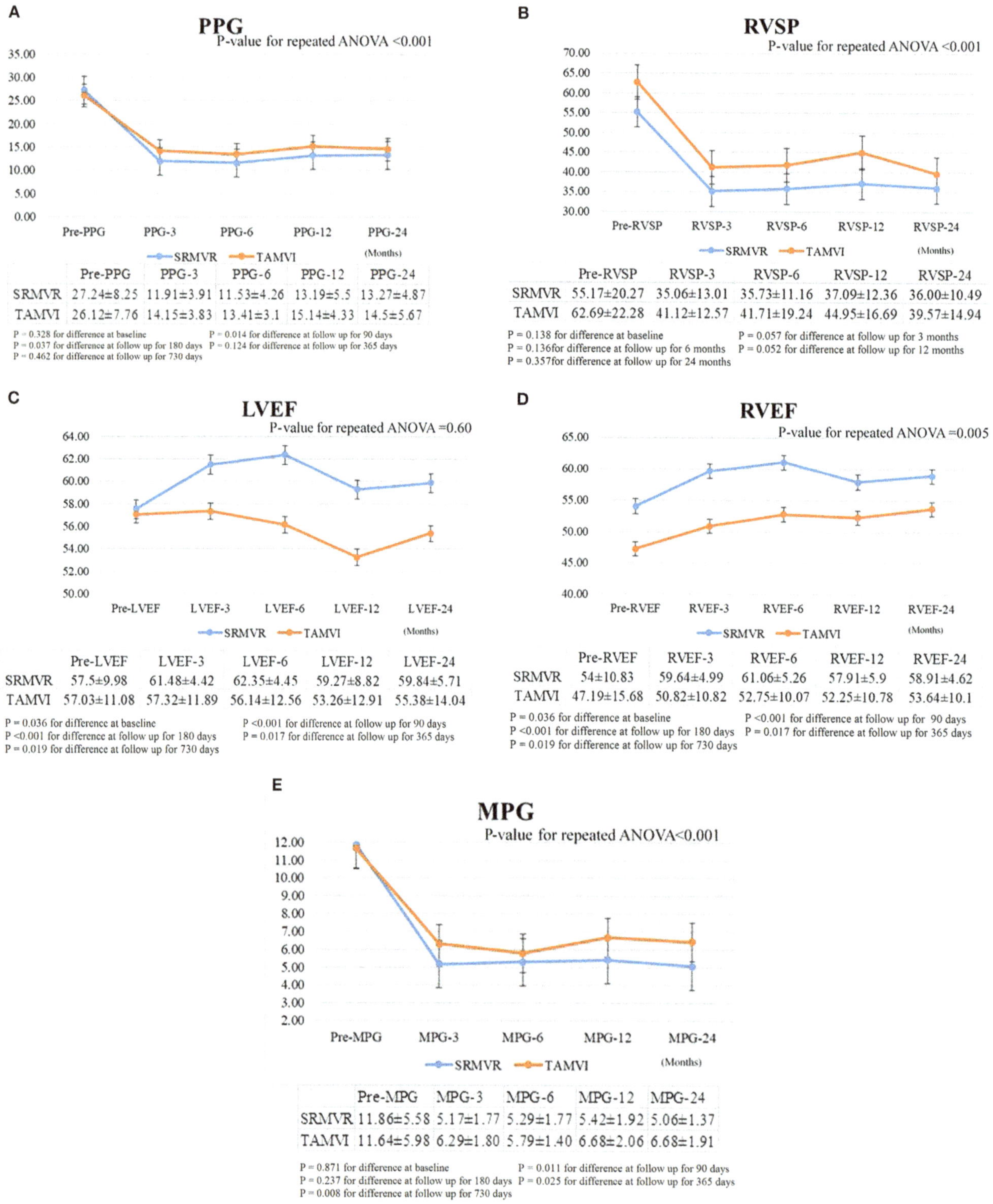


**FIGURE 2 |** The comparison of mean pressure gradient (MPG) **(A)**, transmitral prosthesis gradient (PPG) **(B)**, right ventricular systolic pressure (RVSP) **(C)**, left ventricular ejection fraction (LVEF) **(D)**, right ventricular ejection fraction (RVEF) **(E)** between surgical redo mitral valve replacement (SRMVR) and transapical transcatheter mitral valve-in-valve implantation (TAMVI) ($n = 72$).

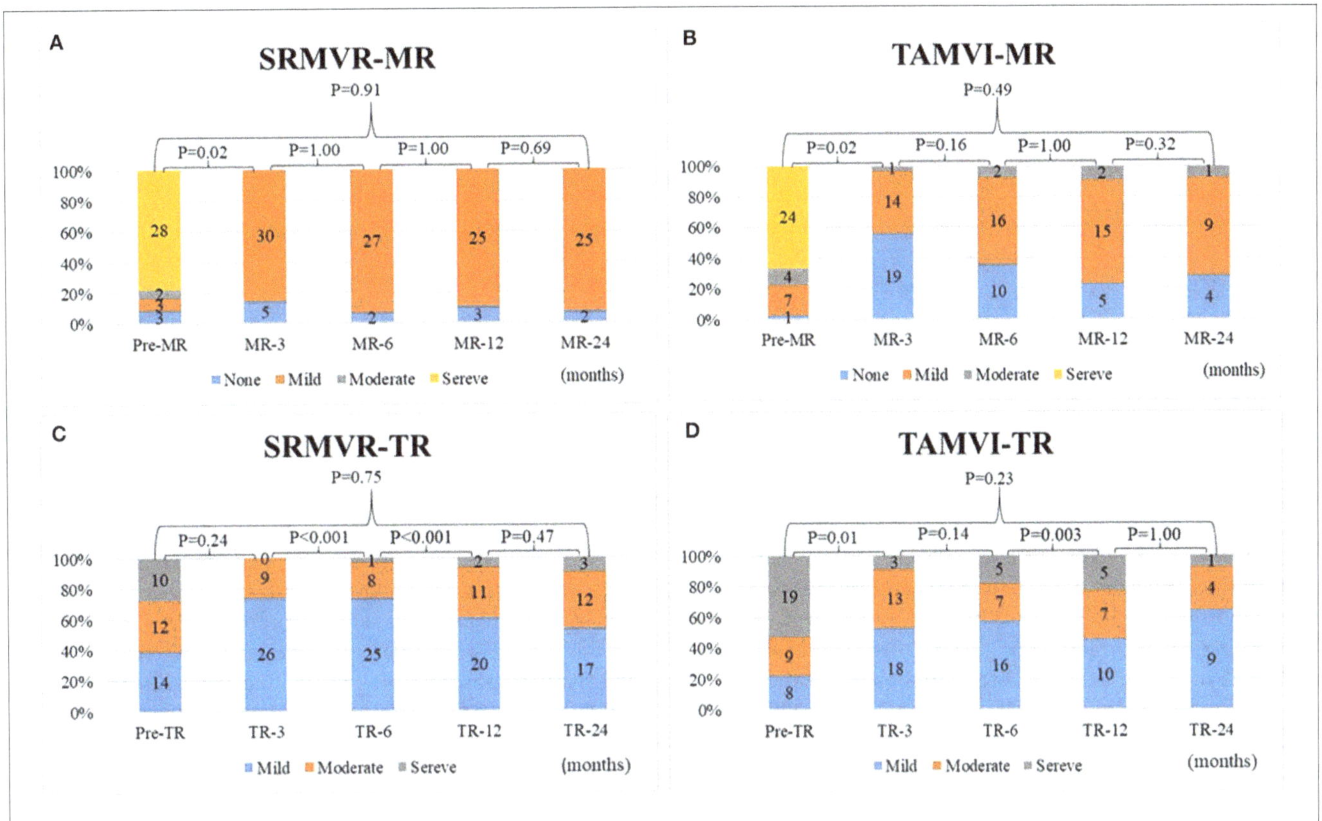


**FIGURE 3 |** The comparison of degrees of mitral regurgitation **(A,B)** and tricuspid regurgitation **(C,D)** in surgical redo mitral valve replacement (SRMVR) and transapical transcatheter mitral valve-in-valve implantation (TAMVI) (*n* = 72).

valve-in-ring, and valve-in-calcification cases. When patients have bleeding problems, the coumadin was stopped and used antiplatelets only. We believe anticoagulation was indicated in these cases due to most of these cases have atrial fibrillation. In additional to these reasons, trans-mitral blood flow is lower and higher residual trans-mitral pressure gradient in these cases.

In addition, **Figures 3A,B** indicates that vast majority of patients after surgical redo MVR appear to have mild regurgitation. The implanted Edwards mitral pericardial valve tend to have mild central valvular regurgitation. In our observation and literatures, this mild regurgitation did not have effect on short-term and long-term outcome (43, 44). We also found the Edwards Sapien valve has the same regurgitation esp. in previous generation of Sapien XT (45). This implies that the central regurgitation is a common finding related to Edwards bovine pericardial valve and does not effect short- and long-term durability of this bioprosthesis.

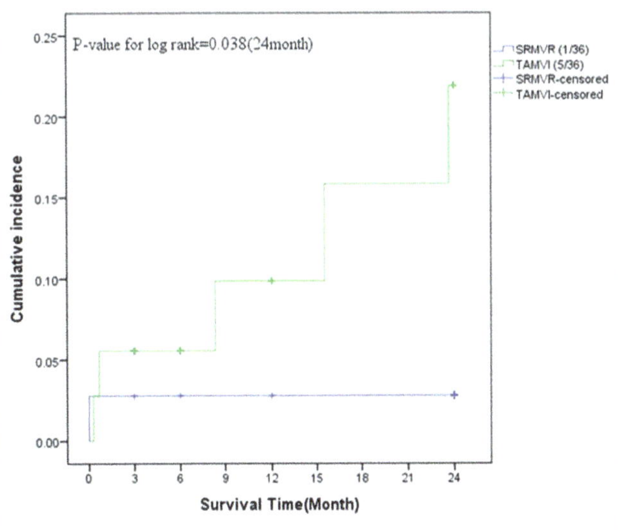


**FIGURE 4 |** The survival analysis between surgical redo mitral valve replacement (SRMVR) and transapical transcatheter mitral valve-in-valve implantation (TAMVI) (*n* = 72).

## Study Limitations

Although the main strength was that we tried to accommodate inherent selection biases with IPTW, the primary limitation of this study was the small number of patients, which may have limited the power to detect significant differences. The decision of whether to adopt TAMVI or SRMVR was made by the heart team in conjunction with the patient. It is likely that this approach introduced bias that could affect outcomes. We made our comparison as homogeneous as possible. However, there are still some differences that may influence the outcomes, including the incidence of new arrhythmias or other side-effects. Second,

**TABLE 7 |** Multivariate analysis using Cox regression model of risk factors associated with the all-cause mortality after adjustment for inverse probability of treatment weighting (IPTW) among patients with SRMVR or TAMVI surgery ($n = 72$).

| Variables | All causes of death (yes vs. no) | | | | |
|---|---|---|---|---|---|
| | β | SE | *P*-value | Hazard ratio | 95% confidence interval |
| STS score | 0.05 | 0.02 | 0.01 | 1.05 | 1.01–1.09 |
| Operation (TAMVI vs. SRMVR) | 2.91 | 1.74 | 0.09 | 18.41 | 0.61–553.92 |
| Procedure time | 0.004 | 0.003 | 0.21 | 1.004 | 0.998–1.011 |
| IPTW | 0.07 | 0.25 | 0.78 | 1.07 | 0.65–1.77 |

our inability to collect details related to the initial SRMVR procedures (many files were missing) may have affected the echocardiographic results and clinical outcomes. Third, fewer SRMVR patients underwent echocardiographic examinations at the time of discharge or during follow-up. The fact that we included patients who underwent SRMVR prior to the advent of TAMVI (80% of SRMVR procedures were performed between 1998 and 2013) meant that we had access to far more follow-up information for SRMVR patients than TAMVI patients. Finally, the perioperative mortality associated with redo mitral surgery is relatively lower than the reiterative mortality seen in the state of New York and Virginia (46, 47). The TAMVI mortality is also lower than that reported by Yoon et al. from the TMVR registry (2). Further long-term studies with a larger number of patients will be required to accurately assess the efficacy of TAMVI.

## CONCLUSIONS

In conclusion, this is a retrospective cohort study from Taiwan examining SRMVR in comparison with TAMVI. Transcatheter techniques will play a large role in the management of SVD in the future with the rapid increase in the use of bioprosthetic valves in younger and younger patients. The statistical analysis is still not robust enough to make a claim that TAMVI is an appropriate alternative. The outcome of the patient appears only to be related to the patient's pre-operative STS score. Equivalence has not been demonstrated, as a non-inferiority study would be required for such a claim to be made. The most that might be able to be said is that at our institution TAMVI has been a viable alternative in patients with adequate access and appropriate LVOT dimensions. For this reason, accumulating single institution reports are an important piece of the overall puzzle that will necessarily include larger scale examinations.

## AUTHOR CONTRIBUTIONS

M-CH, W-HY, P-EC, T-HT, and JW conducted the study and drafted the manuscript. M-CH, P-EC, and T-HT participated in the design of the study and performed statistical analyses. Y-TL, T-PT, K-CL, K-CH, and W-HC conceived the study and participated in its design and coordination. All authors read and approved the final manuscript.

## REFERENCES


1. Spaccarotella C, Mongiardo A, De Rosa S, Indolfi C. Transcatheter aortic valve implantation in patients at intermediate surgical risk. *Int J Cardiol.* (2017) 243:161–8. doi: 10.1016/j.ijcard.2017.04.107
2. Yoon SH, Whisenant BK, Bleiziffer S, Delgado V, Dhoble A, Schofer N, et al. Outcomes of transcatheter mitral valve replacement for degenerated bioprostheses, failed annuloplasty rings, and mitral annular calcification. *Eur Heart J.* (2019) 40:441–51. doi: 10.1093/eurheartj/ehy590
3. Goldstein D, Moskowitz AJ, Gelijns AC, Ailawadi G, Parides MK, Perrault LP, et al. Two-year outcomes of surgical treatment of severe ischemic mitral regurgitation. *N Engl J Med.* (2016) 374:344–53. doi: 10.1056/NEJMoa1512913
4. Whisenant B, Kapadia SR, Eleid MF, Kodali SK, McCabe JM, Krishnaswamy A, et al. One-year outcomes of mitral valve-in-valve using the SAPIEN 3 transcatheter heart valve. *JAMA Cardiol.* (2020) 5:1245–52. doi: 10.1001/jamacardio.2020.2974
5. Urena M, Vahanian A, Brochet E, Ducrocq G, Iung B, Himbert D. Current indications for transcatheter mitral valve replacement using transcatheter aortic valves: valve-in-valve, valve-in-ring, and valve-in-mitral annulus calcification. *Circulation.* (2021) 143:178–96. doi: 10.1161/CIRCULATIONAHA.120.048147
6. Lang RM, Badano LP, Mor-Avi V, Afilalo J, Armstrong A, Ernande L, et al. Recommendations for cardiac chamber quantification by echocardiography in adults: an update from the American Society of echocardiography and the European Association of Cardiovascular Imaging. *Eur Heart J Cardiovasc Imaging.* (2015) 16:233–70. doi: 10.1093/ehjci/jev014
7. Stone GW, Vahanian AS, Adams DH, Abraham WT, Borer JS, Bax JJ, et al. Clinical trial design principles and endpoint definitions for transcatheter mitral valve repair and replacement: part 1: clinical trial design principles a consensus document from the Mitral Valve Academic Research Consortium. *J Am Coll Cardiol.* (2015) 66:278–307. doi: 10.1016/j.jacc.2015.05.046
8. Stone GW, Vahanian AS, Adams DH, Abraham WT, Borer JS, Bax JJ, et al. Clinical trial design principles and endpoint definitions for transcatheter mitral valve repair and replacement: part 2: endpoint definitions a consensus document from the Mitral Valve Academic Research Consortium. *J Am Coll Cardiol.* (2015) 66:308–21. doi: 10.1016/j.jacc.2015.05.049
9. Cerillo AG, Gasbarri T, Celi S, Murzi M, Trianni G, Ravani M, et al. Transapical transcatheter valve-in-valve implantation for failed mitral bioprostheses: gradient, symptoms, and functional status in 18 high-risk patients up to 5 years. *Ann Thorac Surg.* (2016) 102:1289–95. doi: 10.1016/j.athoracsur.2016.03.051
10. Ye J, Cheung A, Yamashita M, Wood D, Peng D, Gao M, et al. Transcatheter aortic and mitral valve-in-valve implantation for failed surgical bioprosthetic valves: an 8-year single-center experience. *JACC Cardiovasc Interv.* (2015) 8:1735–44. doi: 10.1016/j.jcin.2015.08.012
11. Wilbring M, Alexiou K, Tugtekin SM, Sill B, Hammer P, Schmidt T, et al. Transapical Transcatheter Valve-in-Valve Implantation for deteriorated mitral bioprostheses. *Ann Thorac Surg.* (2013) 95:111–7. doi: 10.1016/j.athoracsur.2012.08.004
12. Bapat V, Pirone F, Kapetanakis S, Rajani R, Niederer S. Factors influencing left ventricular outflow tract obstruction following a mitral valve-in-valve or valve-in-ring procedure, part 1. *Catheter Cardiovasc Interv.* (2015) 86:747–

60. doi: 10.1002/ccd.25928

13. Benedetto U, Head SJ, Angelini GD, Blackstone EH. Statistical primer: propensity score matching and its alternatives. *Eur J Cardiothorac Surg.* (2018) 53:1112–7. doi: 10.1093/ejcts/ezy167
14. Murzi M, Berti S, Gasbarri T, Trianni G, Maffei S, Solinas M, et al. Transapical transcatheter mitral valve-in-valve implantation versus minimally invasive surgery for failed mitral bioprostheses. *Interact Cardiovasc Thorac Surg.* (2017) 25:57–61. doi: 10.1093/icvts/ivx067
15. Barnett SD, Ad N. Surgery for aortic and mitral valve disease in the United States: a trend of change in surgical practice between 1998 and 2005. *J Thorac Cardiovasc Surg.* (2009) 137:1422–9. doi: 10.1016/j.jtcvs.2008.08.071
16. Jamieson W, Burr LH, Miyagishima RT, Janusz MT, Fradet GJ, Ling H, et al. Re-operation for bioprosthetic aortic structural failure–risk assessment. *Eur J Cardiothorac Surg.* (2003) 24:873–8. doi: 10.1016/S1010-7940(03)00566-9
17. Jones JM, O'kane H, Gladstone DJ, Sarsam MA, Campalani G, MacGowan SW, et al. Repeat heart valve surgery: risk factors for operative mortality. *J Thorac Cardiovasc Surg.* (2001) 122:913–8. doi: 10.1067/mtc.2001.116470
18. Seeburger J, Borger MA, Falk V, Passage J, Walther T, Doll N, et al. Minimally invasive mitral valve surgery after previous sternotomy: experience in 181 patients. *Ann Thorac Surg.* (2009) 87:709–14. doi: 10.1016/j.athoracsur.2008.11.053
19. Kamioka N, Babaliaros V, Morse MA, Frisoli T, Lerakis S, Iturbe JM, et al. Comparison of clinical and echocardiographic outcomes after surgical redo mitral valve replacement and transcatheter mitral valve-in-valve therapy. *JACC Cardiovasc Interv.* (2018) 11:1131–8. doi: 10.1016/j.jcin.2018.03.011
20. Dai H, Huenges K, Pokorny S, Fischer G, Cremer J, Metzner A, et al. Transcatheter mitral valve implantation: a percutaneous transapical system. *Interact Cardiovasc Thorac Surg.* (2017) 24:527–33. doi: 10.1093/icvts/ivw399
21. Bouleti C, Fassa AA, Himbert D, Brochet E, Ducrocq G, Nejjari M, et al. Transfemoral implantation of transcatheter heart valves after deterioration of mitral bioprosthesis or previous ring annuloplasty. *JACC Cardiovasc Interv.* (2015) 8:83–91. doi: 10.1016/j.jcin.2014.07.026
22. Pieri M, Belletti A, Monaco F, Pisano A, Musu M, Dalessandro V, et al. Outcome of cardiac surgery in patients with low preoperative ejection fraction. *BMC Anesthesiol.* (2016) 16:97. doi: 10.1186/s12871-016-0271-5
23. Akay TH, Gultekin B, Ozkan S, Aslim E, Uguz E, Sezgin A, et al. Mitral valve replacements in redo patients with previous mitral valve procedures: mid-term results and risk factors for survival. *J Card Surg.* (2008) 23:415–21. doi: 10.1111/j.1540-8191.2008.00630.x
24. Eleid MF, Whisenant BK, Cabalka AK, Williams MR, Nejjari M, Attias D, et al. Early outcomes of percutaneous transvenous transseptal transcatheter valve implantation in failed bioprosthetic mitral valves, ring annuloplasty, and severe mitral annular calcification. *JACC Cardiovasc Interv.* (2017) 10:1932–42. doi: 10.1016/j.jcin.2017.08.014
25. Yoon SH, Whisenant BK, Bleiziffer S, Delgado V, Schofer N, Eschenbach L, et al. Transcatheter mitral valve replacement for degenerated bioprosthetic valves and failed annuloplasty rings. *J Am Coll Cardiol.* (2017) 70:1121–31. doi: 10.1016/j.jacc.2017.07.714
26. Gallo M, Dvir D, Demertzis S, Pedrazzini G, Berdajs D, Ferrari E. Transcatheter valve-in-valve implantation for degenerated bioprosthetic aortic and mitral valves. *Expert Rev Med Dev.* (2016) 13:749–58. doi: 10.1080/17434440.2016.1207521
27. Cheung AW, Gurvitch R, Ye J, Wood D, Lichtenstein SV, Thompson C, et al. Transcatheter transapical mitral valve-in-valve implantationsfor a failed bioprosthesis: a case series. *J Thorac Cardiovasc Surg.* (2011) 141:711–5. doi: 10.1016/j.jtcvs.2010.11.026
28. Seiffert M, Conradi L, Baldus S, Schirmer J, Knap M, Blankenberg S, et al. Transcatheter mitral valve-in-valve implantation in patients with degenerated bioprostheses. *JACC Cardiovasc Interv.* (2012) 5:341 9.22. doi: 10.1016/j.jcin.2011.12.008
29. Kamioka N, Corrigan F, Iturbe JM, Caughron H, Lerakis S, Thourani V, et al. Mitral bioprosthetic valve fracture: bail-out procedure for undersized bioprosthesis during mitral valvein- valve procedure with paravalvular leak closure. *JACC Cardiovasc Interv.* (2018) 11:e21–2. doi: 10.1016/j.jcin.2017.10.047
30. Chhatriwalla AK, Allen KB, Saxon JT, Cohen DJ, Aggarwal S, Hart AJ, et al. Bioprosthetic valve fracture improves the hemodynamic results of valve-in-valve transcatheter aortic valve replacement. *Circ Cardiovasc Interv.* (2017) 10:e005216. doi: 10.1161/CIRCINTERVENTIONS.117.005216
31. Dvir D, Webb J. Mitral valve-in-valve and valve-in-ring: technical aspects and procedural outcomes. *EuroIntervention.* (2016) 12:Y93–6. doi: 10.4244/EIJV12SYA25
32. Guerrero M, Salinger M, Pursnani A, Pearson P, Lampert M, Levisay J, et al. Transseptal transcatheter mitral valve-in-valve: A step by step guide from preprocedural planning to postprocedural care. *Catheter Cardiovasc Interv.* (2018) 92:E185–96. doi: 10.1002/ccd.27128
33. Urena M, Himbert D, Brochet E, Carrasco JL, Iung B, Nataf P, et al. Transseptal transcatheter mitral valve replacement using balloon-expandable transcatheter heart valves. *JACC Cardiovasc Interv.* (2017) 10:1905–19. doi: 10.1016/j.jcin.2017.06.069
34. Wilbring M, Alexiou K, Tugtekin SM, Arzt S, Ibrahim K, Matschke K, et al. Pushing the limits—further evolutions of transcatheter valve procedures in the mitral position, including valve-in-valve, valve-in-ring, and valve-in-native-ring. *J Thorac Cardiovasc Surg.* (2014) 147:210–9. doi: 10.1016/j.jtcvs.2013.09.021
35. Urena M, Brochet E, Lecomte M, Kerneis C, Carrasco JL, Ghodbane W, et al. Clinical and haemodynamic outcomes of balloon-expandable transcatheter mitral valve implantation: a 7-year experience. *Eur Heart J.* (2018) 39:2679–89. doi: 10.1093/eurheartj/ehy271
36. Nishimura RA, Otto CM, Bonow RO, Carabello BA, Erwin JP 3rd, Guyton RA, et al. 2014 AHA/ACC guideline for the management of patients with valvular heart disease: executive summary: a report of the American College of Cardiology/American Heart Association Task Force on Practice Guidelines. *J Am Coll Cardiol.* (2014) 63:2438–88. doi: 10.1016/j.jacc.2014.02.537
37. Baumgartner H, Falk V, Bax JJ, De Bonis M, Hamm C, Holm PJ, et al. 2017 ESC/EACTS guidelines for the management of valvular heart disease. *Eur Heart J.* (2017) 38:2739–91. doi: 10.1093/eurheartj/ehx391
38. Badhwar V, Rankin JS, He M, Jacobs JP, Furnary AP, Fazzalari FL, et al. Performing concomitant tricuspid valve repair at the time of mitral valve operations is not associated with increased operative mortality. *Ann Thorac Surg.* (2017) 103:587–93. doi: 10.1016/j.athoracsur.2016.06.004
39. Chan V, Burwash IG, Lam BK, Auyeung T, Tran A, Mesana TG, et al. Clinical and echocardiographic impact of functional tricuspid regurgitation repair at the time of mitral valve replacement. *Ann Thorac Surg.* (2009) 88:1209–15. doi: 10.1016/j.athoracsur.2009.06.034
40. Im JB, Yoo DG, Kim GS, Song H, Jung SH, Choo SJ, et al. Mild-to-moderate functional tricuspid regurgitation in patients undergoing valve replacement for rheumaticmitral disease: the influence of tricuspid valve repair on clinical and echocardiographic outcomes. *Heart.* (2012) 98:24–30. doi: 10.1136/heartjnl-2011-300403
41. Bianchi G, Solinas M, Bevilacqua S, Glauber M. Which patient undergoing mitral valve surgery should also have the tricuspid repair? *Interact Cardiovasc Thorac Surg.* (2009) 9:1009–20. doi: 10.1510/icvts.2009.217570
42. Bapat V. Valve-in-valve apps: why and how they were developed and how to use them. *EuroIntervention.* (2014) 10:U44–51. doi: 10.4244/EIJV10SUA7
43. Goetze S, Brechtken J, Agler DA, Thomas JD, Sabik JF III, Jaber WA. *In vivo* short-term doppler hemodynamic profiles of 189 Carpentier-Edwards perimount pericardial bioprosthetic valves in the mitral position. *J Am Soc Echcardiogr.* (2004) 17:981–7. doi: 10.1016/j.echo.2004.05.006
44. Firstenberg MS, Morehead AJ, Thomas JD, Smedira NG, Cosgrove DM III, Marchand MA. Short-term hemodynamic performance of the mitral Carpentier-Edwards perimount pericardial valve. Carpentier-Edwards PERIMOUNT Investigators. *Ann Thorac Surg.* (2001) 71:S285–8. doi: 10.1016/S0003-4975(01)02514-0
45. Evin M, Guivier-Curien C, Rieu R, Rodés-Cabau J, Pibarot P. Mitral valve-in-valve hemodynamic performance: an *in vitro* study. *J Thorac Cardiovasc Surg.* (2016) 151:1051–59.e6. doi: 10.1016/j.jtcvs.2015.11.039

46. Chikwe J, Chiang YP, Egorova NN, Itagaki S, Adams DH. Survival and outcomes following bioprosthetic vs mechanical mitral valve replacement in patients aged 50 to 69 years. *JAMA.* (2015) 313:1435–42. doi: 10.1001/jama.2015.3164

47. Mehaffey HJ, Hawkins RB, Schubert S, Fonner C, Yarboro LT, Quader M, et al. Contemporary outcomes in reoperative mitral valve surgery. *Heart.* (2018) 104:652–6. doi: 10.1136/heartjnl-2017-312047

# 8

# Benefits and Pitfalls of the Perceval Sutureless Bioprosthesis

*Aleksander Dokollari*[1], *Basel Ramlawi*[2,3], *Gianluca Torregrossa*[2,3], *Michel Pompeu Sá*[2,3], *Serge Sicouri*[2,3], *Edvin Prifti*[4], *Sandro Gelsomino*[5,6] *and Massimo Bonacchi*[7*]

[1] St. Michael's Hospital, Toronto, ON, Canada, [2] Department of Cardiac Surgery, Lankenau Heart Institute, Wynnewood, PA, United States, [3] Department of Cardiac Surgery Research, Lankenau Institute for Medical Research, Wynnewood, PA, United States, [4] Mother Teresa Hospital, University of Tirana, Tirana, Albania, [5] Department of Cardiac Surgery, Maastricht University Medical Center, Maastricht, Netherlands, [6] Department of Cardiothoracic Surgery, Cardiovascular Research Institute Maastricht—CARIM, Maastricht, Netherlands, [7] Cardiac Surgery Unit, Department of Experimental and Clinical Medicine, University of Florence, Florence, Italy

***Correspondence:**
Massimo Bonacchi
mbonacchi@unifi.it

**Objective:** To highlight the main target points covered by clinical studies on the Perceval sutureless valve for surgical aortic valve replacement (SAVR) and raise a point of discussion for further expansion of its use when compared with stented bioprostheses (SB) and transcatheter aortic valve replacement (TAVR).

**Methods:** We reviewed clinical trials and retrospective studies published up to date and compared the outcomes in terms of mortality, myocardial infarction (MI) stroke, paravalvular leak (PVL), permanent pacemaker implantation (PPI), bleeding and long-term outcomes.

**Results:** Clinical studies showed that 30-day mortality ranged from 0–4% for Perceval and 2.9–7% for TAVR. The incidence of PVL (Perceval 1.9–19.4 vs. TAVR 9–53.5%), PPI (Perceval 2–11.2 vs. TAVR 4.9–25.5%), stroke (Perceval 0 vs. TAVR 0–2.8%), MI (Perceval 0 vs. TAVR 0–3.5%), were all higher in the TAVR group. Compared to other SB, mortality ranged from 0–6.4% for Perceval and 0–5.9% for SB. The incidence of PVR (Perceval 1–19.4 vs. SB 0–1%), PPI (Perceval 2–10.7 vs. SB 1.8–8.5%), stroke (Perceval 0–3.7 vs. SB 1.8–7.3%) and MI (Perceval 0–7.8 vs. SB 0–4.3%) were comparable among the groups. In patients with a bicuspid aortic valve, mortality rate was (0–4%) and PVL incidence was (0–2.3%). However, there was a high incidence of PPI (0–20%), and stroke (0–8%). Long-term survival ranged between 96.7–98.6%.

**Conclusions:** The Perceval bioprosthesis has proved to be a reliable prosthesis for surgical aortic valve replacement due to its implantation speed, the reduced cardiopulmonary bypass time, the reduced aortic cross-clamp time and the shorter intensive care unit and hospital length of stay.

**Keywords: benefits, pitfalls, Perceval, sutureless, review, sutureless valve replacement**

## INTRODUCTION

Surgical aortic valve replacement (SAVR) with the sutureless self-expanding Perceval aortic bioprosthesis (LivaNova Group, Milan, Italy) was developed to combine the advantages of the transcatheter aortic valve replacement (TAVR) procedure, allowing for a fast implantation with no need for suturing, with the benefits of a conventional surgical approach owing to the possibility of removing the native valve along with the calcifications. The valve has grown in popularity mostly due to the reduced cardiopulmonary bypass (CPB) time (1), the improved myocardial recovery time and its application in minimally invasive cardiac surgery (MICS) procedures (2). In addition, the three PARTNER clinical trials' (3–5), the SURTAVI trial (6) and other observational cohort studies (7, 8) have evidenced the non-inferiority of TAVR vs. SAVR. In this context, some reports of successful valve-in-valve TAVR in bioprostheses with structural valve deterioration (SVD) have generated enthusiasm particularly for future applications (9, 10). In addition, other outcomes of the valve include improved hemodynamics, a self-expanding radial force, usage in hostile roots, enhanced surgical and recovery speed, and enabling minimally invasive cardiac surgery procedures. However, many points deserve to be highlighted such as the impact of permanent pacemaker implantation (PPI) after SAVR, the application of the sutureless bioprostheses in patients with bicuspid aortic valves (BAV), the impact of thrombocytopenia on the survival rate and the implantation of this bioprostheses in patients with small aortic annuli.

The goal of this review is to highlight the main target points covered by clinical studies and raise a point of discussion for further expansion of the use of Perceval.

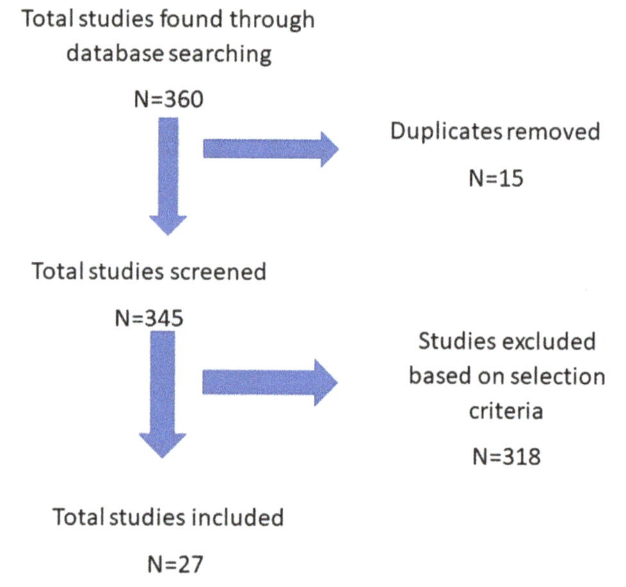


**FIGURE 1** | Flowchart study selection process.

## MATERIALS AND METHODS

### Inclusion Criteria

Studies were included if any of the following criteria were met: (1) reported outcomes of Perceval compared with other heart valve prostheses or procedures; (2) reported analysis of complications using the Perceval; (3) reported off-label experience; (4) reported learning curve analysis; (5) reported one or more case of SAVR with Perceval.

### Exclusion Criteria

Studies were excluded if any of the following criteria were met: (1) reported outcomes of exclusively other sutureless valves; (2) grouped outcomes of Perceval with other prostheses in the same cohort; (3) not published in the English language; (4) not published in a peer-reviewed journal; and (5) was a conference abstract.

### Data Collection

The data collection was done on August 31, 2021. One author (AD) screened the articles and reviewed it three times. The final results were reviewed by another investigator (MPS). The primary reported outcomes of the study included (a) the surgical technique; (b) clinical trials investigating the Perceval valve; (c) the sutureless vs. TAVR; (d) the sutureless vs. other stented bioprostheses (e) Perceval in mini-SAVR; (f) Perceval and bicuspid aortic valves; (g) long-term outcomes of the Perceval valve (valve durability); (h) the incidence of thrombocytopenia after Perceval implantation; (i) the ideal candidate for the prosthesis implantation (**Figure 1**).

## THE MOST APPROPRIATE SURGICAL TECHNIQUE FOR VALVE IMPLANTATION

The aortic incision is performed at the distal portion at the sinotubular junction to preserve a segment of ascending aorta above the prosthetic valve. The aortic valve should be excised at a position corresponding to the incision line of the native leaflets and the aortic annulus should be decalcified to prepare the implant site. A complete decalcification of the aortic annulus is not necessary. To ensure the correct positioning and orientation of the prosthesis, three guiding sutures are placed to act as reference for accurate alignment of the inflow portion of the prosthesis with the insertion plane of the native leaflets. For each valve sinus, one stitch is positioned immediately 2–3 mm below the lowest portion of the native leaflet resection line. On the prosthesis, each guiding suture is passed into a dedicated thread loop located at the midlevel of the inflow ring and aligned to the median part of the prosthetic sinuses. Once the prosthesis is connected to the three guiding suture, the release device is introduced into the aorta (11). In this context, the Perceval Livanova company recommend placing the guiding sutures 2–3 mm below the leaflet insertion line. Using this technique, Yanagawa et al. (12) found a PPI rate of 28%. Therefore, they modified the technique by placing the guiding sutures at the nadir of each cusp and not 2 to 3 mm below. After the modification, the PPI rate dropped to 0%. Nguyen et al. (13), recommend performing the transverse aortotomy ~3.5 cm above the level of the aortic annulus, and 0.5 cm above the sinotubular junction, to leave a free edge for closure of the aortotomy. In bicuspid aortic valves, the surgeon must recreate 3 nadirs that are positioned

---

**Abbreviations:** TAVR, transcatheter aortic valve replacement; CPB, cardiopulmonary bypass; PPI, permanent pacemaker implantation; BAV, bicuspid aortic valve; MI, myocardial infarction; PVL, paravalvular leak; SAVR, surgical aortic valve replacement; MS, mini-sternotomy; RAT, right anterior thoracotomy.

at ~120° to better manage the asymmetry of each cusp. To achieve this, the surgeon can use a commercial sizer with 120° markings to recreate a normal nadir. In addition, a dedicated balloon should be inserted into the prosthesis and inflated at a pressure of 4 atm for 30 sec.

## CLINICAL TRIALS

The "PERCEVAL TRIAL—Perceval S valve pilot study was performed in 30 high-risk patients who were scheduled for isolated SAVR due to severe aortic stenosis (14). This prospective analysis was undertaken at three European Centers from April 2007 to February 2008 and concentrated on perioperative and 1-year outcomes. Operative mortality was 3.3% and moderate paravalvular leak (PVL) was present in two patients. The PERCEVAL-AVR clinical trial evidenced the non-inferiority for the sutureless vs. stented for major adverse cerebral and cardiovascular events at 1 year, whereas aortic valve hemodynamics improved equally in both groups. Perceval significantly reduced surgical times (mean CPB: 71.0 ± 34.1 vs. 87.8 ± 33.9 mins; mean aortic cross-clamp times: 48.5 ± 24.7 vs. 65.2 ± 23.6; both $p$-values <0.001), but resulted in a higher rate of permanent pacemaker implantation (PPI - 11.1 vs. 3.6% at 1 year). Incidences of PVL and central leak were similar.

The CAVALIER clinical trial (15) reported a mean cross-clamp time of 41.5 ± 20.3 mins and a mean CPB time of 39.0 ± 12.5 mins while the mean hospital length of stay was 12.0 ± 7.4 days. There were three reported cardiac valve-related deaths, and eight cases were cardiac related but not valve related. There were five early explanted valves 13.8 days post-implant due to PVL discovered at follow-up.

## PERCEVAL VS. TAVR. WHEN ENEMIES BECOME ALLIES

SVD has been reported in many case series and the treatment in these patients has successfully been delivered through valve-in-valve TAVR using both the Evolut Pro and the Corevalve (16) (**Figure 2**). With respect to Perceval vs. TAVR, the SURTAVI trial (6) showed that TAVR with the self-expanding CoreValve was non-inferior to SAVR for the primary endpoint at 2 years for the treatment of severe aortic stenosis in intermediate-risk patients (STS-PROM, 3–15%; median 4.5%). The Perceval valve benefits, may render ViV-TAVR second procedure easier and safer. This includes a self-expanding nitinol stage, a radio-opaque frame, and sinusoidal struts that "push" coronary ostia and sinuses away from prosthesis leaflets. In addition, eight retrospective clinical studies showed that 30-day mortality was higher in the TAVR group which may be explained with the higher preoperative risk in this population (16–24). The most used prosthesis in TAVR were the Corevalve, Sapien, Lotus and Portico. The CPB and aortic cross-clamp time for the Perceval ranged between 54 and 73.4/SD = 23.1–25 mins and 32–43.4/SD = 13.4–17, respectively. Mortality ranged from 0 to 4% for Perceval and 2.9–7% for TAVR. The incidence of PVL (Perceval 1.9–19.4 vs. TAVR 9–53.5%), PPI (Perceval 2–11.2 vs. TAVR 4.9–25.5%), stroke (Perceval 0 vs. TAVR 0–2.8%), and myocardial infarction (MI) (Perceval 0 vs. TAVR 0–3.5%), were all higher in the TAVR group (**Table 1**).

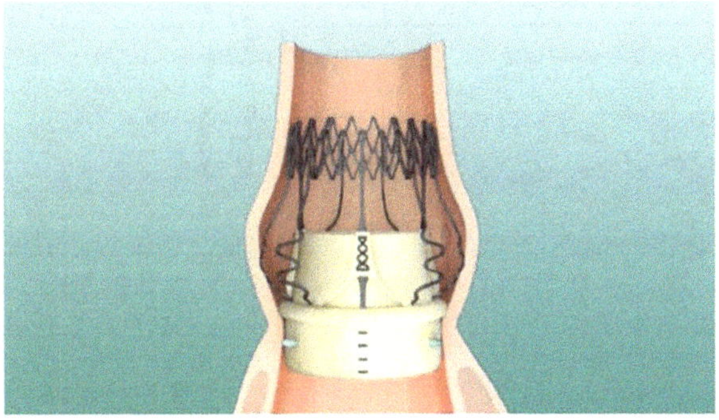

**FIGURE 2** | Sutureless aortic valve in the aortic annulus.

## PERCEVAL VS. OTHER STENTED BIOPROSTHESES. NEW GENERATION VS. OLD STYLE

Compared to other stented bioprostheses (SB), the Perceval valve had similar outcomes. Four prospective and four retrospective clinical studies showed that 30-day mortality was higher in the Perceval group which may be explained with the higher preoperative risk in this population (24–31). Mortality ranged from 0 to 6.4% for Perceval and 0–5.9% for SB. The aortic cross-clamp time in minutes (Perceval 30.8–65.3/SD = 13.6–29.1 vs. SB 59–90/SD = 23–30.3) and CPB time in minutes (Perceval 47–88/SD = 11–34.9 vs. SB 87.8–120/SD = 20.4–37.9) were all significantly higher in the SB group ($p < 0.05$). The incidence of PVL (Perceval 1–19.4 vs. SB 0–1%), PM (Perceval 2–10.7 vs. SB 1.8–8.5%), stroke (Perceval 0–3.7 vs. SB 1.8–7.3%), MI (Perceval 0–7.8 vs. SB 0–4.3%), were comparable among the groups (**Table 2**). The most used stented valves were the CE Perimount, Magna Ease and Triflecta valves.

## PERCEVAL FOR MICS AND MINI-SAVR

One of the benefits of the Perceval bioprosthesis is its widespread usage in mini-SAVR. Perceval has been developed in order to combine the best of two worlds, as they could facilitate the implantation while maintaining the benefits of SAVR. Currently, the upper ministernotomy (MS) and the right anterior thoracotomy (RAT) are the most common approaches for (mini-SAVR). Bonacchi et al. (32) evidenced the benefits of the valve in both MS and RAT. In addition, the international prospective registry (33) comparing MS with RAT showed an aortic cross-clamp time of 43 vs. 55 mins ($p < 0.01$), cardiopulmonary bypass time of 67 vs. 89 mins ($p < 0.01$) and a prosthesis implantation time of 15.5 vs. 12 mins ($p = 0.014$), respectively. In this context, the Sutureless and Rapid Deployment International Registry (34), pointed out the efficacy of the Perceval bioprosthesis in redo

**TABLE 1** | Sutureless aortic valve replacement vs. transcatheter aortic valve replacement.

| Study author | Biancari et al. | | Muneretto et al. | | D'Onofrio et al. | | Santarpino et al. | | Miceli et al. | | Muneretto et al. | | Repossini et al. | | Gerfer et al. | |
|---|---|---|---|---|---|---|---|---|---|---|---|---|---|---|---|---|
| **Type of clinical study** | **Retrospective** | | **Retrospective** | | **Retrospective** | | **Retrospective** | | **Retrospective** | | **Retrospective** | | **Retrospective** | | **Retrospective** | |
| **Valve types and nr. of patients** | **Perceval *N* = 144** | **TAVR *N* = 144** | **Perceval *N* = 53** | **TAVR *N* = 55** | **Perceval *N* = 31** | **TAVR *N* = 143** | **Perceval *N* = 443** | **TAVR *N* = 1,002** | **Perceval *N* = 37** | **TAVR *N* = 37** | **Perceval *N* = 288** | **TAVR = 367** | **Perceval = 158** | **TAVR = 158** | **Perceval = 59** | **TAVR = 59** |
| 30-day Mortality (%) | 1.4 | 6.9 | 0 | 1.8 | 0 | 7 | 4 | 2.9 | 0 | 3 | 5.8 | 9.8 | 1.9 | 5.8 | 5.1 | 1.7 |
| Bleeding (%) | 4.2 | 0 | 7.5 | 0 | NR | NR | NR | NR | 1 | 1 | 4.9 | 1.9 | NR | NR | NR | NR |
| Paravalvular leak (%) | 2.8 | 53.5 | 1.9 | 9 | 19.4 | 28.7 | NR | NR | 2 | 30 | 4 | 18 | 0.5 | 4.3 | 0 | 6.8 |
| Stroke (%) | 0 | 2.1 | 0 | 0 | 0 | 2.8 | NR | NR | 0 | 2 | 1.5 | 5.8 | NR | NR | 1.7 | 0 |
| Myocardial Infarction (%) | 0 | 0 | 0 | 1.8 | 0 | 3.5 | NR | NR | NR | NR | NR | NR | NR | NR | NR | NR |
| Permanent pacemaker implantation (%) | 11.2 | 15.4 | 2 | 25.5 | 3.2 | 4.9 | 5.8 | 11.6 | 2 | 0 | 9.8 | 14.7 | 5.4 | 11.9 | 10.2 | 8.5 |
| Aortic cross-clamp time in minutes ± SD | 42 ± 17 | NA | 32 ± 14 | NA | NR | NA | 43.4 ± 13.4 | NA | NR | NA | 32.8 ± 12.6 | NA | NR | NR | 49 ± 22 | NA |
| Cardiopulmonary bypass time in minutes ± SD | 71 ± 24 | NA | 54 ± 25 | NA | NR | NA | 73.4 ± 23.1 | NA | NR | NA | 50 ± 11.5 | NA | NR | NR | 83 ± 32 | NA |
| TAVR types | NA | CoreValve Sapien Lotus Portico | NA | NR | NA | NR | NA | Sapien | NA | Sapien | NA | Corevalve, Sapien XT, Accurate TA | NA | NR | NA | Accurate NEO |

*TAVR, transcatheter aortic valve replacement; SD, standard deviation; NR, not reported; NA, not applicable.*

**TABLE 2 |** Sutureless aortic valve replacement vs. other stented bioprostheses.

| Study author | Muneretto et al. | | Gilmanov et al. | | Pollari et al. | | D'Onofrio et al. | | Vaquero et al. | | Fischlein et al. | | Dalen et al. | | Forcillo et al. | |
|---|---|---|---|---|---|---|---|---|---|---|---|---|---|---|---|---|
| **Type of clinical study** | **Prospective** | | **Retrospective** | | **Prospective** | | **Retrospective** | | **Prospective** | | **Prospective** | | **Retrospective** | | **Retrospective** | |
| **Valves and patients** | **Perceval *N* = 53** | **Stented *N* = 55** | **Perceval *N* = 133** | **Stented *N* = 133** | **Perceval *N* = 88** | **Stented *N* = 88** | **Perceval *N* = 31** | **Stented *N* = 112** | **Perceval *N* = 140** | **Stented *N* = 409** | **Perceval *N* = 447** | **Stented *N* = 449** | **Perceval = 171** | **Stented = 171** | **Perceval = 76** | **Stented = 319** |
| 30-day Mortality (%) | 0 | 0 | 0.8 | 1.5 | 2.4 | 3.7 | 0 | 1.8 | 6.4 | 5.9 | 1 | 1 | 1.8 | 2.3 | 5 | 6 |
| Bleeding (%) | 7.5 | 10.5 | 6.8 | 3.8 | 2.4 | 6.1 | NR | NR | NR | NR | 4.4 | 6.3 | 4.1 | 6,4 | 8 | 8 |
| Paravalvular leak (%) | 1.9 | 0 | NR | NR | NR | NR | 19.4 | 1 | 3.6 | 0.5 | 1 | 0 | 0 | 1.2 | 0 | 0 |
| Stroke (%) | 0 | 1.8 | NR | NR | 3.7 | 7.3 | 0 | 0 | 2.9 | 2.7 | 1.5 | 1.9 | 2.3 | 1.2 | 0 | 5 |
| Myocardial infarction (%) | 0 | 0 | 1.5 | 0 | NR | NR | 0 | 0.9 | 7.8 | 4.3 | 1 | 1.5 | NR | NR | 0 | 0 |
| Permanent pacemaker implantation (%) | 2 | 1.8 | NR | NR | 6.1 | 8.5 | 3.2 | 0.9 | 10.7 | 2 | 10.6 | 3.2 | 9.9 | 2.9 | 17 | 8 |
| Aortic cross-clamp time in minutes/SD | 30.8 ± 13.6 | 65.3 ± 27.7 | 56 | 90 | 47 ± 16 | 59 ± 23 | NR | NR | 65.3 ± 29.1 | 77.2 ± 30.3 | 48.5 ± 24.7 | 65.2 ± 23.6 | 40 ± 15 | 65 ± 15 | 46 | 68 |
| Cardiopulmonary bypass time in minutes/SD | 47 ± 18.5 | 89.4 ± 20.4 | 88 | 120 | 71 ± 11 | 92 ± 33 | NR | NR | 81.3 ± 34.9 | 95.7 ± 37.9 | 71.0 ± 34.1 | 87.8 ± 33.9 | 69 ± 20 | 87 ± 20 | 60 | 85 |
| Type of stented valves | NA | Perimount, Edwards | NA | CE Edwards, Medtronic, CE standard | NA | NR | NA | NR | NA | Triflecta | NA | NR | NA | CE Perimount | NA | CE, Medtronic, Mitroflow, St. Jude epic, St. Jude Biocor |

*NA, not applicable; SD, standard deviation; NR, not reported.*

operations showing a mean cardiopulmonary bypass time of 95 ± 34.3 mins, an aortic cross-clamp time 57.8 ± 23.2 mins with 0% in hospital mortality, a 3.6% incidence of new PPI and 2.5% incidence of PVL. Recent technological developments have led to endoscopic aortic valve replacement. Vola et al. (35) reported the endoscopic SAVR with Perceval. Exposure was provided by four ports in the second, third, and fifth intercostal spaces with fem-fem CPB. Perceval was implanted with an aortic cross-clamp and CPB time of 80 and 166 mins, respectively. At 5-month follow-up, echocardiography was satisfactory. Balkhy et al. (36) reported the first in human robotic SAVR with Perceval. The patient was a 76-year-old male who underwent a combined procedure of coronary artery bypass surgery and SAVR. Two 8-mm arm ports were placed in the 1st and 3rd intercostal space at the midclavivular line. Aortic cross clamp lasted 86 mins. The patient was discharged on postoperative day 2 and at 6-month follow-up the patient was in good health.

## BICUSPID AORTIC VALVES AND PERCEVAL

This topic remains controversial among surgeons. Many clinical studies, including the PERSIST-AVR clinical trial (37), excluded patients with a congenital bicuspid aortic valve. Some reports suggested that the sutureless valves may increase the risk of PVL and/or potential dislocation related to BAV aortic root asymmetry (38). Nguyen et al. (13) emphasized that the most crucial point during surgery is to recreate three natural nadirs points positioned at 120° with the aim of recreating a circular annulus. Four retrospective clinical studies (13, 34, 39, 40) with a small population ranging between 11 and 88 patients evidenced a low mortality rate (0–4%) and PVL incidence (0–2.3%). However, there was a high incidence of PPI (0–20%), and stroke (0–8%) (**Table 3**). The mean aortic cross clamp time in minutes (39–55/SD = 3.1–14) and CPB time in minutes (54.5–80/SD = 4.4–22) were higher compared to non BAV procedures. These outcomes mean that despite recent surgical technique developments, PPI remain a hurdle for BAV patients undergoing SAVR with sutureless bioprostheses.

## THROMBOCYTOPENIA. DO WE REALLY NEED TO CORRECT IT?

Several causes of platelet dysfunction have been speculated: (1) the detoxification process with homocysteic acid and the storage aldehyde-free solution; (2) the naked alloy stent; and (3) mechanical stress and turbulence, especially in small valve sizes (41). At the end of the day, Vendramin and Bortolotti correctly pose the following questions: Do we really need to solve it and why should we still be worried (42)? In this context, Stegmeier et al. (43) showed that Perceval, when compared to other prostheses, is more prone to causing thrombocytopenia, however, no detrimental clinical effect of this phenomenon was found. The mean minimum platelets count was 47,000 μm and upon discharge the platelets level was 166,000 μm. Can medical therapy have an impact on thrombocytopenia? The result from the study showed a non-significant difference among patients on aspirin and dual antiplatelet medical therapy. In addition, there was no significant change in platelets and red blood cells transfusion. However, the reoperation for bleeding rate (20%) was higher than in the other two groups (Labcor TLPB-A = 4% and Hancock valve = 8%). Moreover, a sub-analysis of the PERSIST-AVR clinical trial evidenced that the Perceval group had a higher platelet reduction than the control group (46 vs. 32%) (44). The phenomenon was transient in both groups, with a slow recovery of the platelet count by hospital discharge. No differences were observed between groups regarding need of transfusions, blood loss, major bleeding and stroke events. While comparing the Intuity valve with its Perceval counterpart, Jiritano et al. (41) found that no risk factors that may have predisposed to platelet dysfunction were found in either group. More red blood cell transfusions were given to the Perceval group as compared with the Intuity group (10 vs. 7 units, $p = 0.012$) as well as platelets (4 vs. 0 units, $P < 0.01$). Platelet count at discharge for Perceval was 102.18 ± 29.34 μm. In addition, mean platelet volume was significantly larger in the Perceval group on postoperative days 1, 3, and 5 ($P = 0.04$, $P = 0.001$, $P = 0.015$), whereas platelet distribution width was significantly larger in the Perceval group on postoperative days 3 and 5 ($P = 0.018$, $P = 0.026$). Looking at the clinical studies outcomes the answer to Vendramin and Bortolotti is the following: "no, we do not need to correct the transient thrombocytopenia, but we should be cautious."

## HEMODYNAMIC CHANGES, VENTRICULAR MASS REGRESSION, AND PORCELAIN AORTA

We found nine clinical studies but only eight were reporting data with standard deviations. Six of the studies were retrospective observational cohort studies and two were prospective non-randomized clinical trials (**Table 4**) (11, 21–23, 35, 36). The effective orifice area (EOA) ranged between 1.5 and 1.7 cm$^2$/SD = 0.3–0.5 since discharge up to 2 years of follow-up. The mean transvalvular gradient ranged between 10.1 and 14 mmHg/ SD = 4.3–6.4 at discharge, 8.9 mmHg/ SD = 3.2–4.2 at 6 months, 8.7–9.9 mmHg/SD = 3.7–5 at 1 year and 8–9 mmHg/SD = 3.4–4.1 at 2 years follow-up. The peak transvalvular gradient was 19.4–27 mmHg/SD = 8.1–11 at discharge, 16.8–19.6 mmHg/SD = 6.7–7.6 at 6 months, 17.1–20.9 mmHg/SD 7.6–9.2 at 1 year, 16.6–18.3 mmHg/SD 5.6–7.2 mmHg at 2 years follow-up. With respect to the ventricular mass regression, Santarpino et al. (45) found that the mean ± SD left ventricular mass index decreased from 148.4 ± 48.4 g/m$^2$ to 119.7 ± 38.5 g/m$^2$ (P = 0.002) whereas interventricular septum and posterior wall thickness decreased from 13.9 ± 2.3 mm to 12.1 ± 2.8 mm ($P = 0.02$) and 12.1 ± 1.6 mm to 11.3 ± 1.3 mm (P = 0.04) at follow-up. In addition, there have been sporadic reports of the implantation of the Perceval in porcelain aortas. Santarpino et al. (46) reported a 72-year-old woman with severe AS, coronary artery disease, and porcelain aorta. The patient underwent CABG, removal of the ascending aorta, and implantation of a 23-mm Perceval

**TABLE 3** | Clinical outcomes of bicuspid aortic valve stenosis treated with sutureless valve.

| Study author | Durdu et al. (mean ± SD) | Nguyen et al. (mean ± SD) | Szecel et al. (mean ± SD) | Miceli et al. (mean ± SD) |
|---|---|---|---|---|
| **Number of patients** | ***N* = 13 patients** | ***N* = 25 patients** | ***N* = 11 patients** | ***N* = 88 patients** |
| Type of clinical study | Retrospective | Retrospective | Retrospective | Retrospective |
| 30-day mortality (%) | 0 | 4 | 0 | 1.6 |
| Bleeding (%) | 7.6 | 1 | NR | 3.1 |
| Paravalvular leak (%) | 0 | 0 | 0 | 2.3 |
| Stroke (%) | 7.6 | 8 | 0 | 4.2 |
| Myocardial infarction (%) | 0 | 0 | 0 | NR |
| Permanent pacemaker implantation (%) | 7.6 | 20 | 0 | 5.7 |
| Aortic cross-clamping time in minutes/SD | 40.3 ± 3.1 | 45.9 ± 14.0 | 39 ± 13 | 55 |
| Cardiopulmonary bypass time in minutes/SD | 54.5 ± 4.4 | 56.1 ± 14.9 | 66 ± 22 | 80 |

*NR, not reported; SD, standard deviation.*

**TABLE 4** | Hemodynamic outcomes.

| Endpoints | Santarpino et al. *N* = 658 (mean ± SD) | Rubino et al. *N* = 314 (mean ± SD) | Mazine et al. *N* = 215 (mean ± SD) | Folliguet et al. *N* = 208 (mean ± SD) | Shrestha et al. *N* = 30 (mean ± SD) | Shrestha et al. *N* = 243 (mean ± SD) | Miceli et al. *N* = 37 (Mean ± SD) | Repossini et al. *N* = 158 |
|---|---|---|---|---|---|---|---|---|
| Type of clinical study | Prospective | Retrospective | Retrospective | Retrospective | Prospective | Retrospective | Retrospective | Retrospective |
| EOA ($cm^2$) at discharge | 1.5 ± 0.4 | NR | 1.56 ± 0.37 | 1.4 ± 0.4 | NR | 1.5 ± 0.4 | NR | NR |
| EOA ($cm^2$) at 6 months | 1.5 ± 0.3 | NR | NR | 1.5 ± 0.4 | NR | 1.5 ± 0.4 | NR | NR |
| EOA ($cm^2$) at 1 year | 1.5 ± 0.4 | NR | NR | 1.5 ± 0.3 | 1.55 ± 0.35 | 1.6 ± 0.4 | NR | NR |
| EOA ($cm^2$) at 2 years | NR | NR | NR | NR | 1.51 ± 0.26 | 1.7 ± 0.5 | NR | NR |
| Mean gradient (mmHg) at discharge | 10.3 ± 4.5 | 14 ± 6 | 13.3 ± 6.4 | 10.4 ± 4.3 | NR | 10.1 ± 4.7 | 11.4 ± 3.7 | 10.9 ± 5.4 |
| Mean gradient (mmHg) at 6 months | 8.9 ± 4.1 | NR | NR | 8.9 ± 3.2 | NR | 8.9 ± 4.2 | NR | NR |
| Mean gradient (mmHg) at 1 year | 9.2 ± 5 | NR | NR | 8.7 ± 3.7 | 9.9 ± 4.6 | 8.9 ± 4.6 | NR | NR |
| Mean gradient (mmHg) at 2 years | NR | NR | NR | NR | 8 ± 4.1 | 9 ± 3.4 | NR | NR |
| Peak gradient (mmHg) at discharge | 19.4 ± 8.1 | 27 ± 11 | 24.5 ± 10.8 | 21.3 ± 8.6 | NR | 20.3 ± 9.9 | 19.2 ± 6.9 | 18.7 ± 9.1 |
| Peak gradient (mmHg) at 6 months | 16.8 ± 7 | NR | NR | 19.6 ± 6.7 | NR | 18 ± 7.6 | NR | NR |
| Peak gradient (mmHg) at 1 year | 17.1 ± 8.7 | NR | NR | 18.8 ± 7.6 | 20.9 ± 9.2 | 17.5 ± 8.2 | NR | NR |
| Peak gradient (mmHg) at 2 years | NR | NR | NR | NR | 16.6 ± 7.2 | 18.3 ± 5.6 | NR | NR |

*EOA, effective orifice area; SD, standard deviation; NR, not reported.*

and FlowWeave Bioseal 24-mm prosthesis (Jotec, Hechingen, Germany). Gatti et al. (47) reported the use of Perceval in four patients with porcelain aorta. All patients were discharged within postoperative day 20 and, at 1 to 6-month, were alive with improvements in symptoms.

## LONG-TERM OUTCOMES OF THE PERCEVAL VALVE

The Perceval aortic valve has proven to be a reliable bioprosthesis with excellent early and midterm outcomes. However, the long-term outcomes of the valve have not been studied and results are coming from some clinical studies. Our literature research found one retrospective study and one clinical trial with a 5-year follow-up period (**Table 5**). Shrestha et al. (48) reported the outcomes of 720 patients evidencing a 1.4% of cardiac deaths, 1,5% of valve explants, 1% of major paravalvular leak, 1.4% of A-V block III and 0.8% of stroke. The 5-year outcomes of a prospective clinical trial (14) with only 30 patients evidenced a cardiac mortality of 3.3%, an A-V block type III of 3.3% but no stroke, paravalvular leak, valve thrombosis or structural valve deterioration was noticed. The echocardiographic outcomes at 3, 4, and 5-year follow-up evidenced an EOA of 1.64–1.68 (SD 0.4–0.42), 1.68 (SD 0.43), 1.69–1.8 (SD 0.3–0.42), respectively. In addition, the mean transvalvular gradient across the valve at 3, 4,

TABLE 5 | Long-term outcomes of the Perceval bioprosthesis.

| Late events> 30 days.studies | Shrestha et al. *N* = 729 patients | Meuris et al. *N* = 30 patients |
|---|---|---|
| Type of study | Retrospective | Prospective clinical trial |
| Follow-up duration | 5 years | 5 years |
| Deaths (%) | 7 | 28.7 |
| Cardiac deaths (%) | 1.4 | 3.3 |
| Valve explants (%) | 1.5 | 0 |
| Major paravalvular leak (%) | 1 | 0 |
| Endocarditis (%) | 1.6 | 6.6 |
| Structural valve deterioration (%) | 0 | 0 |
| Valve thrombosis (%) | 0 | 0 |
| AV block III (%) | 1.4 | 3.3 |
| Stroke | 0.8 | 0 |

TABLE 6 | Long-term echocardiographic outcomes (5-year follow-up) of the Perceval bioprosthesis.

| Study | Shrestha et al. *N* = 729 patients (mean ± SD) | Meuris et al. *N* = 30 (mean ± SD) |
|---|---|---|
| LVEF at 3 years (%) | 67 ± 9 | NR |
| LVEF at 4 years (%) | 66.1 ± 9.1 | NR |
| LVEF at 5 years (%) | 65.8 ± 7.7 | NR |
| Mean transvalvular gradient at 3 years mmHg | 7.7 ± 2.8 | 8.3 ± 2.5 |
| Mean transvalvular gradient at 4 years mmHg | 7.8 ± 3.8 | 7.6 ± 3.6 |
| Mean transvalvular gradient at 5 years mmHg | 8.8 ± 4.6 | 9.3 ± 5.5 |
| Peak transvalvular gradient at 3 years mmHg | 16 ± 5.2 | 16.6 ± 6.2 |
| Peak transvalvular gradient at 4 years mmHg | 17.8 ± 8.1 | 17.5 ± 7.8 |
| Peak transvalvular gradients at 5 years mmHg | 21.1 ± 9.7 | 21.4 ± 11.5 |
| EOA at 3 years (cm$^2$) | 1.64 ± 0.42 | 1.68 ± 0.4 |
| EOA at 4 years (cm$^2$) | 1.68 ± 0.43 | 1.68 ± 0.43 |
| EOA at 5 years (cm$^2$) | 1.8 ± 0.3 | 1.69 ± 0.42 |

and 5 years was 7.7–8.3 mmHg (SD 2.5–2.8), 7.6–7.8 mmHg (SD 3.6–3.8), 8.8–9.3 mmHg (SD 4.6–5.5), respectively. These results once more confirm the usefulness of the Perceval valve (**Table 6**).

## THE IDEAL CANDIDATE FOR SUTURELESS AORTIC VALVE REPLACEMENT

Many studies have evidenced the benefits of Perceval aortic bioprosthesis, especially in the following three situations:

(a) High-risk patients undergoing a combined surgical procedure
(b) Hostile aortic root
(c) A small aortic annulus.

In the first situation, the use of sutureless and rapid-deployment valves allows economy of precious CPB time by alleviating the need to place and tie sutures around the aortic annulus, while still allowing native valve excision and annular decalcification. In a systematic review and meta-analysis that included 12 observational studies, Phan et al. (49) demonstrated that the pooled durations of cardiopulmonary bypass and aortic cross-clamp for isolated SAVR were 57 and 33 min, respectively. These values are nearly half of those reported in the Society of Thoracic Surgeons National Database[1] for conventional SAVR.

In hostile aortic roots and redo operations, Perceval may become the bioprosthesis of choice. In addition to the time-saving procedure and to the non-necessity of complete annular decalcification, it allows valve replacement after graft infection. In the last scenario, the benefits include less foreign material used (pledgets/sutures), less manipulation of friable tissues, and radial force of Perceval solidifies root repair. During reoperations and extensive decalcification of the annulus, clefts in the mitral valve/left atrium can form. In this situation, the Perceval valve can be easily compressed and removed (without the necessity of removing all the sutures as in the stented valves), the cleft repaired, and the valve redeployed again (50). However, neither the CAVALIER nor the PERSISTENT-AVR clinical trials mentioned the hostile aortic root.

Finally, in case of a small aortic annulus, an aortic root enlargement should be performed to implant an adequately sized bioprosthesis. However, this is not always feasible as newly minted surgeons do not have sufficient technical experience to perform these procedures. In this scenario, the sutureless prosthesis have shown good outcomes when implanted with low post-procedural transvalvular gradients (45). In addition, Perceval is a proven option for high-risk patients and for those at risk of prosthesis-patient mismatch (51).

Contraindications for the prosthesis implantation are (a) subjects with aortic root enlargement, where the ratio between observed and expected diameters (calculated as a function of age and patient body surface area) is $\geq$1.3; (b) subjects with known hypersensitivity to nickel alloys, (c) subjects with aneurysmal dilation or dissection of the ascending aortic wall needing surgical correction.

## POTENTIAL PITFALLS OF PERCEVAL

Limitations and drawbacks of the Perceval bioprosthesis are the following;

(a) PVL.
(b) Acquired conduction disorders and PPI.
(c) SVD and need for reintervention.

PVL has shown an increased incidence in the TAVR and the sutureless bioprostheses with the latter being the highest (52). Surgeons came to understand that the Achilles heel of these

[1] https://publicreporting.sts.org/

bioprostheses is the non-coronary sinus which is slightly lower compared to the left and right sinuses. During the deployment phase, the valve must be positioned in a lower angle of 15–30° at the level of the non-coronary sinus, on the side of the surgeon. When the valve is accurately positioned, and no gap exists on visual inspection than it should be deployed. This technique avoids the incidence of PVL. However, it has been shown that these results are related to a learning curve and experienced surgeons tend to have a lower incidence of PVL (53).

The PPI trend has shown a slow but steadily decrease since the introduction by Yanagawa et al. (12) of their modification of the implantation height. They found that a higher implantation of the valve (2–3 mm) decreases the incidence of conduction abnormalities requiring a pacemaker. This is in contrast with the first prescription given from the company to implant the valve below the annular plane. SVD happens continuously and Perceval is not exempt from it.

## CONCLUSIONS

The Perceval bioprosthesis has proved to be a reliable prosthesis for conventional SAVR and mini-SAVR due to its implantation speed, the reduced CPB time, the reduced aortic cross-clamp time and the shorter intensive care unit and hospital length of stay. In addition, its adoption in hostile roots, and the usage in reinterventions coupled with the low profile render it a formidable tool in the surgical armamentarium.

## AUTHOR CONTRIBUTIONS

All authors listed have made a substantial, direct, and intellectual contribution to the work and approved it for publication.

## REFERENCES


1. Santarpino G, Pfeiffer S, Concistre G, Grossmann I, Hinzmann M, Fischlein T. The Perceval S aortic valve has the potential of shortening surgical time: does it also result in improved outcome? *Ann Thorac Surg.* (2013) 96:77–81. doi: 10.1016/j.athoracsur.2013.03.083
2. Solinas M, Bianchi G, Chiaramonti F, Margaryan R, Kallushi E, Gasbarri T, et al. Right anterior mini-thoracotomy and sutureless valves: the perfect marriage. *Ann Cardiothorac Surg.* (2020) 9:305–13. doi: 10.21037/acs-2019-surd-172
3. Leon MB, Smith CR, Mack M, Miller DC, Moses JW, Svensson LG, et al. Transcatheter aortic-valve implantation for aortic stenosis in patients who cannot undergo surgery. *N Engl J Med.* (2010) 363:1597–607. doi: 10.1056/NEJMoa1008232
4. Leon MB, Smith CR, Mack MJ, Makkar RR, Svensson LG, Kodali SK, et al. Transcatheter or surgical aortic-valve replacement in intermediate-risk patients. *N Engl J Med.* (2016) 374:1609–20. doi: 10.1056/NEJMoa15 14616
5. Mack MJ, Leon MB, Thourani VH, Makkar R, Kodali SK, Russo M, et al. Transcatheter aortic-valve replacement with a balloon-expandable valve in low-risk patients. *N Engl J Med.* (2019) 380:1695–705. doi: 10.1056/NEJMoa1814052
6. Reardon MR, Mieghem NMV, Pompa JJ, Kleiman NS, Sondergaard L, Mumtaz M, et al. Surgical or transcatheter aortic-valve replacement in intermediate-risk patients. (2017) 376:1321–31. doi: 10.1056/NEJMoa17 00456
7. Virtanen MPO, Eskola M, Jalava MP, Husso A, Laakso T, Niemela M et al. Comparison of outcomes after transcatheter aortic valve replacement vs. surgical aortic valve replacement among patients with aortic stenosis at low operative risk. *JAMA Netw Open.* (2019) 2:e195742. doi: 10.1001/jamanetworkopen.2019.5742
8. Dokollari A, Cameli M, Mandoli GE, Kalra DS, Poston R, Coku L et al. Early and midterm clinical outcomes of transcatheter valve-in-valve implantation vs. redo surgical aortic valve replacement for aortic bioprosthetic valve degeneration: two faces of the same medal. *J Cardiothorac Vasc Anesth.* (2021) 24:29. doi: 10.1053/j.jvca.2021.05.029
9. Andreas M, Coti J, Laufer G, Kastner J. Valve-in valve transcatheter aortic valve implantation into a novel, sutureless bioprosthesis: technical considerations. *Eurointervention.* (2018) 13:1902–3. doi: 10.4244/EIJ-D-17-00578
10. Suleiman T, Tanseco K, Arunothayaraj S, Michail M, Cockburn J, Hadjivassilev S, et al. Valve-in-valve transcatheter aortic valve implantation for the failing surgical Perceval bioprosthesis. *Cardiovasc Revasc Med.* (2021) 21:S1553-8389. doi: 10.1016/j.carrev.2021.07.023
11. Folliguet TA, Laborde F, Zannis K, Ghorayeb G, Haverich A, Shrestha M. Sutureless perceval aortic valve replacement: results of two European centers. *Ann Thorac Surg.* (2012) 93:1483–8. doi: 10.1016/j.athoracsur.2012.01.071
12. Yanagawa B, Cruz J, Boisvert L, Bonneau D. A simple modification to lower incidence of heart block with sutureless valve implantation. *J Thorac Cardiovasc Surg.* (2016) 152:630–2. doi: 10.1016/j.jtcvs.2016. 02.034
13. Nguyen A, Fortin W, Mazine A, Bouchard D, Carrier M, El-Hamamsy I, et al. Sutureless aortic valve replacement in patients who have bicuspid aortic valve. *J Thorac Cardiovasc Surg.* (2015) 150:851–7. doi: 10.1016/j.jtcvs.2015. 05.071
14. Meuris B, Flameng WJ, Laborde F, Folliguet TA, Haverich A, Shrestha M. Five-year results of the pilot trial of a sutureless valve. *J Thorac Cardiovasc Surg.* (2015) 150:84–8. doi: 10.1016/j.jtcvs.2015.03.040
15. Laborde F, Fischlein T, Hakim-Meibodi K, Misfeld M, Carrel T, Zambala M, et al. Clinical and haemodynamic outcomes in 658 patients receiving the Perceval sutureless aortic valve: early results from a prospective European multicentre study (the Cavalier Trial). *Eur J Cardiothorac Surg.* (2016) 49:978–86. doi: 10.1093/ejcts/ezv257
16. Misfeld M, Abdel-Wahab M, Thiele H, Borger MA, Holzhey D. A series of four transcatheter aortic valve replacement in failed Perceval valves. *Ann Cardiothorac Surg.* (2020) 9:280–8. doi: 10.21037/acs-2020-surd-20
17. Biancari F, Barbanti M, Santarpino G, Deste W, Tamburrino C et al. Immediate outcome after sutureless vs. transcatheter aortic valve replacement. *Heart Vessels.* (2016) 31:427–33. doi: 10.1007/s00380-014-0623-3
18. Muneretto C, Solinas M, Folliguet T, Di Bartolomeo R, Repossini A, Laborde F, et al. Sutureless vs. transcatheter aortic valves in elderly patients with aortic stenosis at intermediate risk: a multi-institutional study. *J Thorac Cardiovasc Surg.* (2020) 4:179. doi: 10.1016/j.jtcvs.2020. 04.179
19. D'Onofrio A, Messina A, Lorusso R, Alfieri O, Fusari M, Rubino P, et al. Sutureless aortic valve replacement as an alternative treatment for patients belonging to the "gray zone" between transcatheter aortic valve implantation and conventional surgery: a propensity-matched, multicenter analysis. *J Thorac Cardiovasc Surg.* (2012) 144:1010–6. doi: 10.1016/j.jtcvs.2012. 07.040
20. Santarpino G, Pfeiffer S, Jessl J, Dell'Aquila AM, Pollari F, Pauschinger M, et al. Sutureless replacement vs. transcatheter valve implantation in aortic valve stenosis: a propensity matched analysis of 2 strategies in high-risk patients. *J Thorac Cardiovasc Surg.* (2014) 147:561–7. doi: 10.1016/j.jtcvs.2013. 10.025
21. Miceli A, Gilmanov D, Murzi M, Marchi F, Ferrarini M, Cerillo AG, et al. Minimally invasive aortic valve replacement with a sutureless valve

through a right anterior mini-thoracotomy vs. transcatheter aortic valve implantation in high-risk patients. *Eur J Cardiothorac Surg.* (2016) 49:960–5. doi: 10.1093/ejcts/ezv210
22. Muneretto C, Alfieri O, Cesana BM, De Bonis M, Di Bartolomeo R, et al. A comparison of conventional surgery, transcatheter aortic valve replacement, and sutureless valves in "real-world" patients with aortic stenosis and intermediate- to high-risk profile. *J Thorac Cardiovasc Surg.* (2015) 150:1570–7; discussion 1577–9. doi: 10.1016/j.jtcvs.2015.08.052
23. Repossini A, Fischlein T, Solinas M, Di Bacco L, Passaretti B, Grubitzsch H, et al. Stentless sutureless and transcatheter valves: a comparison of the hemodynamic performance of different prostheses concept. *Minerva Cardioangiologica.* (2018) 66:180–90. doi: 10.23736/S0026-4725.17.04564-9
24. Gerfer S, Mauri V, Kuhn E, Adam M, Djordevic I, Ivanov B, et al. Comparison of Self-expanding RDV perceval S vs. TAVI ACURATE neo/TF. *Thorac Cardiovasc Surg.* (2021) 69:420–7. doi: 10.1055/s-0040-1722692
25. Muneretto C, Bisleri G, Moggi A, Di Bacco L, Tespili M, Repossini A, et al. Treating the patients in the 'grey-zone' with aortic valve disease: a comparison among conventional surgery, sutureless valves and transcatheter aortic valve replacement. *Interact Cardiovasc Thorac Surg.* (2015) 20:90–5. doi: 10.1093/icvts/ivu340
26. Gilmanov D, Miceli A, Ferrarini M, Farneti P, Murzi M, Solinas M, et al. Aortic valve replacement through right anterior minithoracotomy: can sutureless technology improve clinical outcomes? *Ann Thorac Surg.* (2014) 98:1585–92. doi: 10.1016/j.athoracsur.2014.05.092
27. Pollari F, Santarpino G, Dell'Aquila AM, Gazdag L, Alnahas H, Vogt F, et al. Better short-term outcome by using sutureless valves: a propensity-matched score analysis. *Ann Thorac Surg.* (2014) 98:616–7. doi: 10.1016/j.athoracsur.2014.04.072
28. D'Onofrio A, Rizzoli G, Messina A, Alfieri O, Lorusso R, Salizzoni S, et al. Conventional surgery, sutureless valves, and transapical aortic valve replacement: what is the best option for patients with aortic valve stenosis? a multicenter, propensity-matched analysis. *J Thorac Cardiovasc Surg.* (2013) 146:1065–70; discussion 1070–1. doi: 10.1016/j.jtcvs.2013.06.047
29. Hernandez-Vaquero D, Vigil-Escalera C, Persia Y, Morales C, Pascual I, Dominguez-Rodriguez A, et al. Perceval or trifecta to prevent patient-prosthesis mismatch. *J Clin Med.* (2020) 9:2964. doi: 10.3390/jcm9092964
30. Fischlein T, Folliguet T, Meuris B, Shrestha ML, Roselli EE, McGlothlin A, et al. Sutureless vs. conventional bioprostheses for aortic valve replacement in severe symptomatic aortic valve stenosis. *J Thorac Cardiovasc Surg.* (2021) 161:920–932. doi: 10.1016/j.jtcvs.2020.11.162
31. Dalen M, Biancari F, Rubino AS, Santarpino G, Glaser N, Praetere HD, et al. Aortic valve replacement through full sternotomy with a stented bioprosthesis vs. minimally invasive sternotomy with a sutureless bioprosthesis. *Eur J Cardithorac Surg.* (2016) 49:220–7. doi: 10.1093/ejcts/ezv014
32. Bonacchi M, Dokollari A, Parise O, Sani G, Prifti E, Bisleri G, et al. Ministernotomy compared with right anterior minithoracotomy for aortic valve surgery. *J Thorac Cardiovasc Surg.* (2021) 22:125. doi: 10.1016/j.jtcvs.2021.03.125
33. Glauber M, Di Bacco L, Cuenca J, Di Bartolomeo R, Baghai M, Zakova D, et al. Minimally invasive aortic valve replacement with sutureless valves: results from an international prospective registry. *Innovation.* (2020) 15:120–30. doi: 10.1177/1556984519892585
34. Miceli A, Berretta P, Fiore A, Andreas M, Solinas M, Santarpino G, et al. Sutureless and rapid deployment implantation in bicuspid aortic valve: results from the sutureless and rapid-deployment aortic valve replacement international registry. *Ann Cardiothorac Surg.* (2020) 9:298–304. doi: 10.21037/acs-2020-surd-33
35. Vola M, Fuzellier JF, Campisi S, Grinberg D, Albertini JN, Morel J et al. Total endoscopic sutureless aortic valve replacem rationale, development, perspectives. *Ann Cardiothorac Surg.* (2015) 4:170–4. doi: 10.3978/j.issn.2225-319X.2014.11.04
36. Balkhy S, Kitahara H. First human totally endoscopic robotic-assisted sutureless aortic valve replacement. *Ann Thorac Surg.* (2020) 109:e9–e11. doi: 10.1016/j.athoracsur.2019.04.093
37. Lorusso R, Folliguet T, Shrestha M, Meuris B, Kappetein AP, Roselli E, et al. Sutureless vs. stented bioprostheses for aortic valve replacement: the randomized PERSIST-avr study design. *Thorac Cardiovasc Surg.* (2020) 68:114–23. doi: 10.1055/s-0038-1675847
38. Jug J, Stor Z, Gersak B. Anatomical circumstances and aortic cross-clamp time in minimally invasive aortic valve replacement. *Interact Cardiovasc Thorac Surg.* (2021) 32:204–12. doi: 10.1093/icvts/ivaa251
39. Durdu MS, Gumus F, Ozcinar E, Cakici M, Bermede O, Dincer I et al. Sutureless valve replacement through a right anterior mini-thoracotomy in elderly patients with stenotic bicuspid aortic valve. *Semin Thorac Cardiovasc Surg.* (2019) 31:458–64. doi: 10.1053/j.semtcvs.2018.09.025
40. Szecel D, Eurlings R, Rega F, Verbrugghe P, Meuris B. Perceval sutureless aortic valve implantation: mid-term outcomes. *Ann Thorac Surg.* (2020) 6:64. doi.org/10.1016/j.athoracsur.2020.06.064.
41. Jiritano F, Cristodoro L, Malta E, Mastroroberto P. Thrombocytopenia after sutureless aortic valve implantation: comparison between Intuity and Perceval bioprosthesis. *J Thorac Cardiovasc Surg.* (2016) 152:1631–3. doi: 10.1016/j.jtcvs.2016.07.054
42. Vendramin I, Bortolotti U. The thrombocytopenia conundrum after aortic bioprosthetic implantation: do we really need to solve it? *J Thorac Cardiovasc Surg.* (2021) 161:e21–2. doi: 10.1016/j.jtcvs.2020.06.129
43. Stegmeier P, Schlomicher M, Stiegler H, Straucht JT, Bechtel JFM. Thrombocytopenia after implantation of the Perceval S aortic bioprosthesis. *J Thorac Cardiovasc Surg.* (2020) 160:61–8. doi: 10.1016/j.jtcvs.2019.07.046
44. Lorusso R, Jiritano F, Roselli E, Shrestha M, Folliguet T, Meuris B, et al. Perioperative platelet reduction after sutureless or stented valve implantation: results from the PERSIST-AVR controlled randomized trial. *EJCTS.* (2021) 21:175. doi: 10.1093/ejcts/ezab175
45. Santarpino G, Pfeiffer S, Pollari F, Concistré G, Vogt F, Fischlein F. Left ventricular mass regression after sutureless implantation of the perceval S aortic valve bioprosthesis: preliminary results. *Interact Cardiovasc Thorac Surg.* (2014) 18:38–42. doi: 10.1093/icvts/ivt362
46. Santarpino G, Pfeiffer S, Fischlein T. Perceval sutureless approach in a patient with porcelain aorta unsuitable for transcatheter aortic valve implantation. *Int J Cardiol.* (2012) 155:168–70. doi: 10.1016/j.ijcard.2011.09.025
47. Gatti G, Benussi B, Camerini F, Pappalardo A. Aortic valve replacement within an unexpected porcelain aorta: the sutureless valve option. *Interact Cardiovasc Thorac Surg.* (2014) 18:396–8. doi: 10.1093/icvts/ivt494
48. Shrestha M, Fischlein T, Meuris B, Flameng W, Carrel T, Madonna F, et al. European multicentre experience with the sutureless Perceval valve: clinical and haemodynamic outcomes up to 5 years in over 700 patients. *Eur J Cardiothorac Surg.* (2016) 49:234–41. doi: 10.1093/ejcts/ezv040
49. Phan K, Tsai Y, Ninjaran N, Bouchard D, Carrel T, Dapunt O, et al. Sutureless aortic valve replacement: a systematic review and meta-analysis. *Ann Cardiothorac Surg.* (2015) 4:100–11. doi: 10.3978/j.issn.2225-319X.2014.06.01
50. Mork C, Koechlin L, Schaeffer T, Eckstein F, Ruthebuch O. Long-term follow-up after sutureless Perceval S valve implantation as bail-out strategy in a hostile environment. *Cardiovasc Med.* (2020) 23:w02093. doi: 10.4414/cvm.2020.02093
51. Meco M, Montisci A, Miceli A, Panisi P, Donatelli F, Cirri D, et al. The Perceval valve is a supportive option for high-risk patients and for those at risk of patient–prosthesis mismatch. Sutureless perceval aortic valve vs. conventional stented bioprostheses: meta-analysis of postoperative and midterm results in isolated aortic valve replacement. *J Am Heart Assoc.* (2018) 7:e006091. doi: 10.1161/JAHA.117.006091
52. Genereux P, Head SJ, Hahn R, Deneault B, Kodali S, Williams MR, et al. Paravalvular leak after transcatheter aortic valve replacement: the new Achilles' heel? a comprehensive review of the literature. *J Am Coll Cardiol.* (2013) 61:1125–36. doi: 10.1016/j.jacc.2012.08.1039
53. Murzi M, Cerillo AG, Gilmanov D, Concistre G, Farneti P, Glauber M, et al. Exploring the learning curve for minimally invasive sutureless aortic valve replacement. *J Thorac Cardiovasc Surg.* (2016) 152:1537–46. doi: 10.1016/j.jtcvs.2016.04.094

# 9

# Percutaneous Cementoplasty to Treat Sternal Instability After Cardiac Surgery

*Thaïs Pittet*[1], *Stéphane Cook*[1,2*], *Gregory Khatchatourov*[2] *and Nicolas Theumann*[2]

[1] *Cardiology Department, University Fribourg, Fribourg, Switzerland,* [2] *Hirslanden Clinics Lausanne, Lausanne, Switzerland*

***Correspondence:***
*Stéphane Cook*
*Stephane.cook@unifr.ch*

**Introduction:** Although rare, sternal pseudarthrosis is encountered after cardiac surgery and impacts the quality of life by triggering motion-dependent chest pain. We thought to describe its treatment by percutaneous cementoplasty and report the clinical follow-up of patients treated in our institution.

**Methods:** This case series is a retrospective study based on five patients who benefited from a sternal cementoplasty as a treatment for symptomatic pseudarthrosis after cardiac surgery. The progression of the symptoms was assessed during clinical follow-up using the Quebec back pain disability (QBPD) scale and Visual Analog Scale (VAS).

**Results:** None of the patients presented evidence of local complications or neurological disorders. The intra- et post-operative images show no major leak of the cement, no embolism and no damage to the internal mammary artery or the heart. All patients described an improved quality of life due to reduced pain in all-day clinical activities. The QBPD scores improved from $54.8 \pm 29.3$ to $30.0 \pm 17.4$ ($p = 0.02$) and the VAS from $7.0 \pm 2.8$ to $1.6 \pm 1.6$ ($p = 0.01$). Furthermore, three out of five patients could completely stop taking analgesics.

**Conclusion:** Sternal pseudarthrosis is a debilitating affliction that may complicate sternotomy after cardiac surgery. This series demonstrates that a more conservative approach such as cementoplasty can be successful in terms of reducing pain, and constitutes a promising technique in selected cases.

**Keywords: sternotomy, sternal non-union, percutaneous cementoplasty, heart surgery complications, coronary artery bypass graft (CABG)**

## INTRODUCTION

Median sternotomy is the most common approach for cardiac surgery. This technique is considered safe but pertains a complication rate of 0.5 to 5% (1–3). Sternal instability is the most frequent complication encountered. During the first 2 weeks after surgery, sternal instability is named dehiscence. After 3 months, it is named pseudarthosis (4). Sternal pseudarthrosis (SPA) is defined as a defect of consolidation with no sign of healing and is characterized by sternal instability. This is characterized by sternal clicking, excessive motion discomfort (4), and pain in the absence of infection (5). The incomplete sternal union might be due to scarce sternal stability because of intensified thoracic motions, an exaggerated fibrous tissue covering the osteotomy line, and/or an impaired healing capacity. Patient (diabetes mellitus, obesity, chronic obstructive pulmonary disease, smoking) and procedural (cardiopulmonary bypass, excessive use of bone wax, bilateral internal mammary artery harvesting) risk factors have been considered (1, 4, 6–9). Sternal pseudarthrosis (SPA) significantly impacts the quality of life of suffering patients and increases their risk of pneumonia and mediastinitis (2, 4, 10).

The pain found in SPA is due to the friction of the bone with fibrous tissue. The cement acts in two ways: it reduces the mechanical stress and heats up to 70°C during its polymerisation leading to the destruction of the nerve endings. It already reaches 70% of its solid-state within 20–25 min after injection and is completely compact after 4 h. In SPA, the cement decreases micro-movements and stimulates subsequent bone consolidation. The cement's bridges have good resistance to axial forces, and the remaining sternal wires ensure vertical stability.

We describe hereby the characteristics of five patients suffering from SPA and who underwent percutaneous cementoplasty in our center.

## PATIENTS AND METHODS

All patients treated for SPA in 2017 were included. A *sternal instability scale* (SIS) was used to assess SPA (11). The assessor evaluates the instability by placing two fingers on each side of the incision while the patient performs unilateral and bilateral shoulder flexion and abduction, trunk rotation and lateral flexion, cough and profound inspiration. Indeed, upper limbs' mobilization causes longitudinal shear, whereas cough and deep inspiration put the sternum through lateral and transverse shear (8, 12). Those three distraction forces, particularly lateral shear, are responsible for sternal split (2). The SIS grading ranges from 0 to 4, ranging from no detectable motion to complete instability with up to >1 ½ finger space (11).

The baseline clinical and procedural characteristics were obtained by reviewing the hospital electronic database. Once SPA was considered, its characterization was performed by computed tomography (CT) imaging to delineate the extent of the malunion and the presence or absence of bone bridges.

**TABLE 1** | Patient's characteristics.

| Patients | Gender | Age (years) | Time from operation to cementoplasty (months) | Obesity (> 30 kg/m²) | Diabetes | COPD | Smoking (pack-years) |
|---|---|---|---|---|---|---|---|
| #1 | M | 77 | 11 | − | − | − | Never |
| #2 | F | 74 | 33 | − | − | − | Former, 60 p-y |
| #3 | M | 67 | 60 | + | + | − | Former, 50 p-y |
| #4 | F | 69 | 30 | + | + | + | Former, 45 p-y |
| #5 | F | 78 | 23 | + | + | − | Current, 100 p-y |

*+, present; −, absent.*

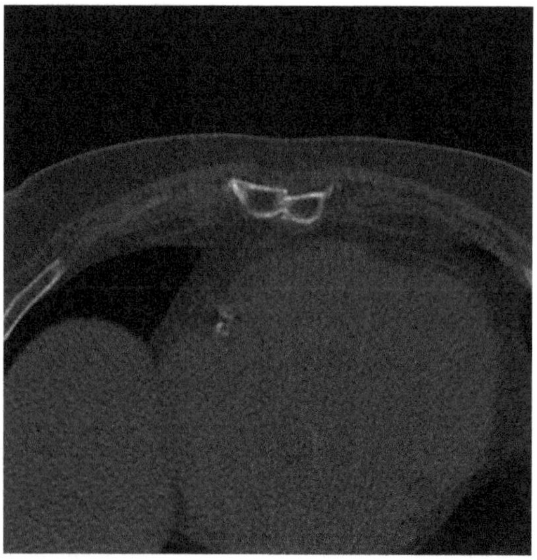

**FIGURE 1** | Pre-operative axial computed-tomography image of patient 1. The diagnosis of pseudarthrosis is clear as we can't see any bone bridges between the two halves.

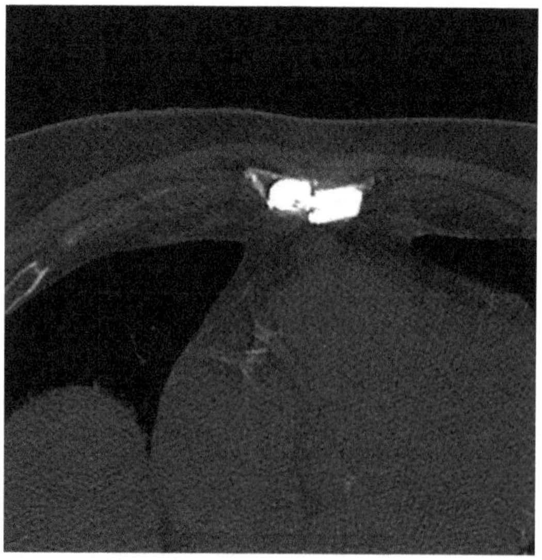

**FIGURE 2** | Post-operative axial computed-tomography image of patient 1. The radiopaque cement fills the pseudathrosic parts of the sternum to reduce the pain and a bridge is created for a better stabilization.

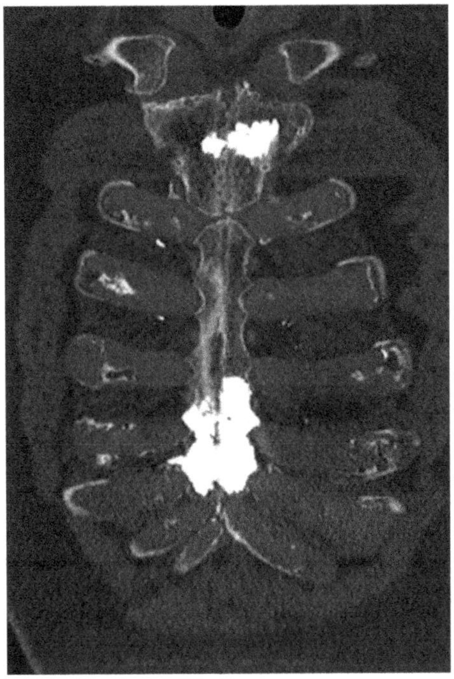

**FIGURE 3** | Post-operative coronal computed-tomography image of patient 1.

## Cementoplasty Technique

After performing local anesthesia with lidocaine, the procedure is executed under sedation-analgesia with morphium, midazolam and intravenous paracetamol. Antibiotic prophylaxis is made with 1.5 g intravenous cefuroxime. The intervention is achieved under CT-scan imaging to verify the correct placement of the needles and the spreading of cement. All CT-guided injections are performed with one 64-channel multidetector CT scanner (Somatom Definition AS; Siemens Healthineers, Erlangen, Germany). A monoplanar CT scout view was obtained in the lateral projection (tube current: 60 mAs, peak voltage: 120 kVp), followed by a spiral CT scan (tube current: 50 mAs, peak voltage: 100 kVp), as preparation for the injection. The pre-injection CT images is limited to the sternal segments of interest to minimize the radiation exposure. The needle puncture site on the skin is selected on the initial spiral CT scan sections.

Spinal Confidence™ combines a highly viscous cement with a hydraulic distribution system. The ultra-viscous radiopaque cement CONFIDENCE™ (DePuy Synthes, Johnson&Johnson) reaches a pasty phase immediately after the cement components have been mixed, thus limiting the risk of intravascular embolization. The amount of cement spread is let at the discretion of the in-charge radiologist. Bedrest is then taken for 4 h to allow the cement to consolidate.

## Follow-Up

As the intervention is made under CT-scan and the cement is almost stiff when the procedure ends, there is no need for a radiological follow-up unless the patient presents new symptoms. One month after the cementoplasty, a clinical appointment is scheduled during which the patient fills the QBPD scale and VAS and some exercises from the sternal instability scale are performed.

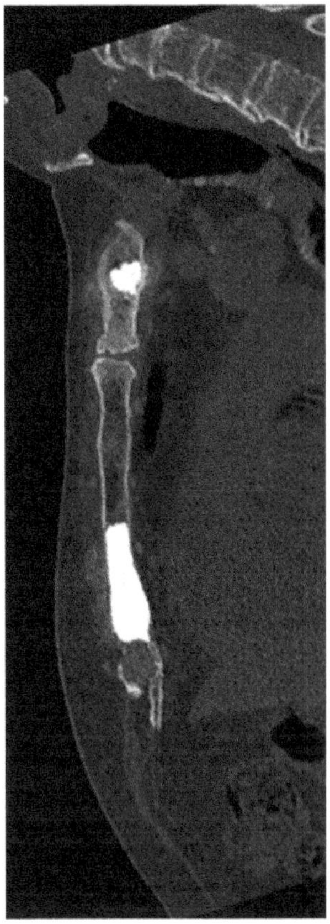

**FIGURE 4** | Post-operative sagittal computed-tomography image of patient 1.

# RESULTS

## Patient Demographics

Three women and two men (age 72 ± 4yo; range: 67–77) suffering from non-infected SPA were treated by percutaneous cementoplasty (**Table 1**). Three of them had a metabolic syndrome with obesity (BMI >30 kg/m$^2$), type-2 diabetes mellitus and dyslipidaemia. One patient suffered from chronic obstructive pulmonary disease (COPD). Four patients were smokers (64 ± 25 pack-years; range: 45–100). All patients underwent coronary artery bypass surgery with left internal mammary artery grafting and three had bilateral internal mammary artery grafting. Two patients suffered from sternal infection after CABG surgery and one patient had a redo operation. SPA was localized in three patients (manubrium $n = 1$; body $n = 2$) and generalized in two.

## Cementoplasty Procedures

The procedure time was 27 ± 12 minutes. The radiation exposure was 0.13 ± 0.04 mGy. During the procedure, 3 ± 3 mL of cement were injected. **Figures 1–4** depict example of pre- and postinterventional CT findings.

**TABLE 2** | Patients' scores from the Quebec back pain disability scale before and after the intervention.

| Patients | QBPD scores before cementoplasty | QBPD scores after cementoplasty | Sites of injection (Manubrium (M) and/or body (B)) |
|---|---|---|---|
| 1 | 64 | 46 | M + B |
| 2 | 5 | 1 | B |
| 3 | 56 | 33 | M |
| 4 | 68 | 40 | B |
| 5 | 81 | 30 | M + B |

No immediate or short-term complication happened. The intra- and post-operative images show no major leak of the cement, no embolism and no damage to the internal mammary artery or the heart.

### Clinical Follow-Up

At one-month follow-up, no patients presented evidence of complications or neurological sensorimotor disorder. Every patient described an improvement in their daily activities and quality of life. The Quebec back pain disability scale score (**Table 2**) improved from 54.8 ± 29.3 to 30.0 ± 17.4 ($p = 0.03$) and concerning the visual analog pain scale, we noted an improvement from 7.0 ± 2.8 to 1.6 ± 1.6 ($p = 0.01$). Furthermore, three out of five patients completely stopped taking painkillers whereas two additional significantly decreased the dose.

## DISCUSSION

Percutaneous cementoplasty was developed for vertebroplasty in 1984 as a treatment for vertebral hemangioma. Its indication has been extended to vertebral fracture due to its capability to tolerate compressive pressures. Here, we report for the first time the possibility of using percutaneous cementoplasty to treat SPA. We demonstrate the feasibility, the safety and the efficacy of this novel and minimally invasive alternative technique to surgery. We are convinced that percutaneous cementoplasty can be used in all type of SPA regardless of its cause.

Postoperative sternal wound infection is found in 0.5–8.4% of cases (13) and could lead to SPA. The classical risk factors for SPA are smoking, metabolic syndrome and COPD (6). In addition to increasing the odds of sternal dehiscence by 3.9 times, obesity seems to be the most critical risk factor for postoperative sternal infection (9). Moreover, Seyfer et al. noted that bilateral mammary artery grafting is at greater risk since every mammary artery harvesting is associated with a 90% drop of the ipsilateral sternal blood flow (14). Therefore, smoking, metabolic syndrome, obesity, COPD and bilateral mammary artery grafting are associated with SPA (1, 15). To limit the incidence of SPA, the modifiable components of these risk factors should be tightly controlled, and the use of steroids and non-steroidal anti-inflammatory drugs minimized during the few weeks before CABG (5). Considering that the separation of the sternal edges usually begins in the caudal third due to the concentration of distraction forces and low blood supply, adding wires at the lower end is an efficient way to lower its incidence (2, 4, 9).

When SPA occurs, a careful physical examination is mandatory during the first year since a large part of non-infectious SPA will resolve spontaneously over time. If not, a CT scan of the sternum should be done. In these patients, surgical closure or percutaneous cementoplasty will be discussed on a case-by-case basis with the in-charge surgeon. In the case of a poor surgical candidate, percutaneous cementoplasty appears to be associated with encouraging preliminary results.

### Limitations

The present study is limited in size with possible selection bias. Given the uncertainty around point estimations, extrapolations should be drawn with caution. The fact that it was performed in a single center with cementoplasty performed by a single experienced operator with uniform procedural strategies makes generalizations to other centers limited.

## CONCLUSION

SPA is a debilitating affliction that may complicate sternotomy after cardiac surgery. Percutaneous cementoplasty constitutes a promising technique in selected cases.

## ETHICS STATEMENT

The studies involving human participants were reviewed and approved by La Commission cantonale d'éthique de la recherche sur l'être humain (CER-VD). The patients/participants provided their written informed consent to participate in this study. All patients gave their written informed consent to the procedure and the work has been performed under the general approval by the Local Ethics Committee (FR-339-14).

## AUTHOR CONTRIBUTIONS

TP: collected the informations in patients' files, interviewed NT, and wrote the article. SC: patients' cardiologist, direct supervisor of TP, and corrected the temporary versions of the article. GK: performed the CABG and corrected the final version of the article. NT: performed the percutaneous cementoplasty and corrected the final version of the article. All authors contributed to the article and approved the submitted version.

## REFERENCES

1. Hamagushi R, Shekar PS, Johnson JA, Orgill DP. Current management of sternal wounds. *Plast Reconstr Surg.* (2021) 148:1012e–25e. doi: 10.1097/PRS.0000000000008510
2. Casha AR, Manche A, Gatt R, Duca E, Gauci M, Schembri-Wismayer P, et al. Mechanism of sternotomy dehiscence. *Interact Cardiovasc Thorac Surg.* (2014) 19:617–21. doi: 10.1093/icvts/ivu184
3. Chase CW, Franklin JD, Guest DP, Barker DE. Internal fixation of the sternum in median sternotomy dehiscence. *Plast Reconstr Surg.* (1999) 103:1667–73. doi: 10.1097/00006534-199905000-00014

4. El-Ansary D, Waddington G, Adams R. Relationship between pain and upper limb movement in patients with chronic sternal instability following cardiac surgery. *Physiother Theory Pract.* (2007) 23:273–80. doi: 10.1080/09593980701209402
5. Gill IP, Montgomery RJ, Wallis J. Successful treatment of sternal non-union by ultrasound. *Interact Cardiovasc Thorac Surg.* (2009) 9:389–90. doi: 10.1510/icvts.2008.196600
6. Truntzer J, Vopat B, Feldstein M, Matityahu A. Smoking cessation and bone healing: optimal cessation timing. *Eur J Orthop Surg Traumatol.* (2014) 25:211–5. doi: 10.1007/s00590-014-1488-y
7. Grechenig S, Pfeifer C, Krutsch W, Hilber F, Nerlich M, Berner A. Komplikationsmanagement bei fehlender Knochenbruchheilung: Pseudarthrosen. *Der Chirurg.* (2015) 86:919–24. doi: 10.1007/s00104-015-0050-8
8. Combes JM, Carrie JM, Soula P, Tricoire JL, Cerene A. Closure of sternotomy with Cotrel staplers. *Ann Chir.* (1993) 47:179–83.
9. Molina JE, Lew RS, Hyland KJ. Postoperative sternal dehiscence in obese patients: incidence and prevention. *Ann Thorac Surg.* (2004) 78:912–7; discussion—7. doi: 10.1016/j.athoracsur.2004.03.038
10. Freidel M, Champsaur A, Champsaur G. Sternal pseudarthrosis in irradiated patients. Repairing by the pectoralis major myocutaneous flap. *Ann Chir Plast Esthet.* (1986) 31:241–4.
11. Fuller LM, El-Ansary D, Button B, Bondarenko J, Marasco S, Snell G et al. Reliability of sternal instability scale (SIS) for transverse sternotomy in lung transplantation (LTX). *Physiother Theory Pract.* (2018) 34:931–4. doi: 10.1080/09593985.2018.1431342
12. Cohen DJ, Griffin LV. A biomechanical comparison of three sternotomy closure techniques. *Ann Thorac Surg.* (2002) 73:563–8. doi: 10.1016/S0003-4975(01)03389-6
13. Grevious MA, Ramaswamy R, Henry GI, Grubb KJ. Sternal Dehiscence Reconstruction, Medscape Drugs & Diseases: Plastic Surgery (2020). Available online at: emedicine.medscape.com/article/1278627 (accessed January 25, 2022).
14. Seyfer AE, Shriver CD, Miller TR, Graeber GM. Sternal blood flow after median sternotomy and mobilization of the internal mammary arteries. *Surgery.* (1988) 104:899–904.
15. Angelini GD, el-Ghamari FA, Butchart EG. Poststernotomy pseudo-arthrosis due to foreign body reaction to bone wax. *Eur J Cardiothorac Surg.* (1987) 1:129–30. doi: 10.1016/1010-7940(87) 90025-X

10

# Endo-Aortic vs. Trans-Thoracic Clamping in Right Mini-Thoracotomy Mitral Valve Surgery: Outcome on Myocardial Protection

*Cristina Barbero [1*], Mauro Rinaldi [1,2], Marco Pocar [1,2], Erik Cura Stura [1], Claudia Calia [1], Viviana Sebastiano [1], Giovanni Marchetto [1], Claudia Filippini [3], Massimo Boffini [1] and Davide Ricci [4,5]*

*[1] Department of Cardiovascular Surgery, Città della Salute e della Scienza, University of Turin, Turin, Italy, [2] Department of Clinical Sciences and Community Health, University of Milan, Milan, Italy, [3] Department of Anesthesia and Critical Care, University of Turin, Turin, Italy, [4] Cardiac Surgery Unit, Scientific Institute for Research, Hospitalization and Healthcare Policlinic Hospital San Martino, Genova, Italy, [5] Department of Integrated Surgical and Diagnostic Sciences, University of Genova, Genova, Italy*

***Correspondence:**
*Cristina Barbero*
*cristina.barbero@unito.it*

**Background:** Perfusion strategies and aortic clamping techniques for right mini-thoracotomy mitral valve (MV) surgery have evolved over time and remarkable short- and long-term results have been reported. However, some concerns have raised about the adequacy of myocardial protection during the minimally invasive approach, particularly with the endo-aortic clamp (EAC). Aim of this study was to compare the efficacy, in terms of myocardial preservation, of the EAC with the trans-thoracic aortic clamp (TTC) in patients undergoing right mini-thoracotomy MV surgery.

**Methods:** A single center, prospective observational study was performed on patients undergoing right mini-thoracotomy MV surgery with retrograde arterial perfusion and EAC or TTC. A propensity matched analysis was performed to compare the two groups. Primary outcome was the comparison between cardiac troponin T levels measured at different time-points after surgery.

**Results:** Eighty EAC patients were compared with 37 TTC patients. No cases of myocardial infarction or low cardiac-output syndrome were overall reported. No differences were recorded in terms of stroke, peri-operative mortality, and in the release of myocardial markers, lactates levels and need for inotropic support at different time-points after surgery. CK-MB peak levels were significantly lower in the EAC group.

**Conclusion:** Despite concerns arising about the EAC, this prospective study shows equivalence in terms of myocardial preservation of the EAC compared with the TTC in patients undergoing right mini-thoracotomy MV surgery.

**Keywords: myocardial protection, minimally invasive cardiac surgery, mitral valve, mitral valve repair, cardioplegia, aortic clamping, cardiopulmonary bypass**

## INTRODUCTION

Perfusion strategies and aortic clamping techniques for right mini-thoracotomy mitral valve (MV) surgery have evolved over time and remarkable short- and long-term results have been reported all over the world (1–5). However, across the years, some concerns have emerged on the adequacy of myocardial protection offered by the minimally invasive approach and on the role of aortic clamping strategies in this context.

The standard right mini-thoracotomy set-up is based on retrograde arterial perfusion (RAP) through the femoral artery and endo-aortic clamp (EAC) or trans-thoracic aortic clamp (TTC). In the former, aortic occlusion is obtained with a balloon catheter inserted through the femoral cannula, and cardioplegia is delivered through the tip of the catheter; in the latter, aortic occlusion is obtained with a trans-thoracic direct clamping and a separate line into the ascending aorta is used for cardioplegia delivery. Efficacy of the EAC setting on myocardial preservation is definitely more debated due to several factors, including the higher risk of instability and possible migration or tearing of the balloon, and the more challenging learning curve for the surgeon (6).

Aim of this prospective observational study was to compare the effectiveness, in terms of myocardial protection, of the EAC vs. the TTC setting in patients undergoing right mini-thoracotomy MV surgery.

## PATIENTS AND METHODS

### Study Design

A single-institution prospective observational study was performed at the University of Turin, Cardio-thoracic Department, between June 2014 and June 2018. The study protocol was reviewed and approved by the Institutional Ethics Committee (protocol number 0095187). Inclusion criteria were diagnosis of MV regurgitation, planned surgery through the right mini-thoracotomy and RAP. Exclusion criteria were non-elective surgery, cardiac ejection fraction lower than 40%, more than mild aortic regurgitation, previous coronary artery bypass grafts, coronary artery disease, severe peripheral vascular disease, and concomitant procedures for atrial fibrillation ablation. Patients admitted at our Department during the study period underwent a full preoperative work-up based upon clinical history and analysis of the vascular anatomy with the aim to be allocated to the most appropriate setting: RAP with EAC, RAP with TTC, or antegrade arterial perfusion with TTC (7–9). All comers were screened for the clinical trial inclusion criteria.

Primary outcome was the comparison between cardiac troponin T (cTn-T) levels measured at different time-points after surgery; secondary outcomes were peri-operative myocardial infarction, creatinine kinase-myocardial band (CK-MB) and lactates levels at different time-points after surgery, the occurrence of low cardiac output syndrome, and the need for post-operative inotropic support.

### Definitions

Peri-operative myocardial infarction was recorded in the case of cTn-T value >10 times the 99th percentile of the upper reference limit during the first 48 h with electrocardiographic (ECG) abnormalities and/or angiographic or imaging evidence of new myocardial ischemia/new loss of myocardial viability (10).

Low cardiac-output syndrome was defined as cardiac index lower than 2 L/min/m$^2$ and systolic blood pressure lower than 90 mmHg, together with signs of tissue hypoperfusion (cold periphery, clammy skin, mental confusion, reduced urine output, elevated lactate levels) in the absence of hypovolemia (11).

Inotropic support was administered with the primary goal of maintaining a mean arterial pressure above 60 mmHg and cardiac index more than 2 L/min/m$^2$. Vasoactive-inotropic score (VIS) indicates the amount of cardiovascular support by various inotropes or vasopressors in the first 24 h after the surgical procedure. The VIS was calculated as: dopamine dose (mg/kg/min) + dobutamine dose (mg/kg/min) + 100 × epinephrine dose (mg/kg/min) + 10 × milrinone dose (mg/kg/min) + 10.000 × vasopressin dose (unit/kg/min) + 100 × norepinephrine dose (mg/kg/min) (12).

Peri-operative mortality was defined as all deaths occurring during hospitalization or within 30 days of the procedure. Post-operative stroke was defined as a new, permanent neurological disability or deficit.

### Surgical Procedure and Myocardial Protection

Right mini-thoracotomy approach with perfusion strategies and aortic clamping techniques used in our Department has been previously described (8, 9). After full heparinization, peripheral cardiopulmonary bypass (CPB) was established with the patient cooled to 30°C. In the EAC setting, arterial cannulation was obtained with a 21F or a 23F cannula with sidearm (Edwards Lifesciences, Irvine, California); in the case of small arteries, a 21F cannula was used for inserting the EAC, while the contralateral artery was used for arterial perfusion by using a standard arterial cannula. In the TTC setting, a standard femoral cannula was used (18F or 20F, Edwards Lifesciences, Irvine, California). Venous return was routinely obtained with a double cannulation (jugular and femoral).

In the EAC setting, clamping and cardioplegia delivery were obtained through a balloon catheter (Intraclude®, Edwards Lifesciences, Irvine, CA) inserted through the sidearm of the arterial cannula; in the TTC setting, a Chitwood clamp, inserted through a first intercostal space port (Scanlan International, Inc., Minneapolis, MN, USA) was used and the cardioplegia was delivered through a 7F cardioplegia needle (CalMed Technologies, CA) placed into the ascending aorta. Antegrade myocardial protection was performed using St Thomas hospital solution 1 (Plegisol™, Hospira Inc., Lake Forest, Illinois, USA) or Bretschneider solution (Custodiol®). At the end of the procedure air venting was obtained, in the EAC group, with the balloon inflated, through the cardioplegia line, while in the TTC group through the aortic line.

All patients receiving Bretschneider solution underwent minimal right atrium incision (<1 cm) in order to remove the crystalloid solution or underwent hemofiltration during cardiopulmonary bypass. No additional topical cooling, nor retrograde cardioplegia through the coronary sinus were used; aortic clamp was released above 33°C in all the patients.

After the surgical procedure, all patients were investigated for ECG abnormalities and for new hypokinetic or akinetic area by echocardiography.

## Biochemical Analysis

Blood samples for biochemical examination were collected immediately after the surgical procedure and at 6, 12, and 24 h post-operatively. Upper reference limit for CK-MB and for cTn-T were 5 ng/mL and 50 ng/L, respectively.

## Statistical Analysis

Continuous data are presented as mean and standard deviation (SD) or median and interquartile range (IQR) depending on data distribution, while categorical data are presented as rate and proportion. In univariate analysis continuous variables were compared using unpaired *t*-test or Wilcoxon-Mann-Whitney according to distribution type. Categorical variables were compared with the use of the Chi-square test or Fisher exact test, when appropriate.

To reduce possible differences between patients receiving EAC or TTC and obtain unbiased estimation of the treatment effect, a matched analysis using propensity score was performed. The propensity score of receiving EAC or TTC was estimated using a multivariable logistic regression analysis with the type of clamping as dependent variable. The priori selected variables were: age, gender, body mass index, pre-operative creatinine, peripheral vasculopathy, EuroSCORE II, previous cardiac surgery, ejection fraction, type of MV disease, length of aortic clamping, type of cardioplegia, and mean pressure during CPB.

The genetic matching method without replacement was used to match patients undergoing surgery with EAC or TTC (13–15). Standard differences were used to test balance and to compare the difference in the covariate between the pre- and post-matched samples, since the calculation is not dependent on sample size. A standardized difference is the difference in means between groups, divided by the (pooled) standard deviation: values <0.1 indicate adequate balance (16).

A mixed-linear regression model for repeated measures was used to examine the temporal effect across groups (EAC and TTC) during the 24-h observation period after surgery. Statistical tests were two-sided, and *p*-values of 0.05 or less were considered statistically significant and were conducted using the following software packages: Stata (Stata-Corp, College Station, Texas), R (R Foundation for Statistical Computing, http://www.r-project.org/) and SAS (SAS Institute, Cary, NC).

A receiver operating characteristic curve (ROC analysis) with peak cTn-T and CK-MB levels was performed. The results were expressed by providing the value of the AUC and relative interval at a 95% confidence level.

# RESULTS

Five-hundred and sixty-six patients underwent right mini-thoracotomy MV surgery at our Department during the study period. One-hundred and eighty-nine patients met the study inclusion criteria. Of these, 81 underwent surgery with the EAC setting and 106 with the TTC setting; two patients did not undergo myocardial protection analysis due to conversion to median sternotomy before CPB onset. Groups were not comparable with respect to age, pre-operative creatinine level, peripheral vascular disease, EuroSCORE II, previous cardiac surgery, and type of MV regurgitation (**Table 1**). After matching, 80 EAC patients were compared with 37 TTC patients (**Table 1**). Standardized difference showed an adequate balance between groups regarding patients' baseline characteristics and intraoperative data apart from age, previous cardiac surgery, and mean pressure during CPB: in these cases, standardized difference between EAC and TTC widely reduced after matching, even if it still remains above 0.2.

No cases of EAC tearing or dislodgement were overall reported. No cases of myocardial infarction or low cardiac-output syndrome were observed. No ECG abnormalities or new hypokinetic or akinetic area were highlighted at the post-operative echocardiogram. No differences were recorded in terms of stroke, intensive care unit and hospital length of stay, and peri-operative mortality (**Table 2**). Two patients undergoing redo MV replacement in the TTC group died in 2nd and in 18th post-operative day, respectively. Cause of death were left ventricle rupture in a severe mitral annulus calcification in the first case, and multi-organ failure in the second case. Levels of myocardial markers in both the patients were below the median of the group.

A significant lower CK-MB peak level was recorded in the EAC group ($p = 0.030$), while no differences were found in the release of myocardial markers, lactates levels and need for inotropic support at different time-points after surgery (**Figure 1**). The ROC analysis showed AUC = 0.56 (95% CI 0.48; 0.63) 95%, and AUC = 0.55 (95% CI 0.48; 0.63) 95% for post-operative peak level of CK-MB and cTn-T, respectively.

# DISCUSSION

Adequate and safe myocardial protection represents the first key requirement in cardiac surgery, regardless of the type of surgical procedure and the approach. When looking at right mini-thoracotomy MV surgery, concerns still remain about the role of aortic clamping strategies, particularly the EAC, on the risk of sub-optimal myocardial protection. The rationale is that it requires consolidated team experience to get the right position and pressure of the balloon in the ascending aorta and to maintain those conditions through all the procedure; migration of the balloon toward the left ventricle or toward the aortic arch, or accidental balloon puncture or tearing could be responsible for inadequate myocardial protection. For these reasons, the TTC is preferred to the EAC in many centers. However, it requires some kind of aortic manipulation, such as dissection around the ascending aorta to allow the external clamp positioning and a separate line

**TABLE 1** | Patients' characteristics and operative data before and after matching.

| | Before matching | | | After matching | | |
|---|---|---|---|---|---|---|
| | **EAC (*n* = 81)** | **TTC (*n* = 106)** | **Standardized difference** | **EAC (*n* = 80)** | **TTC (*n* = 37)** | **Standardized difference** |
| Age years, mean (SD) | 55.5 (12.4) | 68.6 (10.2) | 1.15 | 55.2 (12.4) | 61.8 (9.1) | 0.46 |
| Female, *n* (%) | 29 (35.8) | 46 (43.4) | 0.16 | 28 (35.0) | 11 (29.7) | −0.08 |
| BMI, mean (SD) | 24.5 (3.6) | 24.4 (3.5) | −0.02 | 24.5 (3.6) | 24.2 (3.0) | −0.01 |
| Pre-op creatinine mg/dL, mean (SD) | 0.9 (0.2) | 1 (0.4) | 0.41 | 0.9 (0.2) | 0.9 (0.2) | 0.09 |
| Peripheral arterial disease, *n* (%) | 6 (7.4) | 38 (35.8) | 0.74 | 5 (6.3) | 3 (8.1) | 0.15 |
| Ejection fraction %, mean (SD) | 62.2 (7.2) | 61.8 (7.9) | −0.04 | 62.2 (7.2) | 62.8 (8.1) | 0.11 |
| Previous cardiac surgery, *n (%)* | 9 (11.1) | 1 (0.9) | −0.44 | 8 (10) | 1 (2.7) | −0.26 |
| Log EuroSCORE II, mean (SD) | 4.3 (8.04) | 5.7 (4.4) | 0.20 | 4.0 (7.4) | 3.0 (1.9) | −0.16 |
| MV repair, *n* (%) | 63 (77.7) | 67 (63.2) | 0.32 | 63 (78.8) | 33 (89.2) | −0.20 |
| Aortic clamping min, median (IQR) | 99 (83–115) | 89 (73–106) | −0.37 | 100 (83–115) | 94 (83–113) | −0.19 |
| Custodiol cardioplegia, *n* (%) | 69 (85.2) | 79 (74.5) | −0.27 | 69 (86.2) | 33 (89.2) | −0.10 |
| CPB pressure mmHg, mean (SD) | 60.3 (5.7) | 64.8 (6.2) | 0.75 | 60.3 (5.7) | 62.2 (5.5) | 0.29 |

*EAC, endo-aortic clamp; TTC, trans-thoracic clamp; SD, standard deviation; BMI, body mass index; MV, mitral valve; CPB, cardio-pulmonary by-pass.*

**TABLE 2** | Outcomes in matched cohort.

| | **EAC (*n* = 80)** | **TTC (*n* = 37)** | ***p*** |
|---|---|---|---|
| VF after aortic clamp release, *n* (%) | 11 (13.8) | 8 (21.6) | 0.2830 |
| Ventilation >72 h, *n* (%) | 4 (5.0) | 1 (2.7) | >0.9999 |
| Stroke, n (%) | 2 (2.5) | 0 (0) | >0.9999 |
| Myocardial infarction, *n* (%) | 0 (0) | 0 (0) | – |
| cTn-T peak level, mean (SD) | 1016.8 (654.7) | 1187 (744.5) | 0.1071 |
| CK-MB peak level, mean (SD) | 1394.4 (668.4) | 1775.6 (930) | 0.030 |
| Low cardiac output syndrome, *n* (%) | 0 (0) | 0 (0) | – |
| Dialysis, n (%) | 1 (1.3) | 1 (2.7) | 0.5343 |
| Re-exploration for bleeding, *n* (%) | 0 (0) | 1 (2.7) | 0.3162 |
| Post-op atrial fibrillation, *n* (%) | 23 (28.9) | 12 (32.4) | 0.6858 |
| ICU stay days, mean (SD) | 1.6 (2.5) | 1.3 (0.8) | 0.3121 |
| Hospital stay days, mean (SD) | 7.4 (3.9) | 6.8 (2.0) | 0.3623 |
| Peri-operative mortality, *n* (%) | 0 (0) | 2 (5.4) | 0.0981 |

*EAC, endo-aortic clamp; TTC, trans-thoracic clamp; VF, ventricular fibrillation; cTn-T, cardiac troponin T; CK-MB, creatinine kinase-myocardial band; SD, standard deviation; ICU, intensive care unit.*

for cardioplegia delivery; these maneuvers, compared to the "aortic no touch technique" of the EAC, increase the risk of local damage to the aorta, and some degrees of calcium embolization (6, 17).

A propensity matched analysis comparing the EAC with the TTC in terms of myocardial protection was performed at our Department using established markers of myocardial injury, i.e., cTn-T and CK-MB. Results of the present study do not support concerns existing in the literature regarding the EAC setting: equivalence at each time point after surgery was recorded for cTn-T levels, lactates levels and VIS score; moreover, a significant lower CK-MB post-operative peak level was recorded in the EAC group ($p = 0.030$). The area under the curve for cTn-T has demonstrated excellent linear relationship with the mass of myocardial injury; the area under the curve for CK-MB is also good, although clearly inferior to cTn-T (18). Therefore our results can be read as equivalence between the two aortic clamping techniques.

During the study period and during our every-day clinical practice the choice of one setting in respect to the others is orientated on the patient's aorto/iliac/femoral anatomy and

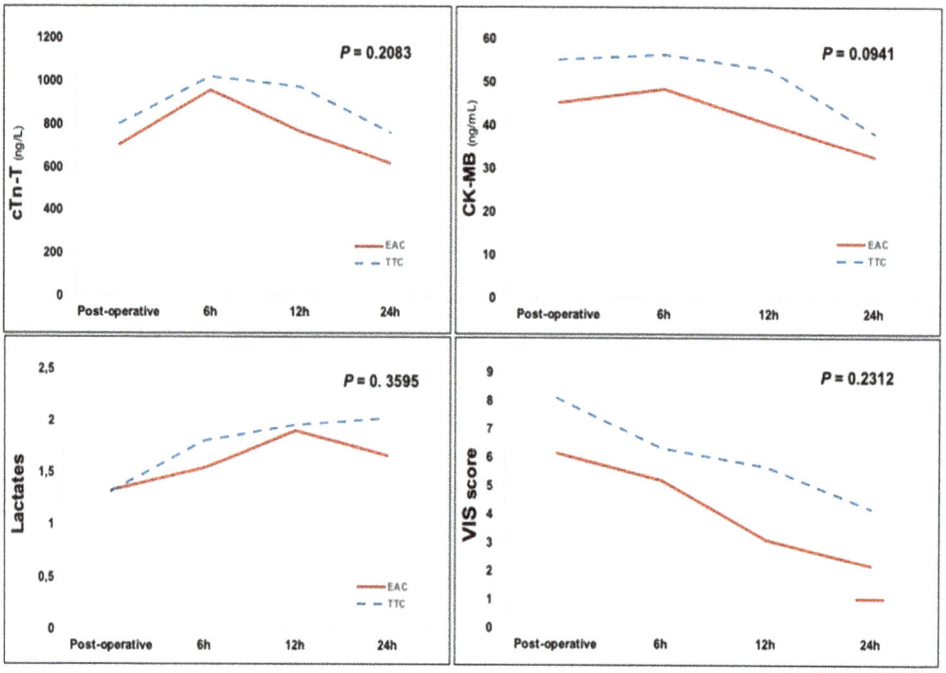


**FIGURE 1 |** Post-operative cTn-T and CK-MB activities, lactates levels and VIS score. EAC, endo-aortic clamp; TTC, trans-thoracic clamp; cTn-T, cardiac Troponin T; CK-MB, creatinine kinase-myocardial band; VIS, vasoactive-inotropic score.

clinical history, regardless of the surgeon's preference. Such as, in case of previous cardiac surgery the EAC setting is used mostly; in case of dilated ascending aorta (diameter >40 mm) the TTC setting was predominantly used; in case of aorto-iliac-femoral arteries disease, an antegrade arterial perfusion with TTC was preferred (8, 19, 20). In cases of patients without peripheral vessel disease or other main comorbidities the setting of choice in our practice is RAP with EAC because it does not require to open extensively the pericardium in order to get a full exposure of the ascending aorta, it does not require to place a cardioplegia/vent needle into the ascending aorta, and it does not require getting a further port in the first intercostals space to introduce and place the aortic clamp (8, 19).

Results of the present study are in contrast with reports of other centers showing superiority of the TTC. Mazine et al., in a retrospective analysis on 243 patients undergoing right mini-thoracotomy MV surgery and EAC or TTC concluded that the TTC setting results in better myocardial protection (6). However, several bias may have influenced this result: longer operative time and several cases of endoclamp dislodgement were reported in the EAC group; cases from both groups were not evenly distributed in time (the balloons were mostly used at the beginning of the experience and thus at the beginning of the learning curve); furthermore only CK-MB plasma levels were taken into consideration for myocardial injury analysis.

More recent experiences show equivalence or even better results with the EAC setting. Bentala et al., in a retrospective analysis on 221 patients undergoing right mini-thoracotomy MV surgery and EAC or TTC showed comparable results in terms of post-operative myocardial infarction and lower maximum post-operative cTn-T levels with the EAC setting (21). A multicentric European study on 500 right mini-thoracotomy MV surgery patients reported a significant lower rate of post-operative myocardial infarction in the EAC group (1.2 vs. 4% in the TTC group, $p = 0.05$) (17). The improvement in myocardial protection in more recent series can be explained considering that these studies have been reported by surgeons with a well-established learning curve and with a consolidated program of patient selection based upon vascular anatomy and clinical history. Another potential influencing factor in the different rate of complications is the type of endo-balloon used: while most of the first reports on right mini-thoracotomy MV surgery with the EAC setting used the Endoclamp, in most recent series either the Endoclamp and the IntraClude devices were used with respect to the time of distribution of the products (Endoclamp at the beginning, Intraclude later). The Intraclude has different new features able to enhance manipulation and stabilization of the balloon in the ascending aorta during the surgical procedure.

The single-center non-randomized study design is clearly the main limitation. However, the reason for not performing a prospective randomized clinical trial was driven by our consolidated practice in minimally invasive surgery based on a tailored approach for each patient. Moreover, the propensity matched analysis reached a suboptimal balance between groups regarding age, previous cardiac surgery, and mean pressure during CPB. Standardized difference for these variables widely reduced after matching, even if it still remains above 0.2: this can be explain considering that in our every-day clinical practice the EAC is the preferred setting in redo cases and in young patients without atheromatous disease. Furthermore, with the EAC setting the mean pressure during CPB is more accurately verified and persistently kept low than 60–65 mmHg because it is one of the determinant factors in maintaining the right position of the balloon during the clamping time; this gives reasons for the different mean CPB pressure recorded between the two groups. It must be said that, from a clinical point of view, there are no differences between 60 and 62 mmHg.

## CONCLUSIONS

Despite concerns arising about the EAC, this prospective study shows equivalence in terms of myocardial protection of the EAC compared with the TTC in patients undergoing right mini-thoracotomy MV surgery.

## ETHICS STATEMENT

The studies involving human participants were reviewed and approved by Institutional Ethics Committee Città della Salute e della Scienza - Torino (protocol number 0095187). The patients/participants provided their written informed consent to participate in this study.

## AUTHOR CONTRIBUTIONS

CB and MR: conceptualization. CB and DR: methodology. CF: software. MR, MB, MP, and GM: validation. CB and CF: formal analysis. ES, CC, and VS: investigation and data curation. CB: writing-original draft preparation and writing-review and editing. MR: supervision and project administration. All authors contributed to the article and approved the submitted version.

## REFERENCES


1. Modi P, Hassan A, Chitwood WR Jr. Minimally invasive mitral valve surgery: a systematic review and meta-analysis. *Eur J Cardiothorac Surg.* (2008) 34:943–52. doi: 10.1016/j.ejcts.2008.07.057
2. Iribarne A, Russo MJ, Easterwood R, Hong KN, Yang J, Cheema FH, et al. Minimally invasive versus sternotomy approach for mitral valve surgery: a propensity analysis. *Ann Thorac Surg.* (2010) 90:1471–7. doi: 10.1016/j.athoracsur.2010.06.034
3. Cheng DC, Martin J, Lal A, Diegeler A, Folliguet TA, Nifong LW, et al. Minimally invasive versus conventional open mitral valve surgery: a meta-analysis and systematic review. *Innovations.* (2011) 6:84–103. doi: 10.1097/imi.0b013e3182167feb
4. Goldstone AB, Atluri P, Szeto WY, Trubelja A, Howard JL, MacArthur JW Jr, et al. Minimally invasive approach provides at least equivalent results for surgical correction of mitral regurgitation: a propensity-matched comparison. *J Thorac Cardiovasc Surg.* (2013) 145:748–56. doi: 10.1016/j.jtcvs.2012.09.093
5. McClure RS, Athanasopoulos LV, McGurk S, Davidson MJ, Couper GS, Cohn LH. One thousand minimally invasive mitral valve operations: early outcomes, late outcomes, and echocardiographic follow-up. *J Thorac Cardiovasc Surg.* (2013) 145:1199–206. doi: 10.1016/j.jtcvs.2012.12.070
6. Mazine A, Pellerin M, Lebon JS, Dionne PO, Jeanmart H, Bouchard D. Minimally invasive mitral valve surgery: influence of aortic clamping technique on early outcomes. *Ann Thorac Surg.* (2013) 96:2116–22. doi: 10.1016/j.athoracsur.2013.07.015
7. Barbero C, Ricci D, El Qarra S, Marchetto G, Boffini M, Rinaldi M. Aortic cannulation system for minimally invasive mitral valve surgery. *J Thorac Cardiovasc Surg.* (2015) 149:1669–72. doi: 10.1016/j.jtcvs.2015.02.040
8. Barbero C, Marchetto G, Ricci D, El Qarra S, Attisani M, Filippini C, et al. Minimal access mitral valve surgery: impact of tailored strategies on early outcome. *Ann Thorac Surg.* (2016) 102:1989–94. doi: 10.1016/j.athoracsur.2016.04.104
9. Barbero C, Rinaldi M. Preoperative vascular screening: a novel breakthrough in minimal invasive mitral valve surgery. *Interact Cardiovasc Thorac Surg.* (2017) 24:368. doi: 10.1093/icvts/ivx063
10. Thygesen K, Alpert JS, Jaffe AS, Chaitman BR, Bax JJ, Morrow DA, et al. The Executive Group on behalf of the Joint European Society of Cardiology (ESC)/American College of Cardiology (ACC)/ American Heart Association (AHA)/World Heart Federation (WHF) Task Force for the Universal Definition of Myocardial Infarction Fourth universal definition of myocardial infarction. *Eur Heart J.* (2019) 40:237–69. doi: 10.1161CIR.0000000000000617
11. Lomivorotov VV, Efremov SM, Kirov MY, Fominskiy EV, Karaskov AM. Low-cardiac-output syndrome after cardiac surgery. *J Cardiothorac Vasc Anesth.* (2017) 31:291–308. doi: 10.1053/j.jvca.2016.05.029
12. Gaies MG, Gurney JG, Yen AH, Napoli ML, Gajarski RJ, Ohye RG. Vasoactive-inotropic score as a predictor of morbidity and mortality in infants after cardiopulmonary bypass. *Pediatr Crit Care Med.* (2010) 11:234–8. doi: 10.1097/PCC.0b013e3181b806fc
13. Sekhon JS, Grieve RD. A matching method for improving covariate balance in cost-effectiveness analyses. *Health Econ.* (2012) 21:695–714. doi: 10.1002/hec.1748
14. Radice R, Ramsahai R, Grieve R, Noemi F, Zia S, Sekhon JS. Evaluating treatment effectiveness in patient subgroups: a comparison of propensity score methods with an automated matching approach. *Int J Biostat.* (2012) 8:25. doi: 10.1515/1557-4679.1382
15. Rosenbaum PR, Rubin DB. Constructing a control group using multivariate matched sampling methods that incorporate the propensity score. *Am Stat.* (1985) 39:33–8.
16. Austin PC. A critical appraisal of propensity-score matching in the medical literature between 1996 and 2003. *Stat Med.* (2008) 27:2037–49. doi: 10.1002/sim.3150
17. Barbero C, Krakor R, Bentala M, Casselman F, Candolfi P, Goldstein J, et al. Comparison of endoaortic and trans-thoracic aortic clamping in less-invasive mitral valve surgery. *Ann Thorac Surg.* (2018) 105:794–8. doi: 10.1016/j.athoracsur.2017.09.054
18. Pegg TJ, Maunsell Z, Karamitsos TD, Taylor RP, James T, Francis JM, et al. Utility of cardiac biomarkers for the diagnosis of type V myocardial infarction after coronary artery bypass grafting: Insights from serial cardiac MRI. *Heart.* (2011) 97:810–6. doi: 10.1136/hrt.2010.213462
19. Barbero C, Marchetto G, Ricci D, Cura Stura E, Clerici A, El Qarra S, et al. Steps forward in minimally invasive cardiac surgery: 10-year experience. *Ann Thorac Surg.* (2019) 108:1922–9. doi: 10.1016/j.athoracsur.2019.04.109
20. Ricci D, Pellegrini C, Aiello M, Alloni A, Cattadori B, D'Armini AM, et al. Port-access surgery as elective approach for mitral valve operation in re-do procedures. *Eur J Cardiothorac Surg.* (2010) 37:920–5. doi: 10.1016/j.ejcts.2009.10.011
21. Bentala M, Heutsb S, Vosc R, Jos M, Scohy TV, Gerritse B, et al. Comparing the endo-aortic balloon and the external aortic clamp in minimally invasive mitral valve surgery. *Interact CardioVasc Thorac Surg.* (2015) 21:359–65. doi: 10.1093/icvts/ivv160

# 11

# Lysophosphatidic Acid May be a Novel Biomarker for Early Acute Aortic Dissection

*Xiaogao Pan*[1,2], *Yang Zhou*[1,2], *Guifang Yang*[1,2], *Zhibiao He*[1,2], *Hongliang Zhang*[1,2], *Zhenyu Peng*[1,2], *Wen Peng*[1,2], *Tuo Guo*[1,2], *Mengping Zeng*[1,2], *Ning Ding*[3] and *Xiangping Chai*[1,2]*

[1] *Department of Emergency Medicine, Second Xiangya Hospital, Central South University, Changsha, China,* [2] *Emergency Medicine and Difficult Diseases Institute, Second Xiangya Hospital, Central South University, Changsha, China,* [3] *Emergency Department, Changsha Central Hospital, University of South China, Changsha, China*

***Correspondence:***
*Xiangping Chai*
*chaixiangping@csu.edu.cn*

**Background:** Misdiagnosis and delayed diagnosis of acute aortic dissection (AAD) significantly increase mortality. Lysophosphatidic acid (LPA) is a biomarker related to coagulation cascade and cardiovascular-injury. The extent of LPA elevation in AAD and whether it can discriminate sudden-onset of acute chest pain are currently unclear.

**Methods:** We measured the plasma concentration of LPA in a cohort of 174 patients with suspected AAD chest pain and 30 healthy participants. Measures to discriminate AAD from other acute-onset thoracalgia were compared and calculated.

**Results:** LPA was significantly higher in AAD than in the AMI, PE, and the healthy (344.69 $\pm$ 59.99 vs. 286.79 $\pm$ 43.01 vs. 286.61 $\pm$ 43.32 vs. 96.08 $\pm$ 11.93, $P < 0.01$) within 48 h of symptom onset. LPA level peaked at 12 h after symptom onset, then gradually decreased from 12 to 48 h in AAD. LPA had an AUC of 0.85 (0.80–0.90), diagnosis threshold of 298.98 mg/dl, a sensitivity of 0.81, specificity of 0.77, and the negative predictive value of 0.85. The ROC curve of LPA is better than D-dimer ($P = 0.041$, Delong test). The decision curve showed that LPA had excellent standardized net benefits.

**Conclusion:** LPA showed superior overall diagnostic performance to D-dimer in early AAD diagnosis may be a potential biomarker, but additional studies are needed to determine the rapid and cost-effective diagnostic tests in the emergency department.

**Keywords: aortic dissection, biomarker, lysophosphatidic acid, diagnosis, chest pain**

## INTRODUCTION

Aortic dissection is a life-threatening cardiovascular disease that causes ~10,000 deaths in the United States each year (21% before admission and 32% in-hospital) (1, 2). Recently, Sweden indicated that the incidence has increased about 7.2/100,000 (3). However, the early identification and diagnosis of high-risk chest pain as acute aortic dissection (AAD) is the major challenge. Treatment measures include coronary angiography and thrombolytic drugs, which may cause poor prognosis in 24.8% of AAD, who are misdiagnosed as acute myocardial infarction (AMI) or acute pulmonary embolism (PE) (4–6). Not only that, chest CT or MRI is time-money-consuming and limited by emergency room conditions compared to biomarkers for the diagnosis of AAD (7, 8).

Several researches have investigated AAD potential biomarkers for faster and more accurate clinical treatment, such as smooth muscle myosin (9), calcium binding protein (10), soluble elastin fragments (11), soluble ST2 (5), and D-dimer (12). While increased values for D-dimers raise suspicion for AAD (4), it is difficult to use it to desciminate AAD from PE in daily practice, and there are nine (2.43%) exhibited negative D-dimer results in 370 AAD patients according to our previous studies (13). Moreover, the younger and smaller thrombosis groups have low specificity. A valuable diagnostic marker should provide information for early identification or elimination to improve the clinical treatment of AAD (12).

Lysophosphatidic acid (LPA) is a small and simple glycerophospholipid (1-acyl-2-hydroxy-3-phosphoglycerol structure) (14), which is an early molecular marker of coagulation cascade activation and cardiovascular-injury (15, 16). Previous researches have shown that lysophosphatidylcholine (LPC) was also involved in aortic aneurysm formation and decreased substantially in AAD, which is hydrolyzed to produce LPA (17, 18). The LPA may be produced earlier than D-dimer, or have a better diagnostic performance than D-dimer and AAD risk scoring system (19, 20), but the relationship between LPA and AAD is unclear. The plasma LPA levels of patients with acute chest pain (AAD, AMI, PE) and healthy participants were measured and compared to evaluate the diagnostic performance in distinguishing AAD from other chest pains.

## METHODS

### Research Sample

This is a single-center retrospective cohort including patients with suspected AAD within 48 h of onset and healthy participants, who came from the emergency department and medical examination center of the Second Xiangya Hospital of Central South University (Changsha, China) between May 2020 and January 2021. All suspected AAD patients were examined for medical imaging and D-dimer for the final diagnosis (19, 21). The exclusion criteria are shown in **Supplementary Table 1**.

About 3–5 ml of whole blood was taken from the brachial vein and placed in a sodium citrate anticoagulant tube immediately after hospital admission. The samples were centrifuged at 1000 r/min for 15 min to process into plasma, and stored at −80°C. All sample processing methods are similar.

The Ethics Committee of the Second Xiangya Hospital of Central South University approved this study. Informed consent was obtained from all patients. However, consent was obtained from a family member in a case of sudden death after admission or during autopsy.

### Outcome

All patients with AAD, characterized by symptoms onset-time within 48 h, had image information from aortic computed tomography to confirm the final diagnosis. AMI diagnosis criteria were: (1) chest pain lasting >20 min, (2) Serial ECG changes with new pathological Q waves or ST-segment and T-wave changes, and (3) a plasma creatine kinase-myocardial band elevation (more than twice the normal level or cardiac troponin I (cTnI) level > 0.1 ng/ml). A positive pulmonary artery computed tomography scan was for PE diagnosis.

### Measurement of LPA

The processed serum was measured by the human lysophosphatidic acid kit (Wuhan Huamei Bioengineering Co., Ltd.), and D-dimer was detected by the TOP700 automatic coagulation analyzer.

### Statistical Analysis

Continuous variables were expressed as mean ± standard deviation or median (IQR). ANOVA and Kruskal-Wallis test

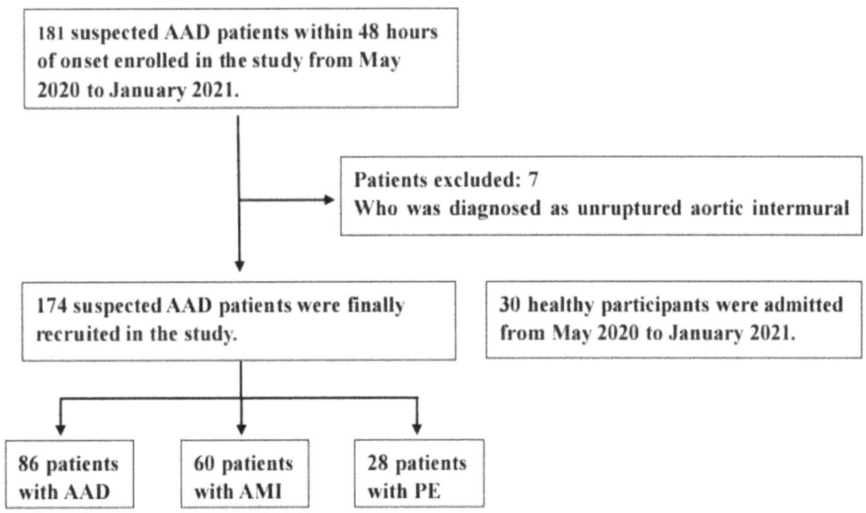


**FIGURE 1** | Flow diagram of exclusion and enrollment of study patients. Describes the exclusion and enrollment of study patients. AAD, acute aortic dissection; AMI, acute myocardial infarction; PE, pulmonary embolism.

were used for parametric and non-parametric data in multiple groups, *T*-test and Mann-Whitney U-test were used as a *post-hoc* analysis. Categorical variables were expressed as frequencies and compared using Fisher's precision probability test or Chi-square analysis. Logistic regression analysis was also used. $P = 0.05$ was considered statistically significant. Pearson correlation and delong test (22) were used to compare the relationship and ROC curve between LPA and D-dimer. The decision curve for a theoretical distribution was given to describe expected net benefit (23, 24).

The R (https://www.r-project.org/), The R Foundation, and EmpowerStats (http://www.empowerstats.com), X&Y Solutions Inc, Boston, MA were used for all statistical analyses.

## RESULTS

A total of 204 patients, including 86 AAD patients, 60 AMI patients, 28 PE patients, and 30 healthy participants (Normal), were selected (**Figure 1**). The patient characteristics after 48 h of onset are shown in **Table 1** and **Supplementary Table 2.** AAD patients were mostly younger males with no significant difference in symptom onset time in all groups than non-AAD patients (**Supplementary Table 3**). The D-dimer and LPA levels were significantly higher in AAD patients than in non-AAD patients on the whole (**Supplementary Table 2**). LPA level (344.69 ± 59.99) was significantly different from AMI, PE, and Normal. However, AMI and PE were not statistically different (**Figure 2A**). D-dimer levels in AAD and PE were

**TABLE 1** | Baseline characteristics of chest pain patients with AAD vs. other groups.

| | AAD | AMI | PE | Normal | *P*-value |
|---|---|---|---|---|---|
| No. of participates | 86 | 60 | 28 | 30 | |
| Gender, male | 58 (67.44)# | 32 (53.33) | 12 (42.86)† | 16 (53.33) | 0.087 |
| Age, year | 53.60 ± 11.46※ | 57.30 ± 5.34† | 55.36 ± 5.15 | 54.67 ± 4.33 | 0.077 |
| Onset time to hospital, hours | 11.45 ± 5.12 | 10.00 ± 4.43 | 11.32 ± 3.84 | - | 0.168 |
| HR,/min | 81.33 ± 18.22 | 79.57 ± 10.57 | 81.57 ± 10.82 | 78.37 ± 11.38 | 0.722 |
| SBP, mmHg | | | | | |
| Left-S | 141.21 ± 38.62 | 136.25 ± 15.99 | 136.32 ± 12.58 | 135.07 ± 15.03 | 0.608 |
| Right-S | 135.58 ± 36.93 | 135.40 ± 15.71 | 136.32 ± 13.21 | 135.50 ± 14.39 | 0.998 |
| Difference-S | 18.00 (7.00–31.00)※#* | 3.00 (2.00–5.00)† | 2.00 (2.00–4.00)† | 3.00 (2.00–4.00)† | <0.001 |
| DBP, mmHg | | | | | |
| Left-D | 79.90 ± 22.31 | 83.42 ± 11.87 | 84.25 ± 9.60 | 79.83 ± 13.53 | 0.473 |
| Right-D | 76.94 ± 20.02※ | 83.83 ± 12.06† | 84.96 ± 11.35 | 81.63 ± 13.25 | 0.030 |
| Difference-D | 10.00 (4.00–13.75)※#* | 3.00 (2.00–4.25)† | 3.00 (1.75–6.00)† | 3.00 (2.00–5.00)† | <0.001 |
| History of | | | | | |
| Hypertension, % | 72 (83.72)※#* | 25 (41.67)†#* | 7 (25.00)†※ | 5 (16.67)†※# | <0.001 |
| Diabetes, % | 5 (5.81)※# | 17 (28.33)†#* | 5 (17.86)† | 3 (10.00)※ | 0.002 |
| Stroke, % | 6 (6.98) | 4 (6.67) | 2 (7.14) | 0 (0) | 0.530 |
| Chronic kidney disease, % | 12 (13.95) | 12 (20.00)# | 3 (10.71)* | 0 (0) | 0.067 |
| OSAS, % | 26 (30.23)※* | 0 (0)†# | 7 (25.00)※* | 0 (0)†# | <0.001 |
| COPD, % | 5 (5.81) | 2 (3.33) | 3 (10.71) | 0 (0) | 0.257 |
| Marfan, % | 2 (2.33) | 0 (0) | 0 (0) | 0 (0) | 0.428 |
| CAD, % | 10 (11.63)※* | 26 (43.33)†#* | 5 (17.86)※* | 0 (0)†※# | <0.001 |
| Valvular heart disease, % | 2 (2.33)※# | 8 (13.33)†* | 3 (10.71)†* | 0 (0)※# | 0.017 |
| Smoking, % | 49 (56.98)#* | 27 (45.00)#* | 4 (14.29)†※ | 7 (23.33)†※ | <0.001 |
| Drinking, % | 21 (24.42)# | 11 (18.33) | 3 (10.71)†* | 6 (20.00)# | 0.056 |
| Medication history | | | | | |
| Aspirin, % | 12 (13.95)* | 11 (18.33) | 5 (17.86) | 0 (0) | 0.100 |
| Clopidogrel, % | 7 (8.14)* | 9 (15.00) | 3 (10.71) | 0 (0) | 0.134 |
| Statin, % | 16 (18.60)* | 10 (16.67) | 3 (10.71) | 0 (0) | 0.075 |
| Hormone, % | 3 (3.49)* | 2 (3.33) | 1 (3.57) | 0 (0) | 0.784 |
| D-dimer, ug/ml | 7.58 ± 4.80※* | 3.14 ± 2.11†#* | 8.49 ± 5.22※* | 0.59 ± 0.43†※# | <0.001 |
| LPA, mg/dl | 344.69 ± 59.99※#* | 286.79 ± 43.01†* | 286.61 ± 43.32†* | 96.08 ± 11.93†※# | <0.001 |

*AAD, acute aortic dissection; AMI, acute myocardial infarction; PE, pulmonary embolism; SBP, systolic blood pressure; DBP, diastolic blood pressure; OSAS, obstructive sleep apnea syndrome; COPD, chronic obstructive pulmonary disease; CAD, coronary artery disease; LPA, lysophosphatidic acid. $P < 0.05$, statistically different. †Significance vs. "AAD," ※Significance vs. "AMI," #Significance vs. "PE," *Significance vs. "Normal."*

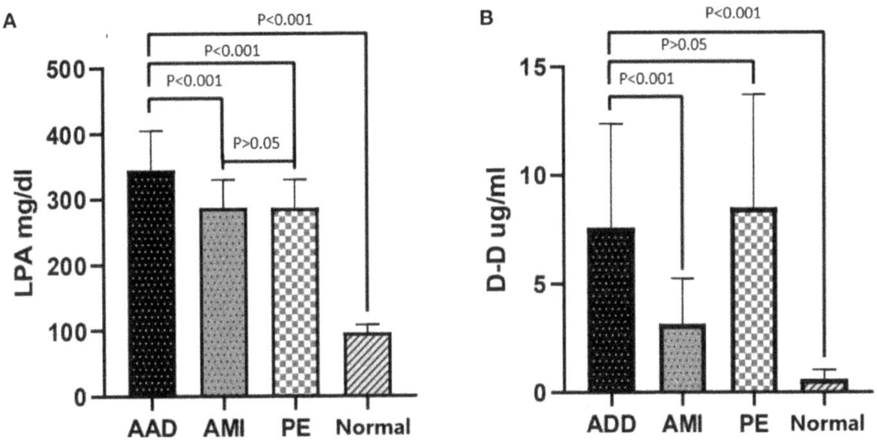


**FIGURE 2** | LPA and D-dimer levels in chest pain patients with AAD vs. other groups. **(A)** LPA distribution (Mean ± standard deviation) in AAD, AMI, PE, and Normal. **(B)** D-dimer distribution (Mean ± standard deviation) in AAD, AMI, PE, and Normal. LPA, lysophosphatidic acid; AAD, acute aortic dissection; AMI, acute myocardial infarction; PE, pulmonary embolism; Normal, healthy participants.

**TABLE 2** | Multivariate regression analysis for AAD diagnosis.

| Exposure | Univariate analysis | | | Multi-factor analysis | | |
|---|---|---|---|---|---|---|
| | OR | 95% CI | *P* | OR | 95% CI | *P* |
| Difference-S, mmHg | 1.56 | 1.33, 1.84 | <0.001 | 1.42 | 1.13, 1.78 | 0.003 |
| Difference-D, mmHg | 1.41 | 1.26, 1.57 | <0.001 | 1.20 | 0.87, 1.67 | 0.272 |
| Right-D, mmHg | 0.97 | 0.96, 0.99 | 0.005 | 0.93 | 0.87, 1.00 | 0.047 |
| Hypertension, % | 11.26 | 5.64, 22.49 | <0.001 | 9.67 | 1.93, 48.32 | 0.006 |
| Diabetes, % | 0.23 | 0.08, 0.63 | 0.004 | 0.04 | 0.00, 0.48 | 0.011 |
| CAD, % | 0.37 | 0.17, 0.80 | 0.012 | 0.15 | 0.01, 2.32 | 0.176 |
| Valvular heart disease, % | 0.23 | 0.05, 1.07 | 0.062 | 0.67 | 0.07, 6.97 | 0.740 |
| Smoking, % | 2.79 | 1.57, 4.96 | 0.001 | 0.41 | 0.07, 2.48 | 0.334 |
| Drinking, % | 2.40 | 1.14, 5.05 | 0.021 | 0.96 | 0.18, 5.10 | 0.962 |
| D-dimer, ug/ml | 1.03 | 1.02, 1.03 | <0.001 | 1.02 | 1.01, 1.03 | 0.043 |
| LPA, mg/dl | 1.23 | 1.13, 1.30 | <0.001 | 1.21 | 1.06, 1.43 | 0.007 |

*AAD, acute aortic dissection; Difference-S, difference of systolic blood pressure; Difference-D, difference of diastolic blood pressure; Right-D, the right diastolic blood pressure; CAD, coronary artery disease; LPA, lysophosphatidic acid. P < 0.05, Statistically different.*

**TABLE 3** | Diagnostic performance of AAD patients vs. others using LPA compared with D-Dimer.

| | AUC | 95% CI | Threshold | Sensitivity | Specificity | PLR | NLR | PPV | NPV |
|---|---|---|---|---|---|---|---|---|---|
| D-D, ug/ml | 0.76 | 0.70–0.82 | 1.87 | 0.90 | 0.55 | 1.82 | 0.11 | 0.57 | 0.91 |
| LPA, mg/dl | 0.86 | 0.80–0.90 | 298.98 | 0.81 | 0.77 | 3.56 | 0.24 | 0.72 | 0.85 |
| *P* for compare | 0.041 | - | - | - | - | - | - | - | - |

*D-D, d dimer; LPA, lysophosphatidic acid. P < 0.05, Statistically different (Delong test).*

higher but no statistical difference between the two (**Figure 2B**). Logistic multiple regression analysis showed that the blood pressure differences, hypertension history, D-dimer, and LPA were independently associated with AAD ($P < 0.001$) (**Table 2**).

Pearson analysis showed that LPA level was positively associated with D-dimer, $p < 0.05$) (coefficient of 0.17 in AAD, 0.15 in AMI, and 0.24 in PE). There was no significant correlation in Normal (**Supplementary Figure 2**).

## LPA Distribution

The box plots were used to analyze LPA levels in AAD patient plasma at different onset times (**Supplementary Figure 3**).

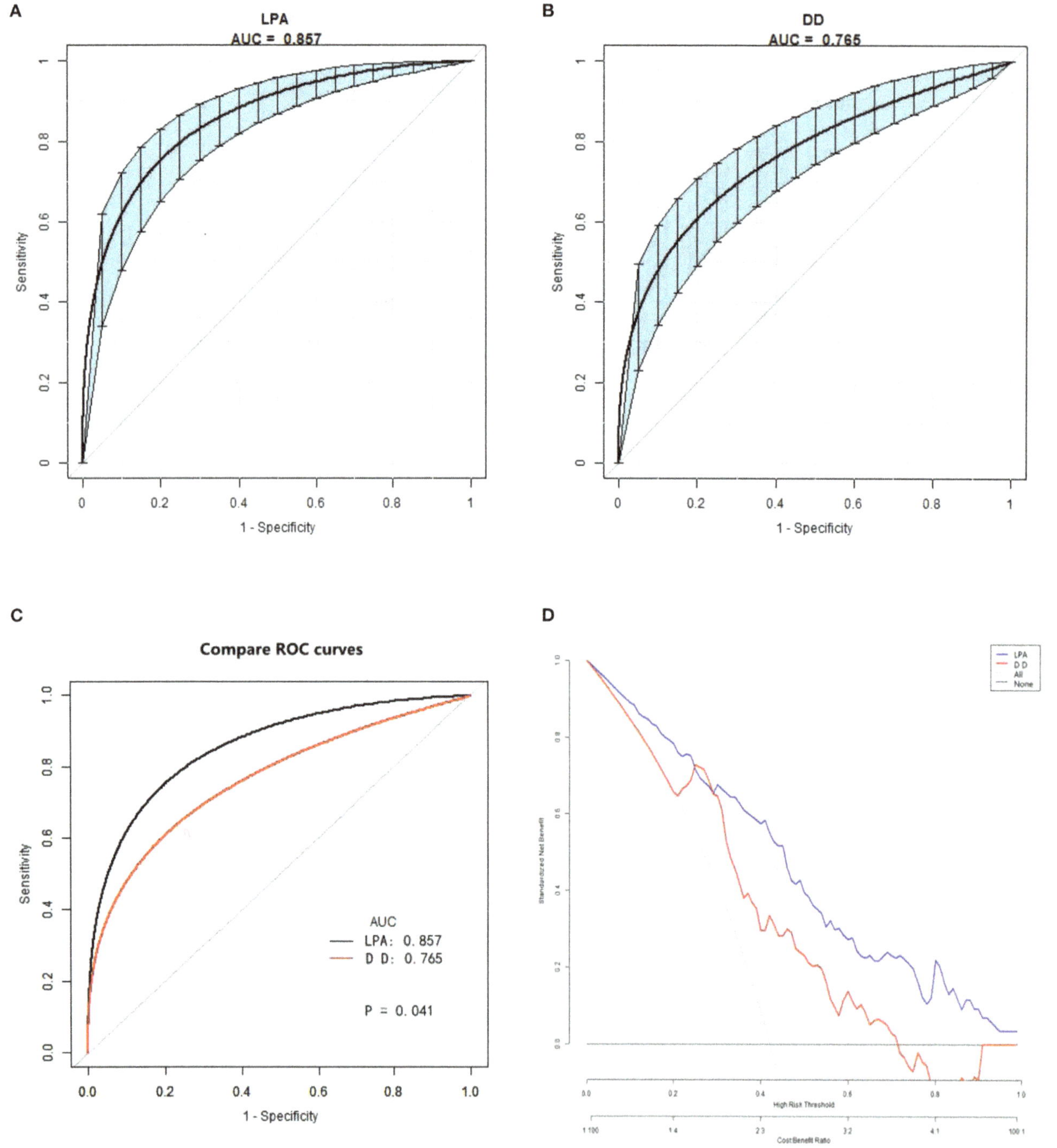


**FIGURE 3** | Receiver operating characteristic and decision curve. **(A)** The AUC value of LPA predicting AAD. **(B)** The AUC value of D-dimer predicting AAD. Blue shading shows the bootstrap estimated 95% CI with AUC. **(C)** Comparison of ROC curves between D-dimer and LPA. The ROC curve of LPA is better than D-dimer (Delong test). **(D)** Decision curve for a theoretical distribution. Solid line: prediction model, LPA = blue, DD = red. Thin gray line: assume all patients have AAD. Black bottom line: assume no patients have AAD. The vertical axis displays standardized net benefit. The two horizontal axes show the correspondence between risk threshold and cost:benefit ratio. The graph gives the expected net benefit per patient associated with LPA and DD, with LPA performing better. LPA, lysophosphatidic acid; AAD, acute aortic dissection; AUC, area under the curve.

Based on the different onsets of symptoms in AAD patients, LPA seems to peak at 12 h and gradually decreased after 12 h, easing after 24 h ($P < 0.05$). The number of chest pain patients at different symptoms onset-time was not statistically significant ($P = 0.148$) (**Supplementary Table 3**).

## Diagnostic Performance for Discriminating AAD

The ROC analysis results indicated that D-dimer had an AUC of 0.76 (0.70–0.82), diagnosis threshold of 1.87 ug/ml, a sensitivity of 0.90, specificity of 0.55, and the negative predictive value of 0.91. LPA had an AUC of 0.85 (0.80–0.90), diagnosis threshold of 298.98 mg/dl, a sensitivity of 0.81, specificity of 0.77, and the negative predictive value of 0.85 (**Table 3**; **Figures 3A,B**). The ROC curve of LPA is better than D-dimer ($P = 0.041$, Delong test) (**Figure 3C**). The decision curve for a theoretical distribution showed that LPA had excellent standardized net benefits (**Figure 3D**).

## DISCUSSION

This study, which included 174 suspected AAD patients and 30 healthy participants, found that LPA may be used for the clinical diagnosis of AAD. LPA, mainly produced by activated platelets, may be an early biomarker of the initiation of thrombosis and coagulation. Researches have shown that coagulation cascade activates platelets to release a large amount of lysophospholipids and autotaxin with phospholipase D activity stored in alpha particles at the same time. The two substances undergo a biochemical reaction to produce LPA, which increases the plasma concentration (14, 25, 26). LPA binding to its receptors (LPA1-6) on platelet surface activates platelets and forms a positive feedback reaction, alters platelet in morphology, promotes aggregation and thrombus stability (27–29). Moreover, LPA activates LPA1 and LPA3 expressed in vascular endothelial cells (30), promotes immune response and aggravate endothelial cell damage via Gαi-RhoA-ROCK-NF-κB dependent pathways (31). LPA also increases the expression of intracellular matrix metalloproteinase-2, which will remodel the extracellular matrix and reduce the aggregation of endothelial cells to promote the migration and aggregation of inflammatory cells, thereby damaging endothelial cells to activate the coagulation cascade (32).

We found that the magnitude of elevated LPA can distinguish patients with AAD from patients with AMI, PE, and the healthy within 48 h after symptom onset. AAD is a disease with high mortality due to severe damage to the aortic structure. There are also some biomarkers showing clinical prognosis including CRP (33), NT-pro BNP (34) and cardiac troponin (35). When aortic dissection occurs, disruption to the aortic media immediately changes aorta hemodynamics, then intramural hematoma expand (especially when the intimal layer is also disrupted) as the blood flow inside media (5). The tissue coagulation factor III directly exposed to the blood in the arterial smooth muscle activates the exogenous coagulation pathway and promotes the coagulation cascade (13). Platelets, an indispensable role in the coagulation cascade, are continuously activated by the LPC-ATX-LPA pathway to produce more LPA before the aortic dissection is surgically repaired (14, 36). Although some studies speculate that the half-life of LPA is only 2–3 min under the action of LPPs, the continuous existence of disruption to the aortic media and positive feedback may be a reasonable explanation for the increase in plasma LPA in AAD patients (37, 38).

Our results suggested that the degree of the elevation of LPA levels is associated with the different magnitudes of vascular injury among AAD, AMI, and PE. Although LPA level in PE and AMI patients was higher than the healthy, there were still lower than AAD in our study. Substantial aortic hemodynamic changes significantly increased the circulating LPA level in the aorta (largest artery) compared with the small and medium blood vessels of pulmonary embolism and acute coronary syndrome. Studies have shown that LPA level is associated with the release location, releasing LPA directly and quickly to the aortic circulation may be another reason for the higher degree of AAD patients (39).

In addition, we speculated that LPA peaks at 12 h according to the symptoms of AAD patients, and our results also found that the threshold of LPA is 298.98 mg/dl, the specificity and AUC are 0.77 and 0.857, respectively, which are better than D-dimer ($P < 0.05$, Delong test). This means that as a marker of platelet activation, LPA $\geq$ 300 mg/dl indicates a high risk of AAD, and may be earlier than D-dimer. However, D-dimer has higher sensitivity and negative predictive value compared to LPA. As a fibrin degradation product in the circulation after thrombolytic fibrinolysis, D-dimer has been found to increase similarly in many diseases, including PE and AAD. In fact, D-dimer aids clinical diagnosis for PE only as a rule-out tool when the test result is negative (5).

To the best of our knowledge, this is the first study showing that LPA is associated with aortic dissection and could be a novel AAD biomarker. However, this study has some limitations. It is still unclear how LPA changes over time in AAD patients, a large-scale prospective multicenter study is needed to confirm the generalizability of the findings, the diagnostic validity, and the accuracy of this novel detection method since this was a single-center study. Second, the assay method used could provide an inconsistent absolute value for the LPA concentration, influencing the recommended cut-off level. Therefore, various detection methods should be accurately calibrated. Thirdly, this study did not include all undifferentiated chest pain patients, hence, patient selection could be biased. Finally, LPA < 300 mg/dl is difficult to rule out AAD in daily practice, and other diseases (ovarian cancer) (40) can also increase LPA levels. Therefore, further confirmatory diagnosis based on medical images is essential to prevent misdiagnosis in clinical practice.

## CONCLUSION

LPA showed superior overall diagnostic performance to D-dimer in early AAD diagnosis may be a potential biomarker, but additional studies are needed to determine the rapid and cost-effective diagnostic tests in the emergency department.

is still some research in progress for the time being. In order not to affect the following research, it is not convenient to disclose the data. Requests to access these datasets should be directed to 188212324@csu.edu.cn.

## ETHICS STATEMENT

The hospital institutional review board of the Second Xiangya Hospital approved the study. The data collection and analysis followed the Ethics Committee of the institution and the Declaration of Helsinki. The Ethics Committee of the institution reviewed the patient consents, and the data were used only for research purposes.

## AUTHOR CONTRIBUTIONS

XP and XC: drafted, revised, and reviewed the article. YZ and GY: conducted statistical analysis. ZH, HZ, ZP, WP, and ND: reviewed and revised the manuscripts. TG and MZ: organized the database. All authors significantly contributed to the conception, study design, execution, data acquisition, analysis, interpretation, approved the final version, agreed on the journal, and are responsible for this study.

## ACKNOWLEDGMENTS

Thanks to the Department of Emergency Medicine and Cardiovascular Surgery, Second Xiangya Hospital, Central South University for the assistance and support.

## REFERENCES


1. Nienaber C, Clough R, Sakalihasan N, Suzuki T, Gibbs R, Mussa F, et al. Aortic dissection. *Nat. Rev. Dis. Primers*. (2016) 2:16071. doi: 10.1038/nrdp.2016.53
2. Mussa F, Horton J, Moridzadeh R, Nicholson J, Trimarchi S, Eagle K. Acute aortic dissection and intramural hematoma: a systematic review. *JAMA*. (2016) 316:754–63. doi: 10.1001/jama.2016.10026
3. Smedberg C, Steuer J, Leander K, Hultgren R. Sex differences and temporal trends in aortic dissection: a population-based study of incidence, treatment strategies, and outcome in Swedish patients during 15 years. *Eur Heart J*. (2020) 41:2430–8. doi: 10.1093/eurheartj/ehaa446
4. Bossone, Eduardo, LaBounty, Troy M, Eagle, Kim A. Acute aortic syndromes: diagnosis and management, an update. *Eur Heart J*. (2018) 39:739–49. doi: 10.1093/eurheartj/ehx319
5. Wang Y, Tan X, Gao H, Yuan H, Hu R, Jia L, et al. Magnitude of Soluble ST2 as a Novel Biomarker for Acute Aortic Dissection. *Circulation*. (2018) 137:259–69. doi: 10.1161/CIRCULATIONAHA.117.030469
6. Pourafkari L, Tajlil A, Ghaffari S, Parvizi R, Chavoshi M, Kolahdouzan K et al. The frequency of initial misdiagnosis of acute aortic dissection in the emergency department and its impact on outcome. *Internal Emerg Med*. (2017) 12:1185–95. doi: 10.1007/s11739-016-1530-7
7. Pape L, Awais M, Woznicki E, Suzuki T, Trimarchi S, Evangelista A et al. Presentation, diagnosis, and outcomes of acute aortic dissection: 17-year trends from the international registry of acute aortic dissection. *J Am Coll Cardiol*. (2015) 66:350–8. doi: 10.1016/j.jacc.2015.05.029
8. Tsai TT, Trimarchi S, Nienaber CA. Acute Aortic Dissection: Perspectives from the International Registry of Acute Aortic Dissection (IRAD). *Eur J Vasc Endovasc Surg*. (2009) 37:149–59. doi: 10.1016/j.ejvs.2008.11.032
9. Suzuki T, Katoh H, Watanabe M, Kurabayashi M, Hiramori K, Hori S, et al. Novel biochemical diagnostic method for aortic dissection. Results of a prospective study using an immunoassay of smooth muscle myosin heavy chain. *Circulation*. (1996) 93:1244–9. doi: 10.1161/01.CIR.93.6.1244
10. Suzuki T, Distante A, Zizza A, Trimarchi S, Villani M, Salerno Uriarte J, et al. Preliminary experience with the smooth muscle troponin-like protein, calponin, as a novel biomarker for diagnosing acute aortic dissection. *Eur Heart J*. (2008) 29:1439–45. doi: 10.1093/eurheartj/ehn162
11. Shinohara T. Soluble elastin fragments in serum are elevated in acute aortic dissection. *Arterioscler Thromb Vasc Biol*. (2003) 23:1839–44. doi: 10.1161/01.ATV.0000085016.02363.80
12. Suzuki T. Eagle KA. Biomarker-assisted diagnosis of acute aortic dissection. *Circulation*. (2018) 137:270–2. doi: 10.1161/CIRCULATIONAHA.117.032048
13. Yang G, Peng W, Zhou Y, He H, Chai X. Characteristics and prognosis of acute type A aortic dissection with negative D-dimer result. *Am J Emerg Med*. (2020) 38:1820–4. doi: 10.1016/j.ajem.2020.05.055
14. Zhao Y, Hasse S, Zhao C, Bourgoin S. Targeting the autotaxin–Lysophosphatidic acid receptor axis in cardiovascular diseases. *Biochem Pharmacol*. (2019) 164:74–81. doi: 10.1016/j.bcp.2019.03.035
15. Moolenaar W. Lysophosphatidic acid, a multifunctional phospholipid messenger. *J Biol Chem*. (1995) 270:12949–52. doi: 10.1074/jbc.270.22.12949
16. Abdel-Latif A, Heron P, Morris A, Smyth S. Lysophospholipids in coronary artery and chronic ischemic heart disease. *Curr Opin Lipidol*. (2015) 26:432–7. doi: 10.1097/MOL.0000000000000226
17. Doppler C, Arnhard K, Dumfarth J, Heinz K, Messner B, Stern C, et al. Metabolomic profiling of ascending thoracic aortic aneurysms and dissections–implications for pathophysiology and biomarker discovery. *PLoS ONE*. (2017) 12:e0176727. doi: 10.1371/journal.pone.0176727
18. Zhou X, Wang R, Zhang T, Liu F, Zhang W, Wang G, et al. Identification of lysophosphatidylcholines and sphingolipids as potential biomarkers for acute aortic dissection via serum metabolomics. *Eur J Vasc Endovasc Surg*. (2018) 57:434–41. doi: 10.1016/j.ejvs.2018.07.004
19. Erbel R, Aboyans V, Boileau C, Bossone E, Bartolomeo R, Eggebrecht H, et al. 2014 ESC Guidelines on the diagnosis and treatment of aortic diseases: document covering acute and chronic aortic diseases of the thoracic and abdominal aorta of the adult. The Task Force for the Diagnosis and Treatment of Aortic Diseases of the European Society of Cardiology (ESC). *Eur Heart J*. (2014) 35:2873–926. doi: 10.1093/eurheartj/ehu281
20. Nazerian P, Mueller C, Soeiro A, Leidel B, Salvadeo S, Giachino F, et al. Diagnostic accuracy of the aortic dissection detection risk score plus d-dimer for acute aortic syndromes: the ADvISED prospective multicenter study. *Circulation*. (2018) 137:250–8. doi: 10.1161/CIRCULATIONAHA.117.029457
21. Hiratzka L, Bakris G, Beckman J, Bersin R, Carr V, Casey D, et al. 2010 ACCF/AHA/AATS/ACR/ASA/SCA/SCAI/SIR/STS/SVM guidelines for the diagnosis and management of patients with Thoracic Aortic Disease: a report of the American College of Cardiology Foundation/American Heart Association Task Force on Practice Guidelines, American Association for Thoracic Surgery, American College of Radiology, American Stroke Association, Society of Cardiovascular Anesthesiologists, Society for Cardiovascular Angiography and Interventions, Society of Interventional Radiology, Society of Thoracic Surgeons, and Society for Vascular Medicine. *Circulation*. (2010) 121: e266–369. doi: 10.1161/CIR.0b013e3181d4739e
22. DeLong E, DeLong D, Clarke-Pearson D. Comparing the areas under two or more correlated receiver operating characteristic curves: a nonparametric approach. *Biometrics*. (1988) 44:837–45. doi: 10.2307/2531595
23. Vickers A, Elkin E. Decision curve analysis: a novel method for evaluating prediction models. *Med Decis Making*. (2006) 26:565–74. doi: 10.1177/0272989X06295361
24. Kerr K, Brown M, Zhu K, Janes H. Assessing the clinical impact of risk prediction models with decision curves: guidance for correct interpretation and appropriate use. *J Clin Oncol*. (2016) 34:2534–40. doi: 10.1200/JCO.2015.65.5654
25. Zhou Y, Little P, Ta H, Xu S, Kamato, D. Lysophosphatidic acid and its receptors: pharmacology and therapeutic potential in atherosclerosis and vascular disease. *Pharmacol Ther*. (2019) 204:107404. doi: 10.1016/j.pharmthera.2019.107404
26. Leblanc R, Lee S, David M, Bordet J, Norman D, Patil R, et al. Interaction of platelet-derived autotaxin with tumor integrin $\alpha V\beta 3$ controls

metastasis of breast cancer cells to bone. *Blood.* (2014) 124:3141–50. doi: 10.1182/blood-2014-04-568683
27. Retzer M, Essler M. Lysophosphatidic acid-induced platelet shape change proceeds via Rho/Rho kinase-mediated myosin light-chain and moesin phosphorylation. *Cell Signal.* (2000)
28. Siess W, Zangl K, Essler M, Bauer M, Brandl R, Corrinth C, et al. Lysophosphatidic acid mediates the rapid activation of platelets and endothelial cells by mildly oxidized low density lipoprotein and accumulates in human atherosclerotic lesions. *Proc Natl Acad Sci U S A.* (1999) 96:6931–6. doi: 10.1073/pnas.96.12.6931
29. Haserück N, Erl W, Pandey D, Tigyi G, Ohlmann P, Ravanat C et al. The plaque lipid lysophosphatidic acid stimulates platelet activation and platelet-monocyte aggregate formation in whole blood: involvement of P2Y1 and P2Y12 receptors. *Blood.* (2004) 103:2585–92. doi: 10.1182/blood-2003-04-1127
30. Shimada H, Rajagopalan L. Rho kinase-2 activation in human endothelial cells drives lysophosphatidic acid-mediated expression of cell adhesion molecules via NF-kappaB p65. *J Biol Chem.* (2010) 285:12536–42. doi: 10.1074/jbc.M109.099630
31. Lin C, Chen C, Chen J, Lee H. Lysophospholipids increase IL-8 and MCP-1 expressions in human umbilical cord vein endothelial cells through an IL-1-dependent mechanism. *J Cell Biochem.* (2006) 99:1216–32. doi: 10.1002/jcb.20963
32. Neidlinger N, Larkin S, Bhagat A, Victorino G, Kuypers F. Hydrolysis of phosphatidylserine-exposing red blood cells by secretory phospholipase A2 generates lysophosphatidic acid and results in vascular dysfunction. *J Biol Chem.* (2006) 281:775–81. doi: 10.1074/jbc.M505790200
33. Vrsalović M. Vrsalović Presečki A. Admission C-reactive protein and outcomes in acute aortic dissection: a systematic review. *Croat Med J.* (2019) 60:309–15. doi: 10.3325/cmj.2019.60.309
34. Vrsalovic M, Vrsalovic Presecki A, Aboyans V. N-terminal pro-brain natriuretic peptide and short-term mortality in acute aortic dissection: a meta-analysis. *Clin Cardiol.* (2020) 43:1255–9. doi: 10.1002/clc.23436
35. Vrsalovic M. Prognostic effect of cardiac troponin elevation in acute aortic dissection: a meta-analysis. *Int J Cardiol.* (2016) 214:277–8. doi: 10.1016/j.ijcard.2016.03.230
36. Smyth S, Kraemer M, Yang L, Van Hoose P, Morris A. Roles for lysophosphatidic acid signaling in vascular development and disease. *Biochim Biophys Acta Mol Cell Biol Lipids.* (2020) 1865:158734. doi: 10.1016/j.bbalip.2020.158734
37. Tomsig J, Snyder A, Berdyshev E, Skobeleva A, Mataya C, Natarajan V, et al. Lipid phosphate phosphohydrolase type 1 (LPP1) degrades extracellular lysophosphatidic acid *in vivo*. *Biochem J.* (2009) 419:611–8. doi: 10.1042/BJ20081888
38. Salous A, Panchatcharam M, Sunkara M, Mueller P, Dong A, Wang Y, et al. Mechanism of rapid elimination of lysophosphatidic acid and related lipids from the circulation of mice. *J Lipid Res.* (2013) 54:2775–84. doi: 10.1194/jlr.M039685
39. Dohi T, Miyauchi K, Ohkawa R, Nakamura K, Kurano M, Kishimoto T, et al. Increased lysophosphatidic acid levels in culprit coronary arteries of patients with acute coronary syndrome. *Atherosclerosis.* (2013) 229:192–7. doi: 10.1016/j.atherosclerosis.2013.03.038
40. Xu Y, Shen Z, Wiper D, Wu M, Morton R, Elson P, et al. Lysophosphatidic acid as a potential biomarker for ovarian and other gynecologic cancers. *JAMA.* (1998) 280:719–23. doi: 10.1001/jama.280.8.719

# 12

# Does a Small Body have a Negative Impact on Minimally Invasive Mitral Valve Surgery?

*Tomonori Shirasaka [1], Shingo Kunioka [1*], Yuta Kikuchi [1], Natsuya Isikawa [1], Hirotsugu Kanda [2] and Hiroyuki Kamiya [1]*

[1] Department of Cardiac Surgery, Asahikawa Medical University, Asahikawa, Japan, [2] Department of Anesthesiology and Critical Care Medicine, Asahikawa Medical University, Asahikawa, Japan

***Correspondence:***
*Shingo Kunioka*
*kyokui090069@gmail.com*

**Backgrounds:** Minimally invasive mitral valve surgery (MIMVS) in patients with a small body presents surgeons with a technically difficult surgical maneuver. We hypothesized that physique might negatively influence the safety and technical complexity of MIMVS.

**Methods:** One hundred and twenty-one patients underwent MIMVS in our institution between May 2014 and April 2020. These patients were categorized into two groups. The first group was the small physique group ($n = 20$) consisting of patients with a stature <150 cm. The second group was the normal physique group ($n = 101$) consisting of patients with a stature >150 cm. The primary endpoint was freedom from death and major adverse cardiovascular and cerebrovascular events (MACCE). The secondary endpoint was freedom from moderate or severe mitral regurgitation.

**Results:** Cardiopulmonary bypass time (130 ± 29 vs. 156 ± 55 min, $p = 0.02$) and aortic cross-clamp time (75 ± 27 vs. 95 ± 39 min, $p = 0.03$) were significantly shorter in the small physique group. Both in the early and midterm periods, there was no significant difference in the mortality (early, 5.0 vs. 1.0%, $p = 0.30$. midterm, 5.0 vs. 1.0%, $p = 0.09$), MACCE (early, 5.0 vs. 6.9%, $p = 0.65$. midterm, 5.0 vs. 5.9%, $p = 0.93$) and the residual MR (early, 0 vs. 1.0%, $p = 0.66$. midterm, 5.0 vs. 4.9%, $p = 0.93$) between the two groups.

**Conclusions:** Small physique is not a hurdle for MIMVS in terms of the safety of the operation.

**Keywords: mitral valve surgery, minimally invasive cardiac surgery, physique, small body, safety**

## INTRODUCTION

Previously, the primary candidates for minimally invasive cardiac surgery (MICS) were young patients who were socially active and had low risk and who expected excellent cosmesis (1). However, the indication for this method has recently expanded to relatively elderly people expecting faster recovery brought about by the preservation of their sternum (2). In the future, other good candidates for MICS will be children or adolescents who are seeking a fast return to social activities and better cosmesis.

Preliminary reports in relation to MICS in congenital cardiac surgery have focused on the clinical success of the operation for atrial septal defect (ASD), ventricular septal defect (VSD), and atrioventricular septal defect *via* right thoracotomy (3, 4). For example, Yoshimura et al. reported excellent operative results for patients with ASD (mean age 7 years, mean body weight 23.9 kg). Mishaly et al. performed ASD or VSD closure and mitral valve repair on young patients, including 60 infants (mean age 9 years, mean body weight 20 kg), and concluded that the establishment of cardiopulmonary bypass (CPB) or the maintenance of good exposure in congenital cardiac surgery *via* right thoracotomy could be achieved in children with a body weight >9 kg.

One of the biggest concerns with MICS in patients with a small body is leg ischemia (5) due to the relatively small vascular diameter required for cannulation and the likelihood of spasticity, especially in young patients. Another concern is the technical difficulty in performing surgical maneuvers in a small pleural cavity (6). These concerns might be the primary reasons for the delay in the introduction of recent technological advances in MICS for congenital heart surgery.

Historically, among all variables with an influence on surgical outcome, body weight and body mass index or body surface area (BSA) have also been investigated (7, 8) to determine whether they significantly influence the outcome. However, in previously published reports, full sternotomy was performed in all documented cases, and none of the studies provided information on the impact of quantitative preoperative variables, such as body height, vascular diameter for cannulation, and the vertical or cross diameter of the pleural cavity on the operative results. Thus, elucidation of the negative factors for the completion of MICS would be of great value.

In this study, the patients who underwent mitral valve surgery were categorized into two groups using the MICS approach (MIMVS), namely, patients with a small physique and those with a normal physique, and the patient characteristics and clinical outcomes between the two groups were compared to elucidate the validity of MIMVS for individuals with a small body.

# METHODS

The institutional review board of Asahikawa Medical University Hospital approved this retrospective study and waived the need for written patient consent (IRB number: 19083).

## Patient Demographics

A total of 121 patients underwent MIMVS in our institution between May 2014 and April 2020. **Figure 1** shows the distribution of body mass index [BMI, 1-(A)], body surface area [BSA, 1-(B)] and height [1-(C)] in these patients. Mean BMI, BSA, and height in male/ female were 22.5 ± 3.1/21.2 ± 3.6 kg/m$^2$, 1.7 ± 0.2/1.5 ± 0.2 m$^2$, and 167 ± 7.2/153 ± 8.3 cm, respectively.

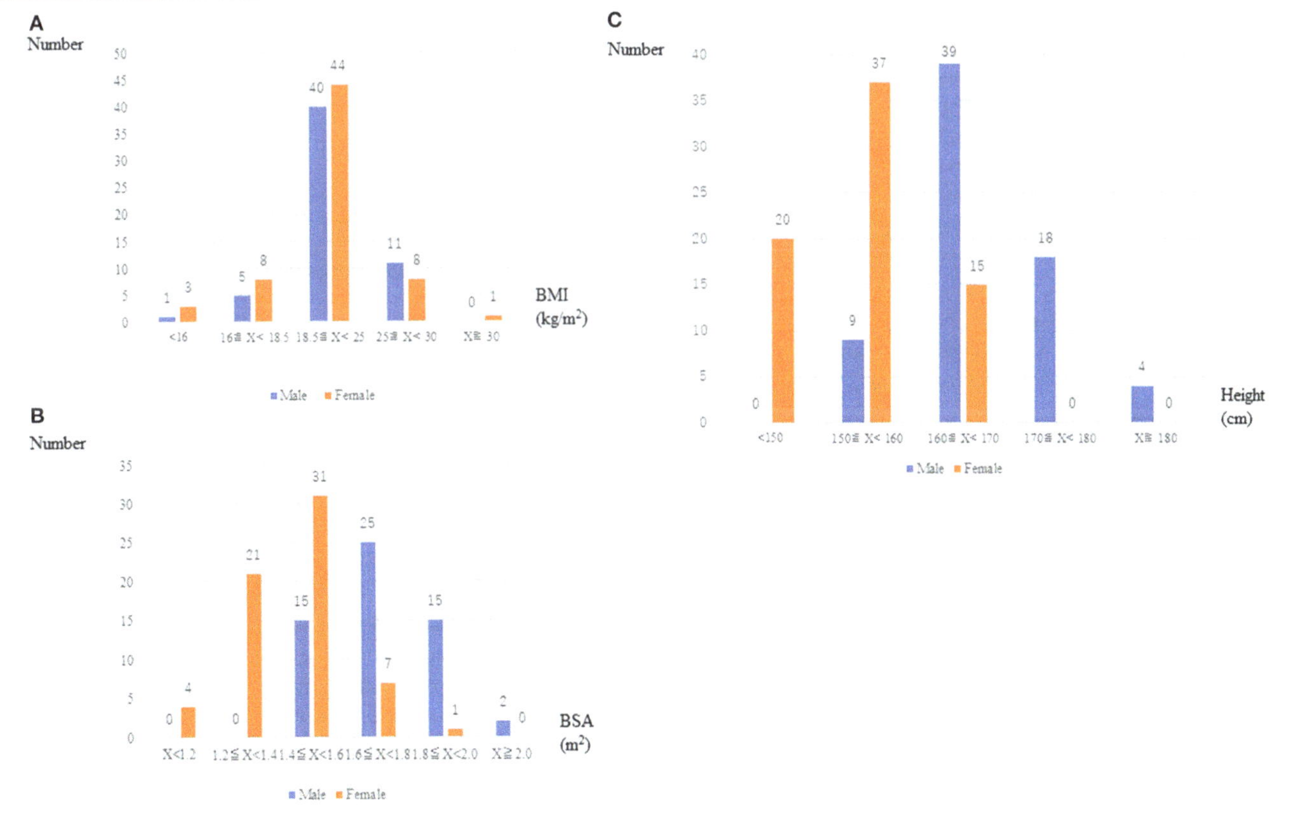


**FIGURE 1 |** Distribution of BMI, BSA, and height in male and female patients.

We categorized these patients into two groups: the small physique group ($n = 20$), which consisted of patients with a stature <150 cm, and the normal physique group ($n = 101$), which consisted of patients with a stature >150 cm.

**Table 1** presents the patient demographics of the two groups. A significant difference in age (79 ± 7 vs. 62 ± 15 years, $p < 0.001$), gender ($p < 0.001$), height (143 ± 4.5 vs. 163 ± 8 cm, $p < 0.001$), body weight (42 ± 7.5 vs. 59 ± 10.7 kg, $p < 0.001$), BSA (1.3 ± 0.1 vs. 1.6 ± 0.1, $p < 0.001$), and the diastolic or systolic dimensions of the left ventricle (LVDd, 49 ± 5 vs. 54 ± 8.0 mm, $p = 0.01$. LVDs, 31 ± 6 vs. 35 ± 8.2 mm, $p = 0.02$) was observed between these two groups. Preoperative computed tomography revealed a significant difference in the axial length of the pleural cavity between the two groups (220 ± 10.6 vs. 242 ± 21.7 mm, $p < 0.001$) but none in the vertebra–sternum distance (97 ± 11.7 vs. 102 ± 196 mm, $p = 0.21$) or diameter of the femoral artery (10 ± 1.6 vs. 11 ± 2.0 mm, $p = 0.15$). Our exclusion criteria for MIMVS are as follows: 1. The existence of calcified or atherothrombotic ascending aorta. 2. The existence of significant coronary artery disease. 3. Severe mitral annular calcification. 4. Very obese patient (BMI ≧ 35) or critical emaciation (BMI ≦ 15). 5. Poor femoral or iliac access.

**TABLE 1** | Patient demographics.

| Variable | Small physique ($n = 20$) | Normal physique ($n = 101$) | *p*-value |
|---|---|---|---|
| Age, y | 79 ± 7 | 62 ± 15 | <0.001* |
| Gender, male | 0 | 57 | <0.001* |
| Height, cm | 143 ± 4.5 | 163 ± 8 | <0.001* |
| Body weight, kg | 42 ± 7.5 | 59 ± 10.7 | <0.001* |
| BMI, kg/ m² | 20.6 ± 3.3 | 22.0 ± 3.4 | 0.22 |
| BSA, m² | 1.3 ± 0.1 | 1.6 ± 0.1 | <0.001* |
| NYHA class | | | |
| 0/I/II/III/IV | 5/10/5/0 | 37/39/20/5 | – |
| ≧III | 5 | 25 | 0.98 |
| Preoperative TTE | | | |
| LVDd, mm | 49 ± 5 | 54 ± 8.0 | 0.01* |
| LVDs, mm | 31 ± 6 | 35 ± 8.2 | 0.02* |
| EF, % | 66 ± 8.1 | 63 ± 10.2 | 0.23 |
| MR grade | | | |
| 0/I/II/III/IV | 0/1/0/0/19 | 0/3/1/4/93 | |
| AR grade | | | |
| 0/I/II/III/IV | 4/7/7/1/0 | 59/19/23/0/0 | |
| Etiology of mitral valve | | | |
| Degenerative | 18 | 88 | 0.73 |
| MS, rheumatic | 1 | 6 | 0.75 |
| IE | 1 | 7 | 0.85 |
| Detail of MR | 19 | 101 | |
| Type I/II/III | 3/15/1 | 14/76/5 | |
| Atrial functional MR | 3 | 14 | 0.89 |
| Preoperative CT | | | |
| Vertebra–sternum distance, mm | 97 ± 11.7 | 102 ± 19.6 | 0.21 |
| Axial length of the pleural cavity, mm | 220 ± 10.6 | 242 ± 21.7 | <0.001* |
| Diameter of the femoral artery, mm | 10 ± 1.6 | 11 ± 2.0 | 0.15 |

*BMI, body mass index; BSA, body surface area; CT, computed tomography; EF, ejection fraction; MR, mitral regurgitation; NYHA, New York Heart Association; TTE, transesophageal echocardiography.*
**Means the existence of significant difference of p-value.*

## Operative Procedure of MICS Mitral Surgery

In this study, 2 surgeons performed MIMVS. In our unit, MIMVS was performed under direct vision with the assistance of thoracoscope routinely for the surgery. Femoral cannulation was performed in surgical cut down technique using a one-stage arterial cannula [PCKC-A 16 French (Fr), 18 Fr, Toyobo, Osaka, Japan] and a single venous cannula (QuickDraw, 25 Fr, Edwards Lifesciences, Irvine, CA, USA) or a two-stage venous cannula (RAP FV cannula 22–25 Fr, LivaNova, Milan, Italy) inserted through the right atrium into the superior vena cava. During CPB, carbon dioxide insufflation of 3 L/min was employed for de-airing of the heart. A 5- to 7-cm right thoracotomy was performed *via* the fourth intercostal space. After establishing a full CPB flow, pericardiotomy was performed. Body temperature was decreased to mild hypothermia of 30–32°C. After aortic cross-clamp using a Cygnet flexible clamp (Vitalitec International, Inc., Plymouth, MA, USA), initial cardioplegia was delivered in an antegrade fashion, followed by left atriotomy with intermittent delivery of blood cardioplegia performed every 30 min.

The left atrium (LA) was exposed by the gentle retraction of the ascending aorta by LA retractor (Adams-Yozu Mini-Valve System, Geister, Tuttlingen, Germany). After mitral valve surgery was completed, LA was closed in a single-layer fashion followed by declamp without terminal hot-shot of cardioplegia. RV pacing lead was placed before routinely releasing the cross-clamp.

## Postoperative Anticoagulation

Postoperative oral anticoagulation was administered. Irrespective of the rhythm pattern, warfarin was routinely administered to all patients, and the prothrombin time–international normalized ratio was controlled between 1.8 and 3.0. If sinus rhythm was stable for longer than 3 months, warfarin therapy was discontinued, except in cases of mitral valve replacement with a mechanical valve.

## Endpoint

The primary endpoint was freedom from death and major cardiac and cerebrovascular event (MACCE). The secondary endpoint was freedom from moderate or severe mitral regurgitation.

## Statistical Analysis

Preoperative, intraoperative, and postoperative data were recorded and retrospectively reviewed. Continuous variables were expressed as mean ± standard deviation, and categorical variables were presented as either absolute numbers or percentages.

Baseline patient characteristics, operative data, postoperative complications, and outcome rates were compared using Pearson's chi-squared test or Fisher's exact test for categorical

**TABLE 2** | The details of operative procedures.

| Variable | Small physique ($n = 20$) | Normal physique ($n = 101$) | $p$-value |
|---|---|---|---|
| Operative time | 177 ± 45 | 210 ± 60 | 0.02* |
| CPB time | 130 ± 29 | 156 ± 55 | 0.02* |
| ACC time | 75 ± 27 | 95 ± 39 | 0.03* |
| Second run of CPB | 0 | 6 | 0.54 |
| Operative procedures | | | |
| Mitral valve | 20 | 101 | – |
| Isolated mitral valve surgery | 16 | 69 | 0.42 |
| Annuloplasty | 18 | 88 | 0.72 |
| Ring | 9 | 41 | 0.81 |
| Band | 9 | 47 | 0.90 |
| Valve repair | 16 | 69 | 0.98 |
| Triangular resection | 4 | 28 | 0.59 |
| Folding plasty | 5 | 22 | 0.77 |
| Indentation closure | 2 | 20 | 0.52 |
| Artificial chordae | 3 | 23 | 0.56 |
| Chordal transplantation | 0 | 3 | 0.44 |
| Central edge to edge | 0 | 1 | 0.66 |
| Commissural closure | 3 | 7 | 0.37 |
| Patch augmentation | 0 | 3 | 0.44 |
| Valve replacement | 2 | 10 | 0.98 |
| Tricuspid valve repair | 4 | 32 | 0.42 |
| Surgical maze procedure | 2 | 28 | 0.15 |

*ACC, aortic cross-clamp; CPB, cardiopulmonary bypass.*

**TABLE 3** | Operative outcomes in the early and midterm periods.

| Variable (percentage) | Small physique ($n = 20$) | Normal physique ($n = 101$) | $p$-value |
|---|---|---|---|
| 30-day mortality | 1 (5.0) | 1 (1.0) | 0.30 |
| In-hospital mortality | 1 (5.0) | 1 (1.0) | 0.30 |
| MACCE (including death) | 1 (5.0) | 7 (6.9) | 0.65 |
| Reexploration for bleeding | 1 (5.0) | 2 (2.0) | 0.42 |
| Reexpansion pulmonary edema | 0 | 0 | – |
| Pulmonary herniation | 0 | 2 (2.0) | 0.53 |
| Stroke | 0 | 0 | – |
| SSI | 0 | 0 | – |
| Reoperation within 12 months | 0 | 3 (3.0) | 0.44 |
| Readmission due to HF | 0 | 0 | – |
| Postoperative TTE at discharge | | | |
| ≧Moderate MR | 0 | 1 (1.0) | 0.66 |
| Mean PG bw LA-LV, mm Hg | 2.5 ± 1.1 | 2.8 ± 1.4 | 0.38 |
| Latest postoperative TTE | | | |
| Follow-up periods, years | 2.1 ± 1.4 | 2.9 ± 1.8 | 0.09 |
| ≧Moderate MR | 1 (5.0) | 5 (4.9) | 0.93 |
| All-cause death | 1 (5.0) | 1 (1.0) | 0.09 |
| MACCE (including death) | 1 (5.0) | 6 (5.9) | 0.93 |
| Reoperation | 0 | 5 (4.9) | 0.31 |

*SSI, surgical site infection; HF, heart failure; MR, mitral regurgitation; TTE, transesophageal echocardiography.*

variables or Student's $t$-test or the Wilcoxon rank-sum test for continuous variables. The significance level was set at $p < 0.05$. For the time-to-event analysis, we employed log-rank tests and the Kaplan–Meier method. The Kaplan–Meier method was employed to demonstrate overall survival, freedom from MACCE and freedom from significant MR defined as moderate or severe MR. Statistical analyses were conducted using STATA version 15.1 (StataCorp LP, College Station, TX, USA).

## RESULTS

Operative time, cardiopulmonary time, and aortic cross-clamp time were significantly shorter in the small physique group than in the normal physique group (operative time, 177 ± 45 vs. 201 ± 60 min, $p = 0.02$; cardiopulmonary time, 130 ± 29 vs. 156 ± 55 min, $p = 0.02$; aortic cross-clamp time, 75 ± 27 vs. 95 ± 39 min, $p = 0.03$; **Table 2**), despite the fact that the percentages of isolated mitral valve surgery in both groups were not significantly different ($p = 0.42$; **Table 2**).

In relation to the details of the operative procedures, no significant difference was observed between the group in the use of materials for mitral annuloplasty ($p = 0.72$), frequency of valve repair ($p = 0.98$), concomitant tricuspid valve repair ($p = 0.42$), and antiarrhythmic operation ($p = 0.15$) (**Table 2**).

In the early postoperative periods, one patient in poor preoperative condition both in the small and normal physique groups died, respectively (30 days mortality, 5.0 vs. 1.0%, $p = 0.30$). There was no significant difference in the rate of MACCE and significant residual MR between two groups (MACCE, 5.0 vs. 6.9%, $p = 0.65$. ≧Moderate MR, 0 vs. 1.0%, $p = 0.66$; **Table 3**).

The postoperative follow-up periods were 2.1 ± 1.4 vs. 2.9 ± 1.8 year, respectively ($p = 0.09$). In the midterm, no significant difference was observed in the rate of overall death (5.0 vs. 1.0%, $p = 0.09$), MACCE (5.0 vs. 5.9%, $p = 0.93$), postoperative significant mitral regurgitation (5.0 vs. 4.9%, $p = 0.93$), and reoperation (0 vs. 4.9%, $p = 0.31$) between the two groups. Kaplan-Meyer curve in relation to overall survival, freedom from MACCE, and freedom from significant MR were not significantly different between the two groups ($p = 0.09$, 0.93, and 0.93, respectively; **Figures 2–4**).

## DISCUSSION

In general, MICS requires performing surgical maneuvers using long-shafted instruments in small spaces, which is not easy due to the technical aspects. Therefore, appropriate patient selection is important, taking into consideration the safety of the procedure, the surgeon's level of comfort performing the surgical maneuvers, and whether the clinical outcome is promising and not compromised as compared with conventional open-heart surgery.

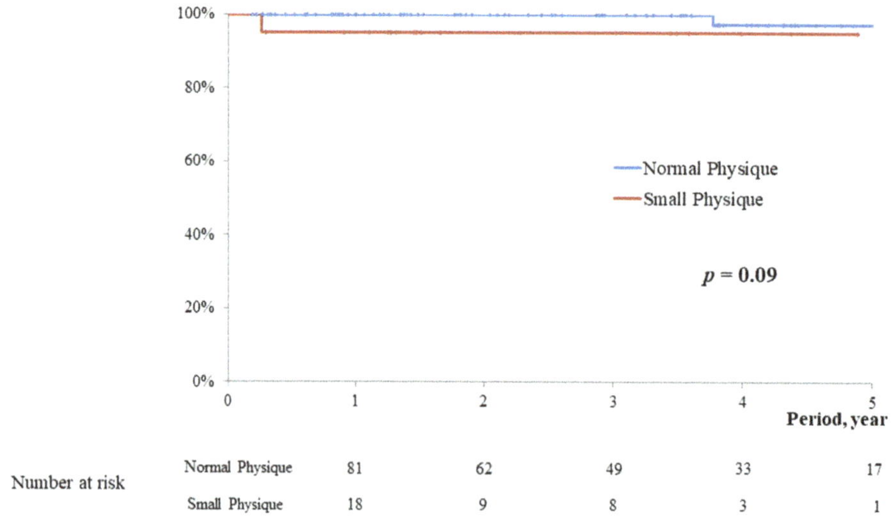


**FIGURE 2** | Survival.

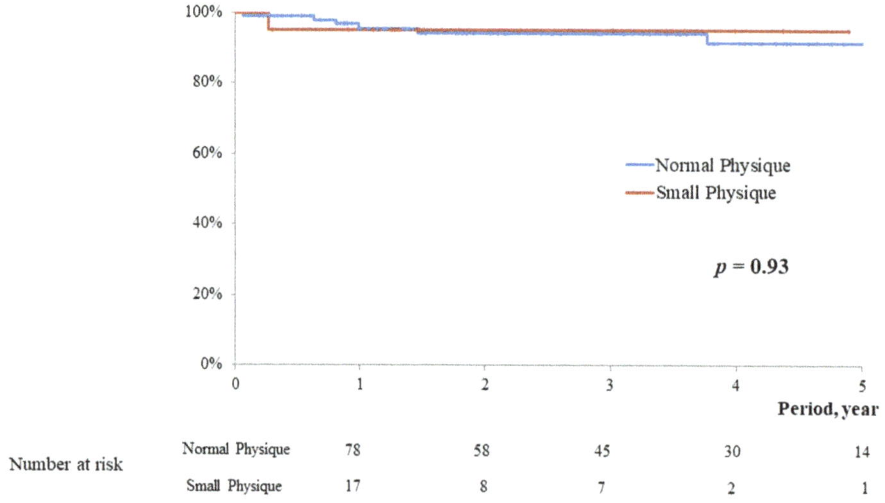


**FIGURE 3** | Freedom from MACCE.

We hypothesized that a small physique might have an influence on the safety or technical complexity of MICS. However, the findings of this study suggest that CPB and aortic cross-clamp time as well as operative time in the small physique group was not longer than that in the normal physique group, although 75% in the small physique group underwent isolated MVP while 64% in the normal physique group and this might be related to the result that CPB and cross clamp time were shorter in the small physique group.

The definition of small stature may vary based on the patient's race. Short stature is defined as an adult height greater than two standard deviations below the mean for age and gender, which corresponds to the shortest 2.3% of individuals (9). Typically, in developed countries, this includes adult men shorter than 158 cm and adult women shorter than 149 cm. A recent national health and nutrition survey in Japan (10) revealed that the mean height of adult men and women in Japan was 168 ± 7.1 and 154.5 ± 7.0 cm, respectively. Taking this into consideration, the definition of small physique in this study was defined as a height <150 cm.

Historically, researchers have discussed how the difference in body size influences the outcomes of cardiac surgery. In their multiple regression analysis, Tarui et al. found significant associations among BMI, cannula size, and operation time and an increase in postoperative creatinine phosphorus kinase (11). Several reports have elucidated the strong association between large BSA or BMI (7, 8, 12) and the inferiority in clinical outcome, indicating that obese individuals typically

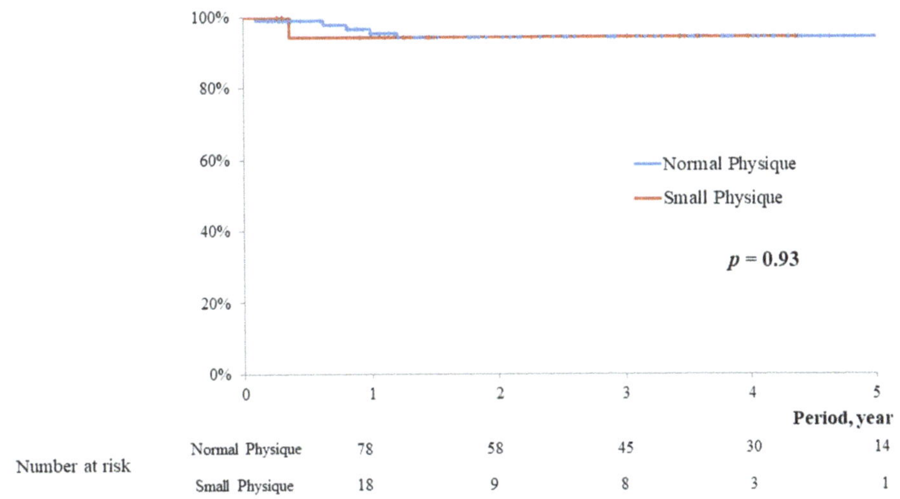


**FIGURE 4** | Freedom from ≧ moderate MR.

have multicomorbidities, such as diabetes, hypertension, and impaired respiratory function. However, all of these studies precluded only conventional cardiac surgery *via* full sternotomy and did not discuss the influence of this factor on the technical complexity in MICS. To the best of our knowledge, this is the first report elucidating whether there is a significant association between small body size and clinical outcome in MIMVS.

Stable perfusion is important in open-heart surgery, especially in MICS. The most typical venous drainage setup in MICS is femoral vein cannulation (13). Poor venous drainage leads to a bad exposure of the mitral valve, making the surgery itself uncomfortable. In addition, venous back pressure results in the washout of cardioplegia, diminishing its cardioprotective effects, which may result in perioperative ventricular dysfunction (14). In the present study, we used low-profile venous cannulas (22 or 25 Fr); thus, we rarely experienced any difficulty in cannulation or in setting the position of the tip of the venous cannula appropriate to the drain under the guidance of intraoperative transesophageal echocardiography, even in patients with small physique. With regard to arterial cannulation in MICS, the common femoral artery (CFA) is the most commonly adopted site. The CFA diameter steadily increases throughout life, and it is significantly correlated with height, weight, and BSA. In addition, the CFA diameter is larger in men than in women (15). Limited to our study, all the patents in the small physique group were elderly women, and the mean diameter of the femoral artery in the two groups was not significantly different from that in the normal physique group. This feature of the current study might have influenced the outcome, which was different from our hypothesis.

As an indicator for the estimation of the actual surgical space in MICS mitral value surgery, the distance between the vertebrae and sternum is regarded as quite important for determining whether the MICS approach is optimal. This distance should preferably be 80 mm or greater for direct vision MICS (6). In fact, in our small physique group, this variable was beyond this threshold. Moreover, none of the patients in the small physique group demonstrated a funnel chest or thorax deformity.

The finding in this study, namely, that physique has no impact on the surgical outcome in MIMVS, contributes to the extension of the indication for the MICS approach in mitral valve surgery to small elderly people or young patients in adolescence who expect a quick recovery *via* preservation of their sternum and subsequent fast return to their daily lives.

## Study Limitations

This study had some limitations. Namely, this was a retrospective study, and the sample size of the two groups was quite small. Patients' selection referred by our exclusion criteria was unavoidable especially early in the series in terms of patient safety.

In this study, small physique group was constituted only by women unexpectedly. It was because that we set the threshold of statue for small physique as 150 cm referring to the national database about physique in Japanese people. We intentionally set only a single parameter (height) as an influencer of the body shape itself on surgical outcome. However, various factors such as BSA or BMI may influence to the clinical outcome of surgery in real practice. Actually, the number of very obese patient whose BMI over 30 was only 1, and that of very slim or skinny patients whose BMI under 16 was 4 in this series (**Figure 1**). Similarly, the number of the patient whose BSA was over 2.0 was only 2 people, and whose BSA under 1.2 was only 4 in this series (**Figure 1**). Moreover, all of them got well soon after MICS uneventfully. So, it is difficult to elucidate the power of very high or low BMI on the clinical outcome in MICS in this study.

Despite these limitations, the strengths of this study include the quite conclusive findings, with complete clinical follow-up examinations performed for all patients, including late echocardiographic follow-up findings.

Our results reconfirm the feasibility of the MICS approach in patients with a small body.

In conclusion, a small physique is not a contraindication for MIMVS.

## ETHICS STATEMENT

The studies involving human participants were reviewed and approved by the Institutional Review Board of Asahikawa Medical University Hospital. The patients/participants provided their written informed consent to participate in this study.

## AUTHOR CONTRIBUTIONS

All authors listed have made a substantial, direct, and intellectual contribution to the work and approved it for publication.

## REFERENCES


1. Sakaguchi T. Minimally invasive mitral valve surgery through a right mini-thoracotomy. *Gen Thorac Cardiovas.* (2016) 64:699–706. doi: 10.1007/s11748-016-0713-5
2. Iribarne A, Easterwood R, Russo MJ, Chan EY, Smith CR, Argenziano M. Comparative effectiveness of minimally invasive versus traditional sternotomy mitral valve surgery in elderly patients. *J Thorac Cardiovasc Surg.* (2012) 143:S86–90. doi: 10.1016/j.jtcvs.2011.10.090
3. Yoshimura N, Yamaguchi M, Oshima Y, Oka S, Ootaki Y, Yoshida M. Repair of Atrial septal defect through a right posterolateral thoracotomy: a cosmetic approach for female patients. *Ann Thorac Surg.* (2001) 72:2103–5. doi: 10.1016/S0003-4975(01)03086-7
4. Mishaly D, Ghosh P, Preisman S. Minimally invasive congenital cardiac surgery through right anterior minithoracotomy approach. *Ann Thorac Surg.* (2008) 85:831–5. doi: 10.1016/j.athoracsur.2007.11.068
5. Toya T, Fujita T, Fukushima S, Shimahara Y, Kume Y, Yamashita K, et al. Efficacy of regional saturation of oxygen monitor using near-infrared spectroscopy for lower limb ischemia during minimally invasive cardiac surgery. *J Artif Organs.* (2018) 21:420–6. doi: 10.1007/s10047-018-1057-y
6. Ito T. Minimally invasive mitral valve surgery through right mini-thoracotomy: recommendations for good exposure, stable cardiopulmonary bypass, and secure myocardial protection. *Gen Thorac Cardiovasc Surg.* (2015) 63:371–8. doi: 10.1007/s11748-015-0541-z
7. Schwann TA, Habib RH, Zacharias A, Parenteau GL, Riordan CJ, Durham SJ, et al. Effects of body size on operative, intermediate, and long-term outcomes after coronary artery bypass operation. *Ann Thorac Surg.* (2001) 71:521–31. doi: 10.1016/S0003-4975(00)02038-5
8. Lio A, Emanuele Bovio E, Nicolò F, Saitto G, Scafuri A, Bassano C, et al. Influence of body mass index on outcomes of patients undergoing surgery for acute aortic dissection: a propensity-matched analysis. *Tex Heart Inst J.* (2019) 46:7–13. doi: 10.14503/THIJ-17-6365
9. Pedicelli S, Peschiaroli E, Violi E, Cianfarani S. Controversies in the definition and treatment of idiopathic short stature (ISS). *J Clin Res Ped Endo.* (2009) 1:105–15. doi: 10.4008/jcrpe.v1i3.53
10. *The National Health and Nutrition Survey in Japan.* (2018). Available online at: http://www.nibiohn.go.jp/eiken/kenkounippon21/en/eiyouchousa/
11. Tarui T, Miyata K, Shigematsu S, Watanabe G. Risk factors to predict leg ischemia in patients undergoing single femoral artery cannulation in minimally invasive cardiac surgery. *Perfusion.* (2018) 33:533–7. doi: 10.1177/0267659118768151
12. Habib RHD, Zacharias A, Schwann TA, Riordan CJ, Durham SJ, Shah A. Effects of obesity and small body size on operative and long-term outcomes of coronary artery bypass surgery: a propensity-matched analysis. *Ann Thorac Surg.* (2005) 79:1976–86. doi: 10.1016/j.athoracsur.2004.11.029
13. Lamelas J, Aberle C, Macias AE, Alnajar A. Cannulation strategies for minimally invasive cardiac surgery. *Innovations.* (2020) 15:261–9. doi: 10.1177/1556984520911917
14. Momin AA, Toth AJ, Gillinov AM, Wierup P, Mick SL. Exploring ventricular dysfunction and poor venous drainage during robotic mitral valve surgery. *J Card Surg.* (2020) 35:1253–7. doi: 10.1111/jocs.14574
15. Sandgren T, Sonesson B, Ahlgren AR, Toste Länne T. The diameter of the common femoral artery in healthy human: influence of sex, age, and body size. *J Vasc Surg.* (1999) 29:503–10. doi: 10.1016/S0741-5214(99)70279-X

# 13

# Post-operative Right Ventricular Failure After Cardiac Surgery: A Cohort Study

*David Levy, Driss Laghlam, Philippe Estagnasie, Alain Brusset, Pierre Squara and Lee S. Nguyen**

*Intensive Care Medicine Department, CMC Ambroise Paré, Neuilly-sur-Seine, France*

***Correspondence:***
*Lee S. Nguyen*
*nguyen.lee@icloud.com*

**Introduction:** Right ventricular failure (RVF) after cardiac surgery is an important risk factor for morbidity and mortality. Its diagnosis is challenging, and thus, its incidence and predictors are not well-established. We investigated the incidence, complications, and variables associated with clinically relevant post-operative RVF.

**Methods:** We included all patients who underwent cardiac surgery with cardiopulmonary bypass between 2016 and 2019 in a cardiac surgery center with standardized diagnostic and therapeutic management of RVF. RVF was considered only if clinically relevant: associated with hemodynamic instability requiring catecholamine support and inhaled nitric oxide relayed by sildenafil.

**Results:** Overall, 3,826 patients were included, of whom, 110 (2.9%) developed post-operative RVF. Mortality was not different among patients who developed post-operative RVF, compared with the rest of the cohort (1.8 vs. 0.7%, $p = 0.17$). Using a composite outcome that combined death, reintubation, stroke, and prolonged intensive care unit stay (more than 14 days) yielded an incidence of 6.6%, and RVF was associated with this composite outcome with an odds ratio of 3.6 (2.2–5.8), $p < 0.001$. In a multivariable model, pre-operative variables independently associated with post-operative RVF were pre-operative atrial fibrillation (AF) {adjusted odds ratio (adjOR) 3.22 [95% confidence interval (95%CI) = 1.94–5.36], $p < 0.001$}, left ventricle ejection fraction below 50% [adjOR = 2.55 (95%CI = 1.52–4.33), $p < 0.001$], systolic pulmonary artery pressure above 55 mmHg [adjOR = 8.64 (95%CI = 5.27–14.1); $p < 0.001$], mitral valve surgery [adjOR = 2.17 CI (95%CI = 1.28–3.66), $p = 0.004$], and tricuspid valve surgery [adjOR = 10.33 (95%CI = 6.14–17.4), $p < 0.001$]. In patients who developed post-operative RVF requiring treatment, 32 (29.1%) showed RV dysfunction before surgery.

**Conclusion:** In this cohort study, 2.9% of patients developed clinically significant post-operative RVF. Moreover, RVF was associated with severe adverse outcomes, including death, strokes, reintubation, and prolonged intensive care unit stay.

**Keywords: right ventricular failure, cardiac surgery, nitric oxide, sildenafil, cohort analyses**

# INTRODUCTION

Right ventricular failure (RVF) after cardiac surgery has been found as a significant cause of morbidity and mortality in several settings (1). Mechanisms of RVF include suboptimal myocardial protection during surgery, long cardiopulmonary bypass (CPB) time, right ventricular (RV) myocardial ischemia or infarction, atrial arrhythmias or loss of atrioventricular synchrony, reperfusion lung injury with secondary pulmonary hypertension (PH), post-operative pulmonary micro- or macro-embolism, pre-existing pulmonary vascular disease, protamine-induced PH, and others (2). An acute increase in PH leads to higher RV afterload, altered RV-pulmonary artery coupling, and then RV failure with compromised hemodynamic (3). Pulmonary vascular resistance (PVR) may increase after CPB because of atelectasis, ischemia–reperfusion injury with inflammatory cytokines, endothelial damage, and reduction of nitric oxide release (4, 5).

Post-operative RVF management includes pulmonary vasodilators, optimal fluid management, inotrope support, and, when necessary, restoring a compromised RV myocardial perfusion pressure, systemic vasopressors. As of yet, these treatments are not supported by robust studies. Inhaled nitric oxide (iNO) has been approved for persistent PH of the newborn but is used off-label in cardiac post-operative RV failure despite poor evidence in hard clinical outcomes (6–8). Similarly, sildenafil showed promise in clinical studies, in post-operative care, by reducing pulmonary pressures and resistance with no alteration in systemic hemodynamic and oxygenation (9, 10).

Another issue lies in the lack of a consensual definition of RVF after surgery (11). Consequently, the incidence of RVF and its risk factors are not well-established. Although some reports described risk scores of RVF after left ventricular assist device implantation, the literature is poor in standard cardiac surgery (12, 13).

This study aimed to characterize the incidence, outcomes, and predictors of RVF after cardiac surgery.

# PATIENTS AND METHODS

## Study Population and Design

From January 1, 2016, to December 31, 2019, the study included all adult patients undergoing cardiac operations with CPB. The exclusion criteria were age below 18 years. We performed a retrospective analysis of data collected prospectively, including perioperative characteristics, post-operative drugs, and outcomes. Data were anonymized as per national regulation and used with the approval of an institutional review board committee (Commission Nationale de l'Informatique et des Libertés, CNIL, declaration number 2109982, 17/10/2017). All the data are part of the Registry for the Improvement of Post-operative Outcomes in Cardiac and Thoracic Surgery database (NCT03209674). Patients' opposition to the use of anonymized data by investigators was systematically sought (i.e., informed consent was obtained from all patients).

## Definitions

Post-operative RVF was defined by the combination of (1) hemodynamic instability requiring administration of vasopressors and/or inotropes and (2) immediate post-operative needs of pulmonary vasodilators (iNO followed by sildenafil® per os). In the post-operative period, patients were systematically explored with echocardiography when presenting with hemodynamic instability. RVF required hypokinesia of the RV free wall or RV/left ventricle (LV) interdependence or enlarged RV with RV/LV ratio $> 1$. Additional optional parameters included tricuspid annular plane systolic excursion (TAPSE) $< 16$ mm and tissue doppler imaging with peak myocardial velocity at the lateral tricuspid annulus (S wave) $< 9.5$ cm/s, also considered if patients did not undergo tricuspid intervention.

## Right Ventricular Failure Management

Inhaled NO was initiated at RVF diagnosis. It was administered at 10 ppm and once hemodynamic stability was achieved for at least 24 h; weaning was achieved by decreasing 1 ppm every hour. Sildenafil was initiated during the first 48 h after surgery, whenever oral intake was possible, with a dosage of 20 mg every 8 h.

## Statistical Analysis

Data distribution was assessed using the Kolmogorov–Smirnov-test with Lilliefors correction. Continuous variables were summarized as mean ± standard deviation or median (interquartile range), as appropriate, and were compared, using the Student *t*-test or Mann–Whitney *U*-test accordingly. Categorical variables were presented as count (percentage) and compared using the chi-square or Fisher exact-test, as appropriate.

Binary logistic regression analysis was performed to assess variables independently associated with RVF. The multivariable model was built by the stepwise selection, with an entry criterion of $p < 0.10$. Variables included in the model were age, sex, previous AF, estimated glomerular filtration rate, systolic pulmonary arterial pressure (sPAP) $> 55$ mmHg, left ventricular ejection fraction (LVEF) $< 50\%$, mitral surgery, tricuspid intervention, and CPB length.

Comparing patients who presented post-operative RVF and those who did not, regarding mortality, was performed using proportion comparison, and using survival analysis, censored at 14 days, with Kaplan–Meier estimates. This censorship was used because 97% of patients were discharged from the intensive care unit (ICU) by day 14, and the remaining 3% presented heterogeneous length of stay, precluding from linear assumptions. For sensitivity, uncensored analyses were performed.

All statistical analyses were performed using IBM SPSS version 26.0 (IBM Corporation, Armonk, New York). A two-sided $p$-value $< 0.05$ was considered to be statistically significant. Figures were drawn using Prism 8.4.3 (GraphPad Software, California, USA) and R software 3.6 (R project, worldwide community software).

**TABLE 1** | Baseline characteristics.

| | Total cohort ($n = 3,716$) | RVF group ($n = 110$) | *p*-value |
|---|---|---|---|
| Age (years) | 68.6 (±10.9) | 71.0 (±9.9) | 0.018 |
| Female | 935 (25.2%) | 40 (36.4%) | 0.008 |
| BMI (kg/m$^2$) | 26.6 (±4.6) | 25.1 (±4.9) | 0.001 |
| COPD | 282 (7.6%) | 13 (11.8%) | 0.1 |
| Hypertension | 2,008 (54.2%) | 41 (37.3%) | <0.001 |
| Type II diabetes | 996 (26.9%) | 22 (20.0%) | 0.1 |
| Previous AF | 287 (8.4%) | 28 (29.2%) | <0.001 |
| eGFR (ml/min) | 69.6 (57.0–82.7) | 57.7 (44.5–71.9) | <0.001 |
| Dialysis (>3 months) | 48 (1.3%) | 5 (4.5%) | 0.017 |
| Previous cardiac surgery | 342 (9.2%) | 23 (20.9%) | <0.001 |
| Euroscore II | 1.7 (0.97–3.2) | 4.1 (2.0–8.0) | <0.001 |
| **Pre-operative LVEF** | | | |
| *30–49%* | 470 (12.7%) | 25 (23.1%) | 0.001 |
| *<30%* | 68 (1.8%) | 3 (2.8%) | 0.45 |
| sPAP 35–55 mmHg | 850 (22.9%) | 30 (33.7%) | 0.017 |
| sPAP > 55 mmHg | 164 (4.4%) | 49 (50.5%) | <0.001 |
| **Type of surgery** | | | |
| CABG | 2,221 (59.9%) | 22 (20.0%) | <0.001 |
| Mitral valve | 621 (16.7%) | 71 (64.5%) | <0.001 |
| Aortic valve | 1,190 (32.1%) | 18 (16.4%) | <0.001 |
| Tricuspid valve | 135 (3.6%) | 55 (50.0%) | <0.001 |
| CPB duration (minutes) | 79.3 (±29.8) | 96.4 (±34.0) | <0.001 |
| Aortic clampage time (minutes) | 61.7 (±23.0) | 63.4 (±24.7) | 0.16 |

*Categorical variables are presented as number (proportion) and continuous variables as mean (standard deviation).*
*AF, atrial fibrillation; BMI, body mass index; CABG, coronary artery bypass graft; CPB, cardiopulmonary bypass; COPD, chronic obstructive pulmonary disease; eGFR, estimated glomerular filtration rate; sPAP, systolic pulmonary arterial pressure.*

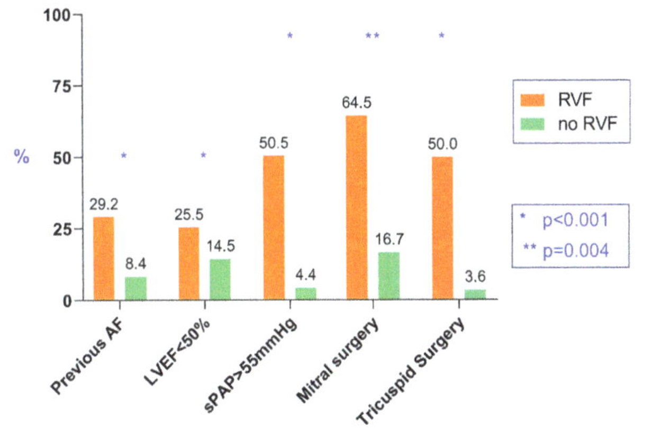


**FIGURE 1** | Variables associated with post-operative right ventricular failure (RVF).

**TABLE 2** | Post-operative outcomes.

| | Total cohort ($n = 3,716$) | RVF group ($n = 110$) | *P* |
|---|---|---|---|
| Death in ICU | 26 (0.7%) | 2 (1.8%) | 0.17 |
| Mechanical ventilation time (hours) | 4 (3–6) | 4 (3–6) | 0.14 |
| VA-ECMO | 11 (0.3%) | 1 (0.9%) | 0.29 |
| Stroke | 63 (1.7%) | 0 | 0.26 |
| Post-operative AF | 973 (26.3%) | 65 (59.1%) | <0.001 |
| ICU length of stay (days) | 3 (3–4) | 4(3–9) | <0.001 |

*Categorical variables are presented as number (proportion) and continuous variables as mean (standard deviation).*
*AF, atrial fibrillation; ICU, intensive care unit; RVF, right ventricular failure; VA-ECMO, veno-arterial extracorporeal membranous oxygenation.*

# RESULTS

## Patients and Baseline Characteristics

We included 3,826 consecutive patients who underwent cardiac surgery with CPB. Baseline characteristics are shown in **Table 1**.

Post-operative RVF occurred in 110 patients (2.9%). Compared with the group who did not develop RVF, patients in the RVF group were older (71.0 ± 9.9 vs. 68.6 ± 10.9 years, $p = 0.018$), had more women (36.4 vs. 25.2%, $p = 0.008$), more history of AF (29.2 vs. 8.4%, $p < 0.001$), lower pre-operative estimated glomerular filtration rate [57.7 (44.5–71.9) vs. 69.6 (57.0- 82.7) ml/min per 1.73 m$^2$, $p < 0.001$], and higher EuroScore II [4.1 (2.0–8.0) vs. 1.7 (0.97–3.2), $p < 0.001$]. Regarding pre-operative echocardiographic data, patient in the RVF group presented more pre-operative LVEF below 50% (25.5 vs. 14.5%, $p = 0.001$) and elevated sPAP above 55 mmHg (50.5 vs. 4.4%, <0.001).

The type of surgical procedure affected the risk of developing RVF. In particular, mitral and tricuspid valve procedures were more at risk (64.5 vs.16.7%, $p < 0.001$, and 50 vs. 3.6%, $p < 0.001$, respectively). CPB time was also higher in patients who developed post-operative RVF (96.4 ± 34.0 vs. 79.3 ± 29.8 min, $p < 0.001$, respectively).

## Clinical Outcomes and Prognosis After Right Ventricular Failure

Post-operative outcomes were similar in patients who presented RVF and those who did not, regarding mortality in ICU (RVF and those without RVF, respectively, 1.8 vs. 0.7%, $p = 0.17$), mechanical ventilation duration [4 (3–6) vs. 4 (3–6) h, $p = 0.14$], veno-arterial extracorporeal membranous oxygenation requirement (0.9 vs. 0.3%, $p = 0.29$), and stroke (0 vs. 1.7%, $p = 0.26$) (see **Figure 1** and **Table 2**).

The outcomes that were different were ICU length of stay (longer in patients with RVF), with 4 (3–9) vs. 3 (3–4) days ($p < 0.001$), and incidence of AF with 59.1 vs. 26.3% ($p < 0.001$).

Focusing on the 14-day in-hospital follow-up, patients who developed post-operative RVF were less likely to be discharged at this point than patients who did not present RVF (log-rank $p < 0.0001$, see **Figure 2**). The uncensored analysis yielded a similar outcome between patients with or without post-operative RVF (log-rank $p = 0.70$).

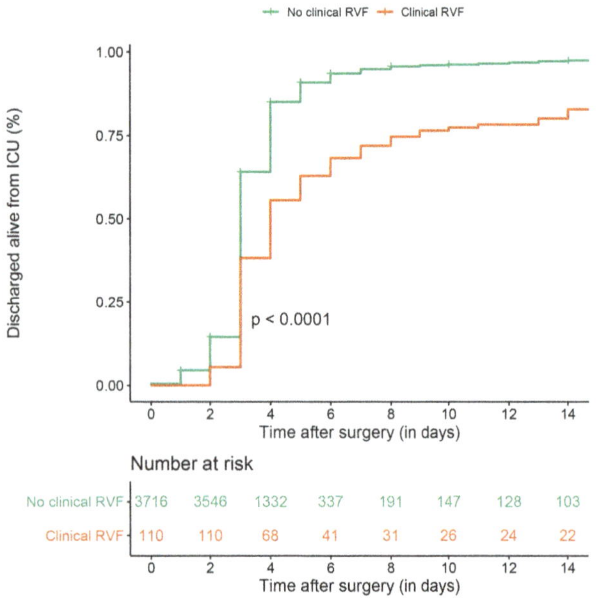


**FIGURE 2 |** Kaplan–Meier estimate of ICU discharge alive, censored at 14 days between clinical post-operative RVF and control patients in the overall surgery cohort.

For sensitivity, we computed a composite outcome that combined death, reintubation, stroke, and prolonged ICU stay (more than 14 days). We found an incidence of 252/3,826 (6.6%), and RVF was associated with this composite outcome (19.1 vs. 6.2%, odds ratio = 3.6 (2.2–5.8), $p < 0.001$).

## Variables Associated With the Incidence of Right Ventricular Failure

In a logistic regression multivariable model, variables independently associated post-operative RVF were pre-operative AF {adjusted odds-ratio (adjOR) 3.22 [95% confidence interval (95%CI) = 1.94–5.36], $p < 0.001$}, left ventricle ejection fraction below 50% [adjOR = 2.55 (95%CI = 1.52–4.33), $p < 0.001$], systolic pulmonary artery pressure above 55 mmHg [adjOR = 8.64 (95%CI = 5.27–14.1); $p < 0.001$], mitral valve surgery [adjOR = 2.17 CI (95%CI = 1.28–3.66), $p = 0.004$], and tricuspid valve surgery [adjOR = 10.33 (95%CI = 6.14–17.4), $p < 0.001$] (see **Table 3**).

## Pre-operative Right Ventricular Function in Patients With Post-operative Right Ventricular Failure

Focusing in patients who presented RVF ($n$ = 110), pre-existing RV dysfunction [with either TAPSE < 16 mm and tissue doppler imaging with peak myocardial velocity at the lateral tricuspid annulus (S wave) < 9.5 cm/s] was found in 32 (29.1%) patients (**Table 4**). Compared with those with preserved pre-operative RV function, those with pre-operative RV dysfunction showed more moderate to severe TR (81.3 vs. 38.2%, $p < 0.001$), larger RA surface [26.5 (22.3–31.8) vs. 21 (14–23) cm$^2$, $p < 0.001$] and underwent more frequently tricuspid procedures (65.6 vs. 43.4%, $p = 0.035$). Inhaled NO tended to used more frequently in patients with pre-operative RVF (87.5 vs. 69.7%, $p = 0.05$).

**TABLE 3 |** Variables associated with post-operative right ventricular failure.

| | Univariate Model OR (95%CI), *p*-value | Multivariate Model OR (95%CI), *p*-value |
|---|---|---|
| Age | 1.02 (1.01–1.04), 0.02 | |
| Female | 1.71 (1.16–2.55), 0.007 | |
| COPD | 1.63 (0.90–2.95), 0.11 | |
| Previous AF | 4.5 (2.88–7.17), <0.001 | 3.22 (1.94–5.36), <0.001 |
| eGFR | 0.98 (0.97–0.99), <0.001 | |
| LVEF < 30% | 1.52 (0.47–4.9), 0.48 | |
| LVEF < 50% | 2.02 (1.30–3.13), 0.002 | 2.55 (1.52–4.33), 0.001 |
| sPAP > 55 mmHg | 23.11 (15.04–35.49), <0.001 | 8.64 (5.27–14.1), <0.001 |
| Mitral surgery | 9.19 (6.16–13.71), <0.001 | 2.17 (1.28–3.66), 0.004 |
| Tricuspid surgery | 28.04 (18.55–42.4), <0.001 | 10.33 (6.14–17.4), <0.001 |
| CPB duration | 1.01 (1.01–1.02), <0.001 | |
| Aortic clampage | 1.00 (0.99–1.01), 0.48 | |

*Variables included in the multivariable model: age, sex, previous AF, eGFR, sPAP > 55 mmHg, LVEF < 50%, mitral surgery, tricuspid intervention, and CPB length.*
*AF, atrial fibrillation; CPB, cardiopulmonary bypass; COPD, chronic obstructive pulmonary disease; eGFR, estimated glomerular filtration rate; LVEF, left ventricular ejection fraction; sPAP, systolic pulmonary artery pressure.*

**TABLE 4 |** Comparison between patients with normal pre-operative RV function and patients with pre-operative RV dysfunction, in the subgroup of patients presenting post-operative RV dysfunction ($n$ = 110).

| | Normal pre-operative RV function ($n$ = 78)[†] | Pre-operative RV dysfunction ($n$ = 32) | *P* |
|---|---|---|---|
| TAPSE (mm) | 22 (21–24) | 15 (14–15.25) | – |
| S wave (cm/s) | 13 (13–14) | 9 (8–10) | – |
| TR, moderate to severe | 29 (38.2%) | 26 (81.3%) | <0.001 |
| Right atrium surface (cm$^2$) | 21 (14–23) | 26.5 (22.3–31.8) | <0.001 |
| Previous AF | 21 (27.6%) | 14 (43.8%) | 0.1 |
| LVEF < 50% | 19 (25%) | 8 (25%) | 1 |
| sPAP > 55 mmHg | 30 (39.5%) | 17 (53.1%) | 0.19 |
| Mitral surgery | 49 (64.5%) | 20 (62.5%) | 0.85 |
| Tricuspid surgery | 33 (43.4%) | 21 (65.6%) | 0.035 |

*[‡]Pre-operative echocardiographic data were incomplete for two patients.*
*Categorical variables are presented as number (proportion) and continuous variables as mean (standard deviation).*
*AF, atrial fibrillation; LVEF, left ventricular ejection fraction; sPAP, systolic pulmonary artery pressure; TR, tricuspid regurgitation; TAPSE, tricuspid annular plane systolic excursion.*

## DISCUSSION

In this study, we described the incidence, risk factors, and prognosis of post-operative RVF. We observed that (1) clinically significant RVF after cardiac surgery is rare, occurring below 3%; (2) despite higher predicted perioperative risk (i.e., EuroScore II), treatment with iNO and sildenafil allowed to reach similar post-operative results regarding hard clinical outcomes when comparing patients with post-operative with and without RVF; (3) independent variables associated with post-operative RVF included the history of AF, pre-operative LVEF below 50%, mitral surgery, tricuspid surgery, and pre-operative sPAP above 55 mmHg; (4) in patients who presented post-operative RVF, its severity was associated with pre-operative RV dysfunction.

Post-operative RVF in cardiac surgery ICU is a major concern because of its challenging diagnosis: sternotomy is an obstacle to procure accurate and reproducible information regarding echocardiographic right heart evaluation. Due to the standard approach in cardiac surgery with pericardial opening, TAPSE may be inherently reduced in the post-operative period without patent clinical RVF (14). Moreover, TAPSE after tricuspid annuloplasty may lead to an underestimation of RV systolic function (15). Definition of RVF is heterogeneous among physicians in the field and the literature, going from only echocardiographic definitions to mild or very severe circulatory failure (16, 17). Although echocardiography is an overall powerful tool, in the post-operative setting, it presents limitations, the first of which is a possible lack of sonographic window allowing for accurate measurements, particularly in mechanically ventilated patients (18). Meanwhile, a single echocardiographic parameter may not be sufficient to define RVF, and as echocardiographic assessment of longitudinal RV systolic function such as TAPSE and S wave may be eyeballed by expert visual assessment (19), we chose a pragmatic endpoint defined as echocardiographic assessment RVF combined with clinical hemodynamic instability requiring immediate treatment.

Our data could not allow for the analysis of the effect of iNO and sildenafil, as RVF treatment, because of a lack of a control group. Recent studies showed interest in sildenafil administration on its own or in association with iNO. In our experience, combining both drugs in the post-operative period seemed to be safe and efficient in decreasing both pressure and resistance in the pulmonary circulation without affecting cardiac output, although, as of yet, no study showed differences in clinical outcomes (20–22).

We confirmed that mitral surgery and previous LVEF $< 50\%$ were associated with post-operative RVF, as already described previously, with a high incidence of low cardiac output state after mitral valve procedures (23, 24). The principal mechanism invoked is an abrupt increase in afterload due to elimination of the reverse flow into the left atrium, all the more so if LV was decreased before correction (25, 26).

As we observed, previous AF could be associated with a complicated post-operative course (27). Gorter et al. showed in patients with heart failure with preserved LVEF that RV and RA functions were more depressed in patients with AF and patients in sinus rhythm but with prior AF, compared with patients without any history of AF (28). Also, they suggested these findings were independent of pulmonary pressures. According to recent studies, functional TR is associated with right atrium (RA) enlargement in the setting of chronic AF (29). Thus, AF, tricuspid regurgitation, and RA enlargement are somehow working together, participating in the development of RVF. Then, TR correction could represent a key therapeutic option, but it has shown to be a major risk factor for post-operative RVF (30, 31). Before surgery, the RV adapted to chronic volume overload, but surgical TR correction could lead to an abrupt increase in afterload with reduced pre-load and then uncoupling RV and pulmonary circulation as an analogy with LV hemodynamics in mitral valve closure, but because of RV anatomy and physiology, it would not support such hemodynamic modification as the LV could accept it. Besides, CPB with induced RH and abnormal septal motion has shown deleterious effect in RV hemodynamics (2). Finally, severe pre-operative RH is a well-known risk factor for post-operative RVF, corresponding to our findings with a threshold of sPAP $> 55$ mmHg in our study. We acknowledge that this study does not solve the issue of whether iNO and sildenafil are appropriate to treat RVF, but it comforts the fact that RVF may be anticipated in some procedures (mainly tricuspid and mitral valve surgery) and that these treatments seem to alleviate the poor prognosis of an RVF outcome.

We acknowledge several limitations. First, although we chose criteria that satisfied clinician need for post-operative RVF (i.e., which required specific treatment, including vasopressors and inhaled NO), there are no consensual and easily obtainable RVF criteria in clinical practice. Secondly, lack of difference in mortality may be imputed to a lack of power; all the more so that the computation of a composite outcome which combined deaths, strokes, prolonged ICU stay, and reintubation showed significantly increased risk in patients who developed post-operative RVF. Third, our center only performed standard cardiac surgery excluding congenital cardiac procedures, heart transplantation, or LVAD implantations, all considered at high risk for post-operative RVF. Fourth, pre-operative RV assessment parameters were only retrievable in patients who developed post-operative RVF; thus, we could not integrate these elements into multivariable analysis regarding pre-operative risk factors of developing post-operative RVF. Nevertheless, we managed to study pre-operative RV function in patients with post-operative RVF, providing important insight into this subgroup in favor of a link between RV dysfunction, AF, TR, and enlarged RA.

Finally, we acknowledge that the lack of a control group (i.e., patients who presented post-operative RVF but were treated with neither iNO nor sildenafil) makes any analysis of treatment efficacy impossible.

Thus, we advocate for the design of a dedicated randomized controlled trial to address this rare but severe issue that is post-operative RVF.

## CONCLUSION

Post-operative RVF occurred in 2.9% of patients after cardiac surgery. Variables significantly associated with RVF were history of AF, LVEF < 50%, sPAP > 55 mmHg, and mitral and tricuspid valve procedures.

## ETHICS STATEMENT

Ethical review and approval was not required for the study on human participants in accordance with the local legislation and institutional requirements. The ethics committee waived the requirement of written informed consent for participation.

## AUTHOR CONTRIBUTIONS

DLe wrote the initial manuscript, participated to data collection, and performed statistical analyses. DLa, PE, AB, and PS participated to data collection and provided critical review. AB also curated the database. LN supervised the study, participated to data collection, analyses, and wrote the final manuscript. All authors contributed to the article and approved the submitted version.

## REFERENCES


1. Denault AY, Pearl RG, Michler RE, Rao V, Tsui SSL, Seitelberger R, et al. Tezosentan and right ventricular failure in patients with pulmonary hypertension undergoing cardiac surgery: the TACTICS trial. *J Cardiothorac Vasc Anesth.* (2013) 27:1212-7. doi: 10.1053/j.jvca.2013.01.023
2. Haddad F, Couture P, Tousignant C, Denault AY. The right ventricle in cardiac surgery, a perioperative perspective: II. *Pathophysiol Clin Import Manage Anesth Analg.* (2009) 108:422-33. doi: 10.1213/ane.0b013e31818d8b92
3. Vonk Noordegraaf A, Chin KM, Haddad F, Hassoun PM, Hemnes AR, Hopkins SR, et al. Pathophysiology of the right ventricle and of the pulmonary circulation in pulmonary hypertension: an update. *Eur Respir J.* (2019) 53:1801900. doi: 10.1183/13993003.01900-2018
4. Morita K, Ihnken K, Buckberg GD, Sherman MP, Ignarro LJ. Pulmonary vasoconstriction due to impaired nitric oxide production after cardiopulmonary bypass. *Ann Thorac Surg.* (1996) 61:1775-80. doi: 10.1016/0003-4975(96)00146-4
5. Gianetti J, Del Sarto P, Bevilacqua S, Vassalle C, De Filippis R, Kacila M, et al. Supplemental nitric oxide and its effect on myocardial injury and function in patients undergoing cardiac surgery with extracorporeal circulation. *J Thorac Cardiovasc Surg.* (2004) 127:44-50. doi: 10.1016/j.jtcvs.2002.08.001
6. Germann P, Braschi A, Della Rocca G, Dinh-Xuan AT, Falke K, Frostell C, et al. Inhaled nitric oxide therapy in adults: European expert recommendations. *Intensive Care Med.* (2005) 31:1029-41. doi: 10.1007/s00134-005-2675-4
7. Pepke-Zaba J, Higenbottam TW, Dinh-Xuan AT, Stone D, Wallwork J. Inhaled nitric oxide as a cause of selective pulmonary vasodilatation in pulmonary hypertension. *Lancet Lond Engl.* (1991) 338:1173-4. doi: 10.1016/0140-6736(91)92033-X
8. Fullerton DA, Jones SD, Jaggers J, Piedalue F, Grover FL, McIntyre RC. Effective control of pulmonary vascular resistance with inhaled nitric oxide after cardiac operation. *Cardiovasc Surg.* (1996) 111:11. doi: 10.1016/S0022-5223(96)70335-5
9. Haché M, Denault A, Bélisle S, Robitaille D, Couture P, Sheridan P, et al. Inhaled epoprostenol (prostacyclin) and pulmonary hypertension before cardiac surgery. *J Thorac Cardiovasc Surg.* (2003) 125:642-9. doi: 10.1067/mtc.2003.107
10. Fattouch K, Sbraga F, Sampognaro R, Bianco G, Gucciardo M, Lavalle C, et al. Treatment of pulmonary hypertension in patients undergoing cardiac surgery with cardiopulmonary bypass: a randomized, prospective, double-blind study. *J Cardiovasc Med Hagerstown Md.* (2006) 7:119-23. doi: 10.2459/01.JCM.0000203850.97890.fe
11. Haddad F, Couture P, Tousignant C, Denault AY. The right ventricle in cardiac surgery, a perioperative perspective: I. *Anat Physiol Assess Anesth Analg.* (2009) 108:407-21. doi: 10.1213/ane.0b013e31818f8623
12. Drakos SG, Janicki L, Horne BD, Kfoury AG, Reid BB, Clayson S, et al. Risk factors predictive of right ventricular failure after left ventricular assist device implantation. *Am J Cardiol.* (2010) 105:1030–5. doi: 10.1016/j.amjcard.2009.11.026
13. Bellavia D, Iacovoni A, Scardulla C, Moja L, Pilato M, Kushwaha SS, et al. Prediction of right ventricular failure after ventricular assist device implant: systematic review and meta-analysis of observational studies. *Eur J Heart Fail.* (2017) 19:926-46. doi: 10.1002/ejhf.733
14. Zanobini M, Saccocci M, Tamborini G, Veglia F, Di Minno A, Poggio P, et al. Postoperative echocardiographic reduction of right ventricular function: is pericardial opening modality the main culprit? *BioMed Res Int.* (2017) 2017:4808757. doi: 10.1155/2017/4808757
15. de Agustin JA, Martinez-Losas P, de Diego JJG, Mahia P, Marcos-Alberca P, Nuñez-Gil IJ, et al. Tricuspid annular plane systolic excursion inaccuracy to assess right ventricular function in patients with previous tricuspid annulopasty. *Int J Cardiol.* (2016) 223:713-6. doi: 10.1016/j.ijcard.2016.08.276
16. Mehra MR, Park MH, Landzberg MJ, Lala A, Waxman AB, International Right Heart Failure Foundation Scientific Working Group. Right heart failure: toward a common language. *J Heart Lung Transplant.* (2014) 33:123-6. doi: 10.1016/j.healun.2013.10.015
17. Vieillard-Baron A, Naeije R, Haddad F, Bogaard HJ, Bull TM, Fletcher N, et al. Diagnostic workup, etiologies and management of acute right ventricle failure: a state-of-the-art paper. *Intensive Care Med.* (2018) 44:774-90. doi: 10.1007/s00134-018-5172-2
18. Price S, Prout J, Jaggar SI, Gibson DG, Pepper JR. 'Tamponade' following cardiac surgery: terminology and echocardiography may both mislead. *Eur J Cardio-Thorac Surg.* (2004) 26:1156-60. doi: 10.1016/j.ejcts.2004.08.020
19. Schneider M, Aschauer S, Mascherbauer J, Ran H, Binder C, Lang I, et al. Echocardiographic assessment of right ventricular function: current clinical practice. *Int J Cardiovasc Imaging.* (2019) 35:49-56. doi: 10.1007/s10554-018-1428-8
20. Ram E, Sternik L, Klempfner R, Eldar M, Goldenberg I, Peled Y, et al. Sildenafil for pulmonary hypertension in the early postoperative period after mitral valve surgery. *J Cardiothorac Vasc Anesth.* (2019) 33:1648-56. doi: 10.1053/j.jvca.2018.12.023
21. Matamis D, Pampori S, Papathanasiou A, Papakonstantinou P, Tsagourias M, Galiatsou E, et al. Inhaled NO and sildenafil combination in cardiac surgery patients with out-of-proportion pulmonary hypertension: acute effects on postoperative gas exchange and hemodynamics. *Circ Heart Fail.* (2012) 5:47-53. doi: 10.1161/CIRCHEARTFAILURE.111.963314
22. Michelakis E, Tymchak W, Lien D, Webster L, Hashimoto K, Archer S. Oral sildenafil is an effective and specific pulmonary vasodilator in patients with pulmonary arterial hypertension: comparison with inhaled nitric oxide. *Circulation.* (2002) 105:2398–403. doi: 10.1161/01.CIR.0000016641.12984.DC
23. Appelbaum A, Kouchoukos NT, Blackstone EH, Kirklin JW. Early risks of open heart surgery for mitral valve disease. *Am J Cardiol.* (1976) 37:201-9. doi: 10.1016/0002-9149(76)90313-1
24. Sethi GK, Miller DC, Souchek J, Oprian C, Henderson WG, Hassan Z, et al. Clinical, hemodynamic, and angiographic predictors of operative mortality in patients undergoing single valve replacement. *J Thorac Cardiovasc Surg.* (1987) 93:884-97. doi: 10.1016/S0022-5223(19)37049-7
25. Ahmadi A, Spillner G, Johannesson T. Hemodynamic changes following experimental production and correction of acute mitral regurgitation with an adjustable ring prosthesis. *Thorac Cardiovasc Surg.* (1988) 36:313-9. doi: 10.1055/s-2007-1022972
26. Rankin JS, Nicholas LM, Kouchoukos NT. Experimental mitral regurgitation: effects on left ventricular function before and after elimination of chronic regurgitation in the dog. *J Thorac Cardiovasc Surg.* (1975) 70:478-88. doi: 10.1016/S0022-5223(19)40322-X
27. Greenberg JW, Lancaster TS, Schuessler RB, Melby SJ. Postoperative atrial fibrillation following cardiac surgery: a persistent complication. *Eur J Cardiothorac Surg.* (2017) 52:665-72. doi: 10.1093/ejcts/ezx039
28. Gorter TM, van Melle JP, Rienstra M, Borlaug BA, Hummel YM, van Gelder IC, et al. Right heart dysfunction in heart failure with preserved ejection fraction: the impact of atrial fibrillation. *J Card Fail.* (2018) 24:177-85. doi: 10.1016/j.cardfail.2017.11.005

29. Cho JY, Kim KH, Kim JY, Sim DS, Yoon HJ, Yoon NS, et al. Predictors of reversible severe functional tricuspid regurgitation in patients with atrial fibrillation. *J Cardiol.* (2016) 68:419-25. doi: 10.1016/j.jjcc.2015.11.010
30. Spratt JA, Olsen CO, Tyson GS, Glower DD, Davis JW, Rankin JS. Experimental mitral regurgitation. Physiological effects of correction on left ventricular dynamics. *J Thorac Cardiovasc Surg.* (1983) 86:479-89. doi: 10.1016/S0022-5223(19)39112-3
31. Suri RM, Schaff HV, Dearani JA, Sundt TM, Daly RC, Mullany CJ, et al. Determinants of early decline in ejection fraction after surgical correction of mitral regurgitation. *J Thorac Cardiovasc Surg.* (2008) 136:442-7. doi: 10.1016/j.jtcvs.2007.10.067

# 14

# Incidence- and In-hospital Mortality-Related Risk Factors of Acute Kidney Injury Requiring Continuous Renal Replacement Therapy in Patients Undergoing Surgery for Acute Type A Aortic Dissection

*Xuelian Chen*[1†], *Jiaojiao Zhou*[2†], *Miao Fang*[3], *Jia Yang*[1], *Xin Wang*[4], *Siwen Wang*[1], *Linji Li*[5], *Tao Zhu*[5], *Ling Ji*[6] *and Lichuan Yang*[6*]

*Division of Nephrology, Department of Medicine, West China Hospital of Sichuan University, Chengdu, China,* [2] *Division of Ultrasound, West China Hospital, Sichuan University, Chengdu, China,* [3] *Department of Orthopedics, Second People's Hospital of Chengdu, Chengdu, China,* [4] *Department of Pediatric Nephrology, West China Second University Hospital, Sichuan University, Chengdu, China,* [5] *Department of Anesthesiology, West China Hospital, Sichuan University, The Research Units of West China (2018RU012), Chinese Academy of Medical Sciences, Chengdu, China,* [6] *Division of Nephrology, West China Hospital of Sichuan University, Chengdu, China*

***Correspondence:***
*Lichuan Yang*
*ylcgh@163.com*

*These authors have contributed equally to this work and share first authorship*

†

**Background:** Few studies on the risk factors for postoperative continuous renal replacement therapy (CRRT) in a homogeneous population of patients with acute type A aortic dissection (AAAD). This retrospective analysis aimed to investigate the risk factors for CRRT and in-hospital mortality in the patients undergoing AAAD surgery and to discuss the perioperative comorbidities and short-term outcomes.

**Methods:** The study collected electronic medical records and laboratory data from 432 patients undergoing surgery for AAAD between March 2009 and June 2021. All the patients were divided into CRRT and non-CRRT groups; those in the CRRT group were divided into the survivor and non-survivor groups. The univariable and multivariable analyses were used to identify the independent risk factors for CRRT and in-hospital mortality.

**Results:** The proportion of requiring CRRT and in-hospital mortality in the patients with CRRT was 14.6 and 46.0%, respectively. Baseline serum creatinine (SCr) [odds ratio (*OR*), 1.006], cystatin C (*OR*, 1.438), lung infection (*OR*, 2.292), second thoracotomy (*OR*, 5.185), diabetes mellitus (*OR*, 6.868), AKI stage 2–3 (*OR*, 22.901) were the independent risk factors for receiving CRRT. In-hospital mortality in the CRRT group (46%) was 4.6 times higher than in the non-CRRT group (10%). In the non-survivor ($n$ = 29) and survivor ($n$ = 34) groups, New York Heart Association (NYHA) class III-IV (*OR*, 10.272, $P = 0.019$), lactic acidosis (*OR*, 10.224, $P = 0.019$) were the independent risk factors for in-hospital mortality in patients receiving CRRT.

**Conclusion:** There was a high rate of CRRT requirement and high in-hospital mortality after AAAD surgery. The risk factors for CRRT and in-hospital mortality in the patients undergoing AAAD surgery were determined to help identify the high-risk patients and make appropriate clinical decisions. Further randomized controlled studies are urgently needed to establish the risk factors for CRRT and in-hospital mortality.

**Keywords: acute type A aortic dissection, surgery, acute kidney injury, continuous renal replacement therapy, CRRT, risk factors**

## INTRODUCTION

Acute kidney injury (AKI) is one of the most common postoperative complications following cardiac surgery and is associated with increased morbidity and mortality (1). There is currently no consensus on the definition of cardiac surgery-associated AKI (CSA-AKI). The Kidney Disease: Improving Global Outcomes criteria (KDIGO) represent the current epidemiological and clinical standard for diagnosing AKI, including CSA-AKI (2, 3). Acute type A aortic dissection (AAAD) is the most dramatic emergency in cardiac surgery due to the high in-hospital mortality rate of ~26% (4). Compared with other heart surgeries, the risk of AKI is higher after aortic dissection surgery (5, 6). Between 1999 and 2008, the incidence of AKI and AKI requiring dialysis (AKI-D) after cardiac surgery has increased from 30 and 5% to 47 and 14%, respectively (7). Continuous renal replacement therapy (CRRT) is widely used for hemodynamically unstable patients with considerable fluid accumulation (3, 8). However, the mortality of receiving CRRT after AKI is 40–70% (9), and second, the high cost of CRRT and the limited medical resources associated with CRRT impose a heavy social burden (10). Early identification of critically ill patients of high risk for CRRT and in-hospital mortality after cardiac surgery can be beneficial in improving the overall prognosis.

Few studies on the risk factors for postoperative CRRT in a homogeneous population of patients with AAAD. This retrospective analysis was designed to describe the incidence of AKI requiring CRRT in the patients undergoing AAAD surgery, evaluate the demographic and perioperative factors associated with the patients with AKI requiring CRRT, identify the association of CRRT with a duration of mechanical ventilation, in-hospital mortality, and 1-year readmission, and analyze the risk factors for CRRT and in-hospital mortality.

**Abbreviations:** AKI, acute kidney injury; CSA-AKI, cardiac surgery-associated acute kidney injury; AAAD, acute type A aortic dissection; KDIGO, Kidney Disease: Improving Global Outcomes; AKI-D, AKI incidence requiring dialysis; eGFR, estimated glomerular filtration rate; SCr, serum creatinine; SD, standard deviations; IQR, interquartile range; BMI, body mass index; CKD, chronic kidney disease; COPD, chronic obstructive pulmonary disease; NYHA, New York Heart Association; AST, aspartate aminotransferase; ALT, alanine aminotransferase; DHCA, Deep hypothermic circulatory arrest; CPB, cardiopulmonary bypass; ALB, albumin; BUN, blood urea nitrogen; UA, uric acid; Cys-C, cystatin C; MAP, mean arterial pressure; AMI, acute myocardial infarction; CVA, acute cerebrovascular accident; ARDS, acute respiratory distress syndrome; CRRT, continuous renal replacement therapy.

## MATERIALS AND METHODS

### Study Population

For this study, in **Figure 1**, we retrospectively collected the electronic medical records and laboratory results of 432 patients aged ≥18 years who underwent cardiac surgery for AAAD diagnosed by echocardiography or enhanced CT at the West China Hospital of Sichuan University (Sichuan, China) between March 2009 and June 2021. The exclusion criteria were as follows: (i) the patients who had received maintenance dialysis within the last month or were on dialysis before surgery ($n = 29$); (ii) the patients who had received kidney transplantation ($n = 5$); (iii) the patients who died within 24 h of admission to the hospital ($n = 23$); and (iv) the patients with incomplete data ($n = 59$). The present study was approved by the Ethics Committees of the West China Hospital of Sichuan University. Sichuan, China.

### Data Collection

The data of the patients included in the present study, including the patient characteristics, perioperative factors, laboratory data, postoperative complications or comorbidities, and outcomes, were extracted from the electronic medical records system of our institution. The laboratory data of the CRRT group were obtained prior to the occurrence of AKI.

### Measurements and Variable Definitions

Acute kidney injury was defined according to the KDIGO criteria (2) as follows: a serum creatinine (SCr) levels increase of ≥0.3 mg/dl within 48 h, or ≥1.5-fold the baseline level, which is known or hypothesized to have occurred within the prior 7 days, or urine output <0.5 ml/kg/h for 6 consecutive h. AKI severity was staged according to the following criteria (2) (**Table 1**).

In this retrospective analysis, the urine output criteria for defining AKI were not used, as 6- and 12-h urine outputs were not reliably recorded, and certain patients were treated with diuretics and CRRT. The decision for CRRT is determined by the assessment of the severity of AKI by the clinician and the comprehensive condition of patients. As some patients with AAAD were referred to our hospital from other hospitals, the lowest SCr level in the 2 days prior to admission was used as the baseline level if data were available; if not, we considered the first SCr available at admission as the baseline value. Drinking is defined as having consumed alcohol at least one time a week in the last year. CKD was defined by past medical history. Preoperative liver insufficiency was defined as a preoperative elevation of >80 U/L of aspartate aminotransferase (AST) or (and) alanine aminotransferase (ALT)

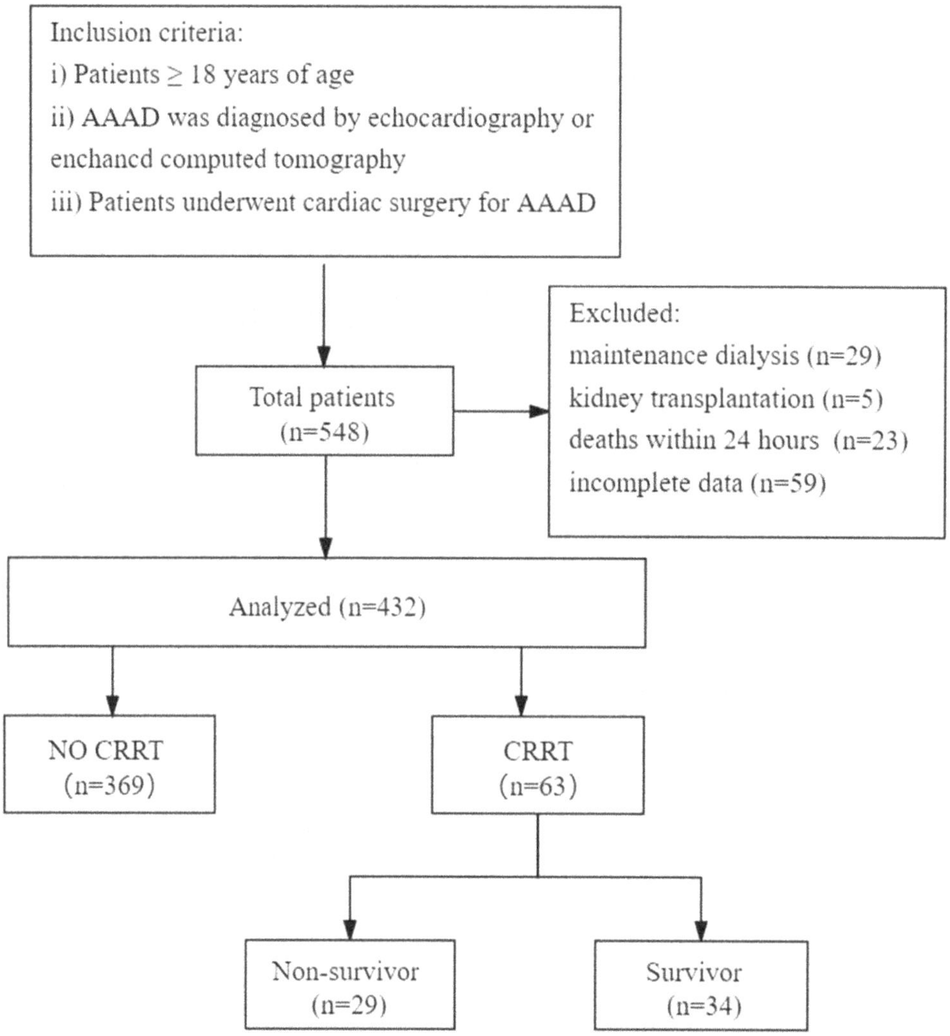


**FIGURE 1** | Flow diagram of the study.

**TABLE 1** | Kidney Disease: Improving Global Outcomes (KDIGO) stages of acute kidney injury (AKI) according to serum creatinine (SCr) levels and urine output.

| Stage | Serum creatinine | Urine output |
|---|---|---|
| 1 | 1.5–1.9 times baseline | <0.5 ml/kg/h for 6–12 h |
| | Or ≥0.3 mg/dl (≥26.5 mmol/l) increase | |
| 2 | 2.0–2.9 times baseline | <0.5 ml/kg/h for ≥12 h |
| 3 | 3.0 times baseline | <0.3 ml/kg/h for ≥24 h Or anuria for ≥12 h |
| | Or increase in serum creatinine to ≥4.0 mg/dl (≥353.6 mmol/l) | |
| | Or initiation of renal replacement therapy or in patients <18 years, decrease in eGFR to <35 ml/min per 1.73 m$^2$ | |

*KDIGO, Kidney Disease: Improving Global Outcomes; eGFR, estimated glomerular filtration rate.*

in the patients. Deep hypothermic circulatory arrest (DHCA) is a measure to protect the brain by arresting extracorporeal circulation after cooling the brain temperature to 14.1–20°C in aortic arch replacement, for brain preservation. The diagnosis of postoperative acute myocardial infarction (AMI) was based on a history of typical chest pain, diagnostic ECG changes, serum cardiac biomarkers, and abnormalities on echocardiography and coronary angiography. Cerebral ischemia or hemorrhage resulting in complete or incomplete loss of brain function was defined as an acute cerebrovascular accident (CVA).

The patients were divided into the CRRT and non-CRRT groups according to whether they required CRRT or not; the patients in the CRRT group were divided into the survivor and non-survivor groups. The independent risk factors and perioperative complications and short-term outcomes were analyzed.

The primary outcomes were the occurrence of severe AKI, requiring CRRT, and in-hospital mortality. The secondary outcomes were the duration of mechanical ventilation, hospitalization costs, and 1-year re-admission.

## Statistical Analysis

The baseline demographic and clinical data of patients were presented as numbers and percentages for categorical variables. The categorical variables were compared using chi-square tests. Data distribution normality was verified using the Kolmogorov–Smirnov test. The normally distributed continuous variables were presented as mean ± SD and the non-normally distributed continuous variables were represented as the median and interquartile range (IQR) and compared accordingly using independent samples $t$-test or Mann–Whitney $U$-test. A stepwise forward binary logistic regression analysis was applied to analyze the risk factors for patients receiving postoperative CRRT and in-hospital mortality. The omnibus tests of model coefficients were used to evaluate the multivariable binary logistic regression model, with $P < 0.05$ indicating that the binary logistic regression model was generally significant. Hosmer and Lemeshow test and −2 log likelihood (−2LL) provided an evaluation of the goodness

**TABLE 2** | Demographics, preoperative factors, and laboratory data of 432 patients.

| | ALL ($n$ = 432) | No CRRT ($n$ = 369) | CRRT ($n$ = 63) | $P$ value |
|---|---|---|---|---|
| Age, year, mean ± SD | 48.19 ± 10.97 | 47.69 ± 10.59 | 51.10 ± 12.63 | **0.023** |
| Gender, n (%) | | | | **0.036** |
| Male | 341 (78.9%) | 285 (77.2%) | 56 (88.9%) | |
| Female | 91 (21.1%) | 84 (22.8%) | 7 (11.1%) | |
| BMI, kg/m$^2$, mean ± SD | 24.85 ± 3.78 | 24.84 ± 3.65 | 24.89 ± 4.53 | 0.916 |
| Smoking, n (%) | 210 (48.6%) | 181 (49.1%) | 29 (46.0%) | 0.658 |
| Drinking, n (%) | 136 (31.5%) | 122 (33.1%) | 14 (22.2%) | 0.087 |
| **Medical history, n (%)** | | | | |
| Hypertension | 250 (57.9%) | 209 (56.6%) | 41 (65.1%) | 0.210 |
| Poor blood pressure control | 92 (21.3%) | 72 (19.5%) | 20 (31.7%) | **0.028** |
| A left ventricular ejection fraction of <35% | 28 (6.5%) | 22 (6.0%) | 6 (9.5%) | 0.289 |
| Marfan syndrome | 18 (4.2%) | 14 (3.8%) | 4 (6.3%) | 0.348 |
| Previous cardiac surgery | 27 (6.3%) | 23 (6.2%) | 4 (6.3%) | 0.972 |
| Aortic regurgitation | 176 (40.7%) | 150 (40.7%) | 26 (41.3%) | 0.926 |
| CKD | 30 (6.9%) | 22 (6.0%) | 8 (12.7%) | 0.052 |
| COPD | 28 (6.5%) | 21 (5.7%) | 7 (11.1%) | 0.106 |
| Diabetes mellitus | 20 (4.6%) | 11 (3.0%) | 9 (14.3%) | **0.000** |
| Chronic liver disease | 22 (5.1%) | 18 (4.9%) | 4 (6.3%) | 0.624 |
| **Preoperative factors** | | | | |
| Hemorrhagic shock, n (%) | 7 (1.6%) | 4 (1.1%) | 3 (4.8%) | 0.094 |
| Pericardial tamponade, n (%) | 20 (4.6%) | 17 (4.6%) | 3 (4.8%) | 0.957 |
| NYHA class III-IV, n (%) | 111 (25.7%) | 85 (23.0%) | 26 (41.3%) | **0.002** |
| Liver insufficiency, n (%) | 51 (11.8%) | 36 (9.8%) | 15 (23.8%) | **0.001** |
| **Renal artery involvement, n (%)** | 184 (42.6%) | 154 (41.7%) | 30 (47.6%) | 0.383 |
| Renal malperfusion, n (%) | 103 (23.8%) | 83 (22.5%) | 20 (31.7%) | 0.113 |
| No renal malperfusion, n (%) | 81 (18.8%) | 71 (19.2%) | 10 (15.9%) | 0.527 |
| **Lab data (mean ± SD) or median (IQR)** | | | | |
| Baseline SCr, μmol/L | 82 (65, 104) | 79 (64, 99) | 97 (83, 131) | **0.000** |
| BUN, mmol/L | 6.32 (4.95, 8.60) | 6.15 (4.90, 8.30) | 7.50 (5.76, 11.41) | **0.000** |
| UA, umol/L | 353 (280, 442) | 349 (276, 430) | 405 (301, 480) | **0.047** |
| Cys-C, mg/L | 1.30 (0.92, 2.08) | 1.2 (0.90, 1.73) | 3.11 (1.54, 4.22) | **0.000** |
| ALB, g/L | 37.90 (34.23, 41.10) | 38.10 (34.35, 41.15) | 36.10 (30.90, 40.30) | 0.056 |
| Proteinuria, n (%) | 178 (41.2%) | 142 (38.5%) | 36 (57.1%) | **0.005** |
| Hematuria, n (%) | 123 (28.5%) | 104 (28.2%) | 19 (30.2%) | 0.748 |

*The continuous variables that follow a normal distribution include age, and BMI which were expressed as mean ± SD. The continuous variables that do not follow a normal distribution were represented as median and IQR. The categorical variables were presented as numbers and percentages. Liver insufficiency was defined as a preoperative elevation of >80 U/L of aspartate aminotransferase (AST) or (and) alanine aminotransferase (ALT) in patients.*

*AKI, acute kidney injury; Scr, serum creatinine; SD, standard deviations; BMI, body mass index; CKD, chronic kidney disease; COPD, chronic obstructive pulmonary disease; NYHA, New York Heart Association; AST, aspartate aminotransferase; ALT, alanine aminotransferase; DHCA, Deep hypothermic circulatory arrest; CPB, cardiopulmonary bypass; ALB, albumin; BUN, blood urea nitrogen; UA, uric acid; Cys-C, cystatin C; CRRT, continuous renal replacement therapy. Bold values represented $P < 0.05$.*

**TABLE 3** | Interoperative factors, postoperative comorbidities, and outcomes of 432 patients.

| | ALL ($n$ = 432) | Non-CRRT ($n$ = 369) | CRRT ($n$ = 63) | $P$ value |
|---|---|---|---|---|
| **Interoperative factors** | | | | |
| Total aortic arch replacement n (%) | 319 (73.8%) | 270 (73.2%) | 49 (77.8%) | 0.442 |
| DHCA n (%) | 105 (24.3%) | 93 (25.2%) | 12 (19.0%) | 0.292 |
| CPB duration ≥180 min n (%) | 387 (89.6%) | 336 (91.1%) | 51 (81.0%) | **0.015** |
| RBC transfusion (units) | 3.0 (1.0, 4.5) | 3.0 (0.0, 4.0) | 3.5 (2.0, 5.5) | 0.150 |
| **Postoperative comorbidities, n (%)** | | | | |
| MAP within 2 h after surgery ≤65 mmHg | 94 (21.8%) | 67 (18.2%) | 27 (42.9%) | **0.000** |
| Second thoracotomy | 22 (5.1%) | 11 (3.0%) | 11 (17.5%) | **0.000** |
| AMI | 14 (3.2%) | 8 (2.2%) | 6 (9.5%) | **0.002** |
| CVA | 39 (9.0%) | 32 (8.7%) | 7 (11.1%) | 0.532 |
| Lung infection | 132 (30.6%) | 94 (25.5%) | 38 (60.3%) | **0.000** |
| Lactic acidosis | 104 (24.1%) | 79 (21.4%) | 25 (39.7%) | **0.002** |
| ARDS | 65 (15.0%) | 50 (13.6%) | 15 (23.8%) | **0.035** |
| Hepatic failure | 40 (9.3%) | 29 (7.9%) | 11 (17.5%) | **0.015** |
| AKI stage 2–3 | 207 (47.9%) | 146 (39.6%) | 61 (96.8%) | **0.000** |
| **Outcomes** | | | | |
| Duration of mechanical ventilation, days | 4 (2, 6) | 3 (2, 5) | 7 (5, 14) | **0.000** |
| Hospitalization costs, \$ | 30410.21 (24734.17, 39734.99) | 29635.79 (24052.40, 36689.51) | 41147.65 (33731.50, 49527.07) | **0.000** |
| 1-year re-admission n (%) | 53 (12.3%) | 46 (12.5%) | 7 (11.1%) | 0.762 |
| In-hospital mortality n (%) | 66 (15.3%) | 37 (10.0%) | 29 (46.0%) | **0.000** |

*The continuous variables and categorical variables were presented as mean ± SD, median and IQR, numbers and percentages, respectively. AKI, acute kidney injury; Scr, serum creatinine; SD, standard deviations; DHCA, deep hypothermic circulatory arrest; CPB, cardiopulmonary bypass; MAP, mean arterial pressure; AMI, acute myocardial infarction; CVA, acute cerebrovascular accident; ARDS, acute respiratory distress syndrome; CRRT, continuous renal replacement therapy. Bold values represented P < 0.05. \$Represents United States Dollar (USD).*

of fit of the logistic regression model, and $P > 0.05$ would indicate a good fit. Only those variables found to be statistically significant in the univariable analysis and with a variance inflation factor (VIF) < 10 in the linear regression analysis were used in logistic regression analysis.

Statistical significance was set at $P \leq 0.05$. Statistical analysis was performed by the SPSS software package, version 26.0 (IBM Corp., Chicago, IL, USA) and GraphPad Prism 8.0 software (GraphPad Software, Inc., San Diego, CA, USA).

## RESULTS

### Demographic and Clinical Characteristics

A total of 432 patients with AAAD were included in the final sample. The demographic and clinical characteristics and laboratory data of patients hospitalized with AAAD are summarized in **Table 2**.

The mean age of all patients included in the study was 48.19 ± 10.97 years. The median body mass index (BMI) was 24.85 ± 3.78 kg/m$^2$. There were 250 (57.9%) patients with hypertension and 92 (21.3%) with poor blood pressure control. A small number of patients had chronic kidney injury (CKD, 6.9%), chronic obstructive pulmonary disease (COPD, 6.5%), diabetes (4.6%), chronic liver disease (5.1%), and other comorbidities. The median of baseline SCr level was 82 (65, 104) μmol/L. The median of cystatin C (Cys-C) level was 1.30 (0.92, 2.08) mg/L. According to aortic computed tomography angiography (CTA) findings, 184 patients were diagnosed with renal artery involvement, 103 of which had coexisting renal malperfusion.

### Primary and Second Outcomes of Patients With AAAD

Among the recorded patients, 47.9% developed postoperative severe AKI (AKI stages 2–3). The total number of in-hospital mortality and requiring for CRRT was 66 (15.3%) and 63 (14.6%), respectively. In-hospital mortality in the CRRT group (46%) was 4.6 times higher than in the non-CRRT group (10%). Compared with the non-CRRT group, the CRRT group had a longer duration of mechanical ventilation and higher hospitalization costs. No statistical difference was observed in the 1-year readmission rate between the two groups ($P$ = 0.762) (**Table 3**).

### Risk Factors for Postoperative AKI With CRRT in Patients With AAAD

The multivariable analysis revealed baseline SCr [odds ratio (*OR*), 1.006; $P$ = 0.011], Cys-C (*OR*, 1.438; $P$ = 0.001), lung infection (*OR*, 2.292; $P$ = 0.017), second thoracotomy (*OR*, 5.185; $P$ = 0.004), diabetes mellitus (*OR*, 6.868; $P$ = 0.001), AKI stage 2–3 (*OR*, 22.901; $P$ = 0.000) were the independent risk factors for receiving CRRT (**Table 4**).

**TABLE 4** | A multivariable analysis of risk factors associated with continuous renal replacement therapy (CRRT).

| Variables | β | Odds ratio | 95% confidence interval | | P value |
|---|---|---|---|---|---|
| | | | Lower | Upper | |
| Baseline SCr | 0.006 | 1.006 | 1.001 | 1.011 | **0.011** |
| Cys-C | 0.364 | 1.438 | 1.167 | 1.774 | **0.001** |
| Lung infection | 0.829 | 2.292 | 1.157 | 4.539 | **0.017** |
| Second thoracotomy | 1.646 | 5.185 | 1.700 | 15.814 | **0.004** |
| Diabetes mellitus | 1.927 | 6.868 | 2.182 | 21.621 | **0.001** |
| AKI stage 2–3 | 3.131 | 22.901 | 5.220 | 100.466 | **0.000** |

*Age, gender, poor blood pressure control, diabetes mellitus, NYHA class III–IV, liver insufficiency, baseline SCr, Cys-C, BUN, UA, proteinuria, MAP within 2 h after surgery ≤ 65 mmHg, second thoracotomy, AMI, lung infection, lactic acidosis, ARDS, hepatic failure, AKI stage 2–3 were included to establish a stepwise forward binary logistic regression (Omnibus tests of model coefficients: $X^2$ = 137.693, P = 0.000; Hosmer–Lemeshow goodness-of-fit test: $X^2$ = 6.711, P = 0.568; −2 log likelihood = 221.224). In the linear regression analysis of these variables, the variance inflation factor (VIF) was <10. Therefore, there were no problems of multicollinearity among these independent variables. The odds ratio (OR) and 95% CI were measured through binary logistic regression. The OR of the continuous variable represented that for a single unit increase, the probability of a positive event will increase by approximately OR-1 times.*

*NYHA, New York Heart Association; PLT, platelet; ALB, albumin; SCr, serum creatinine; Cys-C, cystatin C; CPB, cardiopulmonary bypass; MAP, mean arterial pressure; AMI, acute myocardial infarction; ARDS, acute respiratory distress syndrome; AKI, acute kidney injury. Bold values represented P < 0.05.*

## Risk Factors for In-hospital Mortality in Patients With CRRT After Surgery for AAAD

In this study, 63 patients with CRRT were divided into the survivor (34/63, 54.0%) and non-survivor groups (29/63, 46.0%). The characteristics, perioperative factors, laboratory data, and outcomes of the patients with CRRT are shown in **Table 5**. In the non-survivors and survivors groups, there were statistically significant differences in the history of drinking (41.4 vs. 5.9%), preoperative NYHA class III-IV (75.9 vs. 11.8%), cardiopulmonary bypass (CPB) duration ≥ 180 min (93.1 vs. 70.6%), duration of mechanical ventilation (16.5 vs. 10 days), MAP ≤ 65 mmHg within 2 h postoperatively (62.1 vs. 26.5%), hepatic failure (34.5 vs. 2.9%), acute respiratory distress syndrome (ARDS) (37.9 vs. 11.8%), lactic acidosis (62.1 vs. 20.6%), and CVA (20.7 vs. 2.9%).

In **Table 6**, the multivariable analysis showed that the independent risk factors for in-hospital mortality in the patients with CRRT included preoperative NYHA class III-IV (*OR*, 10.272; *P* = 0.019), lactic acidosis (*OR*, 10.224; *P* = 0.019). The patients with two or more predisposing factors including the history of drinking, CPB duration ≥ 180 min, MAP ≤ 65 mmHg within 2 h postoperatively, ARDS, hepatic failure, and acute cerebrovascular accident (CVA), were high-risk patients for in-hospital death in CRRT (*OR*, 19.816; *P* = 0.002).

## DISCUSSION

This is the first study of independent risk factors for in-hospital mortality in patients with CRRT in a homogenous population of patients with AAAD.

In our study with 432 patients, the incidence of severe AKI (AKI stages 2–3), the overall in-hospital mortality, the proportion for requiring CRRT, and in-hospital mortality after CRRT, was 47.9, 15.3, 14.6, and 46.0%, respectively. Our findings revealed that diabetes, SCr, secondary thoracotomy, pulmonary infection, and severe AKI were the independent risk factors for CRRT. Preoperative severe heart failure, postoperative lactic acidosis, and a combination of any three or more risk factors were the independent risk factors for death in the patients with CRRT. The patients in the CRRT group had longer postoperative mechanical ventilation, higher hospitalization costs, and higher in-hospital mortality. This study supports evidence from the previous observations that 11–27% of patients undergoing surgery for aortic dissection required renal replacement therapy (RRT) (11–13) and the mortality for CRRT was between 40 and 70% (9, 14).

In this study, diabetes was found to be considered as an independent risk factor for CRRT that was consistent with the data published by The Japanese Society for Dialysis Therapy (JSDT), who found that diabetes has become the most common initial diagnosis for end-stage renal disease (ESRD) treated with dialysis (15). This is associated with hyperglycemia causing relative ischemia in the kidney, systemic endothelial cell dysfunction (16), podocyte injury (17), and sterile inflammation, leading to kidney injury and deterioration of kidney function (18).

Pulmonary infection was also an independent risk factor for CRRT. Sepsis (19), non-severe pneumonia (20), can give rise to the development and exacerbation of AKI and an increased risk of death due to the inflammatory response and organ crosstalk between lung and kidney (21).

Our findings were in accord with the recent studies indicating that the baseline SCr levels, second thoracotomy were considered as the independent risk factors for CRRT (11, 22, 23). Increased creatinine levels represent impaired kidney function (24). The second thoracotomy is performed when excessive bleeding occurs, which may cause hypovolemia (22). Perioperative hypotension or poor organ perfusion may lead to deterioration of renal function (25, 26).

Several reports have shown that serum cystatin C is a good indicator for identifying early renal impairment and predicting RRT requirements (27–30). Our study confirms that an elevated Cys-C is an independent risk factor for predicting the CRRT. Since serum cystatin C is not affected by diet, etiology of AKI, or urine output, it is a useful and highly diagnostic marker for AKI (27).

A severe and refractory AKI is an indication for CRRT, and early CRRT is recommended for patients with oliguria or fluid overload (31, 32). In our study, we found that AKI stage 2–3 was an independent risk factor for CRRT. CRRT can maintain water, electrolyte, acid-base balance, uremic solute homeostasis to prevent or delay the deterioration of renal function (32). The patients with AKI stage 2–3 had a 1-year survivability rate of 90% if the renal function was restored within 7 days (33, 34). It remains controversial as to the timing of initiation (35), dose, discontinuation (36), quality assessment indicators (37, 38) of RRT in patients with AKI. The clinicians must formulate and select individual treatment plans for their patients (39).

**TABLE 5** | Demographics, perioperative factors, and outcomes of 63 patients with CRRT.

| | ALL (*n* = 63) | Non-survivor (*n* = 29) | Survivor (*n* = 34) | *P* value |
|---|---|---|---|---|
| Age, year, mean ± SD | 51.10 ± 12.63 | 53.90 ± 12.48 | 48.71 ± 12.45 | 0.104 |
| Gender, n (%) | | | | 0.326 |
| Male | 56 (88.9%) | 27 (93.1%) | 29 (85.3%) | |
| Female | 7 (11.1%) | 2 (6.9%) | 5 (14.7%) | |
| BMI, kg/m$^2$, median (IQR) | 25.06 (22.49, 27.17) | 25.06 (22.49, 27.78) | 24.86 (22.91, 26.45) | 0.610 |
| Smoking, n (%) | 29 (46%) | 14 (48.3%) | 15 (44.1%) | 0.741 |
| Drinking | 14 (22.2%) | 12 (41.4%) | 2 (5.9%) | **0.001** |
| **Medical history, n (%)** | | | | |
| Hypertension | 41 (65.1%) | 19 (65.5%) | 22 (64.7%) | 0.946 |
| Poor blood pressure control | 20 (31.7%) | 11 (37.9%) | 9 (26.5%) | 0.330 |
| A left ventricular ejection fraction of <35% | 6 (9.5%) | 5 (17.2%) | 1 (2.9%) | 0.054 |
| Marfan syndrome | 4 (6.3%) | 1 (3.4%) | 3 (8.8%) | 0.383 |
| Previous cardiac surgery | 4 (6.3%) | 3 (10.3%) | 1 (2.9%) | 0.230 |
| Aortic regurgitation | 26 (41.3%) | 8 (27.6%) | 18 (52.9%) | **0.042** |
| CKD | 8 (12.7%) | 2 (6.9%) | 6 (17.6%) | 0.201 |
| COPD | 7 (11.1%) | 4 (13.8%) | 3 (8.8%) | 0.532 |
| Diabetes mellitus | 9 (14.3%) | 6 (20.7%) | 3 (8.8%) | 0.180 |
| Chronic liver disease | 4 (6.3%) | 2 (6.9%) | 2 (5.9%) | 0.869 |
| **Preoperative factors** | | | | |
| Hemorrhagic shock, n (%) | 3 (4.8%) | 1 (3.4%) | 2 (5.9%) | 1.000 |
| Pericardial tamponade, n (%) | 3 (4.8%) | 2 (6.9%) | 1 (2.9%) | 0.590 |
| NYHA class III-IV n (%) | 26 (41.3%) | 22 (75.9%) | 4 (11.8%) | **0.000** |
| Liver insufficiency, n (%) | 15 (23.8%) | 10 (34.5%) | 5 (14.7%) | 0.066 |
| **Renal artery involvement, n (%)** | 30 (42.7%) | 13 (44.8%) | 17 (50.0%) | 0.682 |
| Renal malperfusion, n (%) | 20 (31.7%) | 7 (24.1%) | 13 (38.2%) | 0.231 |
| No renal malperfusion, n (%) | 10 (15.9%) | 6 (20.7%) | 4 (11.8%) | 0.492 |
| **Lab data (mean ± SD) or median (IQR)** | | | | |
| Baseline Scr, μmol/L | 97 (83, 131) | 97 (86, 111) | 98 (72, 160) | 0.720 |
| BUN, mmol/L | 7.5 (5.76, 11.41) | 8.09 (5.92, 10.75) | 7.40 (5.58, 11.70) | 0.901 |
| UA, umol/L | 390.54 ± 129.90 | 380.25 ± 125.79 | 399.31 ± 134.55 | 0.566 |
| Cys-C, mg/L | 3.11 (1.54, 4.22) | 2.95 (1.87, 4.15) | 3.28 (1.09, 4.33) | 0.940 |
| ALB, g/L | 36.10 (30.90, 40.30) | 36.10 (30.70, 40.80) | 36.10 (30.67, 40.23) | 0.730 |
| Proteinuria, n (%) | 36 (57.1%) | 14 (48.3%) | 22 (64.7%) | 0.189 |
| Hematuria, n (%) | 19 (30.2%) | 9 (31.0%) | 10 (29.4%) | 0.889 |
| **Interoperative factors** | | | | |
| Total aortic arch replacement n (%) | 49 (77.8%) | 21 (72.4%) | 28 (82.4%) | 0.344 |
| DHCA n (%) | 12 (19.0%) | 6 (20.7%) | 6 (17.6%) | 0.759 |
| CPB duration ≥180 min n (%) | 51 (81.0%) | 27 (93.1%) | 24 (70.6%) | **0.023** |
| RBC transfusion (units) | 3.5 (3.0, 5.5) | 3.0 (1.8, 5.5) | 3.8 (2.0, 5.6) | 0.527 |
| **Postoperative comorbidities, n (%)** | | | | |
| MAP within 2 h after surgery ≤ 65 mmHg | 27 (42.9%) | 18 (62.1%) | 9 (26.5%) | **0.004** |
| Second thoracotomy | 11 (17.5%) | 5 (17.2%) | 6 (17.6%) | 0.966 |
| AMI | 6 (9.5%) | 4 (13.8%) | 2 (5.9%) | 0.286 |
| Lung infection | 38 (60.3%) | 21 (72.4%) | 17 (50.0%) | 0.070 |
| Hepatic failure | 11 (17.5%) | 10 (34.5%) | 1 (2.9%) | **0.001** |
| ARDS | 15 (23.8%) | 11 (37.9%) | 4 (11.8%) | **0.015** |
| Lactic acidosis | 25 (39.7%) | 18 (62.1%) | 7 (20.6%) | **0.001** |
| CVA | 7 (11.1%) | 6 (20.7%) | 1 (2.9%) | **0.042** |

*(Continued)*

**TABLE 5** | Continued

| | ALL (*n* = 63) | Non-survivor (*n* = 29) | Survivor (*n* = 34) | *P* value |
|---|---|---|---|---|
| **Outcomes** | | | | |
| Hospitalization costs, $ | 41276.87 ± 14961.75 | 42604.69 ± 15729.64 | 40144.32 ± 14414.22 | 0.520 |
| Duration of mechanical ventilation, days | 7 (5, 14) | 16.5 (9, 21) | 10 (6, 20) | **0.049** |

*The continuous variables that follow a normal distribution include age, uric acid (UA), hospitalization costs were expressed as mean ± SD. The continuous variables that do not follow a normal distribution were represented as median and IQR. The categorical variables were presented as numbers and percentages. Liver insufficiency was defined as a preoperative elevation of >80 U/L of AST or (and) ALT in the patients.*

*AKI, acute kidney injury; Scr, serum creatinine; SD, standard deviations; BMI, body mass index; CKD, chronic kidney disease; COPD, chronic obstructive pulmonary disease; NYHA, New York Heart Association; AST, aspartate aminotransferase; ALT, alanine aminotransferase; DHCA, Deep hypothermic circulatory arrest; CPB, cardiopulmonary bypass; ALB, albumin; BUN, blood urea nitrogen; UA, uric acid; Cys-C, cystatin C; CRRT, continuous renal replacement therapy; DHCA, Deep hypothermic circulatory arrest; CPB, cardiopulmonary bypass; MAP, mean arterial pressure; AMI, acute myocardial infarction; CVA, acute cerebrovascular accident; ARDS, acute respiratory distress syndrome. Bold values represented P < 0.05.*

*$ Represents United States Dollar (USD).*

**TABLE 6** | The multivariable analysis of risk factors associated with in-hospital mortality in the patients with CRRT.

| Variables | β | Odds ratio | 95% confidence interval | | *P* value |
|---|---|---|---|---|---|
| | | | Lower | Upper | |
| Lactic acidosis | 2.325 | 10.224 | 1.459 | 71.641 | **0.019** |
| NYHA class III-IV | 2.329 | 10.272 | 1.469 | 71.802 | **0.019** |
| Risk factors ≥ 2 including | 2.986 | 19.816 | 3.035 | 129.389 | **0.002** |
| Drinking | | | | | |
| CPB duration ≥180 min | | | | | |
| MAP within 2 h after surgery ≤65 mmHg | | | | | |
| Hepatic failure | | | | | |
| ARDS | | | | | |
| CVA | | | | | |

*Drinking history, NYHA class III–IV, CPB duration ≥180 min, duration of mechanical ventilation, MAP within 2 h after surgery ≤ 65 mmHg, CVA, lactic acidosis, ARDS, and hepatic failure were included to establish a stepwise forward binary logistic regression (Omnibus tests of model coefficients: $X^2$ = 48.417, P = 0.000; Hosmer–Lemeshow goodness-of-fit test: $X^2$ = 0.640, P = 0.726; −2 log likelihood = 38.522). In the linear regression analysis of these variables, VIF was <10. There were no problems of multicollinearity among these independent variables. The OR and 95% CI were measured through binary logistic regression.*

*NYHA, New York Heart Association; CPB, cardiopulmonary bypass; MAP, mean arterial pressure; ARDS, acute respiratory distress syndrome; CVA, acute cerebrovascular accident. Bold values represented P < 0.05.*

The results of the current study showed that in-hospital mortality in the CRRT group was 4.6 times higher than in the non-CRRT group. It was reported that close to 40% of the patients in the dialysis mortality population died from the causes, such as heart failure, stroke, and myocardial infarction and infection (15), drinking (40), CPB duration (41, 42), hypotension (43), CVA (44), hepatic failure, and ARDS (45). Our findings were coherent with those of the previous studies. The kidney may induce distant organ crosstalk, including lung, heart, liver, or intestine. The prognosis in complicated AKI is poor when distant organ injury occurs (46, 47). Therefore, to reduce dialysis mortality, it is important to treat the distal organ crosstalk caused by AKI rather than focusing on the renal impairment alone (48).

Previous studies had shown that renal malperfusion was an independent risk factor for AKI, 30-day mortality, and poor prognosis in patients with AAAD (5, 49, 50). In our study, there was no significant increase in the incidence of renal malperfusion and renal artery involvement before surgery in the CRRT group and the post-CRRT in-hospital mortality group relative to the other groups. It is probably because that renal malperfusion improved before surgery or because timely treatment after the occurrence of AKI prevented the progression of AKI and thus reduced the usage of CRRT and in-hospital mortality.

## Study Limitations

There were certain limitations to the present study: (i) data collected by different people over different periods may be affected by confounding factors, thereby affecting the conclusions; (ii) due to the lack of urine data, the creatinine level was used to define AKI; (iii) our study did not include long-term follow-up and did not clarify long-term outcomes, such as long-term mortality, whether the kidney function recovers after the CRRT or whether the condition progresses to chronic or end-stage renal disease after AAAD.

## CONCLUSIONS

In the patients with post-operative AAAD, CRRT was in high demand and in-hospital mortality remained high. Diabetes, baseline SCr, Cys-C, lung infection, second thoracotomy, and severe AKI were independent risk factors for CRRT. Severe cardiac failure and lactic acidosis were independent risk factors for in-hospital mortality in patients with CRRT. The risk factors for CRRT and in-hospital mortality in patients undergoing AAAD surgery were determined to help identify the high-risk patients and make appropriate clinical decisions. Further randomized-controlled studies are urgently needed to establish the risk factors for CRRT and in-hospital mortality.

## ETHICS STATEMENT

The studies involving human participants were reviewed and approved by Ethics Committees of the West China Hospital of Sichuan University. Written informed consent for participation was not required for this study in accordance with the national legislation and the institutional requirements.

## AUTHOR CONTRIBUTIONS

LY, XC, LJ, and JZ: research idea and study design. XC, LL, and TZ: data acquisition. XC, MF, JY, XW, and SW: statistical analysis. LY, JZ, and LJ: supervision or mentorship. All authors contributed to the article and approved the submitted version.

## ACKNOWLEDGMENTS

We thank the staff and participants from the West China Hospital of Sichuan University, Sichuan, China, for providing the clinical data for this research.

## REFERENCES

1. Bove T, Monaco F, Covello RD, Zangrillo A. Acute renal failure and cardiac surgery. *HSR Proc Intensive Care Cardiovasc Anesth.* (2009) 1:13–21.
2. Section 2: AKI definition. *Kidney Int Suppl (2011).* (2012) 2:19–36. doi: 10.1038/kisup.2011.32
3. Wang Y, Bellomo R. Cardiac surgery-associated acute kidney injury: risk factors, pathophysiology and treatment. *Nat Rev Nephrol.* (2017) 13:697–711. doi: 10.1038/nrneph.2017.119
4. Sansone F, Morgante A, Ceresa F, Salamone G, Patanè F. Prognostic implications of acute renal failure after surgery for type A acute aortic dissection. *Aorta (Stamford).* (2015) 3:91–7. doi: 10.12945/j.aorta.2015.14.022
5. Ko T, Higashitani M, Sato A, Uemura Y, Norimatsu T, Mahara K, et al. Impact of acute kidney injury on early to long-term outcomes in patients who underwent surgery for type A acute aortic dissection. *Am J Cardiol.* (2015) 116:463–8. doi: 10.1016/j.amjcard.2015.04.043
6. Hobson CE, Yavas S, Segal MS, Schold JD, Tribble CG, Layon AJ, et al. Acute kidney injury is associated with increased long-term mortality after cardiothoracic surgery. *Circulation.* (2009) 119:2444–53. doi: 10.1161/CIRCULATIONAHA.108.800011
7. Lenihan CR, Montez-Rath ME, Mora Mangano CT, Chertow GM, Winkelmayer WC. Trends in acute kidney injury, associated use of dialysis, and mortality after cardiac surgery, 1999 to 2008. *Ann Thorac Surg.* (2013) 95:20–8. doi: 10.1016/j.athoracsur.2012.05.131
8. Truche AS, Darmon M, Bailly S, Clec'h C, Dupuis C, Misset B, et al. Continuous renal replacement therapy versus intermittent hemodialysis in intensive care patients: impact on mortality and renal recovery. *Intensive Care Med.* (2016) 42:1408–17. doi: 10.1007/s00134-016-4404-6
9. Nadim MK, Forni LG, Bihorac A, Hobson C, Koyner JL, Shaw A, et al. Cardiac and vascular surgery-associated acute kidney injury: the 20th international consensus conference of the ADQI (Acute Disease Quality Initiative) group. *J Am Heart Assoc.* (2018) 7:e008834. doi: 10.1161/JAHA.118.008834
10. Palomba H, Castro I, Yu L, Burdmann EA. The duration of acute kidney injury after cardiac surgery increases the risk of long-term chronic kidney disease. *J Nephrol.* (2017) 30:567–72. doi: 10.1007/s40620-016-0351-0
11. Roh GU, Lee JW, Nam SB, Lee J, Choi JR, Shim YH. Incidence and risk factors of acute kidney injury after thoracic aortic surgery for acute dissection. *Ann Thorac Surg.* (2012) 94:766–71. doi: 10.1016/j.athoracsur.2012.04.057
12. Helgason D, Helgadottir S, Ahlsson A, Gunn J, Hjortdal V, Hansson EC, et al. Acute kidney injury after acute repair of type A aortic dissection. *Ann Thorac Surg.* (2021) 111:1292–8. doi: 10.1016/j.athoracsur.2020.07.019
13. Rice RD, Sandhu HK, Leake SS, Afifi RO, Azizzadeh A, Charlton-Ouw KM, et al. Is total arch replacement associated with worse outcomes during repair of acute type A aortic dissection? *Ann Thorac Surg.* (2015) 100:2159–65. doi: 10.1016/j.athoracsur.2015.06.007
14. Landoni G, Zangrillo A, Franco A, Aletti G, Roberti A, Calabrò MG, et al. Long-term outcome of patients who require renal replacement therapy after cardiac surgery. *Eur J Anaesthesiol.* (2006) 23:17–22. doi: 10.1017/S0265021505001705
15. Hanafusa N, Nakai S, Iseki K, Tsubakihara Y. Japanese society for dialysis therapy renal data registry-a window through which we can view the details of Japanese dialysis population. *Kidney Int Suppl. (2011).* (2015) 5:15–22. doi: 10.1038/kisup.2015.5
16. Goligorsky MS. Vascular endothelium in diabetes. *Am J Physiol Renal Physiol.* (2017) 312:F266–75. doi: 10.1152/ajprenal.00473.2016
17. Stieger N, Worthmann K, Teng B, Engeli S, Das AM, Haller H, et al. Impact of high glucose and transforming growth factor-β on bioenergetic profiles in podocytes. *Metabolism.* (2012) 61:1073–86. doi: 10.1016/j.metabol.2011.12.003
18. Anders HJ, Huber TB, Isermann B, Schiffer M. CKD in diabetes: diabetic kidney disease versus nondiabetic kidney disease. *Nat Rev Nephrol.* (2018) 14:361–77. doi: 10.1038/s41581-018-0001-y
19. Poston JT, Koyner JL. Sepsis associated acute kidney injury. *BMJ.* (2019) 364:k4891. doi: 10.1136/bmj.k4891
20. Murugan R, Karajala-Subramanyam V, Lee M, Yende S, Kong L, Carter M, et al. Acute kidney injury in non-severe pneumonia is associated with an increased immune response and lower survival. *Kidney Int.* (2010) 77:527–35. doi: 10.1038/ki.2009.502
21. Joannidis M, Forni LG, Klein SJ, Honore PM, Kashani K, Ostermann M, et al. Lung-kidney interactions in critically ill patients: consensus report of the Acute Disease Quality Initiative (ADQI) 21 Workgroup. *Intensive Care Med.* (2020) 46:654–72. doi: 10.1007/s00134-019-05869-7
22. Kowalik MM, Lango R, Klajbor K, Musiał-Swiatkiewicz V, Kołaczkowska M, Pawlaczyk R, et al. Incidence- and mortality-related risk factors of acute kidney injury requiring hemofiltration treatment in patients undergoing cardiac surgery: a single-center 6-year experience. *J Cardiothorac Vasc Anesth.* (2011) 25:619–24. doi: 10.1053/j.jvca.2010.12.011
23. Wu HB, Ma WG, Zhao HL, Zheng J, Li JR, Liu O, et al. Risk factors for continuous renal replacement therapy after surgical repair of type A aortic dissection. *J Thorac Dis.* (2017) 9:1126–32. doi: 10.21037/jtd.2017.03.128
24. Brown JR, Cochran RP, Dacey LJ, Ross CS, Kunzelman KS, Dunton RF, et al. Perioperative increases in serum creatinine are predictive of increased 90-day mortality after coronary artery bypass graft surgery. *Circulation.* (2006) 114(1 Suppl.):I409–13. doi: 10.1161/CIRCULATIONAHA.105.000596
25. Chien TM, Wen H, Huang JW, Hsieh CC, Chen HM, Chiu CC, et al. Significance of preoperative acute kidney injury in patients with acute type A aortic dissection. *J Formos Med Assoc.* (2019) 118:815–20. doi: 10.1016/j.jfma.2018.09.003
26. Smischney NJ, Shaw AD, Stapelfeldt WH, Boero IJ, Chen Q, Stevens M, et al. Postoperative hypotension in patients discharged to the intensive care unit after non-cardiac surgery is associated with adverse clinical outcomes. *Crit Care.* (2020) 24:682. doi: 10.1186/s13054-020-03412-5
27. Herget-Rosenthal S, Marggraf G, Hüsing J, Göring F, Pietruck F, Janssen O, et al. Early detection of acute renal failure by serum cystatin C. *Kidney Int.* (2004) 66:1115–22. doi: 10.1111/j.1523-1755.2004.00861.x
28. Royakkers AA, van Suijlen JD, Hofstra LS, Kuiper MA, Bouman CS, Spronk PE, et al. Serum cystatin C-A useful endogenous marker of renal function in intensive care unit patients at risk for or with acute renal failure? *Curr Med Chem.* (2007) 14:2314–7. doi: 10.2174/092986707781696555

29. Villa P, Jiménez M, Soriano MC, Manzanares J, Casasnovas P. Serum cystatin C concentration as a marker of acute renal dysfunction in critically ill patients. *Crit Care.* (2005) 9:R139–43. doi: 10.1186/cc3044
30. White C, Akbari A, Hussain N, Dinh L, Filler G, Lepage N, et al. Estimating glomerular filtration rate in kidney transplantation: a comparison between serum creatinine and cystatin C-based methods. *J Am Soc Nephrol.* (2005) 16:3763–70. doi: 10.1681/ASN.2005050512
31. Jentzer JC, Bihorac A, Brusca SB, Del Rio-Pertuz G, Kashani K, Kazory A, et al. Contemporary management of severe acute kidney injury and refractory cardiorenal syndrome: JACC council perspectives. *J Am Coll Cardiol.* (2020) 76:1084–101. doi: 10.1016/j.jacc.2020.06.070
32. Bagshaw SM, Wald R. Strategies for the optimal timing to start renal replacement therapy in critically ill patients with acute kidney injury. *Kidney Int.* (2017) 91:1022–32. doi: 10.1016/j.kint.2016.09.053
33. Ronco C, Bellomo R, Kellum JA. Acute kidney injury. *Lancet.* (2019) 394:1949–64. doi: 10.1016/S0140-6736(19)32563-2
34. Kellum JA, Sileanu FE, Bihorac A, Hoste EA, Chawla LS. Recovery after acute kidney injury. *Am J Respir Crit Care Med.* (2017) 195:784–91 doi: 10.1164/rccm.201604-0799OC
35. Clark E, Wald R, Levin A, Bouchard J, Adhikari NK, Hladunewich M, et al. Timing the initiation of renal replacement therapy for acute kidney injury in Canadian intensive care units: a multicentre observational study. *Can J Anaesth.* (2012) 59:861–70. doi: 10.1007/s12630-012-9750-4
36. Gibney N, Hoste E, Burdmann EA, Bunchman T, Kher V, Viswanathan R, et al. Timing of initiation and discontinuation of renal replacement therapy in AKI: unanswered key questions. *Clin J Am Soc Nephrol.* (2008) 3:876–80. doi: 10.2215/CJN.04871107
37. Rewa OG, Tolwani A, Mottes T, Juncos LA, Ronco C, Kashani K, et al. Quality of care and safety measures of acute renal replacement therapy: workgroup statements from the 22nd acute disease quality initiative (ADQI) consensus conference. *J Crit Care.* (2019) 54:52–7. doi: 10.1016/j.jcrc.2019.07.003
38. Schiffl H. Discontinuation of renal replacement therapy in critically ill patients with severe acute kidney injury: predictive factors of renal function recovery. *Int Urol Nephrol.* (2018) 50:1845–51. doi: 10.1007/s11255-018-1947-1
39. Forni LG, Chawla L, Ronco C. Precision and improving outcomes in acute kidney injury: personalizing the approach. *J Crit Care.* (2017) 37:244–5. doi: 10.1016/j.jcrc.2016.08.027
40. Gacouin A, Lesouhaitier M, Frerou A, Painvin B, Reizine F, Rafi S, et al. At-risk drinking is independently associated with acute kidney injury in critically ill patients. *Crit Care Med.* (2019) 47:1041–9. doi: 10.1097/CCM.0000000000003801
41. Suen WS, Mok CK, Chiu SW, Cheung KL, Lee WT, Cheung D, et al. Risk factors for development of acute renal failure (ARF) requiring dialysis in patients undergoing cardiac surgery. *Angiology.* (1998) 49:789–800. doi: 10.1177/000331979804900902
42. Axtell AL, Fiedler AG, Melnitchouk S, D'Alessandro DA, Villavicencio MA, Jassar AS, et al. Correlation of cardiopulmonary bypass duration with acute renal failure after cardiac surgery. *J Thorac Cardiovasc Surg.* (2019). doi: 10.1016/j.jtcvs.2019.01.072. [Epub ahead of print].
43. Shawwa K, Kompotiatis P, Jentzer JC, Wiley BM, Williams AW, Dillon JJ, et al. Hypotension within one-hour from starting CRRT is associated with in-hospital mortality. *J Crit Care.* (2019) 54:7–13. doi: 10.1016/j.jcrc.2019.07.004
44. Nadkarni GN, Patel AA, Konstantinidis I, Mahajan A, Agarwal SK, Kamat S, et al. Dialysis requiring acute kidney injury in acute cerebrovascular accident hospitalizations. *Stroke.* (2015) 46:3226–31. doi: 10.1161/STROKEAHA.115.010985
45. Mehta RL, Bouchard J, Soroko SB, Ikizler TA, Paganini EP, Chertow GM, et al. Sepsis as a cause and consequence of acute kidney injury: program to improve care in acute renal disease. *Intensive Care Med.* (2011) 37:241–8. doi: 10.1007/s00134-010-2089-9
46. Husain-Syed F, Rosner MH, Ronco C. Distant organ dysfunction in acute kidney injury. *Acta Physiol (Oxf).* (2020) 228:e13357. doi: 10.1111/apha.13357
47. Lee SA, Cozzi M, Bush EL, Rabb H. Distant organ dysfunction in acute kidney injury: a review. *Am J Kidney Dis.* (2018) 72:846–56. doi: 10.1053/j.ajkd.2018.03.028
48. Doi K, Rabb H. Impact of acute kidney injury on distant organ function: recent findings and potential therapeutic targets. *Kidney Int.* (2016) 89:555–64. doi: 10.1016/j.kint.2015.11.019
49. Englberger L, Suri RM, Li Z, Dearani JA, Park SJ, Sundt TM 3rd, et al. Validation of clinical scores predicting severe acute kidney injury after cardiac surgery. *Am J Kidney Dis.* (2010) 56:623–31. doi: 10.1053/j.ajkd.2010.04.017
50. Zindovic I, Gudbjartsson T, Ahlsson A, Fuglsang S, Gunn J, Hansson EC, et al. Malperfusion in acute type A aortic dissection: an update from the Nordic Consortium for Acute Type A Aortic Dissection. *J Thorac Cardiovasc Surg.* (2019) 157:1324–1333.e6. doi: 10.1016/j.jtcvs.2018.10.134

# 15

# Performance of Sequential Organ Failure Assessment and Simplified Acute Physiology Score II for Post-Cardiac Surgery Patients in Intensive Care Unit

*Fei Xu, Weina Li, Cheng Zhang and Rong Cao**

*Department of Anesthesiology, Chengdu Women's and Children's Central Hospital, Chengdu, China*

***Correspondence:**
Rong Cao
caorong68@163.com*

**Background:** The aim of this study is to assess the performance of Sequential Organ Failure Assessment (SOFA) score and Simplified Acute Physiology Score (SAPS II) on outcomes of patients with cardiac surgery and identify the cutoff values to provide a reference for early intervention.

**Methods:** All data were extracted from MIMIC-III (Medical Information Mart for Intensive Care-III) database. Cutoff values were calculated by the receiver-operating characteristic curve and Youden indexes. Patients were grouped, respectively, according to the cutoff values of SOFA and SAPS II. A non-adjusted model and adjusted model were established to evaluate the prediction of risk. Comparison of clinical efficacy between two scoring systems was made by decision curve analysis (DCA). The primary outcomes of this study were in-hospital mortality, 28-day mortality, 90-day mortality, and 1-year mortality after cardiac surgery. The secondary outcomes included length of hospital stay and intensive care unit (ICU) stay and the incidence of acute kidney injury (AKI) within 7 days after ICU admission.

**Results:** A total of 6,122 patients were collected and divided into the H-SOFA group (SOFA $\geq 7$) and L-SOFA group (SOFA $< 7$) or H-SAPS II group (SAPS II $\geq 43$) and L-SAPS II group (SAPS II $< 43$). In-hospital mortality, 28-day mortality, 90-day mortality, and 1-year mortality were higher, the length of hospital and ICU stay were longer in the H-SOFA group than in the L-SOFA group ($p < 0.05$), while the incidence of AKI was not significantly different. In-hospital mortality, 28-day mortality, 90-day mortality, 1-year mortality, and the incidence of AKI were all significantly higher in the H-SAPS II group than in the L-SAPS II group ($p < 0.05$). Hospital stay and ICU stay were longer in the H-SAPS II group than in the L-SAPS II group ($p < 0.05$). According to DCA, the SAPS II scoring system had more net benefits on assessing the long-term mortality compared with the SOFA scoring system.

**Conclusion:** Exceeding the cutoff values of SOFA and SAPS II scores could lead to increased mortality and extended length of ICU and hospital stay. The SAPS II scoring system had a better discriminative performance of 90-day mortality and 1-year mortality in post-cardiac surgery patients than the SOFA scoring system. Emphasizing the critical value of the scoring system is of significance for timely treatment.

**Keywords: post-cardiac surgery, SOFA, SAPS II, clinic outcome, intensive care unit**

## INTRODUCTION

Prognosis is a common challenge for patients after cardiac surgery. Although some progress has been achieved in the application of cardiac surgery procedures, the mortality rates after surgery remain high. Some scoring systems played an important role in the successful prediction of cardiac surgery-related mortality (1, 2). There was a preoperative risk stratification model, which had been widely accepted for mortality prediction of in-hospital mortality after cardiac surgery (3).

However, the scoring system focused on preoperative indicators without attention to intraoperative or postoperative conditions (4). The severity of surgical stress and inflammatory response to cardiopulmonary surgery could not be ignored (5) in cases that were associated with organ dysfunction and acute physiological changes. Previous studies reported that hyperlactatemia, bicarbonate, heart rate, and creatinine were essential for post-cardiac surgery patients as mortality-predictive variables (6–8). Recent studies had confirmed that the neutrophil/lymphocyte ratio of post 24 h after intensive care unit (ICU) admission is associated with postoperative mortality of cardiac surgery (9). Parameters and physiological indexes of post 24 h after ICU admission may provide a new way to improve prognosis early.

The Sequential Organ Failure Assessment (SOFA) score and Simplified Acute Physiology Score (SAPA II) were composed of organ function and biochemical indexes, which showed excellent predictive performance on many diseases in ICU (10, 11). There were few pieces of small sample literature that explored the role of SAPS II and SOFA scoring systems in predicting poor prognosis after cardiac surgery (12). The purpose of this study was to determine the critical values of the SAPS II and SOFA scoring system and to evaluate their performance in predicting the prognosis of patients undergoing cardiac surgery.

## MATERIALS AND METHODS

### Sources of Data

All data in this study were retrospectively extracted from MIMIC-III (Medical Information Mart for Intensive Care-III) database (13, 14). This is a freely open database for the public, which includes more than 40,000 critically ill patients from Beth Israel Deaconess Medical Center (Boston, Massachusetts, United States) between 2001 and 2012. The application of the database was approved by the institutional review committee of Beth Israel Deaconess Medical Center and Beth Israel Deacons Medical Center (Approval Code 10323541). Patient-related information in the database was anonymous, and personal informed consent was abandoned in this study.

### Data Collection and Definitions

The structure query language (SQL) with code in MIMIC Code Repository (https://github.com/MIT-LCP/Mimic-Website) was used for extracting data. The whole variables involved basic characteristics (age, gender, body mass index), comorbidities (drug abuse, alcohol abuse, coagulopathy, liver disease, hypertension, hypothyroidism, congestive heart failure, diabetes, chronic lung disease, chronic kidney disease), laboratory tests (sodium, potassium, white blood cell counts, hemoglobin, platelet, lactate, creatinine, blood urea nitrogen, prothrombin time, international normalized ratio, glucose), and vital signs (heart rate, respiratory rate, body temperature, pulse oxygen saturation, diastolic pressure, systolic pressure, and mean arterial pressure). The SOFA score and SAPS II score were evaluated within the first 24 h after ICU admission. Variables were reported as the average value within 24 h admitted to ICU.

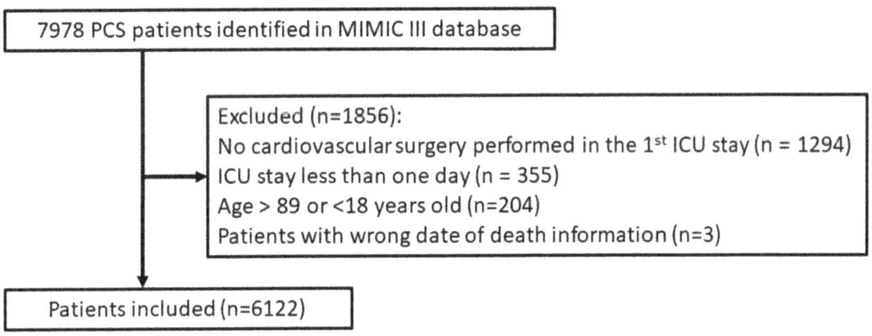


**FIGURE 1** | Flowchart of study cohort selection.

**TABLE 1** | Baseline clinical characteristics between survivors and non-survivors at 1 year.

| Characteristics | Overall ($n = 6,122$) | Survivors ($n = 4,516$) | Non-survivors ($n = 1,606$) | $p$ |
|---|---|---|---|---|
| Age, median (IQR) | 66 (55, 76) | 65.0 (54.0, 74.0) | 69.0 (58.0, 79.0) | <0.001 |
| Male gender, $n$ (%) | 3,704 (60.503) | 2,790 (61.780) | 914 (56.912) | <0.001 |
| BMI, median (IQR) | 27.84 (24.39, 31.84) | 28.04 (24.67, 32.04) | 27.06 (23.55, 31.24) | <0.001 |
| **Comorbidities** | | | | |
| Drug abuse, $n$ (%) | 208 (3.398) | 156 (3.454) | 52 (3.238) | 0.681 |
| Alcohol abuse, $n$ (%) | 474 (7.743) | 331 (7.329) | 143 (8.904) | 0.043 |
| Coagulopathy, $n$ (%) | 1,153 (18.834) | 661 (14.637) | 492 (30.635) | <0.001 |
| Congestive heart failure, $n$ (%) | 816 (13.329) | 384 (8.503) | 432 (26.899) | <0.001 |
| Liver disease, $n$ (%) | 463 (7.563) | 250 (5.536) | 213 (13.263) | <0.001 |
| Renal failure, $n$ (%) | 869 (14.195) | 526 (11.647) | 343 (21.357) | <0.001 |
| hypothyroidism, $n$ (%) | 617 (10.078) | 460 (10.186) | 157 (9.776) | 0.639 |
| Diabetes, $n$ (%) | 1,448 (23.652) | 1,080 (23.915) | 368 (22.914) | 0.418 |
| Chronic pulmonary, $n$ (%) | 1,179 (19.258) | 818 (18.113) | 361 (22.478) | <0.001 |
| hypertension, $n$ (%) | 758 (12.382) | 481 (10.651) | 277 (17.248) | <0.001 |
| **Laboratory test** | | | | |
| WBC mean, median (IQR) | 11.93 (8.9, 15.55) | 11.85 (9.13, 15.2) | 12.3 (8.1, 16.74) | 0.347 |
| BUN mean, median (IQR) | 18.33 (13.0, 29.4) | 16.5 (12.5, 23.5) | 28.5 (18.0, 47.5) | <0.001 |
| Sodium mean, median (IQR) | 138.0 (136.0, 140.2) | 138.0 (136.2, 140.0) | 138.4 (135.33, 141.5) | 0.002 |
| PT mean, median (IQR) | 14.65 (13.6, 16.2) | 14.47 (13.5, 15.7) | 15.6 (13.95, 18.6) | <0.001 |
| INR mean, median (IQR) | 1.3 (1.2, 1.5) | 1.3 (1.2, 1.4) | 1.43 (1.2, 1.8) | <0.001 |
| Potassium mean, median (IQR) | 4.19 (3.87, 4.5) | 4.2 (3.9, 4.49) | 4.15 (3.8, 4.6) | 0.095 |
| Platelet mean, median (IQR) | 175.33 (130.33, 233.33) | 176.33 (136.0, 228.5) | 172.0 (109.67, 253.5) | 0.007 |
| Lactate mean, median (IQR) | 1.93 (1.4, 2.7) | 1.9 (1.4, 2.6) | 2.0 (1.4, 3.1) | <0.001 |
| Hemoglobin mean, median (IQR) | 10.15 (9.15, 11.4) | 10.2 (9.18, 11.4) | 10.0 (9.05, 11.3) | 0.001 |
| Glucose mean, median (IQR) | 130.57 (116.0, 150.89) | 129.67 (116.43, 146.5) | 135.25 (114.4, 166.86) | <0.001 |
| Creatinine mean, median (IQR) | 0.95 (0.72, 1.37) | 0.9 (0.7, 1.18) | 1.27 (0.83, 2.24) | <0.001 |
| PH mean, median (IQR) | 7.38 (7.34, 7.41) | 7.38 (7.34, 7.41) | 7.37 (7.31, 7.42) | <0.001 |
| **Vital sign** | | | | |
| $SpO_2$ mean, median (IQR) | 97.77 (96.52, 98.81) | 97.86 (96.72, 98.86) | 97.47 (95.88, 98.7) | <0.001 |
| BT mean, median (IQR) | 36.81 (36.43, 37.24) | 36.85 (36.47, 37.25) | 36.74 (36.32, 37.21) | <0.001 |
| Resp rate mean, median (IQR) | 18.12 (16.08, 21.17) | 17.7 (15.86, 20.25) | 20.0 (17.19, 23.69) | <0.001 |
| Mean bp mean, median (IQR) | 75.11 (70.17, 81.36) | 75.44 (70.79, 81.27) | 74.02 (68.07, 81.73) | <0.001 |
| Dias bp mean, median (IQR) | 58.39 (53.15, 64.3) | 58.64 (53.77, 64.37) | 57.51 (51.26, 64.07) | <0.001 |
| Sys bp mean, median (IQR) | 112.86 (105.52, 122.26) | 113.35 (106.45, 122.03) | 111.22 (102.62, 123.08) | <0.001 |
| Heartrate mean, median (IQR) | 85.83 (77.53, 96.52) | 84.77 (77.35, 94.74) | 88.91 (78.05, 101.72) | <0.001 |
| **Score system** | | | | |
| SPAS II, median (IQR) | 38 (30, 48) | 35.0 (28.0, 44.0) | 48.0 (38.0, 57.0) | <0.001 |
| SOFA, median (IQR) | 5 (3, 8) | 5.0 (3.0, 7.0) | 7.0 (4.0, 10.0) | <0.001 |
| AKI 7-day, (%) | 4,563 (74.534) | 3,268 (72.365) | 1,295 (80.635) | <0.001 |
| Hospital stay $\geq$ 14 days, $n$ (%) | 2,092 (34.172) | 1,359 (30.093) | 733 (45.641) | <0.001 |
| ICU stay $\geq$ 3 days, $n$ (%) | 3,422 (55.897) | 2,265 (50.155) | 1,157 (72.042) | <0.001 |
| Survival time, median (IQR) | 11.15 (6.26, 27.17) | 9.89 (6.08, 19.68) | 22.2 (8.08, 78.7) | <0.001 |

*BMI, body mass index; WBC, white blood cell count; BUN, Blood urea nitrogen; PT, prothrombin time; INR, international normalized ratio; SOFA, sequential organ failure assessment; SPASII, simplified acute physiology score; AKI, acute kidney injury; ICU, the intensive care unit; $SpO_2$, pulse oxygen saturation; PH, potential of hydrogen; BT, body temperature; Data are represented as median (interquartile range) or n (%).*

Patients with cardiac surgery whose diagnose code ranged from 33,010 to 37,799 were identified using current procedural terminology. Inclusion criteria were patients aged between 18 and 89 years, choosing the first hospitalization for analysis when admitted to hospital or ICU multiple times. Patients hospitalized in ICU <24 h were excluded. The primary outcomes were in-hospital mortality, 28-day mortality, 90-day mortality, and 1-year mortality after cardiac surgery. The secondary outcomes were the length of hospital stay, ICU stay, and the incidence of acute kidney injury (AKI) within 7 days after ICU admission.

The diagnosis of AKI referenced the improving global outcomes guideline (15).

## Statistical Methods

Continuous variables of the study were non-normally distributed and reported as medians along with interquartile ranges (IQRs). Categorical variables were presented as numbers and percentages. Comparison of different groups was made using Kruskal–Wallis test or Mann–Whitney U-test for continuous variables, whereas chi-square or Fisher's exact tests were used for categorical variables. Non-adjusted models and adjusted models were established to investigate the association between scoring systems and outcomes in this study.

The cutoff values of SOFA and SAPS II scoring systems were obtained across receiver-operating characteristic (ROC) curve and Youden Indexes calculation. Based on different cutoff values, patients were divided into two groups. The clinical efficacy of scoring system models for poor outcomes was assessed by decision curve analysis (DCA), which was considered an appropriate method for estimating prognostic strategies (16). Kaplan–Meier curve was used to describe the difference in 1-year survival between different groups of the scoring system.

The SPSS software version 24.0 (IBM Corporation, Armonk, NY, United States) and the R software (version 4.0.3) were used for data processing, statistical analysis, and illustrations. Data missing 30% were removed and data missing <30% were processed by multiple imputations. Statistical differences were set at $p < 0.05$.

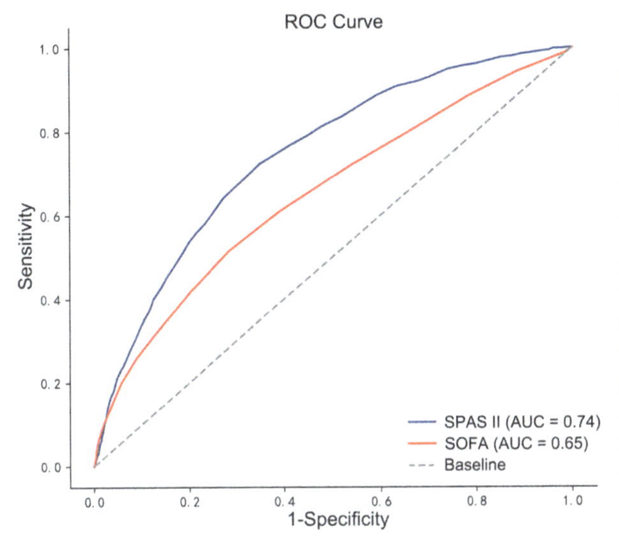


**FIGURE 2** | The ROC curves for SOFA score and SAPS II score with 1-year postoperative mortality. ROC, receiver-operating characteristic.

# RESULTS

## Clinical Characteristics

A total of 6,122 patients admitted to ICU after cardiac surgery were enrolled retrospectively. The procedures and standards for data selection are shown in **Figure 1**. The clinical basic characteristics of the populations are shown in **Table 1**.

The AUC of SOFA and SAPS II scoring systems with 1-year postoperation mortality was 0.649 ($p < 0.001$) and 0.724 ($p < 0.001$), respectively (**Figure 2**). The cutoff value of the SOFA scoring system was 7, whereas the critical value of the SAPS II scoring system was 43. In the SOFA scoring system, the patients were divided into high SOFA group (H-SOFA group, SOFA $\geq 7$, $N = 2{,}114$) and low SOFA group (L-SOFA group, SOFA $< 7$, $N =$

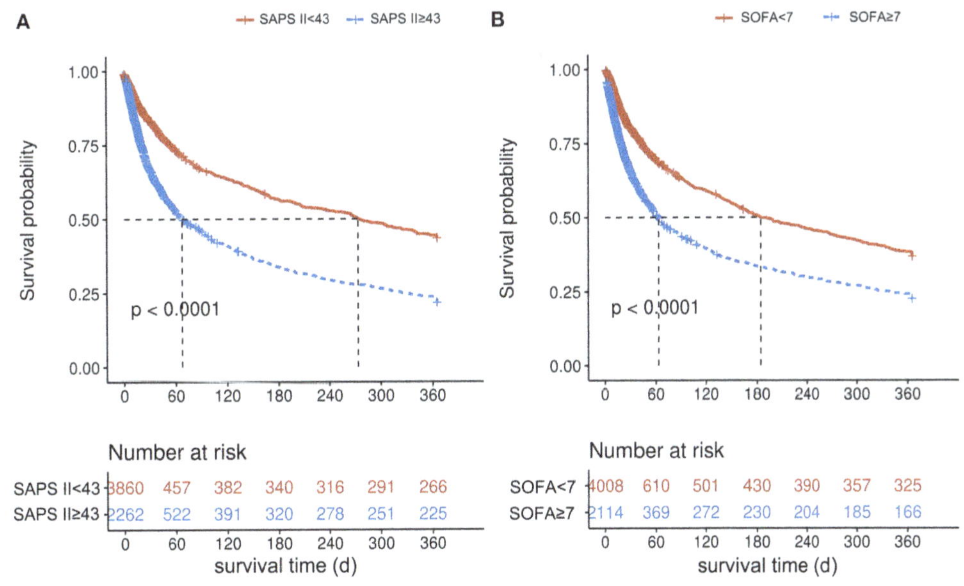


**FIGURE 3** | Kaplan–Meier curves of 1-year mortality by scoring system groups. **(A)** For the SAPS II score, while **(B)** is for the SOFA score.

**TABLE 2** | Basic characteristics of SOFA scoring system.

| Characteristics | Overall ($n$ = 6,122) | SOFA < 7 ($n$ = 4,008) | SOFA≥7 ($n$ = 2,114) | $p$ |
|---|---|---|---|---|
| SOFA, median (IQR) | 5 (3, 8) | 4.0 (2.0, 5.0) | 9.0 (8.0, 11.0) | <0.001 |
| Age, median (IQR) | 66 (55, 76) | 66.0 (55.0, 76.0) | 66.0 (55.0, 76.0) | 0.793 |
| Male gender, $n$ (%) | 3,704 (60.503) | 2,385 (59.506) | 1,319 (62.394) | 0.028 |
| BMI, median (IQR) | 27.84 (24.39, 31.84) | 27.62 (24.22, 31.59) | 28.25 (24.69, 32.28) | <0.001 |
| **Comorbidities** | | | | |
| Drug abuse, $n$ (%) | 208 (3.398) | 126 (3.144) | 82 (3.879) | 0.131 |
| Alcohol abuse, $n$ (%) | 474 (7.743) | 253 (6.312) | 221 (10.454) | <0.001 |
| coagulopathy, $n$ (%) | 1,153 (18.834) | 464 (11.577) | 689 (32.592) | <0.001 |
| Liver disease, $n$ (%) | 463 (7.563) | 193 (4.815) | 270 (12.772) | <0.001 |
| Renal failure, $n$ (%) | 869 (14.195) | 405 (10.105) | 464 (21.949) | <0.001 |
| hypothyroidism, $n$ (%) | 617 (10.078) | 417 (10.404) | 200 (9.461) | 0.244 |
| diabetes, $n$ (%) | 1,448 (23.652) | 934 (23.303) | 514 (24.314) | 0.376 |
| Chronic pulmonary, $n$ (%) | 1,179 (19.258) | 775 (19.336) | 404 (19.111) | 0.831 |
| hypertension, $n$ (%) | 758 (12.382) | 373 (9.306) | 385 (18.212) | <0.001 |
| Congestive heart failure, $n$ (%) | 816 (13.329) | 449 (11.203) | 367 (17.360) | <0.001 |
| **Laboratory test** | | | | |
| WBC mean, median (IQR) | 11.93 (8.9, 15.55) | 11.8 (9.1, 14.9) | 12.23 (8.4, 16.93) | 0.028 |
| BUN mean, median (IQR) | 18.33 (13.0, 29.4) | 16.0 (12.0, 23.0) | 25.5 (16.0, 44.0) | <0.001 |
| Sodium mean, median (IQR) | 138.0 (136.0, 140.2) | 138.0 (136.0, 140.0) | 138.0 (135.8, 140.5) | 0.855 |
| PT mean, median (IQR) | 14.65 (13.6, 16.2) | 14.35 (13.4, 15.55) | 15.45 (14.1, 17.93) | <0.001 |
| INR mean, median (IQR) | 1.3 (1.2, 1.5) | 1.27 (1.17, 1.4) | 1.4 (1.25, 1.7) | <0.001 |
| Potassium mean, median (IQR) | 4.19 (3.87, 4.5) | 4.15 (3.85, 4.45) | 4.26 (3.9, 4.64) | <0.001 |
| Platelet mean, median (IQR) | 175.33 (130.33, 233.33) | 188.67 (147.0, 245.5) | 144.5 (100.5, 203.0) | <0.001 |
| Lactate mean, median (IQR) | 1.93 (1.4, 2.7) | 1.8 (1.36, 2.43) | 2.27 (1.6, 3.33) | <0.001 |
| Hemoglobin mean, median (IQR) | 10.15 (9.15, 11.4) | 10.25 (9.23, 11.5) | 9.95 (9.0, 11.1) | <0.001 |
| PH mean, median (IQR) | 7.38 (7.34, 7.41) | 7.39 (7.35, 7.42) | 7.35 (7.31, 7.4) | <0.001 |
| Glucose mean, median (IQR) | 130.57 (116.0, 150.89) | 128.86 (115.67, 146.17) | 134.57 (116.83, 158.67) | <0.001 |
| Creatinine mean, median (IQR) | 0.95 (0.72, 1.37) | 0.85 (0.7, 1.1) | 1.27 (0.88, 2.37) | <0.001 |
| **Vital sign** | | | | |
| $SpO_2$ mean, median (IQR) | 97.77 (96.52, 98.81) | 97.88 (96.72, 98.92) | 97.54 (96.18, 98.62) | <0.001 |
| BT mean, median (IQR) | 36.81 (36.43, 37.24) | 36.82 (36.44, 37.21) | 36.81 (36.4, 37.3) | 0.975 |
| Resp rate mean, median (IQR) | 18.12 (16.08, 21.17) | 17.71 (15.85, 20.36) | 19.21 (16.68, 22.73) | <0.001 |
| Mean bp mean, median (IQR) | 75.11 (70.17, 81.36) | 76.04 (71.1, 82.55) | 73.55 (68.4, 78.7) | <0.001 |
| Dias bp mean, median (IQR) | 58.39 (53.15, 64.3) | 59.07 (53.88, 65.26) | 56.97 (51.87, 62.63) | <0.001 |
| Sys bp mean, median (IQR) | 112.86 (105.52, 122.26) | 114.87 (107.21, 124.73) | 109.52 (102.82, 118.0) | <0.001 |
| Heartrate mean, median (IQR) | 85.83 (77.53, 96.52) | 84.6 (76.96, 94.64) | 88.25 (79.15, 100.26) | <0.001 |
| **Primary outcome** | | | | |
| Death in hospital, $n$ (%) | 925 (15.109) | 396 (9.880) | 529 (25.024) | <0.001 |
| Death 28-day, $n$ (%) | 1,114 (18.197) | 484 (12.076) | 630 (29.801) | <0.001 |
| Death 90-day, $n$ (%) | 1,301 (21.251) | 585 (14.596) | 716 (33.869) | <0.001 |
| Death 1-year, $n$ (%) | 1,606 (26.233) | 779 (19.436) | 827 (39.120) | <0.001 |
| **Second outcome** | | | | |
| AKI 7-day, $n$ (%) | 4,563 (74.534) | 2,726 (68.014) | 1,837 (86.897) | <0.001 |
| Hospital stay ≥ 14 days, $n$ (%) | 2,092 (34.172) | 1,171 (29.217) | 921 (43.567) | <0.001 |
| ICU stay ≥ 3 days, $n$ (%) | 3,422 (55.897) | 1,935 (48.278) | 1,487 (70.341) | <0.001 |
| Survival time, median (IQR) | 11.15 (6.26, 27.17) | 10.04 (5.95, 23.28) | 14.47 (7.45, 34.13) | <0.001 |

*BMI, body mass index; WBC, white blood cell count; BUN, Blood urea nitrogen; PT, prothrombin time; INR, international normalized ratio; SOFA, sequential organ failure assessment; SPASII, simplified acute physiology score; AKI, acute kidney injury; ICU, the intensive care unit; SPO2, pulse oxygen saturation; PH, potential of hydrogen; BT, body temperature; Data are represented as median (interquartile range) or n (%).*

**TABLE 3** | The logistics regression of SOFA scoring system.

| Outcomes | Non-adjusted model | | | Adjusted model | | |
|---|---|---|---|---|---|---|
| | OR | 95% CL | p | OR | 95% CL | p |
| In-hospital death | 3.044 | 2.64, 3.514 | <0.001 | 2.86 | 2.471, 3.312 | <0.001 |
| 28-day mortality | 3.091 | 2.707, 3.532 | <0.001 | 2.897 | 2.528, 3.323 | <0.001 |
| 90-day mortality | 2.997 | 2.643, 3.399 | <0.001 | 2.817 | 2.475, 3.208 | <0.001 |
| One-year mortality | 2.664 | 2.369, 2,995 | <0.001 | 2.479 | 2.195, 2.8 | <0.001 |
| AKI 7-day | 1.392 | 1.229, 1.578 | <0.001 | 1.122 | 0.981, 1.285 | 0.095 |
| Hospital stay ≥ 14 days day | 1.87 | 1.676, 2.087 | <0.001 | 1.744 | 1.557, 1.954 | <0.001 |
| ICU stay ≥ 3 days | 2.541 | 2.272, 2.843 | <0.001 | 2.444 | 2.18, 2.743 | <0.001 |

*SOFA, sequential organ failure assessment; OR, odds ratio; CI, 95% confidence interval; AKI, acute kidney injury; ICU, intensive care unit; Adjusted for the confounders: resp rate mean, dias BP mean, sys BP mean, heart rate mean, bun mean, INR mean, potassium mean, lactate mean, hemoglobin mean, glucose mean, pH mean, $SpO_2$ mean, BMI, age, renal failure, liver disease, hypertension, alcohol abuse, coagulopathy, congestive heart failure, gender.*

4,008). In the SAPS II scoring system, patients were divided into the high SAPS II group (H-SAPS II group, SAPS II ≥ 43, $N$ = 2,262) and low SAPS II group (L-SAPS II group, SAPS II < 43, $N$ = 3,860). Kaplan–Meier survival curves of scoring system groups were statistically different (log-rank $p < 0.001$, **Figure 3**).

## Correlation Between SOFA Scoring System and Postoperative Outcomes

General comparative data of population are reported in **Table 2** and further explored in **Table 3**. Both short-term and long-term mortality rates were statistically significant in the comparison between SOFA scoring system groups. In-hospital mortality [odds ratio (OR) 2.86, 95% confidence interval (CI) 2.471, 3.312; $p < 0.001$], 28-day mortality (OR 2.897, 95% CI 2.528,3.323; $p < 0.001$), 90-day mortality (OR 2.817, 95% CI 2.475,3.208; $p < 0.001$), 1-year mortality (OR 2.479, 95% CI 2.195, 2.8; $p < 0.001$) all increased in the H-SOFA group compared with the L-SOFA group. In addition, length of in-hospital stay (OR 1.744, 95% CI 1.557, 1.954; $p < 0.001$) and ICU stay (OR 2.444, 95% CI 2.18, 2.743; $p < 0.001$) was extended in the H-SOFA group. However, there were no significant relationships in the incidence of acute renal failure (AKI) within 7 days after ICU admission ($p < 0.05$) between the two groups.

## Correlation Between SAPS II Scoring System and Postoperative Outcomes

The basic general data are summarized in **Table 4** and deeply analyzed in **Table 5**. There were statistical differences between the groups of the SAPS II scoring system. The increased in-hospital mortality (OR 3.544, 95% CI 3.02, 4.164; $p < 0.001$), 28-day mortality (OR 3.92, 95% CI 3.376, 4.558; $p < 0.001$), 90-day mortality (OR 4.069, 95% CI 3.533, 4.693; $p < 0.001$) and 1-year mortality (OR 4.272, 95% CI 3.744, 4.879; $p < 0.001$) were obvious in the H-SAPS II group. The length of in-hospital stay (OR 2.912, 95% CI 2.581, 3.287; $p < 0.001$) and ICU stay (OR 2.997, 95% CI 2.651, 3.392; $p < 0.001$) was longer in the H-SAPS II group than the L-SAPS II group. The incidence of AKI within 7 days admitted to ICU was statistically significant (OR 1.464, 95% CI 1.258, 1.706; $p < 0.001$) in comparison.

## Comparison of Decision Curves

As exhibited in **Figure 4**, the DCA curve of the SAPS II scoring system was higher than that of the SOFA scoring system in predicting 1-year mortality and 90-day mortality. Otherwise, the net benefit was not different between the two scoring systems in in-hospital mortality and 28-day mortality. This suggests that the SAPS-II scoring system is more meaningful than SOFA in assessing long-term mortality.

# DISCUSSION

This retrospective study demonstrated that a score of 7 in the SOFA scoring system and a score of 43 in the SAPS II scoring system with the first 24 h after ICU admission were warning values for predicting the risk of outcomes. Exceeding the warning values of the SOFA score and SAPS II score was associated with elevated mortality, prolonged ICU interval, and hospital interval. Besides, the incidence of AKI was increased in the SAPS II scoring system but not in the SOFA scoring system.

After cardiac surgery, patients have the risk of organ dysfunction or even deterioration, which predicted a poorer prognosis. The aim of the SOFA score was to objectively and quantitatively evaluate the severity of six organ systems dysfunction over time. It consisted of respiratory, circulatory, renal, hematology, hepatic, and central nervous systems, which are related to the recovery of patients with cardiac surgery (17). Although its main role is to predict organ dysfunction, the association between quantification of SOFA score and survival was inevitable (18). A previous systematic review showed that the SOFA model based on 24 h after ICU admission could be used to predict mortality (19). Other types of patients were also effectively evaluated by SOFA score, including post-cardiac arrest syndrome (20), people requiring extracorporeal cardiopulmonary resuscitation (21), critically ill cirrhotic patients with acute decompensation (22), patients with acute respiratory failure in intensive care unit (23), contemporary cardiac intensive care unit population (24), critically ill elderly patients with acute infective endocarditis (25), extracorporeal membrane oxygenation (ECMO)-treated acute myocardial infarction (AMI) patients (26)—some of above

**TABLE 4** | Basic characteristics of SAPS II scoring system.

| Characteristics | Overall ($n$ = 6,122) | SPAS II < 43 ($n$ = 3,860) | SPAS II ≥ 43 ($n$ = 2,262) | $p$ |
|---|---|---|---|---|
| SPASII, median (IQR) | 38 (30, 48) | 32.0 (27.0, 37.0) | 52.0 (47.0, 60.0) | <0.001 |
| Age, median (IQR) | 66 (55, 76) | 63.0 (53.0, 73.0) | 71.0 (61.0, 79.0) | <0.001 |
| Male gender, *n* (%) | 3,704 (60.503) | 2,398 (62.124) | 1,306 (57.737) | <0.001 |
| BMI, median (IQR) | 27.84 (24.39, 31.84) | 27.9 (24.42, 31.98) | 27.77 (24.29, 31.63) | 0.303 |
| **Comorbidities** | | | | |
| Drug abuse, *n* (%) | 208 (3.398) | 152 (3.938) | 56 (2.476) | 0.002 |
| Alcohol abuse, *n* (%) | 474 (7.743) | 301 (7.798) | 173 (7.648) | 0.832 |
| Coagulopathy, *n* (%) | 1,153 (18.834) | 545 (14.119) | 608 (26.879) | <0.001 |
| Liver disease, *n* (%) | 463 (7.563) | 244 (6.321) | 219 (9.682) | <0.001 |
| Renal failure, *n* (%) | 869 (14.195) | 357 (9.249) | 512 (22.635) | <0.001 |
| Hypothyroidism, *n* (%) | 617 (10.078) | 372 (9.637) | 245 (10.831) | 0.134 |
| Diabetes, *n* (%) | 1,448 (23.652) | 883 (22.876) | 565 (24.978) | 0.062 |
| Chronic pulmonary, *n* (%) | 1,179 (19.258) | 714 (18.497) | 465 (20.557) | 0.049 |
| Hypertension, *n* (%) | 758 (12.382) | 326 (8.446) | 432 (19.098) | <0.001 |
| Congestive heart failure, *n* (%) | 816 (13.329) | 353 (9.145) | 463 (20.469) | <0.001 |
| **Laboratory test** | | | | |
| WBC mean, median (IQR) | 11.93 (8.9, 15.55) | 11.7 (9.0, 14.77) | 12.43 (8.72, 17.1) | <0.001 |
| Bun mean, median (IQR) | 18.33 (13.0, 29.4) | 15.67 (12.0, 21.5) | 27.5 (17.0, 44.33) | <0.001 |
| Sodium mean, median (IQR) | 138.0 (136.0, 140.2) | 138.0 (136.2, 140.0) | 138.0 (135.67, 140.71) | 0.720 |
| INR mean, median (IQR) | 1.3 (1.2, 1.5) | 1.3 (1.2, 1.4) | 1.4 (1.2, 1.7) | <0.001 |
| PT mean, median (IQR) | 14.65 (13.6, 16.2) | 14.42 (13.4, 15.65) | 15.25 (13.85, 17.6) | <0.001 |
| Potassium mean, median (IQR) | 4.19 (3.87, 4.5) | 4.15 (3.85, 4.44) | 4.24 (3.9, 4.65) | <0.001 |
| Platelet mean, median (IQR) | 175.33 (130.33, 233.33) | 179.33 (137.0, 233.0) | 168.5 (117.67, 234.0) | <0.001 |
| Lactate mean, median (IQR) | 1.93 (1.4, 2.7) | 1.88 (1.4, 2.5) | 2.12 (1.5, 3.15) | <0.001 |
| Hemoglobin mean, median (IQR) | 10.15 (9.15, 11.4) | 10.3 (9.25, 11.5) | 9.92 (9.0, 11.1) | <0.001 |
| Glucose mean, median (IQR) | 130.57 (116.0, 150.89) | 128.5 (115.33, 145.22) | 134.75 (117.6, 160.33) | <0.001 |
| Creatinine mean, median (IQR) | 0.95 (0.72, 1.37) | 0.87 (0.7, 1.1) | 1.23 (0.85, 2.25) | <0.001 |
| PH mean, median (IQR) | 7.38 (7.34, 7.41) | 7.38 (7.35, 7.42) | 7.36 (7.31, 7.4) | <0.001 |
| **Vital sign** | | | | |
| $SpO_2$ mean, median (IQR) | 97.77 (96.52, 98.81) | 97.82 (96.67, 98.82) | 97.64 (96.28, 98.81) | <0.001 |
| BT mean, median (IQR) | 36.81 (36.43, 37.24) | 36.84 (36.48, 37.24) | 36.77 (36.35, 37.24) | <0.001 |
| Res prate mean, median (IQR) | 18.12 (16.08, 21.17) | 17.72 (15.85, 20.41) | 19.0 (16.57, 22.61) | <0.001 |
| Mean bp mean, median (IQR) | 75.11 (70.17, 81.36) | 76.22 (71.22, 82.61) | 73.4 (68.32, 78.79) | <0.001 |
| Dias bp mean, median (IQR) | 58.39 (53.15, 64.3) | 59.56 (54.39, 65.59) | 56.63 (51.14, 62.15) | <0.001 |
| Sys bp mean, median (IQR) | 112.86 (105.52, 122.26) | 114.55 (107.05, 124.08) | 110.26 (103.03, 119.36) | <0.001 |
| Heart rate mean, median (IQR) | 85.83 (77.53, 96.52) | 84.89 (77.27, 94.66) | 87.35 (78.06, 99.97) | <0.001 |
| **Primary outcome** | | | | |
| Death in-hospital, *n* (%) | 925 (15.109) | 293 (7.591) | 632 (27.940) | <0.001 |
| Death 28-day, *n* (%) | 1,114 (18.197) | 363 (9.404) | 751 (33.201) | <0.001 |
| Death 90-day, *n* (%) | 1,301 (21.251) | 446 (11.554) | 855 (37.798) | <0.001 |
| Death 1-year, *n* (%) | 1,606 (26.233) | 593 (15.363) | 1,013 (44.783) | <0.001 |
| **Second outcome** | | | | |
| AKI 7-day, *n* (%) | 4,563 (74.534) | 2,621 (67.902) | 1,942 (85.853) | <0.001 |
| Hospital stay ≥ 14 days, *n* (%) | 2,092 (34.172) | 950 (24.611) | 1,142 (50.486) | <0.001 |
| ICU stay ≥ 3 days, *n* (%) | 3,422 (55.897) | 1,774 (45.959) | 1,648 (72.856) | <0.001 |
| Survival time, median (IQR) | 11.15 (6.26, 27.17) | 9.82 (5.86, 21.68) | 15.3 (7.94, 41.25) | <0.001 |

*BMI, body mass index; WBC, white blood cell count; BUN, Blood urea nitrogen; PT, prothrombin time; INR, international normalized ratio; SOFA, sequential organ failure assessment; SPASII, simplified acute physiology score; AKI, acute kidney injury; ICU, the intensive care unit; $SPO_2$, pulse oxygen saturation; PH,potential of hydrogen; BT,body temperature; Data are represented as median (interquartile range) or n (%).*

**TABLE 5** | The logistics regression of SAPSII scoring system.

| Outcomes | Non-adjusted model | | | Adjusted model | | |
|---|---|---|---|---|---|---|
| | OR | 95% CL | *p* | OR | 95% CL | *p* |
| In-hospital death | 3.839 | 3.318, 4.45 | <0.001 | 3.544 | 3.02, 4.164 | <0.001 |
| 28-day mortality | 4.292 | 3.744, 4.928 | <0.001 | 3.92 | 3.376, 4.558 | <0.001 |
| 90-day mortality | 4.471 | 3.929, 5.093 | <0.001 | 4.069 | 3.533, 4.693 | <0.001 |
| One-year mortality | 4.748 | 4.208, 5.362 | <0.001 | 4.272 | 3.744, 4.879 | <0.001 |
| AKI 7-day | 2.869 | 2.502, 3.291 | <0.001 | 1.464 | 1.258, 1.706 | <0.001 |
| Hospital stay ≥ 14 days | 3.123 | 2.798, 3.488 | <0.001 | 2.912 | 2.581, 3.287 | <0.001 |
| ICU stay ≥ 3 days | 3.156 | 2.822, 3.533 | <0.001 | 2.997 | 2.651,3.392 | <0.001 |

*SPASII, simplified acute physiology score; OR, odds ratio; CI, 95% confidence interval; AKI, acute kidney injury; ICU: the intensive care unit. Adjusted for the confounders: PT mean, INR mean, platelet mean, lactate mean, hemoglobin mean, glucose mean, creatinine mean, PH mean, $SpO_2$ mean, resp rate mean, mean BP mean, dias bp mean, BMI, congestive heart failure, drug abuse, coagulopathy, liver disease, renal failure, hypertension, gender.*

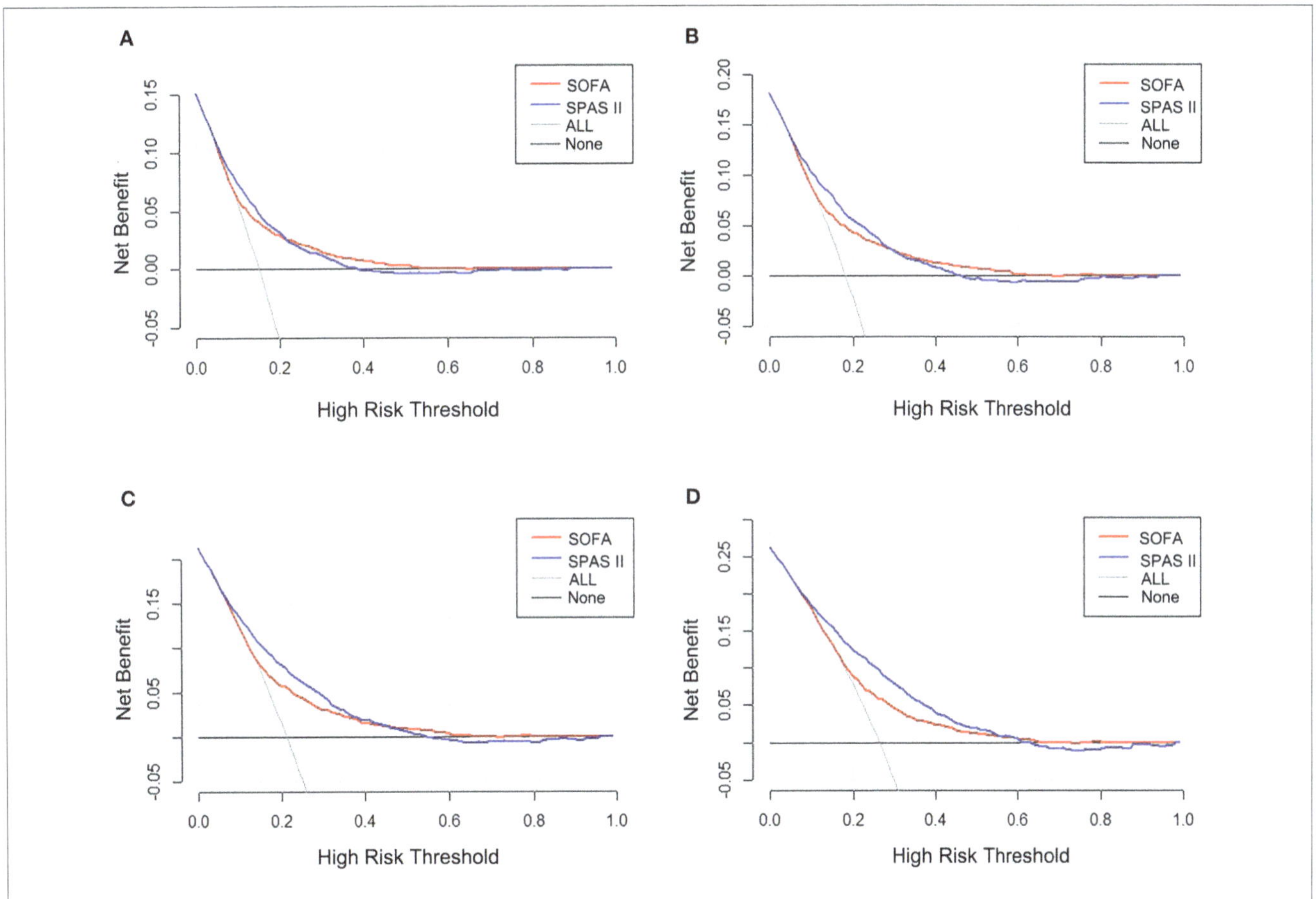


**FIGURE 4** | Decision curve analysis (DCA) of the two scoring systems. **(A)** In-hospital mortality, **(B)** 28-day mortality, **(C)** 90-day mortality, and **(D)** 1-year mortality.

studies behaved even well. In the cardiac surgery population, the previous literature stated that SOFA score had good discriminative power for hospital mortality (27); the same observation was also confirmed in Ceriani et al.'s research (28). Doerr et al.'s study had found that SOFA score could predict 30-day mortality (29). In our study, we used a larger sample size to test the predictive effect of SOFA scores on short-term and long-term mortality. Results are remarkable on the performance of SOFA score as previous studies, especially above the cutoff value. The warning value of the SOFA scoring system is able to assess the risk of outcomes as a new valuable observation index in post-cardiac patients.

The SAPS II scoring system consisted of physiological variables, basic characteristics, and several complications, which could provide an estimate of the risk of death on the basis of large samples with the independence of primary diagnosis, and also was developed for the evaluation of the efficiency of ICUs (30). Recent research established that the SAPS II score could predict the prognosis and in-hospital mortality in AMI patients treated with ECMO with a good performance (26). But it could not ser good predictor for discharged mortality in small sample size studies (31). The result of the previous study of more than 2,000 patients after cardiac surgery showed that the SAPS II score had good discrimination in-hospital mortality (27). The same role was confirmed in another post-cardiac surgery population (32). These researches were consistent with part of our findings. Moreover, previous literature had claimed that the SAPS II scoring system could be implemented reliably while mortality was closely related to the rater's scoring practice (33). This can be interpreted as the diversities of results. Although overestimates of mortality were reported by some researchers (34–37), the objective of our study was for early warning based on the threshold of the SAPS II scoring system.

Decision curve analysis is a method widely used to evaluate the clinical utility of specific models (38). The curve with the highest benefit score at a given threshold was determined to be the best choice (16). A recent study involving multiple scoring systems confirmed the superiority of the SAPS II scoring system in predicting mortality through DCA among sepsis patients (39). Besides, Abraham Schoe et al.'s research including more than 3,600 post-cardiac surgery patients has demonstrated that SOFA score and SAPS II score could predict hospital mortality, while SAPS II was better (32). This tendency is similar to our finding: The SAPS II scoring system had more net benefits on assessing the long-term mortality compared with the SOFA scoring system. As a comprehensive scoring system for postoperative multiple organ physiological function during post-cardiac surgery patients, the SAPS II scoring system may perform better in clinical application.

As for the complexity of progressing in disease, it is hard to find a perfect score of predicting risk comprehensively. The strength of this study lies in identifying warning values of the SOFA score and SAPS II score and giving new insight into the reference value of the SOFA and SAPS II scoring system. Moreover, it enriched the methods of early detecting the prognosis in patients with cardiac surgery and might be used as decision support for clinical intervention. The scoring system was tested in the discrimination of long-term mortality in a large sample of patients with cardiac surgery. However, it was a retrospective observational study which raised possible bias caused by heterogeneous factors. This study focuses on the whole group after cardiac surgery, but we believe that the changes in organ function after different cardiac surgery can also be reflected through the scoring system. Of course, it is also a perfect direction to further explore the differences in the scoring system in different types of cardiac surgery. Moreover, the collected data were from over 10 years ago, these conclusions may not be feasible nowadays with the improvement of surgical technology and ICU treatment level. In this large sample retrospective analysis, the short-term results are consistent with existing studies. There are still few longer-term results. These results can provide clinicians with a warning SOFA and SAPS II value, but the specific implementation should be treated with caution. More retrospective and prospective clinical studies are necessary for verification in the future.

## CONCLUSION

This study suggested that exceeding the cutoff values of the SOFA score and SAPS II score could lead to increased mortality, prolonged length of ICU stay, and in-hospital stay. Score 7 in the SOFA scoring system and score 43 in the SAPS II scoring system with the first 24 h after ICU admission were warning values for worse outcomes. The SAPS II scoring system had a better discriminative performance of 90-day mortality and 1-year mortality in post-cardiac surgery patients than the SOFA scoring system. Focusing on the critical value of the scoring system is of significance for treatment in ICU.

## ETHICS STATEMENT

Access to the database was reviewed and approved by the Institutional Review Committee of Beth Israel Deaconess Medical Center and Beth Israel deacons Medical Center (Approval Code 10323541). Written informed consent was not required for this study, in accordance with the local legislation and institutional requirements.

## AUTHOR CONTRIBUTIONS

FX gathered and processed the data. FX, WL, and CZ prepared the results. FX, WL, and CZ contributed to writing the manuscript. FX and RC put forward the idea. RC revised the manuscript. All the authors read and approved the final manuscript.

## REFERENCES

1. Geissler HJ, Holzl P, Marohl S, Kuhn-Regnier F, Mehlhorn U, Sudkamp M, et al. Risk stratification in heart surgery: comparison of six score systems. *Eur J Cardiothorac Surg.* (2000) 17:400–6. doi: 10.1016/s1010-7940(00)00385-7
2. Nashef SA, Roques F, Michel P, Gauducheau E, Lemeshow S, Salamon R. European system for cardiac operative risk evaluation (EuroSCORE). *Eur J Cardiothorac Surg.* (1999) 16:9–13. doi: 10.1016/s1010-7940(99)00134-7
3. Kunt AG, Kurtcephe M, Hidiroglu M, Cetin L, Kucuker A, Bakuy V, et al. Comparison of original EuroSCORE, EuroSCORE II and STS risk models in a Turkish cardiac surgical cohort. *Interact Cardiovasc Thorac Surg.* (2013) 16:625–9. doi: 10.1093/icvts/ivt022
4. Yalcin M, Godekmerdan E, Tayfur K, Yazman S, Urkmez M, Ata Y. The APACHE II score as a predictor of mortality after open heart surgery. *Turk J Anaesthesiol Reanim.* (2019) 47:41–7. doi: 10.5152/TJAR.2018.44365
5. Tu LN, Hsieh L, Kajimoto M, Charette K, Kibiryeva N, Forero A, et al. Shear stress associated with cardiopulmonary bypass induces expression of inflammatory cytokines and necroptosis in monocytes. *JCI Insight.* (2021) 6:e141341. doi: 10.1172/jci.insight.141341
6. Meregalli A, Oliveira RP, Friedman G. Occult hypoperfusion is associated with increased mortality in hemodynamically stable, high-risk, surgical patients. *Crit Care.* (2004) 8:R60–5. doi: 10.1186/cc2423
7. Ranucci M, De Toffol B, Isgro G, Romitti F, Conti D, Vicentini M. Hyperlactatemia during cardiopulmonary bypass: determinants and impact on postoperative outcome. *Crit Care.* (2006) 10:R167. doi: 10.1186/cc5113

8. Ranucci M, Ballotta A, Castelvecchio S, Baryshnikova E, Brozzi S, Boncilli A, et al. Intensive care unit admission parameters improve the accuracy of operative mortality predictive models in cardiac surgery. *PLoS ONE.* (2010) 5:e13551. doi: 10.1371/journal.pone.0013551
9. Wang Q, Li J, Wang X. The neutrophil-lymphocyte ratio is associated with postoperative mortality of cardiac surgery. *J Thorac Dis.* (2021) 13:67–75. doi: 10.21037/jtd-20-2593
10. Matsuda J, Kato S, Yano H, Nitta G, Kono T, Ikenouchi T, et al. The Sequential Organ Failure Assessment (SOFA) score predicts mortality and neurological outcome in patients with post-cardiac arrest syndrome. *J Cardiol.* (2020) 76:295–302. doi: 10.1016/j.jjcc.2020.03.007
11. Aytuluk HG, Basaran S, Dogan NO, Demir N. Comparison of conventional intensive care scoring systems and prognostic scores specific for intracerebral hemorrhage in predicting one-year mortality. *Neurocrit Care.* (2021) 34:92–101. doi: 10.1007/s12028-020-00987-3
12. Martinez-Alario J, Tuesta ID, Plasencia E, Santana M, Mora ML. Mortality prediction in cardiac surgery patients: comparative performance of Parsonnet and general severity systems. *Circulation.* (1999) 99:2378–82. doi: 10.1161/01.cir.99.18.2378
13. Goldberger AL, Amaral LA, Glass L, Hausdorff JM, Ivanov PC, Mark RG, et al. PhysioBank, PhysioToolkit, and PhysioNet: components of a new research resource for complex physiologic signals. *Circulation.* (2000) 101:E215–20. doi: 10.1161/01.cir.101.23.e215
14. Johnson AE, Pollard TJ, Shen L, Lehman LW, Feng M, Ghassemi M, et al. MIMIC-III, a freely accessible critical care database. *Sci Data.* (2016) 3:160035. doi: 10.1038/sdata.2016.35
15. Stevens PE, Levin A, Kidney Disease: Improving Global Outcomes Chronic Kidney Disease Guideline Development Work Group M. Evaluation and management of chronic kidney disease: synopsis of the kidney disease: improving global outcomes 2012 clinical practice guideline. *Ann Intern Med.* (2013) 158:825–30. doi: 10.7326/0003-4819-158-11-201306040-00007
16. Vickers AJ, Elkin EB. Decision curve analysis: a novel method for evaluating prediction models. *Med Decis Making.* (2006) 26:565–74. doi: 10.1177/0272989X06295361
17. Moreno R, Vincent JL, Matos R, Mendonca A, Cantraine F, Thijs L, et al. The use of maximum SOFA score to quantify organ dysfunction/failure in intensive care. Results of a prospective, multicentre study Working Group on Sepsis related Problems of the ESICM. *Intensive Care Med.* (1999) 25:686–96. doi: 10.1007/s001340050931
18. Arts DG, de Keizer NF, Vroom MB, de Jonge E. Reliability and accuracy of Sequential Organ Failure Assessment (SOFA) scoring. *Crit Care Med.* (2005) 33:1988–93. doi: 10.1097/01.ccm.0000178178.02574.ab
19. Minne L, Abu-Hanna A, de Jonge E. Evaluation of SOFA-based models for predicting mortality in the ICU: A systematic review. *Crit Care.* (2008) 12:R161. doi: 10.1186/cc7160
20. Cour M, Bresson D, Hernu R, Argaud L, SOFA. score to assess the severity of the post-cardiac arrest syndrome. *Resuscitation.* (2016) 102:110–5. doi: 10.1016/j.resuscitation.2016.03.001
21. Bisbal M, Jouve E, Papazian L, de Bourmont S, Perrin G, Eon B, et al. Effectiveness of SAPS III to predict hospital mortality for post-cardiac arrest patients. *Resuscitation.* (2014) 85:939–44. doi: 10.1016/j.resuscitation.2014.03.302
22. Costa ESPP, Codes L, Rios FF, Esteve CP, Valverde Filho MT, Lima DOC, et al. Comparison of general and liver-specific prognostic scores in their ability to predict mortality in cirrhotic patients admitted to the intensive care unit. *Can J Gastroenterol Hepatol.* (2021) 2021:9953106. doi: 10.1155/2021/9953106
23. Huang WC, Xie HJ, Fan HT, Yan MH, Hong YC. Comparison of prognosis predictive value of 4 disease severity scoring systems in patients with acute respiratory failure in intensive care unit: a STROBE report. *Medicine.* (2021) 100:e27380. doi: 10.1097/MD.0000000000027380
24. Jentzer JC, Bennett C, Wiley BM, Murphree DH, Keegan MT, Gajic O, et al. Predictive value of the sequential organ failure assessment score for mortality in a contemporary cardiac intensive care unit population. *J Am Heart Assoc* (2018) 7:8169. doi: 10.1161/JAHA.117.008169
25. Lin Y, Liu F, Gong S, Liao B, Liu H, Yuan J, et al. Validity of SOFA score as a prognostic tool for critically ill elderly patients with acute infective endocarditis. *Rev Cardiovasc Med.* (2021) 22:967–73. doi: 10.31083/j.rcm2203105
26. Kim HS, Park KH, Ha SO, Lee SH, Choi HM, Kim SA, et al. Predictors of survival following veno-arterial extracorporeal membrane oxygenation in patients with acute myocardial infarction-related refractory cardiogenic shock: clinical and coronary angiographic factors. *J Thorac Dis.* (2020) 12:2507–16. doi: 10.21037/jtd.2020.03.51
27. Doerr F, Badreldin AM, Heldwein MB, Bossert T, Richter M, Lehmann T, et al. A comparative study of four intensive care outcome prediction models in cardiac surgery patients. *J Cardiothorac Surg.* (2011) 6:21. doi: 10.1186/1749-8090-6-21
28. Ceriani R, Mazzoni M, Bortone F, Gandini S, Solinas C, Susini G, et al. Application of the sequential organ failure assessment score to cardiac surgical patients. *Chest.* (2003) 123:1229–39. doi: 10.1378/chest.123.4.1229
29. Patila T, Kukkonen S, Vento A, Pettila V, Suojaranta-Ylinen R. Relation of the Sequential Organ Failure Assessment score to morbidity and mortality after cardiac surgery. *Ann Thorac Surg.* (2006) 82:2072–8. doi: 10.1016/j.athoracsur.2006.06.025
30. Le Gall JR, Lemeshow S, Saulnier F. A new Simplified Acute Physiology Score (SAPS II) based on a European/North American multicenter study. *JAMA.* (1993) 270:2957–63. doi: 10.1001/jama.270.24.2957
31. Czajka S, Ziebinska K, Marczenko K, Posmyk B, Szczepanska AJ, Krzych LJ. Validation of APACHE II, APACHE III and SAPS II scores in in-hospital and one year mortality prediction in a mixed intensive care unit in Poland: a cohort study. *BMC Anesthesiol.* (2020) 20:296. doi: 10.1186/s12871-020-0 1203-7
32. Schoe A, Bakhshi-Raiez F, de Keizer N, van Dissel JT, de Jonge E. Mortality prediction by SOFA score in ICU-patients after cardiac surgery; comparison with traditional prognostic-models. *BMC Anesthesiol.* (2020) 20:65. doi: 10.1186/s12871-020-0 0975-2
33. Strand K, Strand LI, Flaatten H. The interrater reliability of SAPS II and SAPS 3. *Intensive Care Med.* (2010) 36:850–3. doi: 10.1007/s00134-010-1772-1
34. Capuzzo M, Scaramuzza A, Vaccarini B, Gilli G, Zannoli S, Farabegoli L, et al. Validation of SAPS 3 Admission Score and comparison with SAPS II. *Acta Anaesthesiol Scand.* (2009) 53:589–94. doi: 10.1111/j.1399-6576.2009.01929.x
35. Desa K, Peric M, Husedzinovic I, Sustic A, Korusic A, Karadza V, et al. Prognostic performance of the Simplified Acute Physiology Score II in major Croatian hospitals: a prospective multicenter study. *Croat Med J.* (2012) 53:442–9. doi: 10.3325/cmj.2012.53.442
36. Haaland OA, Lindemark F, Flaatten H, Kvale R, Johansson KA, A. calibration study of SAPS II with Norwegian intensive care registry data. *Acta Anaesthesiol Scand.* (2014) 58:701–8. doi: 10.1111/aas.12327
37. Nassar AP, Malbouisson LM, Moreno R. Evaluation of Simplified Acute Physiology Score 3 performance: a systematic review of external validation studies. *Crit Care.* (2014) 18:R117. doi: 10.1186/cc13911
38. Fitzgerald M, Saville BR, Lewis RJ. Decision curve analysis. *JAMA.* (2015) 313:409–10. doi: 10.1001/jama.2015.37
39. Hu T, Lv H, Jiang Y. The association between four scoring systems and 30-day mortality among intensive care patients with sepsis: a cohort study. *Sci Rep.* (2021) 11:11214. doi: 10.1038/s41598-021-90806-2

# 16

# Application of a Novel Common-Iliac-Artery Skirt Technology (CST) in Treating Challenge Aorto-Iliac or Isolated Iliac Artery Aneurysms

*Lunchang Wang [1,2], Chang Shu [1,2,3*], Quanming Li [1,2], Ming Li [1,2], Hao He [1,2], Xin Li [1,2], Yin Shi [4], Jian Qiu [1,2], Tun Wang [1,2], Chenzi Yang [1,2], Mo Wang [1,2], Jiehua Li [1,2], Hui Wang [1,2] and Likun Sun [1,2]*

*[1] Department of Vascular Surgery, The Second Xiangya Hospital of Central South University, Changsha, China, [2] Vascular Disease Institute of Central South University, Changsha, China, [3] Department of Vascular Surgery, Fuwai Hospital, Chinese Academy of Medical Sciences & Peking Union Medical College, Beijing, China, [4] Department of Vascular Surgery, Fuwai Yunnan Cardiovascular Hospital, Kunming, China*

***Correspondence:**
*Chang Shu*
*shuchang@csu.edu.cn*

**Purpose:** To report a novel common-iliac-artery skirt technology (CST) in treating challenge iliac artery aneurysms.

**Methods:** When required healthy landing zone of common iliac artery (CIA) is not available, CST is a strategy to exclude the internal iliac artery (IIA) and prevent IIA reflux without need of embolization. Patients who received endovascular aneurysm repair (EVAR) in our center from 2014 to 2020 were retrospectively screened, and patients treated with CST or with IIA embolization (IIAE) were enrolled.

**Results:** After retrospective screen of 524 EVAR patients, 39 CST patients, 26 IIAE patients, and 7 CST + IIAE patients were enrolled in this study. CST group suggested to have more aged, hyperlipemia, and smoking patients than IIAE group. Two groups had comparable maximal diameter of abdominal aorta (AA), CIA, EIA, but larger diameter of IIA (CST 19.82 ± 2.281 vs. IIAE 27.82 ± 3.401, $p = 0.048$), and CIA bifurcation (CST 25.01 ± 1.316 vs. IIAE 29.76 ± 2.775, $p = 0.087$) was found in IIAE group. Anatomy of 79.5% of CST patients and 92.3% of IIAE patients ($p = 0.293$) was not suitable for potential use of iliac branch device. CST group had significant shorter surgery time (CST 97.42 ± 3.891 vs. IIAE 141.0 ± 8.010, $p < 0.001$), shorter hospital stay (CST 15.35 ± 0.873 vs. IIAE 19.32 ± 1.067, $p = 0.009$), lower in-hospital [CST 0% (0/39) vs. IIAE 11.5% (3/26), $p = 0.059$] and 1-year follow-up stent related MAEs [CST 6.7% (2/30) vs. IIAE 28.6% (6/21), $p = 0.052$], but comparable mortality and stent related MAEs for all-cohort follow-up analysis comparing to IIAE group. In our study, a lower in-hospital buttock claudication (BC) rate for CST (CST 20.5% vs. IIAE 46.2%, $p = 0.053$) and a comparable erectile dysfunction (ED) rate (CST 10.3% vs. IIAE 23.1%, $p = 0.352$) were found between CST and IIAE groups. After 1 year, both groups had about one third relief of BC symptoms [CST 33.3% (4/12) vs. IIAE 30.7% (4/13), $p = 1.000$]. Subgroup analysis of 14 patents concomitant with IIA aneurysm in CST group and the 7 CST + IIAE patients were carried out, and no difference was found in mortality, stent MAEs, sac dilation, or reintervention rate. Last, illustration of seven typical CST cases was presented.

**Conclusion:** In selected cases, the CST is a safe, feasible-and-effective choose in treating challenge iliac artery aneurysms and preventing IIA endoleak.

**Keywords: aorto-iliac artery aneurysm, iliac artery aneurysm, internal iliac artery, novel technology, endovascular, aortic surgery**

## INTRODUCTION

Endovascular aneurysm repair (EVAR) has become the preferred way to treat abdominal aortic aneurysms (AAA) with suitable anatomy and life expectancy (1, 2). Iliac artery aneurysms (IAAs) are commonly coexisting with AAAs as aorto-iliac aneurysms in about 10–30% of AAA (3, 4), which poses significant clinical and technical challenges during EVAR (5, 6). Specifically, if the distal common iliac artery (CIA) does not present an adequate healthy landing zone, exclusion of internal iliac artery (IIA) or hypogastric artery is often required. Though benefits of preserving IIAs are now well-acknowledged and different strategies, devices, such as iliac branch device (IBD), are developed (7). Nevertheless, such techniques would significantly increase the surgery time and complexity and could be limited by anatomical constraints, technique experience, and availability of grafts. Remarkably, only 40.9% patients were suitable for use of iliac branch devices in an on-label fashion according to the manufacturer's instructions (8), and IBDs are not available in China until March 2021. And also, aneurysmal patients often complicated with cardiovascular diseases that require a feasible-and-effective procedure, particular for ruptured AAA patients (9, 10).

On the other hand, exclusion of the IIA is widely used and has been proven safe (11–15), and minimal adverse events of possible ischemic complications can be achieved as long as the contralateral IIA is fluent (14, 15). Coil or plug embolization of IIA, direct extension of graft to EIA, or combination of both is the main method for IIA exclusion. Extension of graft to EIA has risk of type II endoleak (16), while coil embolization is challenging and time-consuming with unfeasible anatomy. Here, we described a novel common-iliac-artery skirt technique (CST) in treating challenge aorto-iliac or isolated iliac artery aneurysms, which preserve the advantages of extension of graft to EIA and diminish risk of type II endoleak.

## MATERIALS AND METHODS

### Enrollment and Data Collection

We retrospectively screened patients diagnosed with abdominal or iliac artery aneurysm and treated by endovascular procedures from 2014 to 2020 in our center. Among them, patients treated with CST or IIA embolization (IIAE) were enrolled in this study. Demographic data, risk factors and comorbidity, diagnosis, pre-procedure, procedure and in-hospital data, and follow-up results were analyzed. All patients received informed consent before the surgery, and this study was approved by the Institutional Review Board and the Medical Ethics Committee of our hospital.

A pre-surgical computed tomography angiogram (CTA) was used in all patients to assess extent of aneurysmal disease, tortuosity of the iliac vessels, and patency of the internal and external iliac arteries. Diameter of abdominal aortic and ipsilateral iliac arteries of IIAE or CST were measured from outer-wall to outer-wall of the long-axis. Length of CIA was retrospective collected by DSA with help of centimeter sizing pigtail catheter (Cook Medical Inc). Diameter and length were measured by two authors, and the average value of two authors' was used. Evaluation of erectile dysfunction was only carried out on male patients who are under 70s and had normal erectile function before surgery. Surgery time was calculated from anesthesia induction to the last frame of angiography. Two DSA rooms were routinly used by our group and due to the deficiency of one old-fashion DSA system; unfortunately, not all patients had radiation time and dosage data, so they were not analyzed in this study.

### Indications for CST or IIAE

CIAA without adequate healthy landing zone was the indication for CST or IIAE. Surgical method selection was based on general condition, comorbidities and vascular anatomy of each patient, and also patient's own will. In the IIAE group, embolization was performed preferentially *via* a contralateral approach before EVAR. IIAE was achieved using embolization coils (Cook Medical Inc) at the proximal site of the bifurcation of primary branches.

### Primary and Secondary End Points

Technical successful rate was defined as primary end points, and technique success including complete exclusion of aneurysms and no endoleak from IIA during surgery.

Secondary end points include surgery time, hospital stay, mortality, stent related major adverse events (MAEs), and reintervetion, while stent related MAEs include endoleak, limb occlusion, stent migration, contralateral IIA occlusion, and pelvic ischemia.

### Follow-Up and Statistics

Survival and reintervention events were followed by telephone calls directly with patients regularly. CTA imaging was carried out with available follow-up patients. Data are presented as median (range) or mean ± standard deviation. Data between two groups were analyzed using the Student $t$ test, Chi-square, or Fisher's exact test analysis. A two-tailed $P$ value of <0.05 indicated statistical significance.

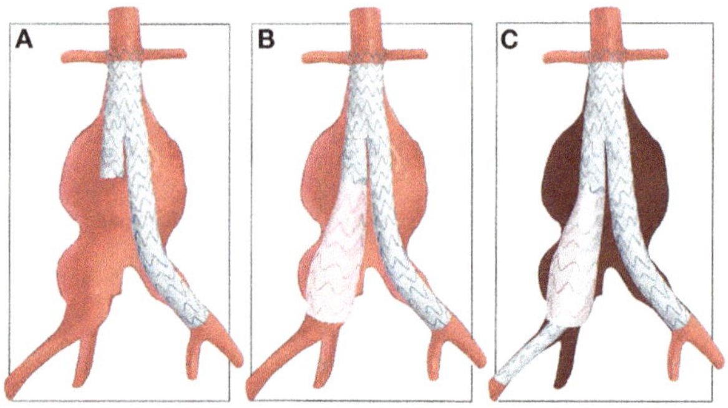


**FIGURE 1 |** Illustration of common-iliac-artery skirt technology. **(A)** An aorto-iliac artery aneurysm and release of the bifurcated main body graft. **(B)** Then, a flared iliac limb is deployed at aneurysmal CIA and with its distal end locating at and sealing the iliac bifurcation, which is named as skirt-limb. **(C)** Another iliac limb with the same proximal diameter of skirt limb is deployed overlap with skirt-limb and elongated to EIA, with IIA excluded and possible reflux of IIA was restricted between the two iliac limbs.

**TABLE 1 |** Demographics and preprocedural data.

| | CST | IIAE | *p* |
|---|---|---|---|
| Male | 97.4% (38/39) | 96.2% (25/26) | 1.000 |
| Age | 70.23 ± 0.969 | 67.54 ± 1.383 | 0.105 |
| Hypertension | 66.7% (26/39) | 65.4% (17/26) | 1.000 |
| Hyperlipidemia | 46.2% (18/39) | 23.1% (6/26) | 0.071 |
| Smoking | 94.8% (33/36) | 61.5% (16/26) | 0.002 |
| CAD | 20.5% (8/39) | 23.1% (6/26) | 1.000 |
| COPD | 23.1% (9/39) | 11.5% (3/26) | 0.334 |
| CKD | 2.56% (1/39) | 0% (0/26) | 1.000 |
| History of CI | 15.4% (6/39) | 3.85% (1/26) | 0.228 |
| Diagnosis | | | 0.253 |
| AAA + CIAA | 30.8% (12/39) | 26.9% (7/26) | / |
| AAA + CIAA + IIAA | 35.8% (14/39) | 19.2% (5/26) | / |
| CIAA | 15.4% (6/39) | 15.4% (4/26) | / |
| CIAA + IIAA | 18% (7/39) | 38.5% (10/26) | / |
| **Diameter of (mm)** | | | |
| AAA | 40.25 ± 2.218 | 34.40 ± 3.203 | 0.129 |
| CIA | 41.22 ± 7.600 | 35.59 ± 2.893 | 0.585 |
| CIA length | 39.45 ± 3.676 | 33.79 ± 3.492 | 0.271 |
| $CIA_b$ | 25.01 ± 1.316 | 29.76 ± 2.775 | 0.087 |
| IIA | 19.82 ± 2.281 | 27.82 ± 3.401 | 0.048 |
| EIA | 9.951 ± 0.174 | 10.34 ± 0.290 | 0.231 |
| Exclusion of IBD | 79.5% (31/39) | 92.3% (24/26) | 0.293 |

*CAD, coronary artery disease; CKD, chronic kidney disease; CI, cerebral infarction; IBD, iliac branch device.*

## RESULTS

### Procedure of a Classical Common-Iliac-Artery Skirt Technique (CST)

As illustrated in **Figure 1**, after deployment of the aortic bifurcated grafts, with the shorter leg placed in aneurysmal CIA side, a flared iliac extension limb (skirt-limb) was deployed at aneurysmal CIA and with its distal end locating at and sealing the iliac bifurcation. The proximal end of skirt-limb with an identical diameter of the bifurcated shorter leg was placed within the leg, the diameter of distal end of skirt-limb should not smaller than the iliac bifurcation, and a 10% oversize of diameter was recommended but not obligatory.

And then, another iliac limb graft with the same proximal diameter of skirt limb was deployed overlap with skirt-limb and elongated to EIA, with IIA excluded and possible reflux of IIA restricted between two iliac limbs (**Figure 1**). Relationship of the two iliac stent grafts was similar with lady's skirt and leg, respectively.

For challenge iliac aneurysm, aortic extension configuration or cuff, or double CST skill can also be used in CST, which will be shown hereinafter.

### Demographics and Pre-Procedural Data

Retrospective screen found 524 patients received EVAR in our center from 2014 to 2020, and 39 CST patients, 26 IIAE patients, and 7 CST + IIAE patients were enrolled in this study. Given the small sample size of CST + IIAE group, regular statistical analysis only carried out between CST and IIAE group and most data of CST + IIAE group was not presented in the text, which but can be provided upon reasonable inquiry.

Demographic data, risk factors and comorbidity analysis suggested that CST group trend to have more aged, hyperlipidemia, and smoking patients than IIAE group, though not all data were statistically significant (**Table 1**). Male patients were overwhelming in both group, 97.4% for CST and 96.2% for IIAE group. Average age was 70.23 ± 0.969 for CST vs. 67.54 ± 1.383 for IIAE group ($p = 0.105$). Hypertension percentage was 66.7% for CST vs. 65.4% for IIAE ($p = 1.000$). CST group had a trend to have more patients with hyperlipidemia (CST 46.2% vs. IIAE 23.1%, $p = 0.07$), but two groups had no difference on coronary artery disease percentage (CST 20.5% vs. IIAE 23.1%, $p = 1.000$). CST group had a significant higher proportion of smoking patients (CST 94.8% vs. IIAE 61.5%, $p = 0.002$) and non-significant higher proportion of COPD patients (CST 23.1% vs. IIAE 11.5%, $p = 0.334$). Both groups had low prevalence of chronic kidney disease, while CST group had more patients with history of cerebral infarction (CST 15.4% vs. IIAE 3.85%, $p = 0.228$), though not significant.

Comparison of diagnosis and vascular anatomy confirmed that all enrolled patients were diagnosed with AAA concomitant with IAA or isolated IAA. Patients were divided into four categories based on diagnosis: AAA + CIAA, AAA + CIAA + IIAA, CIAA, CIAA + IIAA. No significant difference was found on proportion of diagnosis between CST and IIAE group ($p = 0.253$).

Two groups had comparable maximal diameter of AA (CST 40.25 ± 2.218 vs. IIAE 34.40 ± 3.203, $p = 0.129$), CIA (CST 41.22 ± 7.600 vs. IIAE 35.59 ± 2.893, $p = 0.585$), EIA (CST 9.95 ± 0.174 vs. IIAE 10.34 ± 0.290, $p = 0.231$) (**Table 1**), but larger diameter of IIA (CST 19.82 ± 2.281 vs. IIAE 27.82 ± 3.401, $p = 0.048$), and CIA bifurcation (CST 25.01 ± 1.316 vs. IIAE 29.76 ± 2.775, $p = 0.087$) was found in IIAE group. Based on

**TABLE 2** | Procedure and in-hospital data.

| | CST | IIAE | p |
|---|---|---|---|
| **Primary end points** | | | |
| Technique successful rates | 100% | 100% | 1.000 |
| **Secondary end points** | | | |
| In hospital results | | | |
| Surgery time (min) | 97.42 ± 3.891 | 141.0 ± 8.010 | <0.001 |
| Hospital stay (day) | 15.35 ± 0.873 | 19.32 ± 1.067 | 0.009 |
| ICU stay rate | 5.13% (2/39) | 7.69% (2/26) | 1.000 |
| Distal diameter of Skirt stent (mm) | 23.90 ± 0.344 | / | / |
| 20 | 12.8% (5/39) | / | / |
| 24 | 74.4% (29/39) | / | / |
| 28 | 12.8% (5/39) | / | / |
| 28–28 cuff | 7.69% (3/39) | / | / |
| Save of contralateral IIA | 92.3% (36/39) | 76.9% (20/26) | 0.140 |
| All-cause mortality | 0% (0/39) | 0% (0/26) | 1.000 |
| Stent related MAEs | 0% (0/39) | 11.5% (3/26) | 0.059 |
| Endoleak | 0% (0/39) | 0% (0/26) | 1.000 |
| Limb occlusion | 0% (0/39) | 3.8% (1/26) | 0.400 |
| Migration | 0% (0/39) | 0% (0/26) | 1.000 |
| Contralateral IIA occlusion | 0% (0/39) | 3.8% (1/26) | 0.400 |
| Ineffective IIAE | 0% (0/39) | 3.8% (1/26) | 0.400 |
| Reintervetion | 0% (0/39) | 3.8% (1/26) | 0.400 |
| Buttock claudication | 20.5% (8/39) | 46.2% (12/26) | 0.053 |
| Erectile dysfunction | 10.3% (3/29) | 23.1% (3/13) | 0.352 |
| Colonic ischemia | 0% (0/39) | 0% (0/26) | 1.000 |
| Pelvic necrosis | 0% (0/39) | 0% (0/26) | 1.000 |

**TABLE 3** | Follow-up results.

| | CST | IIAE | p |
|---|---|---|---|
| **1-year results** | | | |
| Follow-up rates | 82.1% (32/39) | 92.3% (24/26) | 0.296 |
| All-cause mortality | 6.3% (2/32) | 12.5% (3/24) | 0.639 |
| Stent related MAEs | 6.7% (2/30) | 28.6% (6/21) | 0.052 |
| Endoleak | 0% (0/30) | 0% (0/21) | 1.000 |
| Limb occlusion | 3.3% (1/30) | 14.3% (3/21) | 0.293 |
| Migration | 0% (0/30) | 0% (0/21) | 1.000 |
| Contral IIA occlusion | 3.3% (1/30) | 14.3% (3/21) | 0.293 |
| Endotension or Aneurysm sac dilation | 0% (0/30) | 0% (0/21) | 1.000 |
| Reintervetion | 3.3% (1/30) | 4.8% (1/21) | 1.000 |
| Relived buttock claudication | 37.5% (3/8) | 33.3% (4/12) | 1.000 |
| Relived erectile dysfunction | 0% (0/3) | 33.3% (1/3) | / |
| Colonic ischaemia | 0% (0/30) | 0% (0/21) | 1.000 |
| Pelvic necrosis | 0% (0/30) | 0% (0/21) | 1.000 |
| **All-corhot results** | | | |
| Follow-up (month) | 13–82 m | 12–79 m | 0.203 |
| Median follow-up | 35 | 26 | 0.203 |
| All-cause mortality | 9.38% (3/32) | 12.5% (3/24) | 0.679 |
| Stent related MAEs | 18.8% (6/32) | 25% (6/24) | 0.744 |
| Endoleak | 3.13% (1/32) | 0% (0/24) | 1.000 |
| Limb occlusion | 6.25% (2/32) | 12.5% (3/24) | 0.642 |
| Migration | 3.13% (1/32) | 0% (0/24) | 1.000 |
| Other IIA thrombosis | 6.25% (2/32) | 12.5% (3/24) | 0.642 |
| Endotension or aneurysm sac dilation | 3.13% (1/32) | 0% (0/24) | 1.000 |
| Reintervetion | 6.9% (2/32) | 4.2% (1/24) | 1.000 |

the inclusion/exclusion criteria of the Gore Excluder Iliac Branch Endoprosthesis Trial and the Cook Zenith Iliac Branch Device Clinical Study (17, 18), enrolled patients in our study had a high exclusion rate for potential IBD use (CST 79.5% vs. IIAE 92.3%, $p = 0.293$).

## Procedure and In-Hospital Data

All surgeries were elective and performed under general anesthesia and by the same surgery team. Access was routinely achieved by cut-down femoral artery exposure. For primary end points, both groups had 100% technique successful rates and complete exclusion of aneurysms, though one case of IIAE group only achieved partial IIA embolization, but no endoleak from IIA was found after angiography (**Table 2**). For secondary end points, CST group had significant shorter surgery time (CST 97.42 ± 3.891 vs. IIAE 141.0 ± 8.010, $p < 0.001$) and shorter hospital stay (CST 15.35 ± 0.8734 vs. IIAE 19.32 ± 1.067, $p = 0.009$) compared to IIAE group. Both groups had low rate of Intensive Care Unit stay [CST 5.13% (2/39) vs. IIAE 7.69% (2/26), $p = 1.000$]. By analyzing skirt-limb's distal diameter, we found that 74.4% had a diameter of 24 mm, and 12.8% had a diameter of 28, including three 28–28 mm cuff. Preserve of contralateral IIA was guaranteed as long as suitable anatomy existed, and both groups had high rate of saving contralateral IIA (CST 92.3% vs. IIAE 76.9%, $p = 0.140$).

Analysis of in-hospital results found none mortality for both groups. CST had lower stent related major adverse events compared to IIAE group [CST 0% (0/39) vs. IIAE 11.5% (3/26), $p = 0.059$]. IIAE group had one limb occlusion, one unintended contralateral IIA occlusion, and one ineffective embolization of IIA. No endoleak or stent migration was found in both group. One reintervetion was applied in IIAE group due to limb occlusion. Both groups had pelvic ischemia complications, while CST had lower rate of buttock claudication (BC) (CST 20.5% vs. IIAE 46.2%, $p = 0.053$). Comparable erectile dysfunction (ED) (CST 10.3% vs. IIAE 23.1%, $p = 0.352$) was found, but no severe BC or ED require reintervention existed. No colonic ischemia and pelvic necrosis happened (**Table 2**).

## Follow-Up Results

CST group had 82.1% (32/39) and IIAE group had 92.3% (24/26) ($p = 0.296$) 1-year follow-up (**Table 3**). One-year all cause-mortality rate was 6.3% (2/32) for CST vs. 12.5% (3/24) for IIAE, $p = 0.639$. Stent MAEs increased in both groups after 1 year and IIAE group suggested having higher MAE events [CST 6.7% (2/30) vs. IIAE 28.6% (6/21), $p = 0.052$], which is consistent with in-hospital MAEs. In IIAE group, three limb occlusion and three contralateral IIA occlusion happened. In CST group, one limb occlusion and one contralateral IIA occlusion happened. No endoleak, stent migration, endotension or aneurysm sac

TABLE 4 | Results of different IIAA treatment strategies in CST group.

| | CST | CST + IIAE | p |
|---|---|---|---|
| Diagnosis | | | 0.642 |
| AAA + CIAA + IIAA | 50% (7/14) | 28.6% (2/7) | / |
| CIAA + IIAA | 50% (7/14) | 71.4% (5/7) | / |
| **Diameter of (mm)** | | | |
| CIA | 34.98 ± 4.175 | 46.14 ± 6.244 | 0.146 |
| $CIA_b$ | 29.01 ± 4.179 | 42.40 ± 6.047 | 0.082 |
| IIA | 35.31 ± 3.823 | 48.47 ± 3.230 | 0.038 |
| IIA > 35 mm | 42.9% (6/14) | 100% (7/7) | 0.018 |
| Surgery time (min) | 100.3 ± 5.781 | 120.6 ± 6.962 | 0.047 |
| Save of IIA of other side | 85.7% (12/14) | 42.9% (3/7) | 0.120 |
| Loss of follow-up | 21.4% (3/14) | 14.3% (1/7) | 1.000 |
| Follow-up (month) | 18–70 m | 15–30 m | 0.296 |
| Median FU | 25.5 | 22.5 | 0.296 |
| All-cause mortality | 9.1% (1/11) | 16.7% (1/6) | 1.000 |
| Stent related MAEs | 9.1% (1/11) | 33.3% (2/6) | 0.546 |
| Endoleak | 0% (0/11) | 16.7% (1/6) | 1.000 |
| Limb occlusion | 0% (0/11) | 16.7% (1/6) | 0.353 |
| Migration | 9.1% (1/11) | 0% (0/6) | 1.000 |
| Endotension or Aneurysm sac dilation | 0% (0/11) | 16.7% (1/6) | 0.353 |
| Reintervetion | 9.1% (1/11) | 16.7% (1/6) | 1.000 |

dilation happened for both groups. Both groups only had one reintervetion [CST 3.3% (1/30) vs. IIAE 4.8% (1/21), $p = 1.000$] for symptomatic MAEs. After 1 year, both groups had about one third relief of BC symptoms [CST 33.3% (4/12) vs. IIAE 30.7% (4/13), $p = 1.000$], and IIAE had 33.3% (1/3) relief of erectile dysfunction.

Analysis of all-cohort follow-up data was also carried out. The median follow-up month for CST was 35 (range 13–82), and 26 (range 12–79) for IIAE group ($p = 0.203$). No difference in mortality (CST 9.38% vs. IIAE 12.5%, $p = 0.679$), stent MAEs (CST 18.8% vs. IIAE 25%, $p = 0.744$), and reintervetion rate (CST 6.9% vs. IIAE 4.2%, $p = 1.000$) was found between two groups. CST group had one type II endoleak and sac enlargement of 5 mm from inferior mesenteric artery at 2-year follow-up, and regular follow-up was in process according to patient's willing (**Table 3**).

## Results of Different IIAA Treatment Strategies in CST Group

For patients diagnosed with IIAA, concerns may remain on risk of future IIAA enlargement by only covering the orifice of IIA. So subgroup analysis of 14 patents concomitant with IIA dilation in CST group without IIAE and the 7 CST+IIAE patients were performed (**Table 4**). The proportion of diagnosis was comparable. CST+IIAE group had larger diameter of CIA bifurcation (CST 29.01 ± 4.179 vs. CST+IIAE 42.40 ± 6.047, $p = 0.082$) and IIA (CST 35.31 ± 3.823 vs. CST+IIAE 48.47 ± 3.230, $p = 0.038$) and higher percentage of IIA > 35 mm [CST 42.9% (6/14) vs. CST+IIAE 100% (7/7), $p = 0.018$], and longer surgery time (CST 100.3 ± 5.781 vs. CST+IIAE 120.6 ± 6.962, $p = 0.047$). But all-cohort analysis with a median follow-up of 25.5 months for CST and 22.5 months for CST+IIAE ($p = 0.296$) showed no difference in mortality, stent MAEs, sac dilation, or reintervetion between two groups. Notably, both groups had one sac enlargement event. The one in CST group was described previously, and the sac enlargement in IIAAE group was thought to result from endotension, and open surgery was performed after 5-year follow-up (**Table 4**).

## Illustration of Typical and Challenge Cases With CST

To illustrate the application and advantage of CST, we presented several typical and challenge CST cases. Cases 1–3 showed three cases of AAA concomitant with a huge or short CIAA (**Figure 2**), and cases 1 and 3 were concomitant with IIAA at the same time. A Medtronic 16–28 mm flared skirt-limb placed in CIA and a 16–13 mm iliac limb extended to EIA was used to seal the CIAA and exclusion of one side IIA. From the DSA, we could notice that the reflux of IIA was contained between the skirt graft and the extended iliac limb (white arrow in **Figures 2C,H,M**). One year follow-up results all showed no endoleak or aneurysm sac dilation, and thrombosis formed in space between skirt-limb and extended iliac limb (white arrow in **Figures 2E,J,O**).

Cases 4 and 5 showed application of CST for isolated CIAAs (**Figure 3**). Case 4 showed a satisfactory result of sealing a 50.3 mm CIAA sequentially by a 16–24 mm graft, a 28–28 mm iliac limb, and two 16–16 mm iliac limbs, with the first 16–24 skirt limb located at the orifice of CIA and second 28–28 skirt limb located at the distal bifurcation of CIA. The double skirt-technology fully prevented any potential endoleaks to the aortic sac. Case 5 showed a long and huge CIA with 61 mm maximal diameter, which was also excluded by double CST skill, composed by a graft series of a 16–24, a 16–16, another 16–24 and 16–16 mm graft.

Cases 6 and 7 showed different strategies in treating IIAA in CST group (**Figure 4**). Both cases showed bilateral CIAA concomitant with IIAAs. For case 6, a series of 28–28, 16–13, 16–13 mm grafts were formed a CST for the right side, and a 16–24 followed with a 16–13 mm graft were used for the left side. Post-surgery and 1-year follow-up results showed complete seal of aneurysm, exclusion of IIA blood flow, no endoleak, and no aneurysm sac enlargement. For case 7, both CIAAs were treated by a 28–28 graft combined with a 16–13 mm iliac limb after coil embolization of the IIA. One-year follow-up showed satisfactory seal of aneurysm and complete embolization of IIA, though light type II endoleak from inferior mesenteric artery existed.

## DISCUSSION

Strategies of treating IIA changed during the development of AAA treatment. At the early stage of AAA open surgery, preservation of at least one IIA was thought to be necessary and bypass of IIA to graft was used both in our center and others (19). Then, with the development of endovasular surgery as first line therapy and more and more data of safety on IIA exclusion, save of IIA was secondary to providing adequate landing zone and complete sealing of aneurysms (11, 13, 15). However, with development of new devices and technologies, preservation of

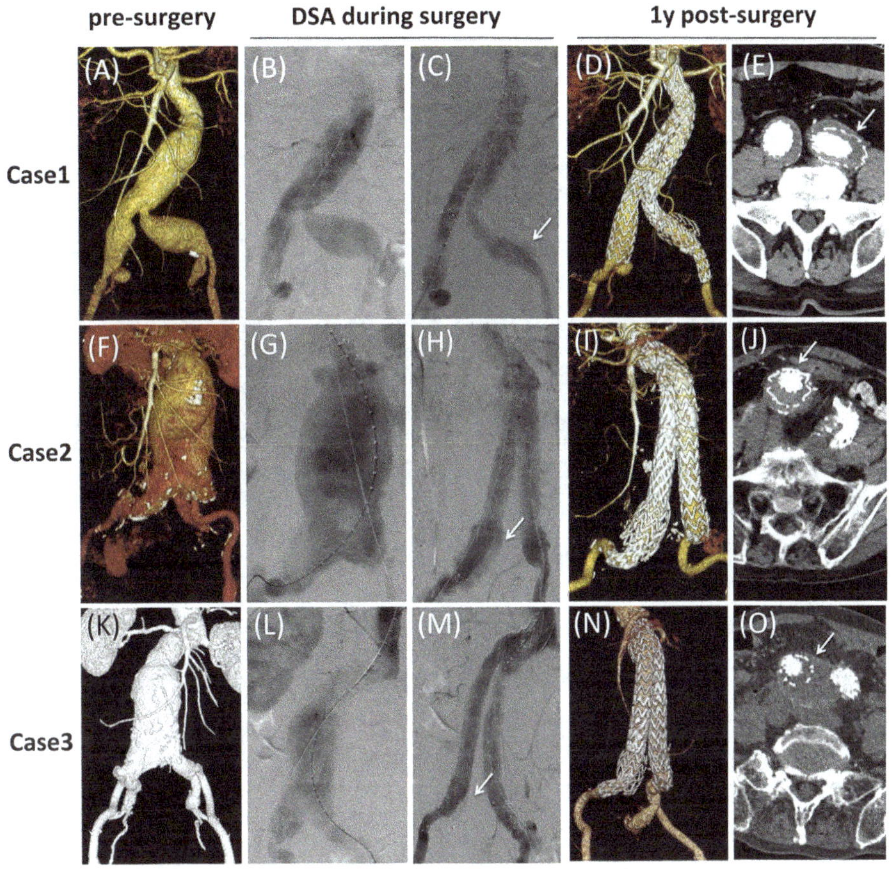


**FIGURE 2** | Typical cases of CST for aorto-iliac aneurysms. **(A,F,K)** Pre-surgical CTA 3D reconstruction. **(B,G,L)** DSA of aneurysms. **(C,H,M)** DSA after CST procedure. The white arrow indicates reflux of IIA was contained between the skirt graft and the extended iliac limb. **(D,I,N)** One-year follow-up CTA 3D reconstruction. **(E,J,O)** Transverse section of 1-year follow-up CTA. The white arrow indicates thrombosis formed in space between skirt graft and extended iliac limb.

IIA and effort to decrease BC and ED become more and more important. With development of IBDs and improved Quality Control of AAA surgery, a preservation era of IIA is thought coming (20).

But, such new techniques still could be limited by anatomical constraints, technique experience, and availability of grafts. For example, IBDs were not available in China until March 2021. After full evaluation of patient condition, activity level, length, tortuosity and thrombus burden of iliac arteries, and cost, exclusion of IIA was still an indispensable technology in selected cases. And here we reported a novel common iliac artery skirt technology for feasible-and-effective IIA exclusion.

Based on retrospective analysis of data from 39 CST and 26 IIAE patients, our experience showed both groups had comparable primary end points and CST had better secondary end points, including significant short surgery time and hospital stay, lower in-hospital and 1-year stent MAEs, comparable mortality, and stent MAEs for all-cohort follow-up. Results of CST showed clear advantages over IIAE in excluding IIA and at the same time preventing the occurrence of type II endoleaks. Actually, the use of a flared grafts in excluding IIA with or without embolization also published in case reports, either with an upside-down or reversed bell-bottom technique (21–24). But, either a manually unsheathed-and-mounted procedure or a contralateral femoral access and crossover process is needed, respectively, which are not necessary for our CST.

Advantages of CST come from its simplicity and which results in short-time surgery and anesthesia, and less endovascular procedures. Ischemia of pelvic is the main concern and complication for exclusion of hypogastric artery. Literature reports of BC rate were 36.5% for bilateral IIA interruption and 27.2% for unilateral IIA interruption (25), and the erectile dysfunction rate was 12.7%. In our study, the in-hospital BC rate was 20.5% for CST vs. 46.2% for IIAE, $p = 0.053$ and the ED rate was 10.3% for CST vs. 23.1% for IIAE, $p = 0.352$. The direct coverage of orifice of IIA was suggested to have lower rate of BC than embolization of IIA in our study, and evidence was also reported in published data (11, 26–28). Nevertheless, the high preserve rate of contralateral IIA in CST should also not be ignored, thought not statistically significant. After 1 year, about one third BC was relived in both groups (CST 37.5% vs. IIAE 33.3%, $p = 1.000$), and which all happened on patients who had a preserved contralateral IAA. Thus, the save of at least one IIA should be guaranteed

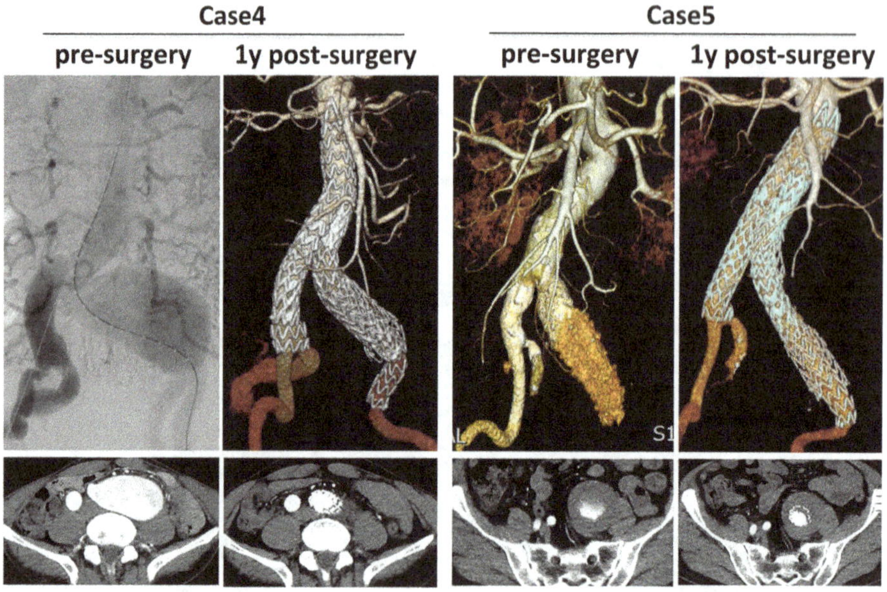


**FIGURE 3 |** Typical cases of CST for isolated iliac aneurysms. 3D CTA pre-surgery and 1-year post-surgery was compared and corresponding transverse section was also presented.

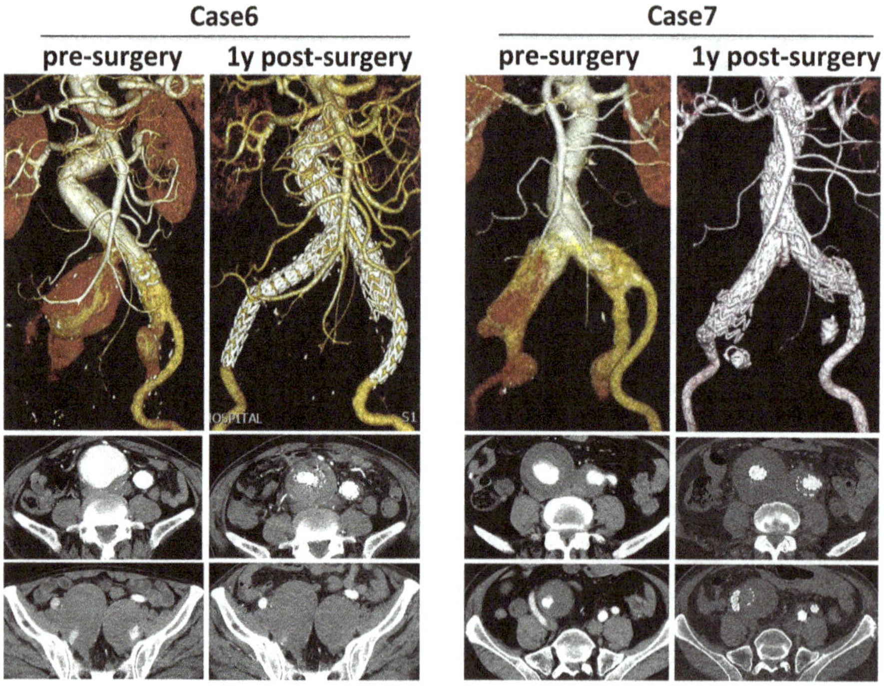


**FIGURE 4 |** Different strategies in treating IIAA in CST group. 3D CTA pre-surgery and 1-year post-surgery was compared and corresponding transverse section was also presented.

as long as possible, as per guidelines (1, 29). And as both CST and IIAE have high and comparable technique successful rate and exclusion of IIA in this study by our group, no difference of mortality and stent MAEs in long term follow-up was found.

Whereas, the critical size for isolated IIAAs treatment is considered to be 3–4 cm (30–32), whether its benefit to treat smaller IIAAs in patients undergoing EVAR for aorta-common iliac aneurysm to avoid the need for secondary interventions is still not clear. And also, for CST group, concerns may remain on risk of future IIAA enlargement by only covering the orifice of IAA. In our study, by subgroup analysis of 14 patents concomitant with IIA dilation in CST group without IIAE and the 7 CST+IIAE patients, no difference was found in mortality, stent MAEs, sac dilation, or reintervetion between two groups. However, considering the challenging of secondary interventions for IIAAs after CST, we recommend that CST plus IIA embolization or other IIAAs procedures should be applied for IIAAs > 35 mm (33).

Overall, the common-iliac-artery skirt technology is simple, since it does not require neither particular endovascular expertise of the operator nor peculiar devices, which has decisive advantage in ruptured patients as a fast and life-saving treatment option. Besides, as the application of CST only restricted by the diameter of CIA bifurcation and the 10% oversize was not strictly needed for the skirt limb, CST was available for majority cases by using available flared iliac limbs and cuffs (maximal 36 mm). Comparing to IIAE, our experience showed CST had advantages in reducing surgery time, hospital stay, stent related MAEs, and BC rates. Satisfying safety and sealing of CIAAs without type II endoleak was also obtained.

Unilateral application of CST plus a patency or preserved contralateral IIA could be a satisfactory solution for most challenge iliac artery aneurysms. Nevertheless, larger sample size and long-term follow-up is warranted to assess the durability of the technology and absence of re-interventions.

As a retrospectively study, limitations of this study may include potential selection bias of patients for surgical method. However, comparable results of majority risk factors were found between groups.

## CONCLUSION

In selected cases, the CST can be used for the complete exclusion of challenge iliac artery aneurysms and preventing type II endoleak from the IIA, especially for those who has advanced age or contralateral health IIA, or cannot tolerate long-time surgery and is limited in activities, or when preservation of IIA does more harm than good or is not practical.

## ETHICS STATEMENT

The studies involving human participants were reviewed and approved by Ethics Committee of the 2nd Xiangya Hospital, Central South University. The patients/participants provided their written informed consent to participate in this study. Written informed consent was obtained from the individual(s) for the publication of any potentially identifiable images or data included in this article.

## AUTHOR CONTRIBUTIONS

CS, LW, QL, ML, HH, and XL contributed to conception and design of the study. LW, YS, JQ, TW, CY, MW, and JL collected data and organized the database. HW and LS performed the statistical analysis. LW wrote the first draft of the manuscript. All authors contributed to manuscript revision, read, and approved the submitted version.

## REFERENCES


1. Wanhainen A, Verzini F, Van Herzeele I, Allaire E, Bown M, Cohnert T, et al. Editor's choice - European Society for Vascular Surgery (ESVS) 2019 clinical practice guidelines on the management of abdominal aorto-iliac artery aneurysms. *Eur J Vasc Endovasc Surg.* (2019) 57:8–93. doi: 10.1016/j.ejvs.2018.09.020
2. Chaikof EL, Dalman RL, Eskandari MK, Jackson BM, Lee WA, Mansour MA, et al. The society for vascular surgery practice guidelines on the care of patients with an abdominal aortic aneurysm. *J Vasc Surg.* (2018) 67:2–77 e2. doi: 10.1016/j.jvs.2017.10.044
3. Krupski WC, Selzman CH, Floridia R, Strecker PK, Nehler MR, Whitehill TA. Contemporary management of isolated iliac aneurysms. *J Vasc Surg.* (1998) 28:1–11; discussion–3. doi: 10.1016/S0741-5214(98)70194-6
4. Armon MP, Wenham PW, Whitaker SC, Gregson RH, Hopkinson BR. Common iliac artery aneurysms in patients with abdominal aortic aneurysms. *Eur J Vasc Endovasc Surg.* (1998) 15:255–7. doi: 10.1016/S1078-5884(98)80186-X
5. Hobo R, Sybrandy JE, Harris PL, Buth J, Collaborators E. Endovascular repair of abdominal aortic aneurysms with concomitant common iliac artery aneurysm: outcome analysis of the EUROSTAR Experience. *J Endovasc Ther.* (2008) 15:12–22. doi: 10.1583/07-2217.1
6. Bannazadeh M, Jenkins C, Forsyth A, Kramer J, Aggarwal A, Somerset AE, et al. Outcomes for concomitant common iliac artery aneurysms after endovascular abdominal aortic aneurysm repair. *J Vasc Surg.* (2017) 66:1390–7. doi: 10.1016/j.jvs.2017.02.058
7. Robalo C, Sousa J, Mansilha A. Internal iliac artery preservation strategies in the endovascular treatment of aortoiliac aneurysms. *Int Angiol.* (2018) 37:346–55. doi: 10.23736/S0392-9590.18.04004-X
8. Gray D, Shahverdyan R, Jakobs C, Brunkwall J, Gawenda M. Endovascular aneurysm repair of aortoiliac aneurysms with an iliac side-branched stent graft: studying the morphological applicability of the Cook device. *Eur J Vasc Endovasc Surg.* (2015) 49:283–8. doi: 10.1016/j.ejvs.2014.12.021
9. Brewster DC, Retana A, Waltman AC, Darling RC. Angiography in the management of aneurysms of the abdominal aorta. Its value and safety. *N Engl J Med.* (1975) 292:822–5. doi: 10.1056/NEJM197504172921602
10. Olin JW, Melia M, Young JR, Graor RA, Risius B. Prevalence of atherosclerotic renal artery stenosis in patients with atherosclerosis elsewhere. *Am J Med.* (1990) 88:46N–51N.
11. Bosanquet DC, Wilcox C, Whitehurst L, Cox A, Williams IM, Twine CP, et al. Systematic review and meta-analysis of the effect of internal iliac artery exclusion for patients undergoing EVAR. *Eur J Vasc Endovasc Surg.* (2017) 53:534–48. doi: 10.1016/j.ejvs.2017.01.009
12. Lee WA, O'Dorisio J, Wolf YG, Hill BB, Fogarty TJ, Zarins CK. Outcome after unilateral hypogastric artery occlusion during endovascular aneurysm repair. *J Vasc Surg.* (2001) 33:921–6. doi: 10.1067/mva.2001.114999
13. Lee C, Dougherty M, Calligaro K. Concomitant unilateral internal iliac artery embolization and endovascular infrarenal aortic aneurysm repair. *J Vasc Surg.* (2006) 43:903–7. doi: 10.1016/j.jvs.2005.12.063
14. Schoder M, Zaunbauer L, Holzenbein T, Fleischmann D, Cejna M, Kretschmer G, et al. Internal iliac artery embolization before endovascular repair of abdominal aortic aneurysms: frequency, efficacy, and clinical results. *AJR Am J Roentgenol.* (2001) 177:599–605. doi: 10.2214/ajr.177.3.1770599
15. Cynamon J, Lerer D, Veith FJ, Taragin BH, Wahl SI, Lautin JL, et al. Hypogastric artery coil embolization prior to endoluminal repair of aneurysms and fistulas: buttock claudication, a recognized but possibly preventable complication. *J Vasc Interv Radiol.* (2000) 11:573–7. doi: 10.1016/S1051-0443(07)61608-X
16. Lo RC, Buck DB, Herrmann J, Hamdan AD, Wyers M, Patel VI, et al. Risk factors and consequences of persistent type II endoleaks. *J Vasc Surg.* (2016) 63:895–901. doi: 10.1016/j.jvs.2015.10.088

17. Pearce BJ, Varu VN, Glocker R, Novak Z, Jordan WD, Lee JT. Anatomic suitability of aortoiliac aneurysms for next generation branched systems. *Ann Vasc Surg.* (2015) 29:69–75. doi: 10.1016/j.avsg.2014.08.003
18. Karthikesalingam A, Hinchliffe RJ, Malkawi AH, Holt PJ, Loftus IM, Thompson MM. Morphological suitability of patients with aortoiliac aneurysms for endovascular preservation of the internal iliac artery using commercially available iliac branch graft devices. *J Endovasc Ther.* (2010) 17:163–71. doi: 10.1583/09-2942.1
19. Unno N, Inuzuka K, Yamamoto N, Sagara D, Suzuki M, Konno H. Preservation of pelvic circulation with hypogastric artery bypass in endovascular repair of abdominal aortic aneurysm with bilateral iliac artery aneurysms. *J Vasc Surg.* (2006) 44:1170–5. doi: 10.1016/j.jvs.2006.08.011
20. Kouvelos G, Nana P, Spanos K. Commentary: time to preserve the iliac arteries during EVAR. *J Endovasc Ther.* (2020) 27:826–7. doi: 10.1177/1526602820940784
21. Leon LR Jr, Mills JL Sr. Successful endovascular exclusion of a common iliac artery aneurysm: off-label use of a reversed Cook Zenith extension limb stent-graft. *Vasc Endovasc Surg.* (2009) 43:76–82. doi: 10.1177/1538574408322661
22. van der Steenhoven TJ, Heyligers JM, Tielliu IF, Zeebregts CJ. The upside down gore excluder contralateral leg without extracorporeal predeployment for aortic or iliac aneurysm exclusion. *J Vasc Surg.* (2011) 53:1738–41. doi: 10.1016/j.jvs.2010.11.108
23. Koike Y, Nishimura J, Hase S, Yamasaki M. The upside down endurant iliac limb stent graft for treatment of a common iliac artery aneurysm. *Vasc Endovasc Surg.* (2014) 48:58–60. doi: 10.1177/1538574413510615
24. Mazzaccaro D, Righini P, Zuccon G, Modafferi A, Malacrida G, Nano G. The reversed bell-bottom technique (ReBel-B) for the endovascular treatment of iliac artery aneurysms. *Catheter Cardiovasc Interv.* (2020) 96:E479–83. doi: 10.1002/ccd.29140
25. Kouvelos GN, Katsargyris A, Antoniou GA, Oikonomou K, Verhoeven EL. Outcome after interruption or preservation of internal iliac artery flow during endovascular repair of abdominal aorto-iliac aneurysms. *Eur J Vasc Endovasc Surg.* (2016) 52:621–34. doi: 10.1016/j.ejvs.2016.07.081
26. Chitragari G, Schlosser FJ, Ochoa Chaar CI, Sumpio BE. Consequences of hypogastric artery ligation, embolization, or coverage. *J Vasc Surg.* (2015) 62:1340–7 e1. doi: 10.1016/j.jvs.2015.08.053
27. Farahmand P, Becquemin JP, Desgranges P, Allaire E, Marzelle J, Roudot-Thoraval F. Is hypogastric artery embolization during endovascular aortoiliac aneurysm repair (EVAR) innocuous and useful? *Eur J Vasc Endovasc Surg.* (2008) 35:429–35. doi: 10.1016/j.ejvs.2007.12.001
28. Jean-Baptiste E, Brizzi S, Bartoli MA, Sadaghianloo N, Baque J, Magnan PE, et al. Pelvic ischemia and quality of life scores after interventional occlusion of the hypogastric artery in patients undergoing endovascular aortic aneurysm repair. *J Vasc Surg.* (2014) 60:40–9, 9 e1. doi: 10.1016/j.jvs.2014.01.039
29. Chaikof EL, Brewster DC, Dalman RL, Makaroun MS, Illig KA, Sicard GA, et al. The care of patients with an abdominal aortic aneurysm: the Society for Vascular Surgery practice guidelines. *J Vasc Surg.* (2009) 50:S2–49. doi: 10.1016/j.jvs.2009.07.001
30. Dix FP, Titi M, Al-Khaffaf H. The isolated internal iliac artery aneurysm–a review. *Eur J Vasc Endovasc Surg.* (2005) 30:119–29. doi: 10.1016/j.ejvs.2005.04.035
31. Rana MA, Kalra M, Oderich GS, de Grandis E, Gloviczki P, Duncan AA, et al. Outcomes of open and endovascular repair for ruptured and nonruptured internal iliac artery aneurysms. *J Vasc Surg.* (2014) 59:634–44. doi: 10.1016/j.jvs.2013.09.060
32. Laine MT, Bjorck M, Beiles CB, Szeberin Z, Thomson I, Altreuther M, et al. Few internal iliac artery aneurysms rupture under 4 cm. *J Vasc Surg.* (2017) 65:76–81. doi: 10.1016/j.jvs.2016.06.109
33. Kliewer M, Plimon M, Taher F, Walter C, Hirsch K, Falkensammer J, et al. Endovascular treatment of hypogastric artery aneurysms. *J Vasc Surg.* (2019) 70:1107–14. doi: 10.1016/j.jvs.2018.12.048

17

# $\Delta PCO_2$ and $\Delta PCO_2/C_{(a-cv)}O_2$ are not Predictive of Organ Dysfunction After Cardiopulmonary Bypass


*Sheng Zhang [1†], Dan Zheng [1†], Xiao-Qiong Chu [1†], Yong-Po Jiang [1], Chun-Guo Wang [2], Qiao-Min Zhang [1], Lin-Zhu Qian [1], Wei-Ying Yang [1], Wen-Yuan Zhang [1], Tao-Hsin Tung [3*] and Rong-Hai Lin [1*]*

[1] *Department of Critical Care Medicine, Taizhou Hospital of Zhejiang Province, Wenzhou Medical University, Linhai, China,*
[2] *Department of Cardiothoracic Surgery, Taizhou Hospital of Zhejiang Province, Wenzhou Medical University, Linhai, China,*
[3] *Evidence-Based Medicine Center, Taizhou Hospital of Zhejiang Province, Wenzhou Medical University, Linhai, China*

***Correspondence:**
*Rong-Hai Lin*
*tylinrh@163.com*
*Tao-Hsin Tung*
*ch2876@yeah.net*

[†] *These authors have contributed equally to this work*



**Background:** Cardiac surgery is associated with a substantial risk of major adverse events. Although carbon dioxide ($CO_2$)-derived variables such as venous-to-arterial $CO_2$ difference ($\Delta PCO_2$), and $PCO_2$ gap to arterial–venous $O_2$ content difference ratio ($\Delta PCO_2/C_{(a-cv)}O_2$) have been successfully used to predict the prognosis of non-cardiac surgery, their prognostic value after cardiopulmonary bypass (CPB) remains controversial. This hospital-based study explored the relationship between $\Delta PCO_2$, $\Delta PCO_2/C_{(a-cv)}O_2$ and organ dysfunction after CPB.

**Methods:** We prospectively enrolled 114 intensive care unit patients after elective cardiac surgery with CPB. Patients were divided into the organ dysfunction group (OI) and non-organ dysfunction group (n-OI) depending on whether organ dysfunction occurred or not at 48 h after CPB. $\Delta PCO_2$ was defined as the difference between central venous and arterial $CO_2$ partial pressure.

**Results:** The OI group has 37 (32.5%) patients, 27 of which (23.7%) had one organ dysfunction and 10 (8.8%) had two or more organ dysfunctions. No statistical significance was found ($P = 0.84$) for $\Delta PCO_2$ in the n-OI group at intensive care unit (ICU) admission (9.0, 7.0–11.0 mmHg), and at 4 (9.0, 7.0–11.0 mmHg), 8 (9.0, 7.0–11.0 mmHg), and 12 h post admission (9.0, 7.0–11.0 mmHg). In the OI group, $\Delta PCO_2$ also showed the same trend [ICU admission (9.0, 8.0–12.8 mmHg) and 4 (10.0, 7.0–11.0 mmHg), 8 (10.0, 8.5–12.5 mmHg), and 12 h post admission (9.0, 7.3–11.0 mmHg), $P = 0.37$]. No statistical difference was found for $\Delta PCO_2/C_{(a-cv)}O_2$ in the n-OI group ($P = 0.46$) and OI group ($P = 0.39$). No difference was detected in $\Delta PCO_2$, $\Delta PCO_2/C_{(a-cv)}O_2$ between groups during the first 12 h after admission ($P > 0.05$). Subgroup analysis of the patients with two or more failing organs compared to the n-OI group showed that the predictive performance of lactate and Base excess (BE) improved, but not of $\Delta PCO_2$ and $\Delta PCO_2/C_{(a-cv)}O_2$. Regression analysis showed that the BE at 8 h after admission (odds ratio = 1.37, 95%CI: 1.08–1.74, $P = 0.009$) was a risk factor for organ dysfunction 48 h after CBP.

**Conclusion :** $\Delta PCO_2$ and $\Delta PCO_2/C_{(a-cv)}O_2$ cannot be used as reliable indicators to predict the occurrence of organ dysfunction at 48 h after CBP due to the pathophysiological process that occurs after CBP.

**Keywords: venous-to-arterial carbon dioxide difference, base excess, lactate, cardiopulmonary bypass, organ dysfunction**

## INTRODUCTION

Despite improvements in surgical technique, anesthesia, management, and postoperative care, cardiac surgery is still associated with a substantial risk of major adverse events (1). Early identification of risk factors and interventions reduce the occurrence of complications. Venous-to-arterial carbon dioxide ($CO_2$) difference ($\Delta PCO_2$) is a parameter that reflects tissue hypoperfusion in critically ill patients who are insufficiently resuscitated (2). The $PCO_2$ gap to arterial–venous $O_2$ content difference ratio ($\Delta PCO_2/C_{(a-cv)}O_2$) has also been described as an indicator of the relationship between oxygen delivery ($DO_2$) and oxygen consumption ($VO_2$) (3). Although they have been successfully used to guide fluid resuscitation in patients with sepsis (4, 5) and predict prognosis of non-cardiac surgery patients (6, 7), the predictive value of $CO_2$-derived variables after cardiopulmonary bypass surgery (CPB) is still controversial (8, 9). $CO_2$-derived variables may be unable to inform on tissue ischemia because they do not track $VO_2$ changes in cardiac surgical patients (10). Hyperlactatemia is related to tissue hypoxia but is also affected by factors such as catecholamines and metabolic rate. A previous study found that base excess (BE) is superior to lactate levels for the prediction of ICU mortality after cardiac surgery (11). Organ dysfunction is central to the pathogenesis of death and disability in critically ill patients, and the prognosis becomes worse as the number of failed organs increases. Therefore, it is more meaningful to use organ dysfunction as a clinical outcome variable because of the potential relationship. Although there are many studies on $CO_2$-derived variables and clinical outcome, few studies have explored the prognostic value of $CO_2$-derived variables basing on organ dysfunction. Organ dysfunction is considered to be an effective new outcome indicator in cardiac surgical patients, especially when the number of cases required is relatively small (12, 13).

The main objective of this study was to investigate relationship between $CO_2$-derived variables and organ dysfunction occurring during the early phases after elective cardiac surgery with CPB. The secondary objective was to compare these variables with BE and lactate, which are usually associated with tissue hypoperfusion.

**Abbreviations:** $\Delta PCO_2/C_{(a-cv)}O_2$, Arterial-venous $O_2$ content difference ratio; $CO_2$, carbon dioxide; CPB, cardiopulmonary bypass; Hb, hemoglobin; ICU, intensive care unit; n-OI, non-organ dysfunction group; OI, organ dysfunction group; $\Delta PCO_2$, venous-to-arterial $CO_2$ difference.

## MATERIALS AND METHODS

We conducted a prospective observational study in a 39-bed mixed intensive care unit (ICU) of a university-affiliated Hospital. Our clinical trial was registered in the China Clinical Trial Registry (registration number: ChiCTR-ROC-17010727). Ethics approval was obtained from the Ethics Committee of Taizhou Hospital, Zhejiang Province. Written informed consent was obtained from all patients. The clinical trial started in February 2017 and ended in August 2018.

Adults ($\geq$18 years old) admitted to ICU immediately after CBP, were included if an arterial line and a central venous catheter (confirmed by X-ray) had been inserted. After initiation of the trial, we removed one of the eligibility criteria: "Factors affecting the accuracy of cardiac output monitoring: aortic regurgitation, atrial fibrillation, aortic balloon counter pulsation, high dose norepinephrine," because it was not necessary and would have reduced our sample size. The exclusion criteria were: emergency surgery, pregnancy, chronic renal insufficiency with dialysis, preoperative acute or chronic liver failure, hematologic diseases, misplacement of the central venous catheter, and death within 48 h.

Intraoperative and ICU management was conducted according to local protocols and international guidelines. Ventilator settings were as follows: control mode, tidal volume 6–8 mL/kg, positive end-expiratory pressure $\leq$5 $cmH_2O$, respirations 14–16 times/min, fraction of inspired oxygen 40%. Analgesia was achieved with continuous infusion of fentanyl (0.5–10 mg/kg/h) targeting Critical Care Pain Observation Tool scores of 0–2. Anesthesia was maintained with a continuous infusion of propofol (1–4 mg/kg/h) targeting Richmond Agitation-Sedation Scale scores of−2–0. Vasoactive drugs and fluid infusions were adjusted according to mean arterial pressure of 60–70 mmHg. Infusion of red blood cells was prescribed as needed to maintain hemoglobin (Hb) concentration $\geq$9.0 g/dL. Crystalloid solution (Lactated Ringer's solution or 0.9% saline) or 20% albumin was added for volume expansion if necessary.

We prospectively collected preoperative, intraoperative, and postoperative variables, including clinical characteristics, duration of surgery, CBP duration, vital signs, fluid balance, vasoactive-inotropic score, routine blood tests, blood gas results, and clinical biochemistry. The specific data collection time points were at ICU admission and 4 h (H4), 8 h (H8), 12 h (H12), 24 h (H24), and 48 h (H48) after ICU admission. White blood cell count, hemoglobin concentration, platelet count, clinical biochemistry, chest X-rays, or CT scans were reviewed to evaluate organ function at ICU admission, H24, and H48. The length of stay in ICU, length of ventilator use,

European System for Cardiac Operative Risk Evaluation II, Acute Physiology and Chronic Health Evaluation Score II (APACHE-II), and sequential organ failure score were recorded at ICU admission, H24, and H48. Paired arterial and central venous blood gases, arterial blood lactate, base excess (BE), and Hb levels were measured at ICU admission, H4, H8, and H12 using an automated analyzer (ABL800 Flex, Radiometer Medical Aps, Aakandevej 21, DK-2700 Bronshoj, Denmark).

Vasoactive-inotropic score (14) and $CO_2$-derived and $O_2$-derived variables were calculated as follows:

$$\text{Vasoactive-inotropic score} = \text{dopamine } (\mu g/kg/min) + \text{dobutamine } (\mu g/kg/min) + 10 \times \text{milrinone } (\mu g/kg/min)$$

$$+ 100 \times \text{epinephrine } (\mu g/kg/min) + 100 \times \text{norepinephrine } (\mu g/kg/min) + 10{,}000 \times \text{vasopressin } (\mu g/kg/min)$$

$$\Delta PCO_2 \,(mmHg) = P_{(cv-a)}CO_2 = P_{cv}CO_2 - P_aCO_2$$

$$C_aO_2(mL/L) = 1.34 \times S_aO_2 \times Hb$$

$$C_{cv}O_2(mL/L) = 1.34 \times S_{cv}O_2 \times Hb$$

$$C_{(a-cv)}O_2 \,(mL/L) = C_aO_2 - C_{cv}O_2$$

$$\Delta PCO_2/C_{(a-cv)}O_2(mmHg/mL) = P_{(cv-a)}CO_2/C_{(a-cv)}O_2 = (P_{cv}CO_2 - P_aCO_2)/\,(C_aO_2 - C_{cv}O_2)$$

$$\text{Oxygen extraction ratio}(O_2ER)(\%) = 1 - S_{cv}O_2/S_aO_2$$

The primary outcome variable was organ dysfunction at H48. Briefly, H48 organ dysfunction included: acute respiratory distress syndrome ($PaO_2$/fraction of inspired oxygen <300 mmHg or $PaO_2$ <60 mmHg requiring non-invasive ventilation or invasive mechanical ventilation support), acute kidney injury [Kidney Disease Improving Global Outcomes (KDIGO) level $\geq$1], acute tissue hypoperfusion (presence of tachycardia and hypotension associated with a central venous oxygen saturation <65%, cardiac index $\leq$2.2 L/min/m$^2$), cardiac arrest (15) (cessation of cardiac mechanical activity, as confirmed by the absence of circulation signs), arrhythmia (15) (atrial fibrillation for $\geq$1 min was recorded, analyzed, and defined as "postoperative atrial fibrillation;" ventricular tachycardia and ventricular fibrillation were recorded by continuous ECG monitoring during the intensive care stay), acute neurologic dysfunction (stroke, seizure, persistent delirium, and Glasgow coma score below 12). According to the presence or absence of organ dysfunction at 48 h after CPB, the patients were divided into organ dysfunction group (OI) and non-organ dysfunction group (n-OI). The OI group was further divided into two subgroups: OI-1 including patients with one organ dysfunction, and OI-2 including patients with two or more organ dysfunctions.

## Sample Size

GPower software version 3.0.10 was applied to estimate required sample size for this study. This study used repeated-measure, between factors for the analysis. The study effect size was set at 0.25, power was set at 90%, alpha value was set at 0.05, and four -time measurements. Based on these, a minimum total sample of 108 subjects is required.

## Statistical Analysis

The statistical analysis was carried out using IBM SPSS 20 software. The Kolmogorov–Smirnoff test evaluated the normality of continuous variables and found that many continuous variables were non-normally distributed. Consequently, all continuous variables were expressed as median. The Mann–Whitney U test or Kruskal–Wallis test was used for group comparison, and repeated-measures ANOVA was used for intragroup comparison. Chi-square test (or Fisher's exact test, when appropriate) was used to compare categorical variables. GraphPad prism version 8.0.2 statistical software was used for boxplot charts.

According to the occurrence of organ dysfunction at H48, the patients were divided into n-OI and OI groups, with the OI group being further subdivided into OI-1 and OI-2 subgroups according to the number of organs with evidence of dysfunction at H48. Comparisons took place within the OI group, within the n-OI group, between the OI and n-OI groups, and between the n-OI and OI-2 subgroups. The ROC curve analysis was carried out to assess the predictive performance of the variables independently associated with H48 organ dysfunction. The area under the curve (AUC) was calculated based on their 95% confidence intervals (CIs).

In a subsequent analysis, variables were introduced into the logistic regression model if significantly associated with H48 organ dysfunction at the univariate analysis, when $P$-value was < 0.05. A Hosmer–Lemeshow test was used to assess the goodness of fit of the model.

# RESULTS

## Clinical Characteristics and Prognosis

A total of 139 patients who fulfilled the criteria were screened and 114 patients were included (**Figure 1**). A total of 77 (67.5%) patients formed the n-OI group, and 37 (32.5%) patients comprised the OI group, of which 23.7% (27/114) had one organ dysfunction, 8.8% (10/114) had two or more organ dysfunctions. Compared to the OI group, the n-OI group had shorter length of stay in hospital [10.0 (8.5–14.0) vs. 13.0 (10.0–18.0) days, $P$ = 0.01], shorter length of ICU stay [42.0 (24.0–48.0) vs. 47.0 (27.0–66.5) h, $P$ = 0.02], and lower H24 and H48 sequential organ failure scores [3 (2–5) vs. 5 (4–7), $P$ = 0.01] and [4 (3–5) vs. 5 (3–6), $P$ = 0.02, respectively]. No statistical difference in the duration of mechanical ventilation was detected between the two groups

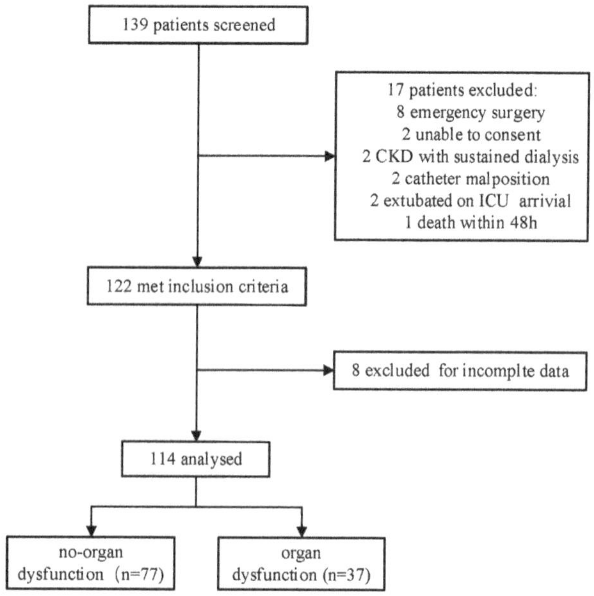


**FIGURE 1** | Study flow-chart. CKD, chronic kidney disease.

of patients [19.0 (16.4–21.0) vs. 20.2 (18.5–22.8) h, $P$ = 0.07] (**Table 1**).

## Dynamic Changes in $CO_2$-Derived Variables in n-OI and OI Groups

The length of ventilator usage in all patients was 19.5 (range: 17.0–21.0) h. In order to reduce the influence of spontaneous breathing on $CO_2$-derived variables after weaning, ICU admission, H4, H8, and H12 time points were selected for analysis.

The $\Delta PCO_2$ of the n-OI group at the four time points were 9.0 (7.0–11.0), 9.0 (7.0–11.0), 9.0 (7.0–11.0), and 9.0 (7.0–11.0) mmHg ($P$ = 0.84), and those of the OI group were 9.0 (8.0–12.8), 10.0 (7.0–11.0), 10.0 (8.5–12.5), and 9.0 (7.3–11.0) mmHg ($P$ = 0.37). The $\Delta PCO_2/C_{(a-cv)}O_2$ of the n-OI group at the four time points were 2.0 (1.6–2.7), 2.1 (1.7–2.8), 2.0 (1.5–2.3), and 2.0 (1.7–2.4) mmHg/mL ($P$ = 0.46), and those of the OI group were 2.1 (1.7–2.9), 2.2 (1.8–2.5), 2.1 (1.8–2.6), and 1.8 (1.6–2.5) mmHg/mL ($P$ = 0.39) (**Table 2**), respectively. There were no statistical differences in the $CO_2$-derived variables at any of the four time points ($P$ > 0.05) between the n-OI and OI groups (**Figure 2**). Statistically significant differences were observed intragroup for pH, $PO_2$, BE, Hb concentration, fraction of inspired oxygen, lactate level, fluid balance, and body temperature at all four time points (**Table 2**).

## The Prognostic Value of $CO_2$-Derived Variables

Regarding specific time point variables, $\Delta PCO_2$, $\Delta PCO_2/C_{(a-cv)}O_2$, lactate and BE had no predictive value (**Table 3**). Comparison of the subgroup OI-2 to the n-OI group demonstrated that lactate and BE had limited predictive value (**Table 4**). After adjusting for age (median, ≤58, >58 years old) and gender, H8 BE (odds ratio = 1.37, 95% CI: 1.08–1.74, $P$ = 0.009) was a risk factor for H48 organ dysfunction after CPB.

# DISCUSSION

## Clinical Implications

We found that the $\Delta PCO_2/C_{(a-cv)}O_2$ and $\Delta PCO_2$ did not differ significantly between the two groups at different time points during the first 12 h after ICU admission. Elevated $\Delta PCO_2$ and $\Delta PCO_2/C_{(a-cv)}O_2$ were common phenomena after CPB. The $\Delta PCO_2/C_{(a-cv)}O_2$ and $\Delta PCO_2$ cannot be used to predict H48 organ dysfunction. The predictive performance of lactate and BE was significantly enhanced as the number of dysfunctioning organs increased, although it was limited.

To the best of our knowledge, this study is the first to analyze the association of both $\Delta PCO_2$ and $\Delta PCO_2/C_{a-cv}O_2$ on 48 h-organ dysfunction after adult cardiac surgery. In our study, the $\Delta PCO_2$ value, CPB time, aortic clamping time, and sequential organ failure score at ICU admission were similar to Guinot et al. study (16). They also found that $\Delta PCO_2$ is not predictive of postoperative complications or mortality. Their research did not provide information on the tidal volume and $pCO_2$, which are thought to affect the accuracy of $\Delta PCO_2$ (17). Our study has very specific ventilator settings, which make up for this deficiency. Additionally, we found that rewarming, Hb dilution, and pH change were universal after CPB, which might have affected the accuracy of our estimations (18, 19). According to the literature, $pCO_2$ may be elevated due to the accumulation of $CO_2$ in tissues caused by reperfusion after CPB (20). Another study with negative results was reported by Morel et al. (21), who believe that $\Delta PCO_2$ is difficult to interpret due to the sudden variation of many parameters interfering with tissue perfusion. Such studies with negative results may have a common feature that outcomes may occur before measurement such as vasoplegia, heart failure, and acute renal failure. Furthermore, the complication itself may lead to an increased $\Delta PCO_2$ and, according to the time of measurement, the arrow of causation could be reversed (22). In our study, the median sequential organ failure score was 5, 4, and 3 at ICU admission, and 24 and 48 h post admission, respectively. Therefore, some of the organ dysfunction was suspected to have occurred during surgery. However, we believe that outcomes to be reliable as organ dysfunction generally results in poor outcomes (prolonged ICU stay, prolonged hospital stay).

A review of the literature also found studies with positive results. Mukai et al. (23) found that the $\Delta PCO_2$ at the end of cardiac surgery was a moderate predictor of postoperative complications (area under the curve [AUC]: 0.731; 95% confidence interval [CI] 0.588–0.874), at a 6.8 mmHg cut off with a sensitivity of 72.0% and specificity of 70.6%. Complications are defined as MMOM (major organ morbidity and mortality) (24), as follows: death, stroke requiring drug treatment, renal failure requiring dialysis, prolonged mechanical ventilation (more than 48 h postoperatively), re-operation, and deep sternal infection. It is worth noting that measurements were obtained at the end of surgery and the definition of complications were easy to identify.

**TABLE 1** | Clinical characteristics and prognosis of patients in the n-OI and OI groups ($N = 114$).

| | All ($N = 114$) | n-OI ($n = 77$) | OI ($n = 37$) | P-value |
|---|---|---|---|---|
| Age (years) | 58 (50–66) | 56 (47–64) | 63 (55–68) | 0.01* |
| **Sex** | | | | 0.32 |
| Male | 52 | 38 | 14 | |
| Female | 62 | 39 | 23 | |
| BMI (kg/m$^2$) | 22.7 (20.7–24.9) | 22.2 (20.1–24.6) | 23.4 (21.7–25.3) | 0.048* |
| **Type of surgery** | | | | 0.58 |
| Valve replacement (or plastic) | 81 | 56 | 25 | |
| CABG | 3 | 1 | 2 | |
| Combined surgery | 13 | 8 | 5 | |
| Other | 17 | 12 | 5 | |
| Duration of surgery (h) | 4.3 (3.5–5.0) | 4.0 (3.5–5.0) | 4.5 (3.6–5.0) | 0.31 |
| CBP duration (min) | 100 (78–135) | 100 (80–135) | 100 (75–145) | 0.90 |
| Aortic clamping duration (min) | 65 (45–80) | 65 (45–80) | 60 (50–80) | 0.94 |
| Pacemaker (yes /no) | 35/79 | 26/51 | 9/28 | 0.39 |
| **Comorbidities** | | | | 0.38 |
| Hypertension | 45 | 27 | 18 | |
| COPD | 3 | 3 | 0 | |
| Diabetes | 8 | 3 | 5 | |
| Stroke | 6 | 4 | 2 | |
| Chronic kidney disease | 2 | 1 | 1 | |
| Malignant cancer | 2 | 0 | 2 | |
| Gastrointestinal disease | 4 | 3 | 1 | |
| Coronary artery disease | 1 | 0 | 1 | |
| Vascular disease | 3 | 2 | 1 | |
| NYHA | | | | 0.93 |
| I | 8 | 5 | 3 | |
| II | 74 | 50 | 24 | |
| III | 30 | 21 | 9 | |
| IV | 2 | 1 | 1 | |
| EuroSCORE | 3 (2–5) | 3 (1–4.5) | 4 (1–5.5) | 0.08 |
| APACHEII (H24) | 6 (4–8) | 6 (4–7) | 7 (4–10) | 0.16 |
| SOFA (H24) | 4 (2–5) | 3 (2–5) | 5 (4–7) | 0.01* |
| APACHEII (H48) | 11 (9–15) | 11 (9–14) | 12 (9–16) | 0.46 |
| SOFA (H48) | 3 (4-5) | 4 (3–5) | 5 (3–6) | 0.02* |
| Length of ventilator (h) | 19.5 (17.0–21.0) | 19.0 (16.4–21.0) | 20.2 (18.5–22.8) | 0.07 |
| LOS in ICU (h) | 44.0 (24.9–48.5) | 42.0 (24.0–48.0) | 47.0 (27.0–66.5) | 0.02* |
| LOS in hospital (days) | 11.0 (9.0–15.0) | 10.0 (8.5–14.0) | 13.0 (10.0–18.0) | 0.01* |

*CABG, coronary artery bypass grafting; COPD, chronic obstructive pulmonary disease; NYHA, New York Heart Association functional classification; Euro SCORE, European system for cardiac operative risk evaluation; APACHE II, acute physiology and chronic health status score II; SOFA, sequential organ failure score; ICU admission, immediately after entering ICU; H24, 24 h after entering ICU; H48, 48 h after entering ICU. Continuous variables are represented by median (IQR). The Mann–Whitney U test was used for intergroup comparison. Categorical variables were used by Fisher's exact test; *$P < 0.05$.*

Hence, we cannot exclude that perioperative $\Delta PCO_2$ could be predictive of outcome (21). A previous study reported that $\Delta PCO_2/C_{(a-cv)}O_2$ is not associated with respiratory quotient (25). In our study, $\Delta PCO_2/C_{(a-cv)}O_2$ was not associated with the existence of tissue hypoxia effectively because of its poor relationship with lactate ($R^2$ =0.067). $\Delta PCO_2/C_{(a-cv)}O_2$ was grouped according to whether it was $\geq$1.4 mmHg/mL, and no statistical significance were detected in the length of the ventilator, LOS in ICU, or the 24 h and 48 h sequential organ failure score (data not provided). That is probably largely because of the influence of CPB on the activation of inflammation *in vivo*, ischemia-reperfusion injury, myocardial suppression, and other factors, thus, a microcirculation disorder exists that can last for 72 h (26). From our research, we have observed many factors that affect $CO_2$-derived indicators after cardiac surgery in the real world, including CBP itself (27), translocation, endothelial dysfunction (28, 29), and microcirculation alterations (30) may directly or indirectly cause complications, making the interpretation of the results more complicated.

**TABLE 2 |** Clinical data on ICU admission and at H4, H8, H12 post admission in n-OI and OI groups.

| | n-OI ($n = 77$) | | | | *P*-value | OI ($n = 37$) | | | | *P*-value |
|---|---|---|---|---|---|---|---|---|---|---|
| | **ICU admission** | **H4** | **H8** | **H12** | | **ICU admission** | **H4** | **H8** | **H12** | |
| pH | 7.40 (7.35–7.45) | 7.37(7.31–7.43)* | 7.38(7.32–7.43) | 7.39 (7.35–7.42) | < 0.01 | 7.39 (7.31–7.43) | 7.35(7.29–7.43) | 7.37(7.30–7.41) | 7.39 (7.33–7.44)† | 0.02 |
| $P_aCO_2$ (mmHg) | 39.0 (35.0–43.0) | 39.0 (35.0–43.0) | 38.0 (34.5–41.5) | 37.0 (34.0–41.0) | 0.15 | 38.0 (35.0–43.0) | 38.0 (35.0–43.5) | 38.0 (33.5–41.0) | 35.0 (32.5–40.0) | 0.10 |
| $P_aO_2$ (mmHg) | 155 (113–186) | 169 (150–190) | 162 (145–181) | 159 (141–180) | 0.04 | 138 (102–163) | 151 (127–175) | 155 (123–179) | 146 (115–170) | 0.24 |
| BE (mmol/L) | −0.3 (−2.2,−1.7) | −2.2 (−5.1,−0.7)* | −2.7 (−5.3,−0.8)** | −2.2 (−3.9,−0.7)¶ | < 0.01 | −1.0 (−4.2–0.5) | −2.6 (−6.8–0.8)* | −3.0 (−6.5,−1.6) | −2.2 (−5.3,−0.7) | 0.01 |
| Hemoglobin (g/L) | 109.0 (101.0–124.0) | 116.5 (105.0–128.8)* | 112.0 (102.5–129.5) | 112.0 (99.3–122.5)† | 0.01 | 116.0 (103.0–125.0) | 121.0(101.0–129.0) | 115.0 (99.0–127.0) | 107.0 (95.5–127.5) | 0.17 |
| $FiO_2$ (%) | 50 (40–54) | 43 (40–50)* | 40 (40–50)** | 40 (40–45)†¶ | < 0.01 | 50 (40–50) | 40 (40–50) | 40 (40–50) | 40 (40–45)¶ | < 0.01 |
| $S_aO_2$ (%) | 99 (99–100) | 99 (99–100) | 99 (99–100) | 99 (99–100) | 0.15 | 99 (98–100) | 99 (98–99) | 99 (98–100) | 99 (99–100) | 0.18 |
| Lactate (mmol/L) | 2.6 (1.7–3.7) | 3.1 (2.0–5.1)* | 3.5 (2.3–5.5)** | 3.3 (2.5–5.3)¶ | < 0.01 | 3.0 (1.9–5.1) | 4.1 (2.0–6.1) | 4.2 (2.6–7.0)** | 3.9 (2.8–6.3) | < 0.01 |
| $S_{cv}O_2$ (%) | 71 (61–79) | 72 (62–78) | 69 (64–76) | 71 (59–78) | 0.80 | 68 (61–79) | 70 (63–79) | 68 (61–75) | 68 (62–73) | 0.57 |
| $\Delta PCO_2$ (mmHg) | 9.0 (7.0–11.0) | 9.0 (7.0–11.0) | 9.0 (7.0–11.0) | 9.0 (7.0–11.0) | 0.84 | 9.0 (8.0–12.8) | 10.0 (7.0–11.0) | 10.0 (8.5–12.5) | 9.0 (7.3–11.0) | 0.37 |
| $S_aO_2$–$S_{cv}O_2$ (%) | 29 (20–38) | 27 (21–35) | 31 (23–36) | 29 (21–39) | 0.71 | 31 (22–40) | 27 (20–38) | 31 (21–39) | 31 (26–38) | 0.52 |
| $C_{a\text{-}cv}O_2$ (mL/ L) | 4.1 (3.1–5.4) | 4.2 (3.0–5.5) | 4.5 (3.7–5.4) | 4.2 (3.2–5.8) | 0.52 | 4.4 (3.8–5.5) | 4.3 (3.3–5.5) | 4.5 (3.4–5.9) | 4.8 (3.8–5.3) | 0.52 |
| $\Delta PCO_2/C_{(a-cv)}O_2$ (mmHg/mL) | 2.0 (1.6–2.7) | 2.1 (1.7–2.8) | 2.0 (1.5–2.3) | 2.0 (1.7–2.4) | 0.46 | 2.1 (1.7–2.9) | 2.2 (1.8–2.5) | 2.1 (1.8–2.6) | 1.8 (1.6–2.5) | 0.39 |
| $O_2ER$ (%) | 29 (20–38) | 27 (21–35) | 31 (23–36) | 29 (21–39) | 0.70 | 31 (23–40) | 27 (20–38) | 31 (22–39) | 40 (27–38) | 0.53 |
| **Ventilator setting** | | | | | | | | | | |
| Tidal volume (mL) | 453 (406–498) | 448 (406–496) | 450 (405–500) | 459 (407–500) | 0.54 | 454 (442–500) | 462 (432–497) | 461 (425–501) | 466 (439–507) | 0.56 |
| Frequency (/min) | 15.0 (15.0–16.0) | 15.0 (15.0–16.0) | 15.0 (15.0–16.0) | 15.0 (15.0–16.0) | 0.96 | 15.0 (15.0–16.0) | 15.0 (15.0–16.0) | 15.0 (15.0–16.0) | 15.0 (15.0–16.0) | 0.72 |
| PEEP ($cmH_2O$) | 5.0 (4.0–5.0) | 5.0 (3.0–5.0) | 5.0 (4.0–5.0) | 5.0 (4.0–5.0) | 0.84 | 5.0 (4.0–5.0) | 5.0 (5.0–5.0) | 5.0 (4.0–5.0) | 5.0 (4.0–5.0) | 0.78 |
| **Fluid challenge** | | | | | | | | | | |
| Intake (mL) | 1845 (1500–2273) | 640 (470–852)* | 1130 (855–1483)‡** | 1470 (1083–1883)¶†ξ | < 0.01 | 1651 (1275–2370) | 530 (385–749)* | 1045 (885–1248)‡** | 1455 (1138–1828)†ξ | < 0.01 |
| Output (mL) | 1300 (1000–2000) | 690 (530–893)* | 1015 (818–1300)‡** | 1285 (1040–1620)†ξ | < 0.01 | 1500 (1075–2275) | 635 (490–968)* | 955 (770–1349)‡** | 1170 (990–1628)†ξ | < 0.01 |
| Fluid balance (mL) | 261 (-25–757) | −66 (-295–250)* | 88 (-180–521)‡ | 140 (-182–541)† | < 0.01 | 350 (-230–900) | −90 (-398–112)* | 15 (-298–327)‡ | 115 (-90–588)†ξ | < 0.01 |
| **VIS** | 4.0 (2.0–6.8) | 4.0 (2.0–8.0) | 4.0 (1.9–9.0) | 4.0 (1.0–9.0) | 0.36 | 4.0 (2.0–6.0) | 5.3 (1.3–10.8) | 5.5 (2.0–11.8) | 5.0 (2.0–11.8) | 0.10 |
| **Vital signs** | | | | | | | | | | |
| SBP (mmHg) | 105 (100–121) | 105 (93–112) | 103 (96–112) | 104 (98–113) | 0.06 | 105 (92–116) | 103 (94–114) | 103 (95–113) | 108 (102–115) | 0.24 |
| DBP (mmHg) | 60 (54–68) | 57 (53–63) | 58 (54–64) | 59 (54–64) | 0.10 | 59 (54–66) | 59 (55–65) | 55 (51–64) | 58 (51–66) | 0.16 |
| MAP (mmHg) | 76 (68–85) | 72 (68–79) | 72 (69–78) | 73 (67–79) | 0.09 | 73 (66–80) | 75 (68–79) | 74 (65–80) | 73 (70–81) | 0.76 |
| CVP (mmHg) | 8 (7–11) | 8 (7–10) | 8 (6–10) | 7 (6–10) | 0.14 | 8 (5–10) | 8 (6–9) | 8 (6–10) | 8 (6–11) | 0.86 |
| Temperature (°C) | 37.0 (36.0–37.0) | 36.7 (36.5–37.0)* | 37.0(36.5–37.3)‡** | 37.1 (36.6–37.4)¶† | < 0.01 | 37.0 (36.0–37.0) | 36.5 (36.25–37.0) | 36.8 (36.5–37.2)** | 37.2 (37.0–37.6)¶† | < 0.01 |
| Respiratory rate (/min) | 15 (15–16) | 15 (15–16) | 15 (15–16) | 15 (15–16) | 0.89 | 15 (15–16) | 15 (15–16) | 15 (15–16) | 15 (15–16) | 0.75 |
| Heart rate (/min) | 85 (78–91) | 83 (76–92) | 83 (74–92) | 81 (74–89) | 0.22 | 89 (79–99) | 86 (75–99) | 84 (71–96) | 84 (80–96) | 0.42 |

*$P_aCO_2$, arterial partial pressure of carbon dioxide; $P_aO_2$, arterial partial pressure of oxygen; BE, base excess; $FiO_2$, fraction of inspiration $O_2$; $S_aO_2$, arterial oxygen saturation; $S_{cv}O_2$, central venous oxygen saturation; $\Delta PCO_2$, central venous-to-arterial carbon dioxide difference; $\Delta PCO_2/C_{(a-cv)}O_2$, $\Delta PCO_2$ to arterial-central venous oxygen content difference rate; $O_2ER$, oxygen extraction ratio; VIS, vasoactive-inotropic score; SBP, systolic pressure; DBP, diastolic pressure; MAP, mean arterial pressure; CVP, central venous pressure. Continuous variables are represented by median (IQR). Repeated-measures ANOVA was used for intragroup comparison. *$P < 0.05$ for groups H0 vs. H4, **$P < 0.05$ for groups H0 vs. H8, ¶$P < 0.05$ for groups H0 vs. H12, ‡ $P < 0.05$ for groups H4 vs. H8, †$P < 0.05$ for groups H4 vs. H12, ξ $P < 0.05$ for groups H8 vs. H12.*

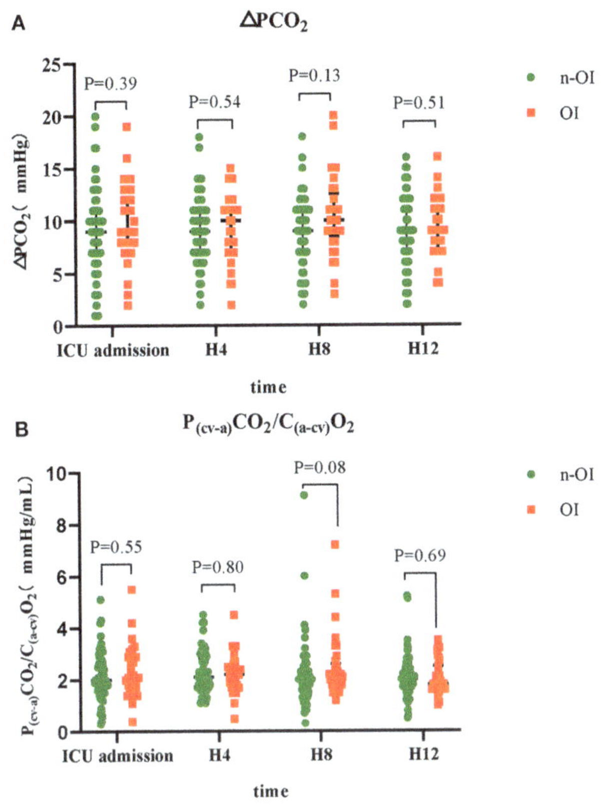


**FIGURE 2 |** Dynamic changes of carbon dioxide-derived variables of n-OI and OI groups at the four time points. **(A)** central venous-to-arterial carbon dioxide difference ($\Delta PCO_2$) **(B)** $\Delta PCO_2$ to arterial-central venous oxygen content difference rate ($\Delta PCO_2/C_{(a-cv)}O_2$). GraphPad prism version 8.0.2 statistical software was used to construct box charts (median with interquartile range). The Mann–Whitney U test was used for intergroup comparison.

Hyperlactatemia is common after cardiopulmonary bypass, and it can be influenced by many factors. Patients undergoing CPB are exposed to the "elution effect," i.e., the release of lactic acid from the lungs (31) and the liver due to organ malfunction associated with CPB (32). A recent study has demonstrated that hyperlactatemia may be also in relation to tissue metabolic uncoupling (33). Therefore, lactic acid does not always reflect tissue hypoxia. The predictive value of lactate after CPB surgery is limited. This study demonstrated that postoperative lactic acidemia is common, with progressively decreasing levels of lactic acid observed in both groups. After adjustment for confounding factors, compared to $\Delta PCO_2$ and $\Delta PCO_2/C(a\text{-}cv)O_2$, lactic acid has a moderate ability to predict two or more organ dysfunction. In addition, BE is the amount of base in mmol required to titrate 1 L of whole arterial blood to a pH of 7.40, with the sample fully saturated with oxygen at 37°C and a $P_aCO_2$ of 40 mmHg. We also found that BE was a more robust predictor of H48 organ dysfunction than lactic acid, and H8 BE was a risk factor for dysfunction of two or more organs (odds ratio = 1.37), whereas lactic acid was not. A high negative value of BE may be associated with renal dysfunction, metabolic acidosis, and shock, but the factors associated with the reduced systemic BE in patients after cardiac surgery are yet to be clarified (34). We speculated that lactic acidosis might be one of the main

**TABLE 3 |** Area under the ROC curve of variables grouped into n-OI and OI.

| Variable | AUC | Standard error | *P*-value | 95% CI |
|---|---|---|---|---|
| ICU admission$\Delta PCO_2$ | 0.571 | 0.072 | 0.334 | 0.430–0.711 |
| H4$\Delta PCO_2$ | 0.514 | 0.076 | 0.843 | 0.366–0.663 |
| H8$\Delta PCO_2$ | 0.588 | 0.072 | 0.230 | 0.447–0.729 |
| H12$\Delta PCO_2$ | 0.566 | 0.070 | 0.366 | 0.429–0.704 |
| ICU admission $\Delta PCO_2/C_{(a-cv)}O_2$ | 0.510 | 0.075 | 0.892 | 0.363–0.658 |
| H4$\Delta PCO_2/C_{(a-cv)}O_2$ | 0.479 | 0.074 | 0.776 | 0.333–0.625 |
| H8$\Delta PCO_2/C_{(a-cv)}O_2$ | 0.588 | 0.071 | 0.236 | 0.449–0.728 |
| H12$\Delta PCO_2/C_{(a-cv)}O_2$ | 0.443 | 0.076 | 0.448 | 0.295–0.592 |
| ICU admission Lactate | 0.586 | 0.063 | 0.150 | 0.463–0.710 |
| H4 Lactate | 0.569 | 0.063 | 0.254 | 0.446–0.691 |
| H8 Lactate | 0.567 | 0.060 | 0.265 | 0.449–0.685 |
| H12 Lactate | 0.574 | 0.063 | 0.219 | 0.451–0.697 |
| ICU admission Base excess | 0.608 | 0.058 | 0.069 | 0.494–0.722 |
| H4 Base excess | 0.578 | 0.059 | 0.190 | 0.463–0.693 |
| H8 Base excess | 0.594 | 0.058 | 0.112 | 0.481–0.708 |
| H12 Base excess | 0.544 | 0.061 | 0.462 | 0.423–0.664 |

*$\Delta PCO_2$, central venous-to-arterial carbon dioxide difference; $\Delta PCO_2/C_{(a-cv)}O_2$, $\Delta PCO_2$ to arterial-central venous oxygen content difference rate. SPSS 20 statistical software.*

**TABLE 4 |** Area under the ROC curve of variables grouped into n-OI and OI-2.

| Variable | AUC | Standard error | *P*-value | 95% CI |
|---|---|---|---|---|
| ICU admission$\Delta PCO_2$ | 0.538 | 0.105 | 0.713 | 0.333–0.744 |
| H4$\Delta PCO_2$ | 0.549 | 0.118 | 0.636 | 0.318–0.780 |
| H8$\Delta PCO_2$ | 0.591 | 0.118 | 0.380 | 0.360–0.822 |
| H12$\Delta PCO_2$ | 0.456 | 0.119 | 0.674 | 0.224–0.689 |
| ICU admission $\Delta PCO_2/C_{(a-cv)}O_2$ | 0.562 | 0.109 | 0.550 | 0.348–0.777 |
| H4$\Delta PCO_2/C_{(a-cv)}O_2$ | 0.670 | 0.100 | 0.104 | 0.473–0.866 |
| H8$\Delta PCO_2/C_{(a-cv)}O_2$ | 0.700 | 0.104 | 0.055 | 0.497–0.903 |
| H12$\Delta PCO_2/C_{(a-cv)}O_2$ | 0.557 | 0.119 | 0.581 | 0.324–0.791 |
| ICU admission Lactate | 0.635 | 0.103 | 0.195 | 0.434–0.837 |
| H4 Lactate | 0.634 | 0.098 | 0.198 | 0.442–0.826 |
| H8 Lactate | 0.715 | 0.099 | 0.039* | 0.521–0.908 |
| H12 Lactate | 0.634 | 0.123 | 0.198 | 0.393–0.875 |
| ICU admission Base excess | 0.662 | 0.103 | 0.093 | 0.459–0.864 |
| H4 Base excess | 0.723 | 0.104 | 0.021* | 0.519–0.926 |
| H8 Base excess | 0.831 | 0.061 | 0.001* | 0.710–0.951 |
| H12 Base excess | 0.703 | 0.103 | 0.035* | 0.501–0.904 |

*$\Delta PCO_2$, central venous-to-arterial carbon dioxide difference; $\Delta PCO_2/C_{(a-cv)}O_2$, $\Delta PCO_2$ to arterial-central venous oxygen content difference rate. SPSS 20 statistical software. *$P < 0.05$.*

reasons leading to the high negative value of BE because a good correlation was established between BE and lactic acid ($R2 = 0.599$, $P < 0.05$), which could also explain the low susceptibility of BE to interference from other factors.

## Methodological Considerations

This study has some limitations. First, this was a single-center study, and its results may not be generalizable. Second, the sample size was relatively small, and no deaths occurred among the study patients. Third, because the group classification was based solely on the occurrence of organ dysfunction, a misclassification bias may have occurred. However, our subgroup analysis was based on the number of failing organs and resulted in similar conclusions. Fourth, $P_{cv-a}CO_2/C_{(a-cv)}O_2$ cannot replace $P_{mv-a}CO_2/C_{(a-cv)}O_2$ (mv: mixed venous blood) and might have underestimated the $CO_2$ exchange from splanchnic circulation. Finally, it was not easy to detect when the outcome of interest, i.e., organ dysfunction, first occurred relative to the measurement. Continuous measurements or change over time may have more prognostic value than a single time point. However, the dynamic changes of $\Delta PCO_2$ at t0 and T6 time points were not found to be associated with postoperative complications or mortality in children after CPB (16).

# CONCLUSION

In conclusion, $\Delta PCO_2$ and $\Delta PCO_2/C_{(a-cv)}O_2$ cannot be used as reliable indicators to predict the occurrence of organ dysfunction at 48 h after CBP, which is due to the complex pathophysiological processes after CBP.

# ETHICS STATEMENT

The studies involving human participants were reviewed and approved by Ethics Committee of Taizhou Hospital, Zhejiang Province. The patients/participants provided their written informed consent to participate in this study. Written informed consent was obtained from the individual(s) for the publication of any potentially identifiable images or data included in this article.

# AUTHOR CONTRIBUTIONS

SZ: data curation, investigation, resources, writing—original draft, validation, and funding acquisition. DZ: data curation, investigation, and methodology. X-QC: data curation, investigation, methodology, and software. Y-PJ, L-ZQ, W-YY, and W-YZ: data curation, investigation, and resources. C-GW: data curation and formal analysis. Q-MZ: data curation and resources. T-HT: design of the study and performed data synthesis of the revised stage. R-HL: conceptualization, data curation, formal analysis, funding acquisition, software, validation, writing—review, and editing. All authors have read and approved the manuscript.

# ACKNOWLEDGMENTS

The authors kindly thank Dr. Zhang Meixian for her contribution to establishing the database.

# REFERENCES

1. D'Agostino RS, Jacobs JP, Badhwar V, Fernandez FG, Paone G, Wormuth DW, et al. The society of thoracic surgeons adult cardiac surgery database: 2018 update on outcomes and quality. *Ann Thorac Surg.* (2018) 105:15–23. doi: 10.1016/j.athoracsur.2017.10.035
2. Mallat J, Lemyze M, Tronchon L, Vallet B, Thevenin D. Use of venous-to-arterial carbon dioxide tension difference to guide resuscitation therapy in septic shock. *World J Crit Care Med.* (2016) 5:47–56. doi: 10.5492/wjccm.v5.i1.47
3. Mekontso-Dessap A, Castelain V, Anguel N, Bahloul M, Schauvliege F, Richard C, et al. Combination of venoarterial $PCO_2$ difference with arteriovenous O2 content difference to detect anaerobic metabolism in patients. *Intensive Care Med.* (2002) 28:272–7. doi: 10.1007/s00134-002-1215-8
4. Ospina-Tascón GA, Umaña M, Bermúdez W, Bautista-Rincón DF, Hernandez G, Bruhn A, et al. Combination of arterial lactate levels and venous-arterial $CO_2$ to arterial-venous $O_2$ content difference ratio as markers of resuscitation in patients with septic shock. *Intensive Care Med.* (2015) 41:796–805. doi: 10.1007/s00134-015-3720-6
5. Ospina-Tascón GA, Bautista-Rincón DF, Umaña M, Tafur JD, Gutiérrez A, García AF, et al. Persistently high venous-to-arterial carbon dioxide differences during early resuscitation are associated with poor outcomes in septic shock. *Crit Care.* (2013) 17:R294. doi: 10.1186/cc13160
6. Robin E, Futier E, Pires O, Fleyfel M, Tavernier B, Lebuffe G, et al. Central venous-to-arterial carbon dioxide difference as a prognostic tool in high-risk surgical patients. *Crit Care.* (2015) 19:227. doi: 10.1186/s13054-015-0917-6
7. Futier E, Robin E, Jabaudon M, Guerin R, Petit A, Bazin JE, et al. Central venous $O_2$ saturation and venous-to-arterial $CO_2$ difference as complementary tools for goal-directed therapy during high-risk surgery. *Crit Care.* (2010) 14:R193. doi: 10.1186/cc9310
8. Ospina-Tascón GA, Calderón Tapia LE. Venous-arterial $CO_2$ to arterial-venous $O_2$ differences: a physiological meaning debate. *J Crit Care.* (2018) 48:443–4. doi: 10.1016/j.jcrc.2018.09.030
9. Huette P, Ellouze O, Abou-Arab O, Guinot PG. Venous-to-arterial $pCO_2$ difference in high-risk surgical patients. *J Thorac Dis.* (2019) 11:S1551–7. doi: 10.21037/jtd.2019.01.109
10. Abou-Arab O, Braik R, Huette P, Bouhemad B, Lorne E, Guinot PG. The ratios of central venous to arterial carbon dioxide content and tension to arteriovenous oxygen content are not associated with overall anaerobic metabolism in postoperative cardiac surgery patients. *PLoS ONE.* (2018) 13:e0205950. doi: 10.1371/journal.pone.0205950
11. O'Connor E, Fraser JF. The interpretation of perioperative lactate abnormalities in patients undergoing cardiac surgery. *Anaesth Intensive Care.* (2012) 40:598–603. doi: 10.1177/0310057X1204000404
12. Stoppe C, McDonald B, Benstoem C, Elke G, Meybohm P, Whitlock R, et al. Evaluation of persistent organ dysfunction plus death as a novel composite outcome in cardiac surgical patients. *J Cardiothorac Vasc Anesth.* (2016) 30:30–8. doi: 10.1053/j.jvca.2015.07.035
13. Heyland DK, Muscedere J, Drover J, Jiang X, Day AG, Canadian Critical Care Trials Group. Persistent organ dysfunction plus death: a novel, composite outcome measure for critical care trials. *Crit Care.* (2011) 15:R98. doi: 10.1186/cc10110
14. Gaies MG, Gurney JG, Yen AH, Napoli ML, Gajarski RJ, Ohye RG, et al. Vasoactive-inotropic score as a predictor of morbidity and mortality in infants after cardiopulmonary bypass. *Pediatr Crit Care Med.* (2010) 11:234–8. doi: 10.1097/PCC.0b013e3181b806fc
15. Jammer I, Wickboldt N, Sander M, Smith A, Schultz MJ, Pelosi P, et al. Standards for definitions and use of outcome measures for clinical effectiveness research in perioperative medicine: European perioperative clinical outcome (EPCO) definitions: a statement from the ESA-ESICM joint

taskforce on perioperative outcome measures. *Eur J Anaesthesiol.* (2015) 32:88–105. doi: 10.1097/EJA.0000000000000118

16. Guinot PG, Badoux L, Bernard E, Abou-Arab O, Lorne E, Dupont H. Central venous-to-arterial carbon dioxide partial pressure difference in patients undergoing cardiac surgery is not related to postoperative outcomes. *J Cardiothorac Vasc Anesth.* (2017) 31:1190–6. doi: 10.1053/j.jvca.2017.02.015
17. Mallat J, Mohammad U, Lemyze M, Meddour M, Jonard M, Pepy F, et al. Acute hyperventilation increases the central venous-to-arterial $PCO_2$ difference in stable septic shock patients. *Ann Intensive Care.* (2017) 7:31. doi: 10.1186/s13613-017-0258-5
18. Dubin A, Ferrara G, Kanoore Edul VS, Martins E, Canales HS, Canullán C, et al. Venoarterial $PCO_2$-to-arteriovenous oxygen content difference ratio is a poor surrogate for anaerobic metabolism in hemodilution: an experimental study. *Ann Intensive Care.* (2017) 7:65. doi: 10.1186/s13613-017-0288-z
19. Ospina-Tascón GA, Hernández G, Cecconi M. Understanding the venous-arterial $CO_2$ to arterial-venous $O_2$ content difference ratio. *Intensive Care Med.* (2016) 42:1801–4. doi: 10.1007/s00134-016-4233-7
20. Jakob SM, Groeneveld AB, Teboul JL. Venous-arterial $CO_2$ to arterial-venous $O_2$ difference ratio as a resuscitation target in shock states? *Intensive Care Med.* (2015) 41:936–8. doi: 10.1007/s00134-015-3778-1
21. Morel J, Grand N, Axiotis G, Bouchet JB, Faure M, Auboyer C, et al. High veno-arterial carbon dioxide gradient is not predictive of worst outcome after an elective cardiac surgery: a retrospective cohort study. *J Clin Monit Comput.* (2016) 30:783–9. doi: 10.1007/s10877-016-9855-3
22. Huette P, Beyls C, Mallat J, Martineau L, Besserve P, Haye G, et al. Central venous-to-arterial $CO_2$ difference is a poor tool to predict adverse outcomes after cardiac surgery: a retrospective study. *Can J Anaesth.* (2021) 68:467–76. doi: 10.1007/s12630-020-01881-4
23. Mukai A, Suehiro K, Kimura A, Funai Y, Matsuura T, Tanaka K, et al. Comparison of the venous-arterial $CO_2$ to arterial-venous $O_2$ content difference ratio with the venous-arterial $CO_2$ gradient for the predictability of adverse outcomes after cardiac surgery. *J Clin Monit Comput.* (2020) 34:41–53. doi: 10.1007/s10877-019-00286-z
24. Shroyer AL, Coombs LP, Peterson ED, Eiken MC, DeLong ER, Chen A, et al. The society of thoracic surgeons: 30-day operative mortality and morbidity risk models. *Ann Thorac Surg.* (2003) 75:1856–64. doi: 10.1016/S0003-4975(03)00179-6
25. Bar S, Grenez C, Nguyen M, de Broca B, Bernard E, Abou-Arab O, et al. Predicting postoperative complications with the respiratory exchange ratio after high-risk noncardiac surgery: a prospective cohort study. *Eur J Anaesthesiol.* (2020) 37:1050–7. doi: 10.1097/EJA.0000000000001111
26. Dekker NAM, Veerhoek D, Koning NJ, van Leeuwen ALI, Elbers PWG, van den Brom CE, et al. Postoperative microcirculatory perfusion and endothelial glycocalyx shedding following cardiac surgery with cardiopulmonary bypass. *Anaesthesia.* (2019) 74:609–18. doi: 10.1111/anae.14577
27. McGuinness J, Bouchier-Hayes D, Redmond JM. Understanding the inflammatory response to cardiac surgery. *Surgeon.* (2008) 6:162–71. doi: 10.1016/S1479-666X(08)80113-8
28. Magoon R, Makhija N. Endothelial glycocalyx and cardiac surgery: newer insights. *J Cardiothorac Vasc Anesth.* (2020) 34:310–1. doi: 10.1053/j.jvca.2019.07.003
29. Brettner F, Chappell D, Schwartz L, Lukasz A, Kümpers P, Becker BF, et al. Vascular endothelial dysfunction during cardiac surgery: on-pump versus off-pump coronary surgery. *Eur Surg Res.* (2017) 58:354–68. doi: 10.1159/000480431
30. Kara A, Akin S, Ince C. The response of the microcirculation to cardiac surgery. *Curr Opin Anaesthesiol.* (2016) 29:85–93. doi: 10.1097/ACO.0000000000000280
31. Gasparovic H, Plestina S, Sutlic Z, Husedzinovic I, Coric V, Ivancan V, et al. Pulmonary lactate release following cardiopulmonary bypass. *Eur J Cardiothorac Surg.* (2007) 32:882–7. doi: 10.1016/j.ejcts.2007.09.001
32. Mustafa I, Roth H, Hanafiah A, Hakim T, Anwar M, Siregar E, et al. Effect of cardiopulmonary bypass on lactate metabolism. *Intensive Care Med.* (2003) 29:1279–85. doi: 10.1007/s00134-003-1860-6
33. Bar S, Nguyen M, de Broca B, Bernard E, Dupont H, Guinot PG. Risk factors and determinants of intraoperative hyperlactatemia in major non-cardiac surgery. *J Clin Anesth.* (2021) 74:110359. doi: 10.1016/j.jclinane.2021.110359
34. Zante B, Reichenspurner H, Kubik M, Kluge S, Schefold JC, Pfortmueller CA. Base excess is superior to lactate-levels in prediction of ICU mortality after cardiac surgery. *PLoS ONE.* (2018) 13:e0205309. doi: 10.1371/journal.pone.0205309

# 18

# Concomitant Atrial Fibrillation Procedures During Cardiac Surgery in a UK Center: Reflection of Worldwide Practice?

*Alina-Adriana Mistirian, Martin T. Yates and Wael I. Awad**

*Department of Cardiothoracic Surgery, St Bartholomew's Hospital, London, United Kingdom*

***Correspondence:**
*Wael I. Awad*
*wael.awad@nhs.net*

**Background:** Guidelines recommend concomitant atrial fibrillation (AF) ablation during cardiac surgery to restore normal sinus rhythm (NSR). The study determines, to what extent patients with AF undergoing cardiac surgery at our institution received a concomitant AF procedure, what these procedures entailed, and short-term outcomes.

**Methods:** A retrospective study of 2,984 patients undergoing cardiac surgery over 18 months. Patients who were in preoperative AF were identified and those who underwent a concomitant AF procedure (Group 1) were compared with those who did not (Group 2).

**Results:** Three hundred and thirteen (10.5%) patients had pre-operative AF; paroxysmal (19.5%), persistent (11.8%), longstanding (63%), unknown (5.8%). 116/313 (37.1%) patients had a concomitant AF procedure: 7.7% patients had a concomitant AF ablation and 29.4% had only a Left Atrial Appendage Occlusion (LAAO). Fewer patients with paroxysmal and persistent AF underwent concomitant AF procedures compared with the ones who had no AF procedures (6.7 vs. 12.8% and 17.6 vs. 31%, respectively). Greater in-hospital survival (99.1 vs. 93.9%, $p = 0.025$) and survival at a mean follow up of 6 weeks (97.4 vs. 89.3%, $p = 0.09$) was probably determined by patient's preoperative comorbidities. There were no differences in readmission rates, permanent pacemaker insertion, cerebral events or NSR at discharge or follow-up, between groups.

**Conclusions:** In our center, concomitant AF ablation is performed only in 7.7% of cases, 29.4% had only an LAAO performed at the time of surgery. There was no difference in restoring NSR, cerebral events, or readmission rates compared with patients who had nothing done for their preoperative AF.

**Keywords: atrial fibrillation, concomitant ablation, cardiac surgery, Cox-Maze, left atrial appendage occlusion**

## INTRODUCTION

Atrial fibrillation (AF) is a common supraventricular arrhythmia, with increased prevalence with increasing age. The incidence of AF is greater in patients who have significant coronary artery disease or valvular heart pathology (1). AF is associated with a five-fold risk of stroke, a three-fold incidence of congestive heart failure, higher hospitalization and mortality (2). It significantly impairs patients' quality of life and reduces long-term survival. Management strategies include rate and rhythm control, anticoagulation following risk assessment for stroke and bleeding, and AF ablation.

AF ablation can be performed as a stand-alone surgical procedure, on a beating heart, via thoracotomy or sub-xiphoid approach or using cardio-pulmonary bypass, through mini or full midline sternotomy or concomitantly with other cardiac surgery, with good results reported (2). Concomitant AF ablation can vary from pulmonary vein isolation to a bi-atrial ablation or a full Cox-Maze procedure. The Cox-Maze (CM) procedure is considered the gold standard surgical AF ablation technique. Clinical results have shown that the CM IV achieves equivalent success rate of the original CM procedure while significantly reducing operative time and lowering complication rates (3).

Left atrial appendage occlusion (LAAO) in patients with AF, although not an ablation procedure has been shown to reduce perioperative stroke and the long-term risks of thromboembolic complications (4). The most recent 2017 guidelines from the Society of Thoracic Surgeons (STS) recommend concomitant AF ablation for patients undergoing all types of cardiac procedures but particularly during mitral valve (MV) surgery, with good results in restoring normal sinus rhythm (NSR) (5).

There is increasing evidence demonstrating reduced stroke rates (6), fewer bleeding incidents (7), fewer readmissions for AF or heart failure (8, 9), but also improved long term survival and quality of life (10, 11), for patients who have a concomitant AF ablation procedure. The best outcomes following concomitant AF ablation during cardiac surgery depend on good patient selection. Higher chances in restoring NSR after concomitant AF ablation, are seen in patients with preoperative AF duration <1 year (paroxysmal or persistent) (12). Other studies show that the echocardiographic dimensions of the left atrium (LA) are also important to determine the chances of restoring normal sinus rhythm, with best results achieved if LA dimensions are <55 mm (13). Other factors such as diabetes, hypertension, or smoking are associated with worse results after AF ablation (13, 14).

Despite strong evidence for concomitant AF ablation, surgeons are still reluctant to offer this treatment during cardiac surgery for a variety of reasons including increased operative time, the need to open the left or right atria and concerns regarding intraoperative complications. However, patients may be missing a unique opportunity to have their AF treated at the time of their cardiac surgery.

The aim of this study is to determine to what extent patients with AF undergoing cardiac surgery at our institution received a concomitant AF procedure, what these procedures entailed, and whether these procedures are adequate in restoring NSR and maintaining it at short term follow up. Through this study we aim to raise awareness about the potential advantage of concomitant AF ablation during cardiac surgery. Finally, we aim to provide some recommendations to improve the management of patients with atrial fibrillation undergoing cardiac surgery.

## METHODS

A retrospective study of all patients who underwent cardiac surgery at our institution between June 2017 and January 2019. Our hospital is a large tertiary cardiac center undertaking around 2,500 cardiac cases per annum. Study cohort were patients presenting with preoperative AF. The types of AF were stratified further and defined as following: (i) Paroxysmal AF- recurrent AF (≥2 episodes) that terminates spontaneously within 7 days or episodes of AF ≤48 h duration, ended with electrical or pharmacologic conversion; (ii) Persistent AF- continuous AF, sustained beyond 7 days or episodes of AF in which the decision of electrical or pharmacological cardioversion is made after ≥48 h, but prior to 7 days; (iii) Longstanding persistent AF-continuous AF of >12 months (15).

Patients with preoperative AF were divided into two groups: Group 1 patients underwent a concomitant AF procedure at the time of cardiac surgery and Group 2 patients did not. The two groups were compared with respect to patient characteristics and comorbidity, postoperative complications, hospital stay, and early outcomes (in-hospital and at routine follow-up at 6–8 weeks following discharge from hospital).

*Definitions:* severe renal impairment: patient on dialysis or creatinine clearance <30 mls/min; extracardiac arteriopathy: claudication, carotid occlusion or >50% stenosis, amputation for arterial disease or previous or planned intervention on the abdominal aorta, limb arteries, or carotids; chronic pulmonary disease: long term use of bronchodilators or steroids for lung disease; pulmonary hypertension: systolic pressure >55 mg Hg.

The following procedures were considered as AF ablation procedures: Cox-Maze procedure, pulmonary vein (PV) isolation (radiofrequency or cryoablation) and left atrium (LA) ablation (radiofrequency or cryoablation). We included left atrial appendage occlusion (LAAO) as an AF procedure and not an ablation.

We recorded patient's rhythm before the surgical procedure, postoperatively, at discharge from hospital and in the out-patient clinic, 6–8 weeks from discharge. The ECG was the main tool used to record the rhythm. Only a few patients had a 24 h ECG at follow up review. The duration of preoperative AF was documented from patient's medical records.

Continuous variables were expressed as mean ± 1 standard deviation. Differences between the two Groups were analyzed with Chi-squared test and $T$-test for Independent Means. A $p < 0.05$ was considered significant.

## RESULTS

A total of 2,984 patients underwent a cardiac surgical procedure over this 18 month period at our institution. Three hundred and thirteen (10.4%) had preoperative AF: 61 (19.5%) paroxysmal, 37 (11.8%) persistent, 45 (14.4%) longstanding, 152 (48.5%) permanent, and 18 (5.8%) could not be classified. **Table 1** shows the characteristics of Group 1 and Group 2 patients with preoperative AF. Overall the characteristics of the two groups of patients were similar, except for two of them: the presence of infective endocarditis (0.9 vs. 6.1%, $p = 0.025$) and previous cardiac surgery (1.7 vs. 14.2%, $p = 0.001$), both significantly higher in Group 2 patients.

**Table 2** shows the type of AF in both Group 1 and Group 2 patients. The majority 77 (66.4%) of patients in Group 1 (who had a concomitant AF procedure performed) mainly presented with

**TABLE 1** | Patients characteristics.

| | Group 1: AF procedure $n = 116$ | Group 2: No AF procedure $n = 197$ | *P*-value |
|---|---|---|---|
| Male gender | 70 (60.3%) | 123 (62.4%) | 0.713 |
| Age at operation (years) | 71 ± 9.67 | 70 ± 10.39 | 0.984 |
| Severe renal impairment | 27(23.3%) | 59 (29.9%) | 0.206 |
| **Active IE** | **1 (0.9%)** | **12 (6.1%)** | **0.025** |
| Extracardiac arteriopathy | 3 (2.6%) | 11 (5.6%) | 0.215 |
| Chronic pulmonary disease | 17 (14.6%) | 26 (13.2%) | 0.717 |
| MI within 30 days | 5 (4.3%) | 8 (4.1%) | 0.914 |
| Previous TIA or CVA | 18 (15.5%) | 20 (10.1%) | 0.160 |
| IDDM | 2 (1.7%) | 8 (4.1%) | 0.256 |
| HTN | 90 (77.6%) | 158 (80.2%) | 0.581 |
| Smoking history | 6 (5.2%) | 13 (6.6%) | 0.609 |
| Pulmonary HTN | 23 (19.8%) | 54 (27.4%) | 0.132 |
| Poor LV function preop (LVEF<30%) | 6 (5.2%) | 19 (9.6%) | 0.158 |
| NYHA III/IV preop | 19 (16.4%) | 23 (11.7%) | 0.238 |
| Preop PPM | 6 (5.2%) | 14 (7.1%) | 0.499 |
| **Previous cardiac surgery** | **2 (1.7%)** | **28 (14.2%)** | **<0.001** |

*IE, infective endocarditis; MI, myocardial infarction; IDDM, insulin-dependent diabetes mellitus; HTN, hypertension; TIA, transient ischemic attack; CVA, cerebrovascular accident; LV, left ventricle; NYHA, New York Heart Association classification; PPM, permanent pacemaker. Bold value indicate that the difference between the values was statistically significant.*

**TABLE 2** | Type of AF in group 1 and group 2 patients.

| AF type | Group 1: AF procedure $n = 116$ | Group 2: No AF procedure $n = 197$ | *P*-value |
|---|---|---|---|
| Paroxysmal 61 (19.5%) | 21 (18.1%) | 40 (20.3%) | 0.634 |
| Persistent 37 (11.8%) | 15 (12.9%) | 22 (11.2%) | 0.640 |
| Longstanding 197 (62.9%) | 77 (66.4%) | 120 (60.9%) | 0.333 |
| Unknown 18 (5.8%) | 3 (2.6%) | 15 (7.6%) | – |

*AF, atrial fibrillation.*

longstanding AF. Only 27 (31%) of patients who presented with AF duration <1 year before cardiac surgery (paroxysmal and persistent) had a concomitant AF procedure (ablation procedure or just a LAAO).

**Table 3** illustrates the types of cardiac procedures which the patients included in Group 1 underwent. The cardiac procedures performed for patients included both in Group 1 and Group 2 were similar. Most commonly performed procedures were: isolated valve replacement/repair (aortic/mitral), double or triple valve replacement, coronary artery bypass graft surgery (CABG), major aortic surgery (aortic root replacement, ascending aorta, or hemiarch replacement) and combined procedures. Of those patients undergoing a concomitant atrial fibrillation procedure, 92 (79%) underwent isolated left atrial appendage occlusion. Two (1.7%) further patients had isolated pulmonary vein isolation. Twenty two (19%) patients who had left atrial appendage occlusion combined with an ablation procedure as follows: Cox-Maze 5 (4.3%), LA ablation 10 (8.6%) and PV Isolation 7 (6%). **Table 4** shows the exact AF procedures undertaken in relation to the type of AF: paroxysmal, persistent, and longstanding. **Figure 1** shows the type of concomitant AF procedures undertaken at the time of the respective cardiac procedure performed.

Patients in Group 1 and Group 2 were classified into three categories based on preoperative cardiac echocardiography dimensions of the left atrium [dilated (LA < 55 mm), significantly dilated (LA > 55 mm) and severely dilated (≥65 mm)] and the preoperative duration of AF as illustrated in **Table 5**. Of 79 patients with longstanding AF and severely dilated LA, 37 (46.8%) patients had a concomitant AF procedure and 42 (53.2%) did not ($p = 0.987$).

Postoperative complications in both patient groups are shown in **Table 6**. Group 1 patients had a significantly lower return to theater compared with Group 2 patients (2.6 vs. 9.1%, $p = 0.026$), a shorter hospital stay (11.9 ± 6 vs. 16.6 ± 19, $p = 0.013$) and better in-hospital survival (99.1 vs. 93.9%, $p = 0.025$). The majority of patients were discharged on antiarrhythmic medication (amiodarone, beta-blockers, or calcium channels blockers), except for a few cases where patients were bradycardiac and could not be discharged on any antiarrhythmic medications. Group 1 patients were more likely to be discharged on antiarrhythmic drugs compared with Group 2 patients, 85.3 vs. 73.1%, $p = 0.012$), respectively.

In Group 1, patients who had an AF procedure done, 114/116 pts (98.3%) had a LAAO.

In 79/114 pts (69.3%) with LAAO the rhythm identified at discharge was AF. The rhythm identified for the other 2 pts with isolated PVI at discharge was AF, as well. Overall, in Group 1 the rate of postoperative AF at discharge was 69.8%. Looking at Group 2, 110/197 pts (55.8%) were discharged in AF. Postoperative AF was significantly higher at discharge for Group 1 compared with Group 2 (69.8 vs. 55.8%, $p = 0.01$).

In addition to antiarrhythmic therapy, patients were discharged on oral anticoagulant therapy [warfarin or direct oral anticoagulants (DOACs)]. The majority [74 (68%)] of patients without a mechanical valve replacement and in AF at discharge were discharged on DOACs. Patients undergoing an AF procedure (even just an LAAO procedure) were more likely to be discharged on anticoagulation therapy compared with those who did not (93.9 vs. 82.2%, $p = 0.033$).

277/313 patients (88.5%) had a mean follow up of 6.09 ± 1.57 weeks, excluding the 22 patients who died and another 14 patients who were lost to follow up. Patients in Group 1 with a concomitant AF procedure had better survival compared with patients in Group 2, although this did not reach significance (97.4 vs. 89.3%, $p = 0.09$). There were no differences between the two Groups in the incidence of normal sinus rhythm (58.7 vs. 56.9%, $p = 0.759$) or hospital readmissions for AF or anticoagulation issues (7.7 vs. 6%, $p = 0.569$), at follow up.

At follow up, 47/114 pts (41.2%) with LAAO were identified as being in AF, and overall 41.4% pts were in AF in Group 1. In Group 2, 73/197 pts (37.1%) were identified as being in AF. There is a small difference between the 2 groups with

**TABLE 3** | Cardiac procedures performed in n=116 patients undergoing concomitant AF procedure.

| Isolated procedures | | | | Mixed procedures | | | | | | |
|---|---|---|---|---|---|---|---|---|---|---|
| **CABG** $n = 12$ | **Valve repair/replacement** $n = 46$ | | | **Double/triple valve procedures** $n = 31$ | | | **Other procedures** $n = 27$ | | | |
| | Mitral $n = 34$ | Aortic $n = 11$ | Tricuspid $n = 1$ | AVR+ MVR/+ TV repair $n = 10$ | MVR +TV repair $n = 14$ | MV repair +TV repair/+ AVR $n = 7$ | VR/ repair + CABG $n = 16$ | VR+ SM $n = 5$ | AAR/hemiarch+ VR/CABG $n = 4$ | AM + CABG $n = 2$ |

*AAR, ascending aorta replacement; AM, atrial myxoma; CABG, coronary artery bypass graft; AVR, aortic valve replacement; MVR, mitral valve replacement; MV, mitral valve; SM, septal myectomy; TV, tricuspid valve; VR, valve replacement.*

**TABLE 4** | Concomitant AF procedure performed in different types of AF.

| **AF type** | **Concomitant AF procedure** $n = 116$ | | | | |
|---|---|---|---|---|---|
| | **Cox-Maze + LAAO** $n = 5$ | **LAa + LAAO** $n = 10$ | **PVI + LAAO** $n = 7$ | **PVI** $n = 2$ | **LAAO** $n = 92$ |
| Paroxysmal | 2 (1.7%) | 3 (2.6%) | 2 (1.7%) | 1 (0.9%) | 13 (11.2%) |
| Persistent | 2 (1.7%) | 1 (0.9%) | 0 | 0 | 12 (10.3%) |
| Longstanding | 1 (0.9%) | 5 (4.3%) | 5 (4.3%) | 1 (0.9%) | 65 (56%) |
| Unknown | 0 | 1 (0.9%) | 0 | 0 | 2 (1.7%) |

*AF, atrial fibrillation; LAa, left atrial ablation; LAAO, left atrial appendage occlusion; PVI, pulmonary vein isolation.*

more pts with postoperative AF at follow up in Group 1 (41.4 vs. 37.1%, $p = 0.44$).

## DISCUSSION

Concomitant AF ablation during cardiac surgery is strongly supported by the most recent 2017 guidelines from the STS. Studies confirm that restoring NSR through concomitant AF ablation reduces the risk of stroke (5), bleeding (6), rate of readmissions for AF (7), risk of heart failure in addition to improving long term survival of patients and their quality of life (8–11). We have shown that adherence to these guidelines remains low, even in a high volume cardiac surgery center. In our study, out of 313 patients who presented with preoperative AF, and undergoing cardiac surgery, 37% had an AF procedure performed, of whom only 7.7% had an AF ablation. The majority of patients having a concomitant AF procedure only had a LAA clip, despite evidence showing that when a more complex ablation procedure was performed, there was a higher chance of restoring NSR and improved outcomes.

Despite evidence-backed guidelines regarding the safety and efficacy of concomitant AF ablation, this was not routinely performed in our cohort of patients. One frequent explanation provided for this is that in the presence of comorbidities, the risk to the patient is increased. In our study, both Groups (patients who had a concomitant AF ablation and those who did not) were similar regarding patient characteristics and co-morbidity, except the presence of preoperative infective endocarditis and previous cardiac surgery, which are both indeed associated with increased procedure risks. Hypertension, diabetes, and smoking are major independent predictors for AF ablation failure (1), however this did not appear to play a role in selection of our patients (**Table 1**).

Patients undergoing all types of cardiac surgery will benefit from a concomitant AF ablation, but those undergoing procedures on the mitral valve are most likely to benefit and given that the left atrium is opened, no extra incisions are required (5). In our study, 34 patients with preoperative AF and undergoing an isolated MV procedure had a concomitant AF procedure however only three had a full Cox-Maze procedure. Further investigation would be required to understand why this group of patients does not gain the benefit of an ablation.

Concomitant AF ablation is effective restoring sinus rhythm in patients undergoing aortic valve replacement (AVR) or coronary artery bypass surgery (CABG), only one patient had a concomitant Cox-Maze procedure performed in this cohort of our study (16). This may be explained by reluctance to open the heart purely to perform an ablation.

Preoperative AF duration and left atrial dimensions predict the time until AF recurrences after concomitant left atrial ablation (17). The authors report that the sinus rhythm conversion rate was superior when preoperative AF duration was 2 years or less. Forlani et al. report that preoperative AF <1 year (paroxysmal/ persistent) is more likely to convert back to sinus rhythm after AF ablation (11). In our study, of the 98 patients most likely to benefit from a concomitant AF procedure (with paroxysmal / persistent AF), only one third had a concomitant AF procedure performed, and paradoxically, more than half of the patients with longstanding AF (patients who are least likely to benefit) had a concomitant AF procedure. The nature of an individual's AF history together with education of the cardiologist and surgeon is critical to perioperative decision making.

Preoperative LA dimensions predict AF recurrence after an ablation procedure (18). LA dimensions <55 mm predict a higher rate of success in restoring NSR after a concomitant AF

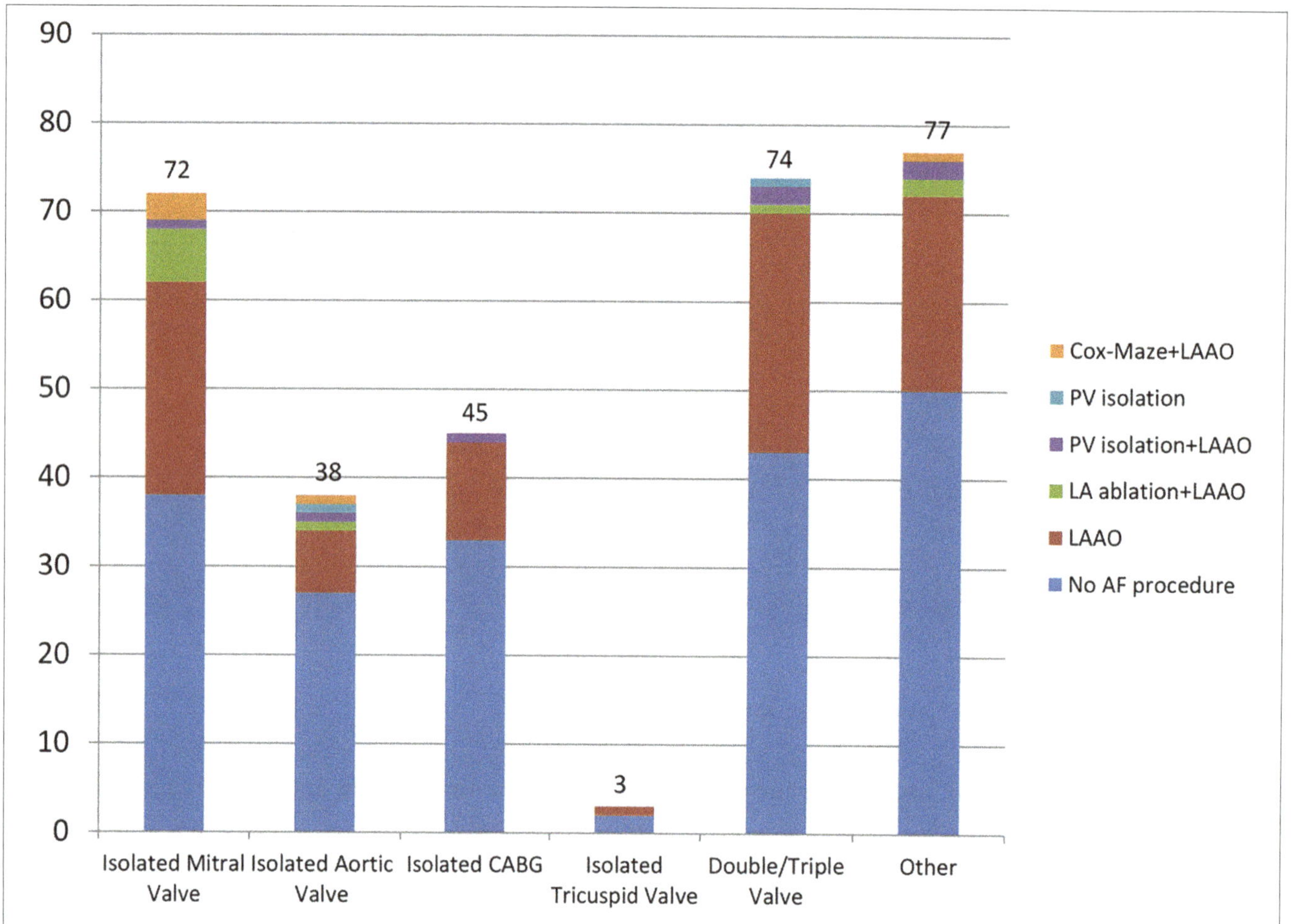


**FIGURE 1** | Cardiac procedures and concomitant AF procedures performed. AF, atrial fibrillation; PV, pulmonary vein; LAAO, left atrial appendage occlusion; LA, left atrium; CABG, coronary artery bypass graft; "Other" procedures category includes: Valve replacement + CABG, Valve replacement + septal myectomy, Ascending aorta/hemiarch replacement + CABG/valve replacement, myxoma + CABG.

**TABLE 5** | LA dimensions and type of AF in group1 vs. group 2 patients.

| **AF type** | **Preoperative LA dimensions** | | | | | | | | |
|---|---|---|---|---|---|---|---|---|---|
| | **Dilated (<55 mm)** | | | **Significantly dilated (>55 mm)** | | | **Severely dilated (≥65mm)** | | |
| | **Group 1 *n* (%)** | **Group 2 *n* (%)** | ***P*=** | **Group 1 *n* (%)** | **Group 2 *n* (%)** | ***P*=** | **Group 1 *n* (%)** | **Group 2 *n* (%)** | ***P*=** |
| Paroxysmal | 9 (2.9) | 25 (8) | 0.442 | 2 (0.6) | 3 (1) | 0.701 | 6 (1.9) | 6 (1.9) | 0.813 |
| Persistent | 5 (1.6) | 6 (1.9) | 0.300 | 3 (1) | 7 (2.2) | 0.845 | 7 (2.2) | 6 (1.9) | 0.586 |
| Longstanding | 22 (7) | 44 (14) | 0.651 | 7 (2.2) | 16 (5.2) | 0.745 | **37 (4.2)** | **42 (1.6)** | **0.987** |
| Unknown | 1 (0.3) | 5 (1.6) | 0.418 | 1 (0.3) | 1 (0.3) | 0.586 | 1 (0.3) | 4 (1.3) | 0.219 |

*LA, left atrium; AF, atrial fibrillation. Bold value indicate that the difference between the values was statistically significant.*

ablation. In our patients with preoperative AF duration <1 year and LA dimensions <55 mm only a third had a concomitant AF procedure. Thus, almost 70% of the patients with the greatest chance of maintaining NSR after concomitant AF procedure did not have specific treatment for their AF. Pecha et al. (18) showed that the duration of AF and a preoperative smaller left atrial diameter are statistically significant predictors of long term ablation success. The authors investigated whether performing a concomitant AF ablation on patients with an enlarged LA >55 mm is successful and showed freedom from AF in 64.4% of patients at 1-year follow-up. However, they concluded that these patients need more interventions (medical or electrical cardioversion) and additional catheter-based ablation to achieve satisfactory results.

**TABLE 6 |** In-hospital outcomes.

| | Group 1: concomitant AF procedure $n = 116$ | Group 2: no AF procedure $n = 197$ | $P =$ |
|---|---|---|---|
| **Return to theater** | **3 (2.6%)** | **18 (9.1%)** | **0.026** |
| Mean ITU LOS (nights) | 4.7 ± 6 | 6.5 ± 11 | 0.120 |
| Post-op cerebral events | 3 (2.6%) | 12 (6.1%) | 0.161 |
| Post-op PPM insertion | 16 (13.8%) | 29 (14.7%) | 0.821 |
| **Mean hospital LOS (days)** | **11.9 ± 6** | **16.6 ± 19** | **0.013** |
| NSR at discharge | 35 (30.2%) | 61 (31%) | 0.883 |
| **In-hospital survival** | **115 (99.1%)** | **185 (93.9%)** | **0.025** |

*Continuous variables are listed as mean ± standard deviation; AF, atrial fibrillation; n, number; P, p-value; ITU, intensive therapy unit; LOS, length of stay; post-op, postoperative; PPM, permanent pacemaker; NSR, normal sinus rhythm. Bold value indicate that the difference between the values was statistically significant.*

In our study, both Group 1 and Group 2 patients had similar rates of sinus rhythm at discharge and at short-term follow-up. More patients who had an AF procedure (98.3% had a LAAO) performed for their preoperative AF (Group 1) compared with those who had noting done, presented postoperative AF at discharge, as was highlighted by Yao et al. (19). Similar incidences of postoperative cerebral events, PPM insertion, and readmissions for AF or anticoagulation issues were also observed in both Groups. These findings may be explained by inconsistent patient selection and incomplete AF ablation (a full Cox-Maze was performed in only 4.3% of cases and majority of patients didn't have an AF ablation performed, but only a clip on their LAA), but does not address the effectiveness of the AF ablation procedures.

Patients who had an AF procedure performed were less likely to return to theater, had a shorter hospital stay, and improved survival. These findings can be explained by the patient's selection and inclusion in our cohort group. The patients included in Group 1, who had an AF procedure performed, were identified as lower risk for surgery compared with Group 2, which may explain the shorter hospital stay and improved survival, related to their comorbidities and not to have or not an AF procedure performed.

There are multiple ways to encourage surgeons to perform concomitant AF ablation in addition to education of the benefits as per international guidelines. This study, for example, was performed in a public health system where concomitant ablation attracts no additional reimbursement. Adherence to guidelines can be encouraged with increased reimbursement for additional procedures of proven benefit, such as AF ablation and application of a LAAO device, or withholding of reimbursement from those who do not follow guidelines or at least recommendations by a multi-disciplinary heart team.

## STUDY LIMITATIONS

During data collection, we encountered limited information in some patients' records regarding the duration of the preoperative AF and were, thus, unable to classify the type of AF. There was an absence of standardized echocardiography reporting with respect to LA dimensions, as our patient population came from many different referring centers, making the pre-operative assessment of LA size and the preoperative selection of patients for AF ablation, variable. In addition, our patient follow up has been incomplete, with only a small number of patients having a 24 h tape ECG to determine rhythm, some just a 12 lead ECG in out-patient clinic and some only a clinical determination of the heart rhythm and review by a trainee surgeon.

Our small cohort size does not allow for adjusted comparisons such as with propensity matching which requires large samples, with substantial overlap between treatment and control groups.

## CONCLUSIONS

Despite strong recommendations for, concomitant AF ablation is still not undertaken in most patients with preoperative AF undergoing cardiac surgery (in our center, AF ablation is performed in 7.7% of cases). The patients from both groups had similar rates of sinus rhythm at discharge and at short-term follow-up, but also similar incidences of postoperative cerebral events and readmissions for AF, which may be explained by inconsistent patient selection and incomplete AF ablation.

## RECOMMENDATIONS

As a consequence of these findings, we have made and implemented the following recommendations: establishing a dedicated multidisciplinary team meeting attended by cardiac electrophysiologists, general cardiologists and cardiac surgeons; identified a group of surgeons dedicated to and experienced in the surgical management of AF to champion this treatment; establishment of an AF register to improve the accuracy of patient data collection; standardized the reporting of cardiac investigations and the post-operative follow-up of patients undergoing AF procedures; employment of a specialist AF nurse.

## ETHICS STATEMENT

The studies involving human participants were reviewed and approved by Barts Health Clinical Effectiveness Unit Audit ID 10421 11/07/2019. The Ethics Committee waived the requirement of written informed consent for participation.

## AUTHOR CONTRIBUTIONS

A-AM, MY, and WA have contributed in different but equal ways to this work. All authors contributed to the article and approved the submitted version.

## REFERENCES

1. Gu W, Guo H, Lu C, Huang H, Liu J, Xie B, et al. Surgical ablation for persistent atrial fibrillation in concomitant cardiac surgery: mid-long-term result. *Eur J Cardio-Thorac Surg.* (2017) 52:888–94. doi: 10.1093/ejcts/ezx179

2. Camm J, Lip G, De Caterina R, Savelieva I, Atar D, Hohnloser S, et al. 2012 focused update of the ESC Guidelines for the management of atrial fibrillation. An update of the 2010 ESC Guidelines for the management of atrial fibrillation. Developed with the special contribution of the European Heart Rhythm Association. *Eur Heart J.* (2012) 33:2719–47. doi: 10.1093/eurheartj/ehs253
3. Lall SC, Melby SJ, Voeller RK, Zierer A, Bailey MS, Guthrie TJ, et al. The effect of ablation technology on surgical outcomes after the Cox-maze procedure: a propensity analysis. *J Thorac Cardiovasc Surg.* (2007) 133:389–96. doi: 10.1016/j.jtcvs.2006.10.009
4. Park-Hasen J, Holme SJV, Irmukhamedov A, Carranza CL, Greve AM, Al-Farra G, et al. Adding left atrial appendage closure to open heart surgery provides protection from ischemic brain injury six years after surgery independently of atrial fibrillation history: the LAACS randomized surgery. *J Cardiothoracic Surgery.* (2018) 13:1–8. doi: 10.1186/s13019-018-0740-7
5. Badhwar V, Rankin JS, Damiano RJ, Gillinov AM, Bakaeen FG, Edgerton JR, et al. The Society of Thoracic Surgeons 2017 clinical practice guidelines for the surgical treatment of atrial fibrillation. *Ann Thorac Surg.* (2017) 103:329–41. doi: 10.1016/j.athoracsur.2016.10.076
6. Cox JL, Ad N, Palazzo T. Impact of the maze procedure on the stroke rate in patients with atrial fibrillation. *J Thorac Cardiovasc Surg.* (1999) 118:833–40. doi: 10.1016/S0022-5223(99)70052-8
7. Alikhan R, Lefevre C, Menown I, Lister S, Bird A, You M, et al. Risk of recurrent bleeding events in nonvalvular atrial fibrillation treated with vitamin k antagonists: a clinical practice research datalink study. *TH Open.* (2019) 3:e316–24. doi: 10.1055/s-0039-1698413
8. Joy PS, Gopinathannair R, Olshansky B. Effect of ablation for atrial fibrillation on heart failure readmission rates. *Am J Cardiol.* (2017) 120:1572–7. doi: 10.1016/j.amjcard.2017.07.057
9. Liang JJ, Callans DJ. Ablation for atrial fibrillation in heart failure with reduced ejection fraction. *CFR.* (2018) 4:33–7. doi: 10.15420/cfr.2018:3:1
10. Musharbash FN, Schill MR, Sinn LA, Schuessler RB, Maniar HS, Moon MR, et al. Performance of the Cox-maze IV procedure is associated with improved long term survival in patients with AF undergoing cardiac surgery. *J Thorac Cardiovasc Surg.* (2018) 155:159–70. doi: 10.1016/j.jtcvs.2017.09.095
11. Forlani S, De Paulis R, Guerrieri Wolf L, Greco R, Polisca P, Moscarelli M, et al. Conversion to sinus rhythm by ablation improves quality of life in patients submitted to mitral valve surgery. *Ann Thorac Surg.* (2006) 81:863–7. doi: 10.1016/j.athoracsur.2005.09.004
12. Raissouni K, Petrosyan A, Malapert G, Jazayeri S, Morgant MC, Bouchot O. Concomitant cardiac surgery and radiofrequency ablation of atrial fibrillation: a retrospective single center study. *J Cardiothorac Vasc Anesth.* (2020) 34:401–8. doi: 10.1053/j.jvca.2019.09.021
13. Damiano RJ Jr, Badhwar V, Acker MA, Veeragandham RS, Kress DC, Robertson JO, et al. The CURE-AF trial: a prospective, multicenter trial of irrigated radiofrequency ablation for the treatment of persistent atrial fibrillation during concomitant cardiac surgery. *Heart Rhythm.* (2014) 11:39–45. doi: 10.1016/j.hrthm.2013.10.004
14. Pecha S, Ghandili S, Hakmi S, Willems S, Reichenspurner H, Wagner FM. Predictors of long-term success after concomitant surgical ablation for atrial fibrillation. *Semin Thorac Cardiovasc Surg.* (2017) 29:294–8. doi: 10.1053/j.semtcvs.2017.08.015
15. Calkins H, Cappato R, Heinz Kuck K, Brugada J, Camm AJ, Chen SA, et al. 2012 HRS/EHRA/ECAS expert consensus statement on catheter and surgical ablation of atrial fibrillation: recommendations for patient selection, procedural techniques, patient management and follow-up, definitions, endpoints, and research trial design. *EP Europace.* (2012) 14:528–606. doi: 10.1093/europace/eus027
16. Geidel S, Ostermeyer J, Lass M, Geisler M, Kotetishvili N, Aslanacier HA, et al. Permanent atrial fibrillation ablation surgery in CABG and aortic valve patients is at least as effective as in mitral valve disease. *Thorac Cardiovasc Surg.* (2006) 54:91–5. doi: 10.1055/s-2005-872860
17. Grubitzsch H, Grabow C, Orawa H, Konertz W. Factors predicting the time until atrial fibrillation recurrence after concomitant left atrial ablation. *Eur J Cardiothorac Surg.* (2008) 34:67–72. doi: 10.1016/j.ejcts.2008.03.054
18. Pecha S, Hakmi S, Subbotina I, Willems S, Reichenspurner H, Wagner FM. Concomitant surgical ablation for atrial fibrillation (AF) in patients with significant atrial dilation >55 mm. Worth the effort? *J Cardiothorac Surg.* (2015) 10:1–5. doi: 10.1186/s13019-015-0337-3
19. Yao X, Gersh B, Holmes D Jr, Melduni R, Johnsrud D, Sangaralingham L, et al. Association of surgical left atrial appendage occlusion with subsequent stroke and mortality among patients undergoing cardiac surgery. *JAMA.* (2018) 319:2116–26. doi: 10.1001/jama.2018.6024

# 19

# Association of Post-operative Systolic Blood Pressure Variability with Mortality After Coronary Artery Bypass Grafting

*Zhuoming Zhou [1,2†], Jiantao Chen [1,2†], Guangguo Fu [1,2], Xiaodong Zhuang [2,3,4], Jian Hou [1,2], Sida Chen [1,2], Suiqing Huang [1,2], Yuan Yue [1,2], Liqun Shang [1,2], Keke Wang [5], Linhua Lv [1,2], Mengya Liang [1,2*] and Zhongkai Wu [1,2*]*

*[1] Department of Cardiac Surgery, The First Affiliated Hospital of Sun Yat-Sen University, Guangzhou, China, [2] NHC Key Laboratory of Assisted Circulation, Sun Yat-Sen University, Guangzhou, China, [3] Department of Cardiology, The First Affiliated Hospital of Sun Yat-Sen University, Guangzhou, China, [4] Center for Information Technology & Statistics, The First Affiliated Hospital of Sun Yat-Sen University, Guangzhou, China, [5] Department of Emergency, The First Affiliated Hospital of Sun Yat-Sen University, Guangzhou, China*

***Correspondence:**
*Zhongkai Wu*
*wuzhk@mail.sysu.edu.cn*
*Mengya Liang*
*infisdsums@163.com*

*† These authors have contributed equally to this work*

**Background:** Blood pressure variability (BPV) has long been considered a risk factor for cardiovascular events. We aimed to investigate whether post-operative systolic BPV was associated with early and late all-cause mortality in patients undergoing coronary artery bypass grafting (CABG).

**Methods:** Clinical variables and blood pressure records within the first 24 h in the post-operative intensive care unit stay from 4,509 patients operated on between 2001 and 2012 were extracted from the Medical Information Mart for Intensive Care III (MIMIC-III) database. BPV was measured as the coefficient of the variability of systolic blood pressure, and we compared patients in the highest quartile with patients in the other three quartiles.

**Results:** After full adjustment, patients in the highest quartile of BPV were at a higher risk of intensive care unit mortality (OR = 2.02, 95% CI: 1.11–3.69), 30-day mortality (OR = 1.92, 95% CI: 1.22–3.02), and 90-day mortality (HR = 1.64, 95% CI: 1.19–2.27). For 2,892 patients with a 4-year follow-up, the association between a higher post-operative BPV and the risk of 4-year mortality was not significant (HR = 1.17, 95% CI: 0.96–1.42). The results were supported by the comparison of survival curves and remained generally consistent in the subgroup analyses and sensitivity analyses.

**Conclusions:** Our findings demonstrated that in patients undergoing CABG, a higher post-operative BPV was associated with a higher risk of early mortality while the association was not significant for late mortality. Post-operative BPV can support doctors in identifying patients with potential hemodynamic instability and making timely clinical decisions.

**Keywords: coronary artery bypass grafting, blood pressure, variability, mortality, intensive care**

## INTRODUCTION

Elevated blood pressure (BP) has been demonstrated to be a dominant contributor and risk factor for a poor cardiovascular prognosis (1–3). However, BP is a dynamic physiological parameter, and the average of multiple BP readings over a period of time is insufficient to reflect the real risks of patients (4). A growing number of studies have indicated that blood pressure variability (BPV) over hours, days, and years is associated with cardiovascular events, including heart failure (5), atrial fibrillation (6), coronary artery disease, stroke, and both cardiovascular and all-cause mortality in different non-surgical populations (7–9), independent of the corresponding mean BP. The underlying mechanisms remain incompletely understood, but arterial compliance and endothelial dysfunction may be involved (10).

Coronary artery bypass grafting (CABG) is a surgical treatment for patients with severe coronary artery disease, and many of them have concomitant diseases such as hypertension, diabetes mellitus, and congestive heart failure (CHF) (11). Therefore, fluctuations of BP due to cardiac insufficiency, unsatisfactory vascular quality, and inappropriate BP management frequently occur pre- and post-operatively. Previous publications have shown that preoperative long-term BPV and intraoperative oscillation of BP can predict short-term outcomes in patients undergoing CABG (12, 13). However, it is difficult to regularly measure and control preoperative long-term BP, while post-operative BP can be routinely monitored and adjusted in the intensive care unit (ICU) after surgery.

As systolic blood pressure (SBP) has been considered to have more clinical significance than diastolic blood pressure (DBP) (14, 15), the aim of our study was to further explore the association between post-operative systolic BPV and early and late all-cause mortality in patients undergoing CABG and discuss its prognostic and therapeutic implications for optimizing post-operative BP management.

## METHODS

### Data Source and Study Population

Data were obtained from the Medical Information Mart for Intensive Care III (MIMIC-III) database, which is a large, freely available database with information from more than 40,000 patients who had critical care unit stays at the Beth Israel Deaconess Medical Center between 2001 and 2012 (16). Our right to access the database and acquire the data was approved by the institutional review board of the Massachusetts Institute of Technology (Cambridge, MA, USA) after one of our authors (Zhou) finished the online training for the Collaborative Institutional Training Initiative program of the National Institutes of Health (Record ID 35971811).

Among all of the patients in the MIMIC-III database, 5,007 consecutive patients undergoing CABG between 2001 and 2012 were included. The exclusion criteria were as follows: (1) missing BP measurement records ($n = 274$); (2) death within the first 24 h of post-operative ICU admission ($n = 6$); (3) length of ICU stay <24 h ($n = 188$); (4) BP measured <10 times within the first 24 h of post-operative ICU admission ($n = 28$); and (5) Patients with abnormal times (more than 1,000 times) of BP measurement ($n = 2$). Finally, a total of 4,509 patients were included in the study population.

### Data Extraction

All data were obtained and extracted using the Structured Query Language (SQL), and pgAdmin4 for Post-greSQL was used as the administrative platform. The extracted data included: (1) demographics: age, sex, and ethnicity; (2) comorbidities defined using the International Classification of Diseases, Ninth Revision, Clinical Modification (ICD-9-CM) codes, including CHF, hypertension, acute myocardial infarction (AMI), diabetes mellitus, respiratory failure, peripheral vascular disease, and end stage renal disease (ESRD); (3) concomitant surgical procedures: cardiopulmonary bypass, number of revascularized arteries, single internal thoracic artery (SITA) grafting, and concomitant valvular surgery; (4) intensive care scores: Sequential Organ Failure Assessment (SOFA) and Simplified Acute Physiology Score II (SAPS II); (5) vital signs: SBP, DBP, heart rate, and percutaneous oxygen saturation ($SpO_2$); (6) antihypertensive medication including angiotensin-converting enzyme inhibitors (ACEIs), angiotensin receptor blockers (ARBs), calcium channel blockers (CCBs), beta-blockers, and diuretics; and (7) vasoactive medication including dobutamine, dopamine, epinephrine, norepinephrine, phenylephrine, and vasopressin.

### BP Measurement and the Definition of BPV

Post-operative BP was continuously measured and recorded with a bedside BP monitor (Component Monitoring System IntelliVue MP-70; Philips Healthcare, Andover, MA) via an invasive arterial line within the first 24 h in the ICU. BP data was extracted from the database, and systolic and diastolic BPV was calculated and evaluated using the following parameters: (1) the coefficient of variation (CV) of BP, defined as the standardized deviation (SD) of SBP or DBP divided by the mean and expressed as a percentage; and (2) the SD of BP, defined as the SD of all SBP or DBP records for a patient within the first 24 h of ICU admission. Patients in the highest quartile group were defined as patients with higher BPV, and were compared with patients from the three lowest quartiles of variability.

### Definition of Outcomes and Follow-Up

All patients were followed up for at least 90 days, and the primary outcome was all-cause mortality occurring within 30 days after the CABG operation. ICU and 90-day mortality were considered secondary outcomes. For the 2,892 consecutive patients who underwent surgery between 2001 and 2008, they were followed up for at least 4 years; thus, 4-year all-cause mortality was set as an additional outcome for those patients.

### Statistical Analysis

The study population was categorized into two groups according to the highest and the other three CV quartiles of SBP. Continuous variables were presented as the mean ± SD and were compared by Student $t$-test. Categorical data were presented as numbers with proportions and were analyzed by $\chi^2$-tests.

Logistic regression models and Cox proportional hazards models were applied for the univariable and multivariable analyses to identify the association between the highest BPV quartile and mortality. Model 1 was adjusted for key demographic characteristics like age and sex; Model 2 was adjusted for age, sex, and comorbidities including CHF, hypertension, AMI, diabetes mellitus, respiratory failure, peripheral vascular disease, and ESRD. To account for the post-operative antihypertensive and vasoactive medication within the first 24 h, they were adjusted in Model 3. Model 4 was adjusted for the variables in Model 3 plus the number of BP measurements within the first 24 h. The results were presented as odds ratios (ORs) or hazard ratios (HRs) and 95% confidence intervals (CIs). Survival curves at 30 days, 90 days, and 4 years were estimated using the Kaplan-Meier method and compared by the log-rank test. Subgroup analyses were performed with a logistic regression model in Model 4, according to age strata ($<70$ and $\geq 70$ years), sex, CHF, hypertension, AMI, diabetes mellitus, and antihypertensive and vasoactive medication. The *P* for interaction was derived from a multivariable logistic regression model. Sensitivity analyses were performed by measuring BPV as SD quartiles of SBP, CV quartiles of DBP, and SD quartiles of DBP. Then, patients who were discharged or died within the first 12 h were excluded, and analyses of BPV within the first 12 h based on the remaining 4,670 patients were performed. Finally, we included patients who were discharged within 24 h or had BP measured $<10$ times to assess the robustness of our analysis. All tests were two-sided, and $P < 0.05$ were considered significant. All statistical analyses were performed using STATA, version 14.0 (StataCorp, College Station, TX).

## RESULTS

### Characteristics of the Patients

In total, 4,509 patients who met the selection criteria were enrolled in our study, all of whom were followed for 90 days, and among these, 2,892 patients were followed for 4 years. The baseline characteristics of the patients grouped by CV quartiles of SBP are briefly summarized in **Table 1**. Compared with the other three quartiles, patients in the highest BPV group were older, tend to be female, and were more likely to have CHF, diabetes mellitus and ESRD, higher BP, more BP measurements, higher intensive care scores, and less antihypertensive medication usage. The ICD-9-CM codes of the included comorbidities were summarized in **Supplementary Table 1**.

### Systolic BPV and the Risk of ICU and 30-day Mortality

Higher ICU mortality and 30-day mortality in the highest CV quartile of SBP were found in the unadjusted and adjusted models (Models 1–4). After adjusting for age, sex, comorbidities, medications, and the number of BP measurements (Model 4), patients in the highest BPV group were still at higher risk of ICU mortality ($Q_4$ vs. $Q_{1-3}$: OR = 2.02, 95% CI: 1.11–3.69) and 30-day mortality ($Q_4$ vs. $Q_{1-3}$: OR = 1.92, 95% CI: 1.22–3.02) (**Table 2**).

**TABLE 1** | Baseline characteristics of patients undergoing CABG, categorized by the coefficient of variation quartiles of post-operative SBP.

| Variables | Coefficient of variation of SBP | | *P*-value |
|---|---|---|---|
| | **Q1–3 (*n* = 3,382)** | **Q4 (*n* = 1,127)** | |
| **Demographics** | | | |
| Age, years | 67.46 (10.89) | 70.02 (10.36) | <0.001 |
| Sex, female, *n* (%) | 826 (24.4) | 350 (31.1) | <0.001 |
| **Ethnicity, *n* (%)** | | | |
| White | 2,377 (70.3) | 793 (70.4) | 0.256 |
| Black | 82 (2.4) | 39 (3.5) | |
| Asian | 68 (2.0) | 19 (1.7) | |
| Others | 855 (25.3) | 276 (24.5) | |
| CV of SBP | 11.59 (2.14) | 18.31 (3.15) | <0.001 |
| **Comorbidities, *n* (%)** | | | |
| Congestive heart failure | 874 (25.8) | 350 (31.1) | 0.001 |
| Hypertension | 2,305 (68.2) | 773 (68.6) | 0.786 |
| Acute myocardial infarction | 267 (7.9) | 104 (9.2) | 0.158 |
| Diabetes mellitus | 1,304 (38.6) | 487 (43.2) | 0.006 |
| Respiratory failure | 136 (4.0) | 65 (5.8) | 0.014 |
| Peripheral vascular disease | 185 (5.5) | 92 (8.2) | 0.001 |
| End-stage renal disease | 121 (3.6) | 67 (5.9) | 0.001 |
| **Concomitant surgical procedures** | | | |
| Concomitant valvular surgery, *n* (%) | 690 (20.4) | 251 (22.3) | 0.181 |
| Cardiopulmonary bypass, *n* (%) | 3,195 (94.5) | 1,045 (92.7) | 0.032 |
| SITA grafting, *n* (%) | 3,003 (88.8) | 969 (86.0) | 0.012 |
| Number of revascularized arteries | 2.24 (0.92) | 2.20 (0.88) | 0.195 |
| **Scores** | | | |
| SOFA | 4.76 (2.48) | 5.37 (2.66) | <0.001 |
| SAPSII | 35.10 (11.31) | 39.61 (12.39) | <0.001 |
| **Vital signs** | | | |
| Number of BP measurement, times | 37.15 (11.45) | 42.65 (14.40) | <0.001 |
| Mean SBP, mmHg | 112.35 (9.72) | 113.12 (9.62) | 0.020 |
| Mean DBP, mmHg | 56.90 (7.60) | 56.54 (7.02) | 0.159 |
| Heart rate, beats/minute | 85.28 (9.83) | 85.46 (9.42) | 0.593 |
| $SpO_2$, % | 98.02 (1.23) | 98.05 (1.72) | 0.532 |
| **Medication** | | | |
| **Antihypertensive, *n* (%)** | 2,599 (76.8) | 784 (69.6) | <0.001 |
| ACEI | 141 (4.2) | 33 (2.9) | 0.061 |
| ARB | 23 (0.7) | 10 (0.9) | 0.480 |
| Beta-blocker | 2,013 (59.5) | 534 (47.4) | <0.001 |
| CCB | 135 (4.0) | 34 (3.0) | 0.136 |
| Diuretics | 2,331 (68.9) | 714 (63.4) | 0.001 |
| **Vasoactive, *n* (%)** | 2,164 (64.0) | 723 (64.2) | 0.920 |
| Dobutamine | 68 (2.0) | 31 (2.8) | 0.142 |
| Dopamine | 71 (2.1) | 34 (3.0) | 0.077 |
| Epinephrine | 439 (13.0) | 220 (19.5) | <0.001 |
| Norepinephrine | 275 (8.1) | 128 (11.4) | 0.001 |
| Phenylephrine | 2,089 (61.8) | 691 (61.3) | 0.786 |
| Vasopressin | 135 (4.0) | 72 (6.4) | 0.001 |

*The highest quartile (Q4) was compared with Q1–3. Continuous variables are presented as the mean (SD), and categorical variables are presented as numbers (%).*

*ACEI, angiotensin-converting enzyme inhibitor; ARB, angiotensin receptor blocker; CABG, coronary artery bypass grafting; CCB, calcium channel blocker; CV, coefficient of variation; DBP, diastolic blood pressure; Q, quartile; SAPS II, Simplified Acute Physiology Score II; SBP, systolic blood pressure; SITA, single internal thoracic artery; SOFA, Sequential Organ Failure Assessment; $SpO_2$, percutaneous oxygen saturation.*

**TABLE 2** | Association between the highest quartile (Q4) vs. Q1–3 for the coefficient of variation of SBP within the first 24 h of post-operative ICU admission and mortality.

| Events | No. of events (%) | Univariable analysis | Multivariable analysis | | | |
|---|---|---|---|---|---|---|
| | | | Model 1 | Model 2 | Model 3 | Model 4 |
| | | | | **OR (95% CI)** | | |
| **ICU mortality** | | | | | | |
| Q1–3 | 27 (0.80) | | | 1.00 (Reference) | | |
| Q4 | 23 (2.04) | 2.59 (1.48–4.53) | 2.40 (1.36–4.22) | 2.19 (1.21–3.94) | 2.17 (1.20–3.94) | 2.02 (1.11–3.69) |
| **30-day mortality** | | | | | | |
| Q1–3 | 49 (1.45) | | | 1.00 (Reference) | | |
| Q4 | 39 (3.46) | 2.44 (1.59–3.73) | 2.28 (1.48–3.5) | 2.11 (1.35–3.28) | 2.07 (1.33–3.23) | 1.92 (1.22–3.02) |
| | | | | **HR (95% CI)** | | |
| **90-day mortality** | | | | | | |
| Q1–3 | 96 (2.84) | | | 1.00 (Reference) | | |
| Q4 | 64 (5.68) | 2.04 (1.48–2.79) | 1.81 (1.32–2.49) | 1.70 (1.24–2.34) | 1.66 (1.21–2.29) | 1.64 (1.19–2.27) |
| **4-year mortality** | | | | | | |
| Q1–3 | 313 (15.03) | | | 1.00 (Reference) | | |
| Q4 | 159 (19.63) | 1.32 (1.09–1.61) | 1.19 (0.98–1.45) | 1.17 (0.96–1.41) | 1.16 (0.96–1.41) | 1.17 (0.96–1.42) |

*Model 1 was adjusted for age and sex.*
*Model 2 was adjusted for age, sex, congestive heart failure, hypertension, acute myocardial infarction, diabetes mellitus, respiratory failure, peripheral vascular disease, and end-stage renal disease.*
*Model 3 was adjusted for the variables in Model 2 plus post-operative antihypertensive and vasoactive medication within the first 24 h.*
*Model 4 was adjusted for the variables in Model 3 plus the number of blood pressure measurements within the first 24 h.*
*ICU, intensive care unit; Q, quartile; SBP, systolic blood pressure.*

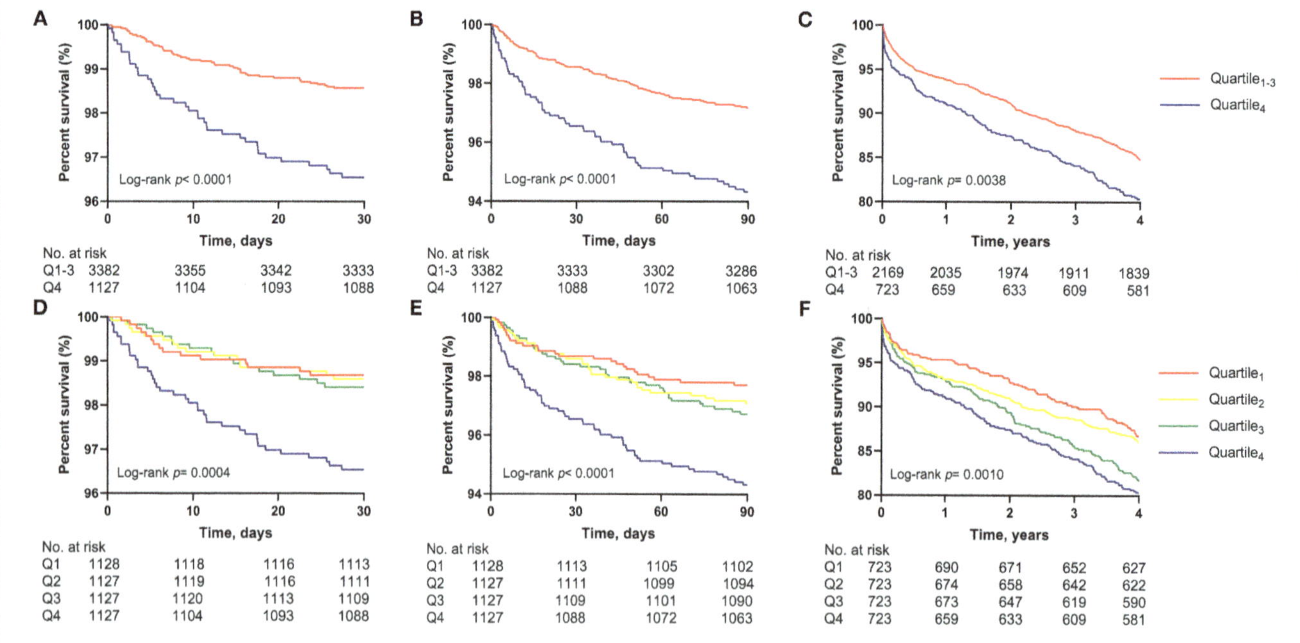


**FIGURE 1** | Kaplan-Meier survival analysis among patients stratified by quartiles of the coefficient of variation of post-operative systolic BPV. Comparison of **(A)** 30-day, **(B)** 90-day, and **(C)** 4-year survival of the highest quartile (Q4) vs. the other three quartiles (Q1–3); Comparison of **(D)** 30-day, **(E)** 90-day, and **(F)** 4-year survival of the four quartiles; BPV, blood pressure variability; Q, quartile.

## Systolic BPV and the Risk of 90-day and 4-year Mortality

The highest quartile of systolic BPV was significantly associated with a higher risk of 90-day morality in all models. The correlation remained unchanged after fully adjusting for the variables in Model 4 ($Q_4$ vs. $Q_{1-3}$: HR = 1.64, 95% CI: 1.19–2.27) (**Table 2**).

In the 2,892 consecutive patients who were followed up for 4 years, the univariate analysis indicated that patients with the highest systolic BPV were at higher risk of 4-year mortality.

**TABLE 3** | Risk of 30-day mortality for the highest quartile (Q4) vs. Q1–3 for the coefficient of variation of SBP in different subgroups.

| Variables | Group | Number of patients | OR (95% CI) | *P* for interaction |
|---|---|---|---|---|
| Age | <70 years | 2,325 | 2.38 (1.15–4.94) | 0.573 |
| | ≥70 years | 2,052 | 1.73 (0.97–3.10) | |
| Sex | Male | 3,333 | 2.50 (1.44–4.34) | 0.134 |
| | Female | 1,176 | 1.07 (0.47–2.42) | |
| CHF | Yes | 1,224 | 1.44 (0.78–2.69) | 0.203 |
| | No | 3,285 | 2.29 (1.17–4.48) | |
| Hypertension | Yes | 3,078 | 1.76 (0.88–3.50) | 0.998 |
| | No | 1,431 | 2.18 (1.18–4.02) | |
| AMI | Yes | 371 | 1.29 (0.40–4.18) | 0.415 |
| | No | 4,138 | 2.06 (1.24–3.41) | |
| Diabetes mellitus | Yes | 1,791 | 1.25 (0.61–2.56) | 0.076 |
| | No | 2,718 | 2.72 (1.47–5.03) | |
| Antihypertensive medication | Yes | 3,383 | 1.78 (0.99–3.22) | 0.787 |
| | No | 1,126 | 2.04 (0.97–4.30) | |
| Vasoactive medication | Yes | 2,887 | 1.71 (1.01–2.90) | 0.466 |
| | No | 1,622 | 3.36 (1.30–8.66) | |

*ORs (95% CIs) were derived from a logistic regression model adjusted for age, sex, CHF, hypertension, AMI, diabetes mellitus, respiratory failure, peripheral vascular disease, end-stage renal disease, antihypertensive medication, vasoactive medication, and the number of blood pressure measurements.*

*AMI, acute myocardial infarction; CHF, congestive heart failure; Q, quartile; SBP, systolic blood pressure.*

However, after fully adjusting for variables in the multivariable analyses, this association became statistically insignificant, although the trend still favored a higher risk in Q4 ($Q_4$ vs. $Q_{1-3}$: HR = 1.17, 95% CI: 0.96–1.42) (**Table 2**).

The Kaplan-Meier survival curves comparing patients in $Q_4$ and patients in $Q_{1-3}$ also demonstrated that a higher systolic BPV was significantly associated with higher 30-day, 90-day, and 4-year mortality (**Figure 1**).

## Subgroup Analyses and Sensitivity Analyses

In general, after full adjustment, patients with a higher CV of SBP were associated with a higher risk of 30-day mortality across the various subgroups (**Table 3**).

In the sensitivity analyses, similar patterns can be observed when evaluating BPV as the SD of SBP, but the difference was not significant for ICU mortality or 4-year mortality (**Supplementary Table 2**). When we estimated BPV as the CV or SD of DBP, the results remained generally consistent, but most of the results were statistically insignificant after adjustment (**Supplementary Tables 3, 4**). Then, patients who were discharged or died within 12 h were excluded, and analyses based on BP records within 12 h were performed. The results revealed a similar association, with no significant difference observed for ICU, 30-day or 4-year mortality when fully adjusted (**Supplementary Table 5**). In addition, patients who were discharged within the first 24 h or had BP measured <10 times were also included in the analysis and the results remained consistent. Finally, we compared the survival curves of different BPV quartiles, and the difference was not significant between Q1 and Q3 for 30- and 90-day survival, while an obviously higher mortality was seen for Q4. For 4-year survival, a significant difference was observed between the four groups (**Figure 1**).

# DISCUSSION

To the best of our knowledge, this is the first study with a large dataset to demonstrate an association between post-operative BPV and the prognosis of patients undergoing CABG. Higher systolic BPV was associated with a higher risk of early mortality, including ICU, 30- and 90-day mortality. However, the association between higher BPV and 4-year mortality was not significant.

As early as 2010, Aronson et al. reported that intraoperative BPV was associated with 30-day mortality in patients undergoing CABG (13). Early outcomes can be predicted from intraoperative BPV, but its clinical significance is limited, as cardiopulmonary bypass and vasoactive agents are routinely used to stabilize the BP and maintain organic perfusion when the heart is not beating. In 2019, Dyke et al. analyzed 405 patients and demonstrated that preoperative 3-year visit-to-visit BPV was a risk factor for adverse outcomes after CABG (12). However, the prognostic value of preoperative visit-to-visit BPV is restricted by the inconvenience of follow-up prior to surgery, patient non-compliance, and the uncertainty of surgical timing while post-operative short-term BPV based on ICU monitoring records is a clinically applicable prognostic factor with practical clinical utility for patients undergoing CABG.

Although various studies have reported the relationship between higher BPV and the risk of cardiovascular events, the measurement, and assessment of BPV have not been standardized, and BPV could be measured in various ways, including visit-to-visit, day-to-day and beat-to-beat variability (17). Each has its strength and limits. For healthy individuals or patients with chronic diseases such as chronic kidney disease that require long-term follow-up, visit-to-visit BPV could provide additional predictive value for long-term cardiovascular events (6, 18). For patients with acute illnesses such as intracerebral hemorrhage and patients undergoing surgical treatment, short-term post-admission or post-operative BPV is easier to acquire and more appropriate to be considered as a risk factor (19, 20). In addition, BPV is commonly evaluated based on CV and SD, while the average real variability and variation independent of the mean have also been suggested (21, 22). Regardless of which approach is selected for evaluation, methodological problems, including mortal time bias, informatics censors, inappropriate adjustment, and inconsistent equipment, can inevitably lead to potential bias (23).

In our study, systolic BPV within the first post-operative 24-h was evaluated by CV, and sensitivity analyses were performed by measuring BPV as SD quartiles of SBP and CV or SD quartiles of DBP. In addition, logistic and Cox regression analyses based on different models and subgroup analyses were conducted, and the results of the sensitivity analyses were generally consistent, though the results based on DBP were statistically insignificant. To evaluate whether post-operative 12-h BPV was associated with the prognosis, we conducted an analysis based on the post-operative 12-h CV of SBP. Although similar trends could be observed, the results were statistically insignificant when fully adjusted. One possible explanation was that within the first 12 h, patients were in unstable conditions and primarily affected by the surgical operation and intraoperative anesthesia, analgesia, and vasoactive medication usage. In addition, volume adjustment and medical titration at the beginning of ICU admission also influences the fluctuation of BP (24). As SBP is considered to be more sensitive than DBP (14, 15) and CV can better balance the difference of baseline BP compared with SD, the first 24-h systolic BPV evaluated by CV was chosen as a more rational parameter to demonstrate the association between post-operative BPV and the prognosis in patients undergoing CABG.

Compared with 4-year mortality, the association between BPV and ICU, 30- and 90-day mortality were more replicable in the analyses, indicating that the prognostic value of BPV was more prominent for short-term outcomes. For long-term survival, although the results of the Cox regression analyses demonstrated no significant difference between the two groups, the trend still favored a higher risk in the highest quartile, and the survival curves of different quartiles were separated from each other with a $P < 0.01$. The insignificance was clinically reasonable since more death attributed to other unknown confounding factors occurred as time went on, and of note is that if patients could survive the initial hemodynamic instability, they were unlikely to have long-term outcome issues.

On the basis of evidence proposed by the guidelines (25), short-term 24-h BPV is considered for risk stratification in populations or cohorts while this parameter has not come into routine usage in the current clinical practice. For better observation and treatment after the CABG operation, patients are sent to the ICU where their vital signs can be monitored and recorded in the electronic health records. The evaluation of BPV supports doctors in identifying potential patients with hemodynamic instability, which might be reflective of other issues like multi-system organ dysfunction syndrome, and making timely clinical decisions based on the oscillations of BP. Although limited therapeutic strategy targeting post-operative BPV was reported, long-acting antihypertensive drugs like amlodipine and chlorthalidone were recommended to reduce long-term BPV (26, 27). However, the optimal approaches in BPV management and whether these approaches indeed bring benefits to patients, namely, an independent reduction in adverse events and mortality, need further investigations.

The current study must be interpreted within the context of its limitation. Considering most of our included patients have received medications that limit the natural variation of BP, this would be expected to bias our results toward statistical insignificance. However, analyses based on different models and parameters consistently yielded confirmatory results. Additionally, the definition of comorbidities based on the ICD-9-CM codes would be potentially not specific enough, and certain important information including preoperative risk scores, urgent or emergent surgery, intraoperative details, and cardiovascular events were not available in the database. Finally, the nature of single-center-based cohort limits the generalizability of our conclusions and further well-designed studies should be conducted to further investigate the cause-effect relationship, prognostic, and therapeutic implication of post-operative BPV.

## CONCLUSIONS

In conclusion, our findings demonstrated that a higher systolic BPV within the first post-operative 24 h was associated with a higher risk of early mortality in patients undergoing CABG while the correlation was not significant for late mortality. Post-operative BPV can support doctors in identifying patients with potential hemodynamic instability and making timely clinical decisions.

## ETHICS STATEMENT

The studies involving human participants were reviewed and approved by the Massachusetts Institute of Technology (Cambridge, MA) and the Institutional Review Boards of Beth Israel Deaconess Medical Center (Boston, MA). Written informed consent for participation was not required for this study in accordance with the national legislation and the institutional requirements.

## AUTHOR CONTRIBUTIONS

ML and XZ: conception and design. ZW and LL: administrative support. ZZ, JH, and GF: provision of study materials or patients. SC, SH, YY, LS, and KW: selection and assembly of data. ZZ, JC, and ML: data analysis and interpretation. All authors contributed to the article and approved the submitted version.

## REFERENCES

1. Lewington S, Clarke R, Qizilbash N, Peto R, Collins R. Age-specific relevance of usual blood pressure to vascular mortality: a meta-analysis of individual data for one million adults in 61 prospective studies. *Lancet.* (2002) 360:1903–13. doi: 10.1016/S0140-6736(02)11911-8
2. Kannel WB. Blood pressure as a cardiovascular risk factor: prevention and treatment. *JAMA.* (1996) 275:1571–6. doi: 10.1001/jama.275.20.1571
3. James PA, Oparil S, Carter BL, Cushman WC, Dennison-Himmelfarb C, Handler J, et al. 2014 evidence-based guideline for the management of high blood pressure in adults: report from the panel members appointed to the Eighth Joint National Committee (JNC 8). *JAMA.* (2014) 311:507–20. doi: 10.1001/jama.2013.284427
4. Parati G, Ochoa JE, Salvi P, Lombardi C, Bilo G. Prognostic value of blood pressure variability and average blood pressure levels in patients with hypertension and diabetes. *Diabetes Care.* (2013) 36 (Suppl. 2):S312–24. doi: 10.2337/dcS13-2043
5. Nuyujukian DS, Koska J, Bahn G, Reaven PD, Zhou JJ. Blood pressure variability and risk of heart failure in ACCORD and the VADT. *Diabetes Care.* (2020) 43:1471–8. doi: 10.2337/dc19-2540

6. Lee SR, Choi YJ, Choi EK, Han KD, Lee E, Cha MJ, et al. Blood pressure variability and incidence of new-onset atrial fibrillation: a nationwide population-based study. *Hypertension.* (2020) 75:309–15. doi: 10.1161/HYPERTENSIONAHA.119.13708
7. Ernst ME, Chowdhury EK, Beilin LJ, Margolis KL, Nelson MR, Wolfe R, et al. Long-term blood pressure variability and risk of cardiovascular disease events among community-dwelling elderly. *Hypertension.* (2020) 76:1945–52. doi: 10.1161/HYPERTENSIONAHA.120.16209
8. Mehlum MH, Liestøl K, Kjeldsen SE, Julius S, Hua TA, Rothwell PM, et al. Blood pressure variability and risk of cardiovascular events and death in patients with hypertension and different baseline risks. *Eur Heart J.* (2018) 39:2243–51. doi: 10.1093/eurheartj/ehx760
9. Gosmanova EO, Mikkelsen MK, Molnar MZ, Lu JL, Yessayan LT, Kalantar-Zadeh K, et al. Association of systolic blood pressure variability with mortality, coronary heart disease, stroke, and renal disease. *J Am Coll Cardiol.* (2016) 68:1375–86. doi: 10.1016/j.jacc.2016.06.054
10. Parati G, Ochoa JE, Lombardi C, Bilo G. Assessment and management of blood-pressure variability. *Nat Rev Cardiol.* (2013) 10:143–55. doi: 10.1038/nrcardio.2013.1
11. LaPar DJ, Crosby IK, Rich JB, Quader MA, Speir AM, Kern JA, et al. Bilateral internal mammary artery use for coronary artery bypass grafting remains underutilized: a propensity-matched multi-institution analysis. *Ann Thorac Surg.* (2015) 100:8–14; discussion: 5. doi: 10.1016/j.athoracsur.2015.02.088
12. Dyke CM, Benz CL, Taggart CM, Klug MG, Basson MD. Systolic and diastolic blood pressure variability as risk factors for adverse events after coronary artery bypass grafting. *JAMA Surg.* (2019) 154:92–4. doi: 10.1001/jamasurg.2018.3233
13. Aronson S, Stafford-Smith M, Phillips-Bute B, Shaw A, Gaca J, Newman M. Intraoperative systolic blood pressure variability predicts 30-day mortality in aortocoronary bypass surgery patients. *Anesthesiology.* (2010) 113:305–12. doi: 10.1097/ALN.0b013e3181e07ee9
14. Haider AW, Larson MG, Franklin SS, Levy D. Systolic blood pressure, diastolic blood pressure, and pulse pressure as predictors of risk for congestive heart failure in the Framingham Heart Study. *Ann Int Med.* (2003) 138:10–6. doi: 10.7326/0003-4819-138-1-200301070-00006
15. Kannel WB, Gordon T, Schwartz MJ. Systolic versus diastolic blood pressure and risk of coronary heart disease. The Framingham study. *Am J Cardiol.* (1971) 27:335–46. doi: 10.1016/0002-9149(71)90428-0
16. Johnson AE, Pollard TJ, Shen L, Lehman LW, Feng M, Ghassemi M, et al. MIMIC-III, a freely accessible critical care database. *Sci Data.* (2016) 3:160035. doi: 10.1038/sdata.2016.35
17. Webb AJS, Lawson A, Wartolowska K, Mazzucco S, Rothwell PM. Progression of beat-to-beat blood pressure variability despite best medical management. *Hypertension.* (2021) 77:193–201. doi: 10.1161/HYPERTENSIONAHA.120.16290
18. Gregg LP, Hedayati SS, Yang H, Van Buren PN, Banerjee S, Navaneethan SD, et al. Association of blood pressure variability and diuretics with cardiovascular events in patients with chronic kidney disease stages 1-5. *Hypertension.* (2021) 77:948–59. doi: 10.1161/HYPERTENSIONAHA.120.16117
19. de Havenon A, Majersik JJ, Stoddard G, Wong KH, McNally JS, Smith AG, et al. Increased blood pressure variability contributes to worse outcome after intracerebral hemorrhage. *Stroke.* (2018) 49:1981–4. doi: 10.1161/STROKEAHA.118.022133
20. Divani AA, Liu X, Di Napoli M, Lattanzi S, Ziai W, James ML, et al. Blood pressure variability predicts poor in-hospital outcome in spontaneous intracerebral hemorrhage. *Stroke.* (2019) 50:2023–9. doi: 10.1161/STROKEAHA.119.025514
21. Mena L, Pintos S, Queipo NV, Aizpúrua JA, Maestre G, Sulbarán T. A reliable index for the prognostic significance of blood pressure variability. *J Hypertens.* (2005) 23:505–11. doi: 10.1097/01.hjh.0000160205.81652.5a
22. Yano Y. Visit-to-visit blood pressure variability-what is the current challenge? *Am J Hypertens.* (2017) 30:112–4. doi: 10.1093/ajh/hpw124
23. Stevens SL, Wood S, Koshiaris C, Law K, Glasziou P, Stevens RJ, et al. Blood pressure variability and cardiovascular disease: systematic review and meta-analysis. *BMJ.* (2016) 354:i4098. doi: 10.1136/bmj.i4098
24. Costa AS, Costa PH, de Lima CE, Pádua LE, Campos LA, Baltatu OC. ICU blood pressure variability may predict nadir of respiratory depression after coronary artery bypass surgery. *Front Neurosci.* (2015) 9:506. doi: 10.3389/fnins.2015.00506
25. Schutte R, Thijs L, Liu YP, Asayama K, Jin Y, Odili A, et al. Within-subject blood pressure level–not variability–predicts fatal and nonfatal outcomes in a general population. *Hypertension.* (2012) 60:1138–47. doi: 10.1161/HYPERTENSIONAHA.112.202143
26. Webb AJ, Fischer U, Mehta Z, Rothwell PM. Effects of antihypertensive-drug class on interindividual variation in blood pressure and risk of stroke: a systematic review and meta-analysis. *Lancet.* (2010) 375:906–15. doi: 10.1016/S0140-6736(10)60235-8
27. Kollias A, Stergiou GS, Kyriakoulis KG, Bilo G, Parati G. Treating visit-to-visit blood pressure variability to improve prognosis: is amlodipine the drug of choice? *Hypertension.* (2017) 70:862–6. doi: 10.1161/HYPERTENSIONAHA.117.10087

# Nitric Oxide in Selective Cerebral Perfusion Could Enhance Neuroprotection During Aortic Arch Surgery

*Daniele Linardi*[1*], *Romel Mani*[1], *Angela Murari*[1], *Sissi Dolci*[2], *Loris Mannino*[2], *Ilaria Decimo*[2], *Maddalena Tessari*[1], *Sara Martinazzi*[1], *Leonardo Gottin*[3], *Giovanni B. Luciani*[1], *Giuseppe Faggian*[1] and *Alessio Rungatscher*[1]

[1] *Division of Cardiac Surgery, Department of Surgery, University of Verona, Verona, Italy,* [2] *Department of Pharmacology, University of Verona, Verona, Italy,* [3] *Division of Cardio-Thoracic Anesthesiology and Intensive Care, Department of Surgery, University of Verona, Verona, Italy*

***Correspondence:***
*Daniele Linardi*
*daniele.linardi@aovr.veneto.it*

**Background:** Hypothermic circulatory arrest (HCA) in aortic arch surgery has a significant risk of neurological injury despite the newest protective techniques and strategies. Nitric oxide (NO) could exert a protective role, reduce infarct area and increase cerebral perfusion. This study aims to investigate the possible neuroprotective effects of NO administered in the oxygenator of selective antegrade cerebral perfusion (SCP) during HCA.

**Methods:** Thirty male SD adult rats (450–550 g) underwent cardiopulmonary bypass (CPB), cooling to 22°C body core temperature followed by 30 min of HCA. Rats were randomized to receive SCP or SCP added with NO (20 ppm) administered through the oxygenator (SCP-NO). All animals underwent CPB-assisted rewarming to a target temperature of 35°C in 60 min. At the end of the experiment, rats were sacrificed, and brain collected. Immunofluorescence analysis was performed in blind conditions.

**Results:** Neuroinflammation assessed by allograft inflammatory factor 1 or ionized calcium-binding adapter molecule 1 expression, a microglia activation marker was lower in SCP-NO compared to SCP ($4.11 \pm 0.59$ vs. $6.02 \pm 0.18\%$; $p < 0.05$). Oxidative stress measured by 8oxodG, was reduced in SCP-NO ($0.37 \pm 0.01$ vs. $1.03 \pm 0.16\%$; $p < 0.05$). Brain hypoxic area extent, analyzed by thiols oxidation was attenuated in SCP-NO ($1.85 \pm 0.10$ vs. $2.74 \pm 0.19\%$; $p < 0.05$). Furthermore, the apoptotic marker caspases 3 was significantly reduced in SCP-NO ($10.64 \pm 0.37$ vs. $12.61 \pm 0.88\%$; $p < 0.05$).

**Conclusions:** Nitric oxide administration in the oxygenator during SCP and HCA improves neuroprotection by decreasing neuroinflammation, optimizing oxygen delivery by reducing oxidative stress and hypoxic areas, finally decreasing apoptosis.

**Keywords: hypothermic circulatory arrest (HCA), nitric oxide (NO), selective cerebral perfusion, neuroprotection, aortic arch surgery/hemiarch repair**

## INTRODUCTION

Hypothermic circulatory arrest (HCA) is required during aortic arch surgery (1). Since the 1990's, selective brain perfusion (SCP) techniques have become increasingly common (2, 3). Despite these advancements, neurological damage of different severity develops in 5–20% of patients, mainly in urgent interventions for aortic dissection (4).

Neurological damage comprises permanent neurological dysfunction (PND) and temporary neurological dysfunction (TND). These two types of damage differ for etiopathogenesis, histological and clinical manifestation. PND manifests itself clinically as a neurological deficit secondary to perfusion deficit (embolism, vascular occlusion, and absence of blood flow). Risk factors for PND include an atheromatous disease and vasculopathy of the epiaortic vessels and the cerebral circulation (5, 6). TND is a reversible and widespread lesion attributed primarily to a global brain ischemic lesion consequence of inadequate brain protection (7).

Although techniques advancements and developments have reduced PND, the percentage of patients with TND is still exceedingly high (8). A combination of hypothermia and SCP could expose the brain to an excess of oxygen delivery related to reduced demand during hypothermia (9). This could impair cerebral microvascular autoregulation with the production of reactive oxygen species (ROS), oxidative stress, and inflammation that could contribute to TND development (**Figure 1**).

Nitric oxide (NO) has been recognized for its cardioprotective and neuroprotective effects (10). Since constitutive NO synthase (cNOS) is impaired during hypothermia (11), NO administration could effectively optimize cerebral microvascular blood flow, attenuating ischemia-reperfusion injury, neuroinflammation, and neuronal death (12). This preclinical study aims to investigate the neuroprotective effects of NO administered through SCP in HCA.

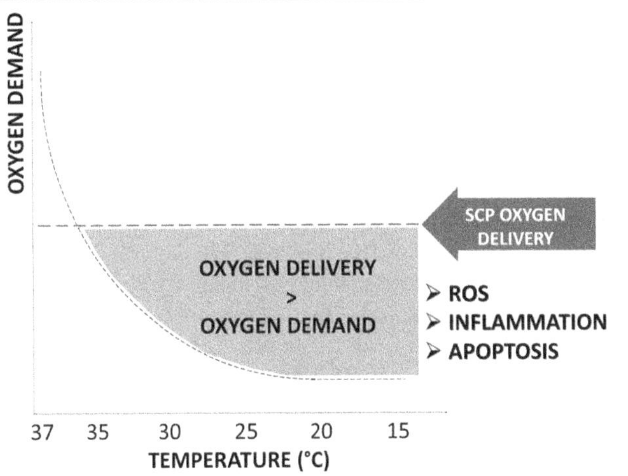


**FIGURE 1 |** Oxygen delivery in hypothermia. The excess of oxygen delivered by selective cerebral perfusion (SCP) compared to decreased oxygen demand at the different grades of hypothermia is represented by the gray area under "SCP oxygen dysfunction." An excess in oxygen delivery increases reactive oxygen species (ROS), oxidative stress, inflammation, and apoptosis and promotes temporary neurologic deficit (TND) development. SCP flow rate, oxygen content, temperature, and blood gas management of the perfusate have not been clearly defined and vary considerably among centers.

## METHODS

All experiments were performed according to the Guide for the Care and Use of Laboratory Animals (National Institutes of Health Publication No. 85-23, revised 1996). The experimental protocol was validated by the scientific committee for experimental research of the University of Verona and approved by the National Ministry of Health (Ministerial Authorization Number 568/2020-PR, Protocol Number 56DC9.54).

A total of 30 male Sprague Dawley rats weighing 450 ± 50 g, aged 6–7 months, were used for the experiments.

### Surgical Procedure

Anesthesia was induced with Sevoflurane 6% (Forene; Abbott, Baar, Switzerland), rats were orotracheal intubated and ventilated by mechanical respirator for rodents (Harvard Model 687, Harvard Apparatus, Holliston, MA, USA). Tidal volume was 10 ml/kg and respiratory frequency 70 breaths per minute, animals were kept sedated with a mixture of oxygen and sevoflurane 2%, ketoprofen 2 mg/kg was injected subcutaneously to maintain analgesia, and 2 mg/kg of pancuronium-bromide was infused through the right femoral vein to obtain muscle relaxation. Electrocardiogram and body temperature through a rectal probe were monitored throughout the entire experiment. Furthermore, a miniaturized 2-Fr-diameter catheter (model SPR 838, Millar Instruments, Houston, TX, USA) was inserted into the right femoral artery to monitor systemic arterial pressure.

Animals were surgically prepared for cardiopulmonary bypass (CPB). Rat CPB model was previously described in detail (13–15). The circuit was modified to permit selective cerebral perfusion. After right external jugular isolation, a 5-Fr-diameter cannula was inserted and advanced in the right atrium, and 500 IU/kg of heparin was administered. The left common carotid artery was cannulated with a 24 G catheter advanced to the aortic arch, and another 26 G catheter was inserted in the upper left carotid artery and directed to the brain. The two cannulas were connected through a three-way stopcock to the arterial perfusion line.

The extracorporeal circulation circuit was constituted by an outflow tube connected to the right jugular vein, a venous reservoir connected to vacuum (maintained between −40 and −60 $cmH_2O$), a connection tube that runs through a roller pump (Stockert SIII, Sorin, Germany) and ends in a hollow

**Abbreviations:** CPB, Cardiopulmonary bypass; DAPI, 4′,6-Diamidine-2′-phenylindole dihydrochloride; HCA, Hypothermic circulatory arrest; Iba1, Allograft inflammatory factor 1 or ionized calcium-binding adapter molecule 1; NO, Nitric oxide; NOS, Nitric oxide synthase; PND, Permanent neurological dysfunction; ROS, Reactive oxygen species; SCP, Selective cerebral perfusion; TND, Temporary neurological dysfunction.

fiber oxygenator with industrial standard characteristics (Sorin, Mirandola, MO, Italy), and an inflow tube connected through a three-way stopcock to upper and lower left carotid artery. The total length of the extracorporeal circuit was 90 cm, outflow tube had 2 mm inside diameter whereas the remaining circuit had 1.6 mm inside diameter; total filling volume was 6.5 ml and constituted by 50% lactated Ringer's solution and 50% colloid solution (Voluven, Fresenius Kabi Italia Srl, VR, Italy). The oxygenator exchange surface area was 450 $cm^2$. A flow rate of 110–130 ml/kg/min and a range of mean arterial pressure of 70–80 mmHg was assured. The temperature was adjusted by a heat exchanger (Sarns cardioplegic set, Terumo Cardiovascular System Corp., Ann Arbor, MI, USA) incorporated in the circuit, and it was modulated upon rectal temperature monitoring.

## Experimental Protocol

Hypothermia (22°C) was induced in 25 min. CPB was conducted with the total assisted flow (110–130 ml/kg). When the temperature was 22 ± 1°C, the aorta was clamped, and rats were left in a state of HCA. Immediately the three-way stopcock on the arterial line was turned to direct the oxygenated blood flow only to the cannula inserted in the upper left carotid and, therefore, to the brain. In its gaseous form, NO could be administered to the patient through the CPB, connecting the NO delivery system directly to the oxygenator (16, 17).

Animals were randomized to receive unilateral SCP (10 ml/kg/min) with oxygenated blood (group SCP; $n = 15$) or with the addition of NO (20 ppm) using a gas delivery system (iNOmax, Mallinckrodt Staines-upon-Thames, United Kingdom) connected directly to the oxygenator (group SCP-NO; $n = 15$).

The experimental model has been evaluated in preliminary experiments to measure the blood flow through the cannula inserted in the superior left carotid artery, the cerebral electrical activity measured by continuous EEG, and methemoglobin production on right jugular vein blood samples.

The dose regimen of 20 ppm of NO has been selected considering the highest dosage with a cumulative methemoglobin production minor or equal to 4% in pilot experiments. After 30 min, the aortic clamp was removed, and total CPB was re-established. After 60 min of reperfusion and rewarming to 35°C, the animals were weaned from CPB (**Figure 2**).

## Arterial Blood Gas Analysis

Arterial samples were collected for blood gas analysis (pH, $pO_2$, $pCO_2$, hematocrit, and lactate) before the procedure (T0), before HCA (T1), after HCA (T2), and at the end of the experiment (T3).

## Tissue Analysis

After injection of a lethal bolus of KCl, phosphate-buffered saline (PBS 1X, 10 ml) was injected in the cannula inserted in the upper left carotid, followed by 10 ml paraformaldehyde 4% (PFA)-4% sucrose. A posterior craniotomy was performed, and the whole brain was removed and placed in PFA 4–4% sucrose overnight. The next day brains were placed in 30% sucrose solution and kept at 4°C. About 70 slides were prepared for each sample, each with 4–5 slices (35-μm-thick) and stored at −20°C. Cryosections were incubated overnight at 4°C in the primary antibody solution. The following day, slides were left in incubation with the secondary antibody conjugated with fluorophores. Slides were kept in the dark to avoid the photobleaching of the fluorophore.

Ionized calcium binding adapter molecule 1 (Iba1) (Wako Chemicals, USA) is specific for microglia cells and macrophages that are determinants of the central nervous system's first and primary immune defense (18–20). To analyze the degree of oxidative stress and apoptosis, we evaluate the expression of 8-oxo-2′-deoxyguanosine (8oxodG) (ABCAM, UK) and caspases 3 (Cell Signaling, USA) (21–23).

After incubation with the primary and secondary antibody solution, slides were incubated with DAPI (4′,6-diamidine-2′-phenylindole dihydrochloride, molecular probes—Thermo Fisher Scientific, 1:3,000) for nucleus staining.

To detect hypoxic regions in the brain, reduced thiols were labeled (24). After perfusion with a solution containing N-ethylmaleimide (NEM) and iodoacetic acid (IAA) to block free thiols, brains were fixed with 4% PFA containing NEM and IAA. Finally, brains were dissected and kept overnight in the same solution and then processed for cryosectioning as described before. After cryosectioning, samples were washed with a solution containing tris(2-carboxyethyl) phosphine hydrochloride in PBS to reduce free disulfides. Samples were then labeled with 0.1% CPM (7-diethylamino-3-(4'-maleimidylphenyl)-4-methylcoumarin) and mounted with DABCO (1,4-diazabicyclo[2.2.2]octane).

Slides were examined with a fluorescence microscope (Eclipse Ti, Nikon, objective 20X); images obtained for each region considered were then transferred to a computer for analysis using a custom-designed ImageJ macro (US National Institutes of Health) in blind conditions.

## Statistical Analysis

Data analysis was performed using SPSS software version 21 (SPSS Inc., Chicago, Illinois), mean ± SD was calculated for all the measurements. The average percentage of cells positive for specific markers: Iba1, 8oxodG, and caspases 3 expressions were quantified in randomly selected brain regions comprising the sensory-motor cortex. The number of marker positive cells (Iba1, 8oxodG, and caspases 3) was normalized to the total number of nuclei of the regions considered (429 images were quantified across the different conditions, each image was acquired as a single image). For the hypoxic area analysis, the sensory-motor cortex was delimited, and hypoxic areas were quantified as the percentage of the mean gray level of each brain slice. The percentage of positive pixels for the hypoxic areas were normalized for the total pixel in the region considered (121 images were quantified across the different conditions, each image was acquired as a large image constituted by 6 × 20 fields).

Student *t*-test or Mann–Whitney non-parametric tests were applied to compare the immunofluorescent analysis and the blood gas values of the two groups; $p < 0.05$ was considered statistically significant.

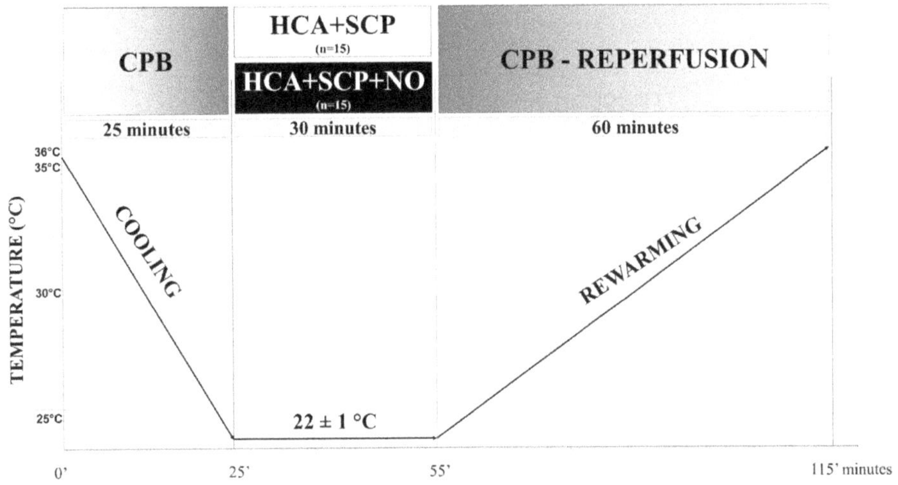


**FIGURE 2** | Experimental protocol. Timeline of the experimental protocol. CPB, cardiopulmonary bypass; HCA, hypothermic circulatory arrest; SCP, selective cerebral perfusion.

# RESULTS

## Arterial Blood Gas Analysis

Blood gas analysis showed an increase in lactates during HCA, followed by a gradual normalization during rewarming. The pH returned normal during rewarming after the development of acidosis in the circulatory arrest phase. No significant differences were identified between SCP and SCP-NO groups (**Table 1**).

## Inflammation

Ionized calcium binding adapter molecule 1 (Iba1) expression is specific for microglia cells and macrophages and indicates an inflammatory activation, and its amount correlates with the degree of neuroinflammation. Expression of Iba1 in different brain areas of the sensory-motor cortex in the SCP-NO group was lower compared to SCP (4.11 ± 0.59 vs. 6.02 ± 0.18%; $p < 0.05$), indicating decreased microglia activation and neuroinflammation (**Figure 3**).

## Oxidative Stress

Hypothermic circulatory arrest (HCA) and SCP contribute to ROS production and oxidative stress, which determine cell death by lipid peroxidation and DNA oxidation. The latter is associated with the conversion of the deoxyguanosine into 8-oxo-2'-deoxyguanosine (8oxoDG) that is recognized as a marker of oxidative stress. In the SCP-NO group, the 8oxoDG content was lower compared to SCP (0.37 ± 0.01 vs. 1.03 ± 0.16%; $p < 0.05$), indicating attenuated oxidative stress (**Figure 4**).

## Hypoxia

Thiols are a functional group of cysteine amino acids, which on the base of the oxidoreductive state could exist either as a reduced form of free thiols (-SH) or an oxidized form (-S-S-). In states of higher tissue oxygenation, thiols exist as oxidized disulfides; on the contrary, lower oxygen tissue oxygenation (hypoxia condition) leads to an increased free thiols presence. The latter indicate hypoxic brain areas, which were lower in SCP-NO compared to SCP (1.85 ± 0.10 vs. 2.74 ± 0.19%; $p < 0.01$), indicating a beneficial effect on NO in promoting the oxygen delivery counteracting impaired cerebral microcirculation (**Figure 5**).

## Apoptosis

The expression of caspases 3 identifies cells where the apoptotic process is initiated. The apoptotic index (% of apoptotic cells) was lower in SCP-NO compared to SCP (10.64 ± 0.37 vs. 12.61 ± 0.88%; $p < 0.05$), demonstrating an attenuated cell death (**Figure 6**).

# DISCUSSION

Hypothermic circulatory arrest (HCA) is still necessary to safely perform aortic arch surgery. Nowadays, SCP is the primary technique for brain protection in large aortic centers, while the HCA temperature has been rising progressively over the last few years (25, 26). There is a certain degree of consensus in the use of SCP and HCA; however, the temperatures and flow of perfusion vary from center to center, and there are no consensus statements, no clinical guidelines (4). Although HCA reduces brain metabolism and assures neuroprotection while permitting intervention in a clear surgical field, it can induce oxidative stress, inflammatory response, endothelial swelling, cerebral edema, and vasospasm (27). The critical role of reperfusion and simultaneous rewarming should not be underestimated since they have been demonstrated to be the main responsible for neuroinflammation and neuronal apoptosis, resulting in TND and cognitive dysfunction (28, 29).

To maximize the neurological outcome, efforts to identify possible neuroprotective agents combined with SCP should be pursued similarly to what has been done for cardioplegic solutions. The ideal pharmacological agent to add to SCP should improve perfusion distribution overcoming impaired cerebral autoregulation during hypothermia. Moreover, it

**TABLE 1** | Blood gas parameters.

| | | | SCP | SCP-NO | SCP | SCP-NO |
|---|---|---|---|---|---|---|
| | **T0 (35°C)** | **T1 (22°C)** | **T2 (22°C)** | **T2 (22°C)** | **T3 (35°C)** | **T3 (35°C)** |
| pH | 7.40 ± 0.05 | 7.36 ± 0.04 | 7.23 ± 0.10 | 7.22 ± 0.12 | 7.38 ± 0.03 | 7.38 ± 0.05 |
| $pCO_2$ (mmHg) | 39 ± 2.5 | 32 ± 3 | 48 ± 5.3 | 48 ± 3.7 | 32 ± 4.3 | 30 ± 5.8 |
| $pO_2$ (mmHg) | 140 ± 10 | 305 ± 20 | 90 ± 15 | 87 ± 12 | 210 ± 33 | 213 ± 43 |
| Hematocrit (%) | 45 ± 2.5 | 47.6 ± 2.3 | 31 ± 2.5 | 32 ± 2.5 | 29 ± 2.8 | 30 ± 2.8 |
| Lactate (mmol/l) | 1.0 ± 0.2 | 2.5 ± 0.5 | 8.5 ± 2.5 | 8.3 ± 2.4 | 4.1 ± 1.6 | 4.6 ± 2 |

*SCP, selective cerebral perfusion; SCP-NO, selective cerebral perfusion plus nitric oxide. T0, baseline; T1, before hypothermic circulatory arrest (HCA); T2, after HCA; T3, end of reperfusion.*

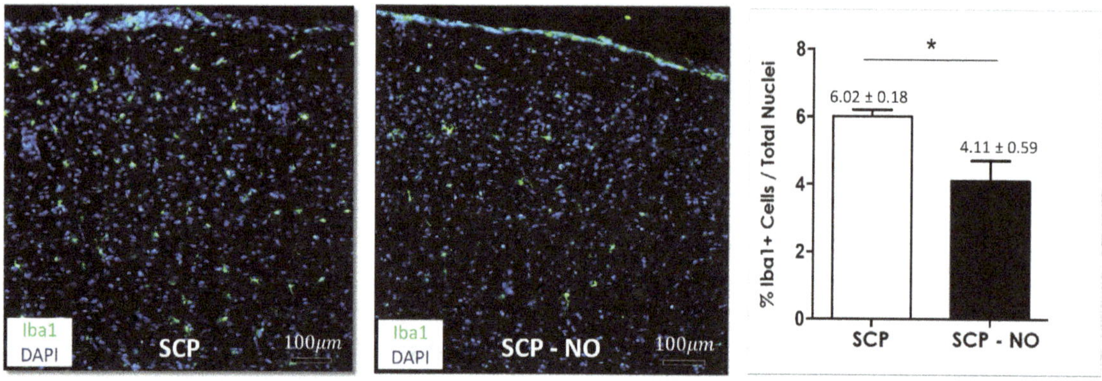


**FIGURE 3** | Inflammation: Iba1. Representative images of Iba1 expression at the cortical level, between the selective cerebral perfusion (SCP) group compared to selective cerebral perfusion with nitric oxide 20 ppm (SCP-NO). In the graph, blind quantification was performed to calculate the average percentage of Iba1 expression in the brain regions considered (*$p < 0.05$). The average percentage of Iba1 positive cells was normalized to the total number of nuclei in the regions of interest considered (170 images quantified across the different conditions) (magnification ×20). Iba1, ionized calcium-binding adapter molecule 1; DAPI, 4′,6-diamidine-2′-phenylindole dihydrochloride.

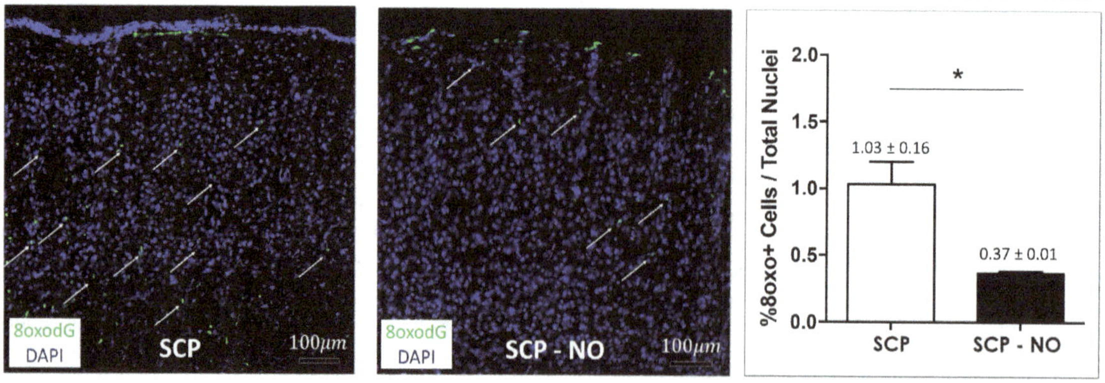


**FIGURE 4** | Oxidative stress: 8oxodG. Representative images of 8oxodG expression at the cortical level (arrows), in selective cerebral perfusion (SCP) group compared to selective cerebral perfusion with nitric oxide 20 ppm (SCP-NO). In the graph, blind quantification was performed to calculate the average percentage of 8oxodG expression in the brain regions considered (*$p < 0.05$). The average percentage of 8oxodG positive cells was normalized to the total number of nuclei in the regions of interest considered (85 images quantified across the different conditions) (magnification ×20). 8oxodG, 8-oxo-2′-deoxyguanosine. DAPI, 4′,6-diamidine-2′-phenylindole dihydrochloride.

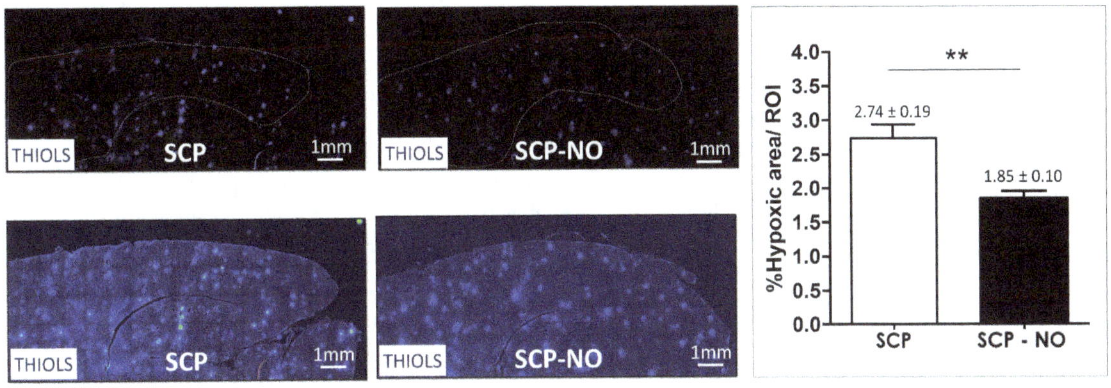


**FIGURE 5 |** Hypoxia: thiols. Representative images of hypoxic areas at the cortical level, in selective cerebral perfusion (SCP) group compared to selective cerebral perfusion with nitric oxide 20 ppm (SCP-NO). In the graph, blind quantification was performed to calculate the average percentage of the hypoxic area extension in the brain regions considered (**$p < 0.01$). The average percentage of the positive pixels for the hypoxic area was normalized to the total number of pixels of the regions of interest considered (121 images quantified across the different conditions) (magnification ×20). DAPI, 4′,6-diamidine-2′-phenylindole dihydrochloride.

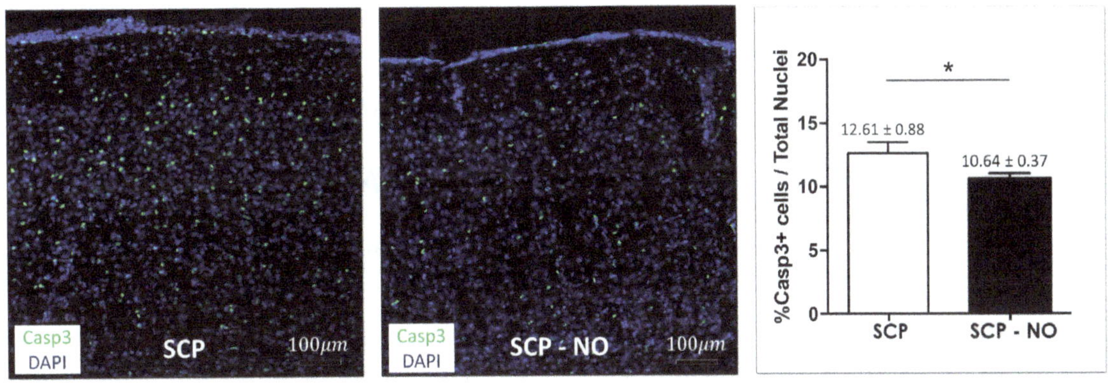


**FIGURE 6 |** Apoptosis: caspases 3. Representative images of caspase 3 expression at the cortical level, in selective cerebral perfusion (SCP) group compared to selective cerebral perfusion with nitric oxide 20 ppm (SCP-NO). In the graph, blind quantification was performed to calculate the average percentage of caspase 3 expression in the brain regions considered (*$p < 0.05$). The average percentage of caspase 3 positive cells was normalized to the total number of nuclei in the regions of interest considered (174 images quantified across the different conditions) (magnification ×20). Casp3, caspases 3. DAPI, 4′,6-diamidine-2′-phenylindole dihydrochloride.

should minimize ischemia-reperfusion injury responsible for neuroinflammation and apoptosis (30).

Nitric oxide (NO) administration has been studied after focal cerebral ischemia and has been demonstrated to decrease nuclear factor kappa B activation, oxidative and nitrosative stress, inflammation, and apoptosis, resulting in reduced infarct size and increased cerebral blood flow. The basal concentration is mainly due to constitutive isoforms of NO synthase (eNOS and nNOS). It is essential for regulating cerebrovascular hemodynamic and protecting endothelium integrity from inflammatory, oxidative, and procoagulant stimuli. Total suppression of eNOS activity in knockout mice makes them hypertensive and more susceptible to ischemia-reperfusion injury, with larger infarcts than in controls and severe reduction in cerebral blood flow. Conversely, nNOS gene deficiencies or nNOS inhibition decrease infarct volume and neuronal death (12).

During ischemia and hypothermia, the production of NO by constitutive NO synthase decreases. This is followed by a late burst of NO produced by inducible NO synthase (iNOS) that further increases its concentration to toxic concentrations (10). The primary sources of iNOS include microglia, astrocytes, and endothelial cells, infiltrating leukocytes, and can influence the evolution of brain damage after an ischemic injury. To the same extent microglia and macrophages express Iba1 when activated by a proinflammatory stimulus or by hypothermia (20, 31).

In this study, NO administration in SCP resulted in a reduced expression of Iba1, corresponding to lower neuroinflammation. Indeed, less activation of microglia leads to lower production of inflammatory cytokines, and prevents the expression of iNOS, thus attenuating cell damage resulting from inflammatory activation (32). This is consistent with the results obtained investigating the effects of inhaled NO on microglia after deep HCA (33).

In this study, NO administration during circulatory arrest reduced oxidative stress, as shown by the lower 8oxodG content. Cerebrovascular ischemia induces an inflammatory response and associated increased cytokine release and iNOS activity. NO, generated mainly by iNOS, reacts with superoxide and forms peroxynitrite. Peroxynitrite causes cellular necrosis with other ROS by lipid peroxidation, DNA damaging, disrupting mitochondrial respiratory chain, and ATP production (10).

Changes in eNOS expression, increased ROS production, and eNOS uncoupling are the principal reasons behind endothelial dysfunction. NADPH oxidase catalyzes the transfer of electrons from NADPH to oxygen to produce superoxide. The mitochondrial electron transport chain is another important source of superoxide in the cerebral vasculature. Oxidative stress and related cytotoxicity result in mitochondrial dysfunction, further accelerating superoxide production and neuronal death (12).

Nitric oxide (NO) administration reduces iNOS activation and eNOS uncoupling (10). In this situation, the production of peroxynitrite and superoxide is lowered, and oxidative stress on neuronal cells decreases.

In addition to the reduced neuroinflammation and oxidative stress, the reduction in hypoxic areas in animals treated with NO-enriched SCP could contribute to neuronal cell survival. Thiols groups are oxidized more uniformly, and the hypoxic area extension, detected by reduced thiols, decreases. The reduction of oxidative stress and hypoxic areas are indicative of preserved coupling between oxygen delivery and consumption. Administration of NO downregulates neuronal apoptosis by inhibiting increased phosphorylation of JNK, c-Jun, and Bcl-2. Furthermore, NO can nytrosilate caspases 3 directly and prevent the activation of apoptosis (12). These effects, along with an increase in cerebral blood flow, reduce brain damage after the ischemia-reperfusion event (21).

All these elements with an attenuated inflammatory milieu explain the reduced apoptosis index demonstrated in brains perfused by SCP added with NO. Indeed, NO significantly decreased caspases 3 positive cells, demonstrating a positive effect of NO administration on cell survival.

A possible limitation of this study is that it was performed on a small animal model constituted of healthy rats and with data collected in an early phase (1 h) after hypothermic circulatory arrest.

However, the protocol is clinically relevant and assured continuous SCP during 30-min HCA. The two groups studied were equivalent, and there were no vascular alterations; the consequence was diffuse and non-focal brain damage. The latter was measured by immunofluorescence analysis, and it is not possible to diagnose through current clinical techniques. Clinical manifestations can range from a slow awakening after anesthesia to delirium and psychomotor agitation resulting in TND. This study aimed to address this type of neurological damage, which negatively impacts neurologic outcomes and prognosis after aortic arch surgery.

The results of this study could inspire prospective randomized clinical studies to investigate NO application as a neuroprotective agent during SCP and HCA.

## CONCLUSIONS

Nitric oxide (NO) administration in the oxygenator during SCP and HCA may improve neuroprotection decreasing neuroinflammation, optimize oxygen delivery by reducing oxidative stress and hypoxic areas finally decrease apoptosis.

Further experiments are needed to investigate the effects on neurological outcomes.

## ETHICS STATEMENT

The animal study was reviewed and approved by the Scientific Committee for Experimental Research of the University of Verona and approved by the National Ministry of Health (Ministerial Authorization Number 568/2020-PR, Protocol Number 56DC9.54).

## AUTHOR CONTRIBUTIONS

DL: conceptualization, methodology, investigation, and writing-original draft. AR: conceptualization project administration, writing-review, and editing. GF and GL: funding acquisition and supervision. LG: resources acquisition (nitric oxide). SM and MT: methodology and investigation (cardiopulmonary bypass technician). ID, LM, and SD: formal analysis (immunofluorescence). AM and RM: methodology, investigation, and experiment execution. All authors contributed to the article and approved the submitted version.

## REFERENCES


1. Englum BR, Andersen ND, Husain AM, Mathew JP, Hughes GC. Degree of hypothermia in aortic arch surgery - optimal temperature for cerebral and spinal protection: deep hypothermia remains the gold standard in the absence of randomized data. *Ann Cardiothorac Surg.* (2013) 2:184–93. doi: 10.3978/j.issn.2225-319X.2013.03.01
2. Kazui T, Inoue N, Yamada O, Komatsu S. Selective cerebral perfusion during operation for aneurysms of the aortic arch: a reassessment. *Ann Thorac Surg.* (1992) 53:109–14. doi: 10.1016/0003-4975(92)90767-X
3. Griepp RB. Cerebral protection during aortic arch surgery. *J Thorac Cardiovasc Surg.* (2001) 121:425–7. doi: 10.1067/mtc.2001.113594
4. Linardi D, Faggian G, Rungatscher A. Temperature management during circulatory arrest in cardiac surgery. *Ther Hypothermia Temp Manag.* (2016) 6:9–16. doi: 10.1089/ther.2015.0026
5. Okada T, Shimamoto M, Yamazaki F, Nakai M, Miura Y, Itonaga T, et al. Insights of stroke in aortic arch surgery: identification of significant risk factors and surgical implication. *Gen Thorac Cardiovasc Surg.* (2012) 60:268–74. doi: 10.1007/s11748-011-0884-z
6. Goldstein LJ, Davies RR, Rizzo JA, Davila JJ, Cooperberg MR, Shaw RK, et al. Stroke in surgery of the thoracic aorta: incidence, impact, etiology, and prevention. *J Thorac Cardiovasc Surg.* (2001) 122:935–45. doi: 10.1067/mtc.2001.117276
7. Ergin MA, Griepp EB, Lansman SL, Galla JD, Levy M, Griepp RB. Hypothermic circulatory arrest and other methods of cerebral protection

during operations on the thoracic aorta. *J Card Surg.* (1994) 9:525–37. doi: 10.1111/j.1540-8191.1994.tb00886.x

8. Okita Y. Neuro-protection in open arch surgery. *Ann Cardiothorac Surg.* (2018) 7:389–96. doi: 10.21037/acs.2018.04.01
9. Mavroudis CD, Ko T, Volk LE, Smood B, Morgan RW, Lynch JM, et al. Does supply meet demand? A comparison of perfusion strategies on cerebral metabolism in a neonatal swine model. *J Thorac Cardiovasc Surg.* (2022) 163:e47–58. doi: 10.1016/j.jtcvs.2020.12.005
10. Darra E, Rungatscher A, Carcereri de Prati A, Podesser BK, Faggian G, Scarabelli T, et al. Dual modulation of nitric oxide production in the heart during ischaemia/reperfusion injury and inflammation. *Thromb Haemost.* (2010) 104:200–6. doi: 10.1160/TH09-08-0554
11. Chatzipanteli K, Wada K, Busto R, Dietrich WD. Effects of moderate hypothermia on constitutive and inducible nitric oxide synthase activities after traumatic brain injury in the rat. *J Neurochem.* (1999) 72:2047–52. doi: 10.1046/j.1471-4159.1999.0722047.x
12. Godínez-Rubí M, Rojas-Mayorquín AE, Ortuño-Sahagún D. Nitric oxide donors as neuroprotective agents after an ischemic stroke-related inflammatory reaction. *Oxid Med Cell Longev.* (2013) 2013:297357. doi: 10.1155/2013/297357
13. Rungatscher A, Tessari M, Stranieri C, Solani E, Linardi D, Milani E, et al. Oxygenator is the main responsible for leukocyte activation in experimental model of extracorporeal circulation: a cautionary tale. *Mediators Inflamm.* (2015) 2015:484979. doi: 10.1155/2015/484979
14. Rungatscher A, Linardi D, Tessari M, Menon T, Luciani GB, Mazzucco A, et al. Levosimendan is superior to epinephrine in improving myocardial function after cardiopulmonary bypass with deep hypothermic circulatory arrest in rats. *J Thorac Cardiovasc Surg.* (2012) 143:209–14. doi: 10.1016/j.jtcvs.2011.09.020
15. Rungatscher A, Linardi D, Giacomazzi A, Tessari M, Menon T, Mazzucco A, et al. Cardioprotective effect of ??-opioid receptor agonist vs. mild therapeutic hypothermia in a rat model of cardiac arrest with extracorporeal life support. *Resuscitation.* (2013) 84:244–8. doi: 10.1016/j.resuscitation.2012.06.016
16. Checchia PA, Bronicki RA, Muenzer JT, Dixon D, Raithel S, Gandhi SK, et al. Nitric oxide delivery during cardiopulmonary bypass reduces postoperative morbidity in children - a randomized trial. *J Thorac Cardiovasc Surg.* (2013) 146:530–6. doi: 10.1016/j.jtcvs.2012.09.100
17. James C, Millar J, Horton S, Brizard C, Molesworth C, Butt W. Nitric oxide administration during paediatric cardiopulmonary bypass: a randomised controlled trial. *Intensive Care Med.* (2016) 42:1744–52. doi: 10.1007/s00134-016-4420-6
18. Imai Y, Ibata I, Ito D, Oshawa K, Kohsaka S. A novel gene iba1 in the major histocompatibility complex class III region encoding an EF hand protein expressed in a monocytic lineage. *Biochem Biophys Res Commun.* (1996) 224:855–62. doi: 10.1006/bbrc.1996.1112
19. Jeong HK, Ji KM, Kim J, Jou I, Joe EH. Repair of astrocytes, blood vessels, and myelin in the injured brain: possible roles of blood monocytes. *Mol Brain.* (2013) 6:28. doi: 10.1186/1756-6606-6-28
20. Zhao SC, Ma LS, Chu ZH, Xu H, Wu WQ, Liu F. Regulation of microglial activation in stroke. *Acta Pharmacol Sin.* (2017) 38:445–58. doi: 10.1038/aps.2016.162
21. Olmez I, Ozyurt H. Reactive oxygen species and ischemic cerebrovascular disease. *Neurochem Int.* (2012) 60:208–12. doi: 10.1016/j.neuint.2011.11.009
22. Ock CY, Kim EH, Choi DJ, Lee HJ, Hahm KB, Chung MH. 8-Hydroxydeoxyguanosine: not mere biomarker for oxidative stress, but remedy for oxidative stress-implicated gastrointestinal diseases. *World J Gastroenterol.* (2012) 18:302–8. doi: 10.3748/wjg.v18.i4.302
23. Hyun JW, Jung YC, Kim HS, Choi EY, Kim JE, Yoon BH, et al. 8-Hydroxydeoxyguanosine causes death of human leukemia cells deficient in 8-oxoguanine glycosylase 1 activity by inducing apoptosis. *Mol Cancer Res.* (2003) 1:290–9.
24. Shah SR, Esni F, Jakub A, Paredes AJ, Lath N, Malek M, et al. Embryonic mouse blood flow and oxygen correlate with early pancreatic differentiation. *Dev Biol.* (2011) 349:342–9. doi: 10.1016/j.ydbio.2010.10.033
25. Minatoya K, Ogino H, Matsuda H, Sasaki H, Tanaka H, Kobayashi J, et al. Evolving selective cerebral perfusion for aortic arch replacement: high flow rate with moderate hypothermic circulatory arrest. *Ann Thorac Surg.* (2008) 86:1827–31. doi: 10.1016/j.athoracsur.2008.07.024
26. Leshnower BG, Kilgo PD, Chen EP. Total arch replacement using moderate hypothermic circulatory arrest and unilateral selective antegrade cerebral perfusion. *J Thorac Cardiovasc Surg.* (2014) 147:1488–92. doi: 10.1016/j.jtcvs.2014.01.044
27. Dong SB, Xiong JX, Zhang K, Zheng J, Xu SD, Liu YM, et al. Different hypothermic and cerebral perfusion strategies in extended arch replacement for acute type A aortic dissection: a retrospective comparative study. *J Cardiothorac Surg.* (2020) 15:236. doi: 10.1186/s13019-020-01284-y
28. Rungatscher A, Luciani GB, Linardi D, Milani E, Gottin L, Walpoth B, et al. Temperature variation after rewarming from deep hypothermic circulatory arrest is associated with survival and neurologic outcome. *Ther Hypothermia Temp Manag.* (2017) 7:101–6. doi: 10.1089/ther.2016.0037
29. Linardi D, Walpoth B, Mani R, Murari A, Tessari M, Hoxha S, et al. Slow versus fast rewarming after hypothermic circulatory arrest: effects on neuroinflammation and cerebral oedema. *Eur J Cardiothorac Surg.* (2020) 58:792–800. doi: 10.1093/ejcts/ezaa143
30. Giuliano K, Torres-Odio S, Etchill E, Carr P, Talbot CC Jr, Blueet BE, et al. Inflammatory profile in a canine model of hypothermic circulatory arrest. *J Surg Res.* (2021) 264:260–73. doi: 10.1016/j.jss.2021.02.014
31. Liu M, Li Y, Gao S, Yan S, Zhang Q, Liuet G, et al. A novel target to reduce microglial inflammation and neuronal damage after deep hypothermic circulatory arrest. *J Thorac Cardiovasc Surg.* (2020) 159:2431–44.e7. doi: 10.1016/j.jtcvs.2019.06.115
32. Rodríguez-Gómez JA, Kavanagh E, Engskog-Vlachos P, Engskog MKR, Herrera AJ, Espinosa-Oliva AM, et al. Microglia: agents of the CNS pro-inflammatory response. *Cells.* (2020) 9:1717. doi: 10.3390/cells9071717
33. Kajimoto M, Nuri M, Sleasman JR, Charette KA, Nelson BR, Portman MA. Inhaled nitric oxide reduces injury and microglia activation in porcine hippocampus after deep hypothermic circulatory arrest. *J Thorac Cardiovasc Surg.* (2021) 161:e485–98. doi: 10.1016/j.jtcvs.2019.12.075

# 21

# Comparison of Single Axillary vs. Dual Arterial Cannulation for Acute Type A Aortic Dissection: A Propensity Score Matching Analysis

*Yi Chang, Hongyuan Lin, Xiangyang Qian*, Hongwei Guo, Cuntao Yu, Xiaogang Sun, Bo Wei, Qiong Ma, Yizhen Wei and Yi Shi*

*Department of Vascular Surgery, National Center for Cardiovascular Diseases, Fuwai Hospital, Cardiovascular Institute, Chinese Academy of Medical Science & Peking Union Medical College, Beijing, China*

***Correspondence:**
*Xiangyang Qian*
*m13701097213@163.com*

**Background:** The optimal arterial cannulation site for acute aortic dissection repair is unclear, especially for complex arch surgery. Axillary artery cannulation is widely accepted but adding femoral artery cannulation to it was considered to potentially improve perfusion and early outcomes. To clarify this point, a comparison of perioperative outcomes for these two different cannulation strategies was conducted regarding the pathological features of dissection.

**Methods:** From January 2010 to December 2019, 927 consecutive patients underwent a total arch replacement combined with frozen elephant trunk for acute type A aortic dissection. The data, including detailed pathological features, were retrospectively collected and analyzed. Propensity score matching and multivariate logistic regression analysis were used for adjusting confounders that are potentially related to the outcome.

**Results:** A total of 523 patients (56.3%) accepted a dual arterial cannulation (DAC group), and 406 patients (43.7%) received a single axillary artery cannulation (SAC group). In total, 388 pairs of patients were well-matched. Whether before or after adjusting the preoperative characteristics by matching, there were no significant differences in operative mortality (6.7 vs. 5.4%, $P = 0.420$ before matching; 5.4 vs. 5.4%, $P = 1$ after matching), stroke (6.7 vs. 5.4%, $P = 0.420$ before matching; 6.4 vs. 5.2%, $P = 0.435$ after matching), spinal cord injury (5 vs. 5.7%, $P = 0.640$ before matching; 5.4 vs. 5.7%, $P = 1$. After matching), and acute renal failure requiring dialysis (13.8 vs. 9.6%, $P = 0.050$ before matching; 12.6 vs. 9.5%, $P = 0.174$) between the two groups. Dual arterial cannulation was not an independent protective factor of operative mortality (odds ratio [OR] 1.01, 95% confidence interval [CI] 0.55–1.86), stroke (OR 1.17, 95% CI 0.65–2.11), spinal cord injury (OR 1.17, 95% CI 0.65–2.11), and acute renal failure requiring continuous renal replacement therapy (CRRT) (OR 1.24, 95% CI 0.78–1.97) after adjusting for confounding factors by multivariable logistic regression analysis. In the subgroup analysis, no advantage of dual arterial cannulation was found for a particular population.

**Conclusions:** Single axillary artery cannulation was competent in the complex arch repair for acute aortic dissection, presenting with a satisfactory result as dual arterial cannulation. Adding femoral artery cannulation was necessary when a sufficient flow volume could not be achieved by axillary artery cannulation or when a lower limb malperfusion existed.

**Keywords: aortic dissection, total arch replacement, frozen elephant trunk, cannulation, propensity adjustment**

## INTRODUCTION

Nowadays on China, there is a tendency to perform a total arch replacement (TAR) with frozen elephant trunk (FET) as a standard approach for acute type A aortic dissection (ATAAD), involving arch or more distally. The TAR combined with FET is more invasive and complex so that more evidence is needed to prove the optimal management for each step of this procedure. Regarding the arterial cannulation site, although the latest expert consensus of AATS (1) recommended kinds of options, controversy always exists and high-level evidence is absent. In the past years, we had attempted to apply a dual arterial cannulation to reduce the malperfusion-related mortality and morbidities by extrapolation based on clinical experience. We sought to compare dual arterial cannulation and single axillary artery cannulation on early outcomes by rigorous statistical analysis.

## MATERIALS AND METHODS

### Study Cohort

The institutional database of aortic dissection was retrospectively reviewed. All consecutive patients who were surgically treated for ATAAD using TAR and FET from January 2010 to December 2019 were included. The patients, who were not appropriate for axillary cannulation (for example, the vessel was too thin or was dissected), accepted a single femoral cannulation and they were excluded from this study (flowchart of enrollment can be seen in **Supplementary Figure I**). The Ethics Committee of Fuwai Hospital (Beijing, China) approved this retrospective study, and the need for informed consent was waived. The data of demographics, clinical features, imaging materials, surgical characteristics, and postoperative outcomes were collected.

### Institution-Specific Definition

To identify the special conditions and scenarios that would influence the progress and outcome of ATAAD, we defined some institution-specific terms to describe them. Hemodynamic instability was defined as persistent pre-anesthesia hypotension (systolic blood pressure <90 mmHg) that is preoperative for any reason. Innominate artery stenosis (IAS) was defined as severe stenosis of the true lumen caused by thrombus compression. Innominate artery, originating from the false lumen (IA-FL), as the name suggests, referred to the detachment or complete avulsion of its orifice. All the malperfusion mentioned in this study referred to the obviously disrupted blood flow of main branches of the aorta with radiographical evidence. Because superior mesenteric artery malperfusion had particular importance in ATAAD, it was identified and categorized into three types according to prior studies (2–4). Similarly, lower limb malperfusion was determined as mentioned above. Selective antegrade cerebral perfusion duration usually started from distal circulatory arrest initiation (at this moment three brachiocephalic arteries were clamped) until the anastomosis of the left common carotid artery was completed.

### Clinical Endpoints

Operative mortality, stroke, spinal cord injury, and acute renal failure requiring continuous renal replacement therapy (CRRT) were primary endpoints of interest. Operative mortality was defined as any death, regardless of cause, occurring within 30 days after surgery in or out of the hospital, and after 30 days during the same hospitalization subsequent to the operation. For stroke, spinal cord injury, and renal failure, only the new onsets were considered as complications. Spinal cord injury included permanent or transient paresis and paraplegia. All the outcomes were defined using the Society of Thoracic Surgeons definitions (see http://www.sts.org/sts-national-database/database-managers/adultcardiac-surgery-database/data-collection).

### Operative Methods

All procedures were implemented by a median sternotomy and cardiopulmonary bypass (CPB). Eight surgeons finished these operations (QXY, GHW, YCT, SXG, WB, MQ, WYZ, and SY). Arterial cannulation was manipulated as follows: (1) right axillary artery: it was exposed by subclavian incision and a purse-string suture was made on it, then a cannula (Bio-Medicus, Medtronic, Minneapolis, MN, USA) with a tapered core was directly inserted through a small incision inside the purse-string; and (2) femoral artery: it was exposed by an incision parallel to the inguinal ligament and cannulated in the same manner as described above. We used axillary artery cannula according to body weight and axillary artery size, cannula size ranged from 17Fr- 21Fr, median size was 19 Fr. We usually selected the 19 Fr–21Fr cannula for the femoral artery.

After distal anastomosis of the arch was accomplished, the femoral artery cannula was removed and the perfusion conduit was shifted to 1 limb of the 4-branch prosthetic graft. In our institute, dual arterial cannulation (right axillary artery+ femoral artery) was individually selected, mainly according to the preference and judgment of the surgeon. In rare cases, we selected femoral artery cannulation as a supplement to

**TABLE 1** | Baseline characteristics.

| Variable | Unmatched | | | P | Missing | Matched | | | P |
|---|---|---|---|---|---|---|---|---|---|
| | Overall n = 929 | DAC n = 523 | SAC n = 406 | | | Overall n = 776 | DAC n = 388 | SAC n = 388 | |
| Age, year ($\bar{X}$ ± SD) | 46.8 ± 10.1 | 47.3 ± 10.2 | 46.2 ± 9.8 | 0.09 | 0 (0.0) | 46.4 ± 10.0 | 46.4 ±10.1 | 46.3 ± 9.8 | 0.92 |
| Male (*n*, %) | 757 (81.5) | 424 (81.1) | 333 (82.0) | 0.71 | 0 (0.0) | 633 (81.6) | 316 (81.4) | 317 (81.7) | 0.92 |
| BMI, Kg/m$^2$ ($\bar{X}$ ± SD) | 26.4 ±4.1 | 26.6 ± 4.1 | 26.2 ± 4.0 | 0.17 | 2 (0.2) | 26.2 ± 4.0 | 26.2 ± 3.9 | 26.2 ± 4.1 | 0.91 |
| HT (*n*, %) | 589 (63.4) | 327 (62.5) | 262 (64.5) | 0.53 | 0 (0.0) | 497 (64.0) | 249 (64.2) | 248 (63.9) | 0.94 |
| CAD (*n*, %) | 58 (6.2) | 37 (7.1) | 21 (5.2) | 0.23 | 0 (0.0) | 43 (5.5) | 22 (5.7) | 21 (5.4) | 0.88 |
| AF (*n*, %) | 8 (0.9) | 3 (0.6) | 5 (1.2) | 0.31* | 0 (0.0) | 6 (0.8) | 3 (0.8) | 3 (0.8) | 1.00 |
| DM (*n*, %) | 22 (2.4) | 10 (1.9) | 12 (3.0) | 0.30 | 0 (0.0) | 21 (2.7) | 9 (2.3) | 12 (3.1) | 0.66 |
| Marfan syndrome (*n*, %) | 68 (7.3) | 38 (7.3) | 30 (7.4) | 0.94 | 0 (0.0) | 59 (7.6) | 30 (7.7) | 29 (7.5) | 0.89 |
| Previous stroke (*n*, %) | 35 (3.8) | 22 (4.2) | 13 (3.2) | 0.42 | 0 (0.0) | 22 (2.8) | 9 (2.3) | 13 (3.4) | 0.50 |
| CRI (*n*, %) | 7 (0.8) | 3 (0.6) | 4 (1.0) | 0.71* | 0 (0.0) | 6 (0.8) | 3 (0.8) | 3 (0.8) | 1.00 |
| Scr, μmol/L ($\bar{X}$ ± SD) | 99.09 ± 40.80 | 102.09 ± 46.14 | 95.24 ± 32.35 | 0.008 | 2 (0.2) | 98.80 ± 41.84 | 102.55 ± 49.27 | 95.04 ± 32.40 | 0.012 |
| Previous heart surgery (*n*, %) | | | | 0.20 | 0 (0.0) | | | | 1.00 |
| No | 895 (96.3) | 502 (96.0) | 393 (96.8) | | | 757 (97.6) | 380 (97.9) | 377 (97.2) | |
| TEVAR | 12 (1.3) | 9 (1.7) | 3 (0.7) | | | 0 (0.0) | 0 (0.0) | 0 (0.0) | |
| AVR | 9 (1.0) | 3 (0.6) | 6 (1.5) | | | 7 (0.9) | 3 (0.8) | 4 (1.0) | |
| Others | 13 (1.4) | 9 (1.7) | 4 (1.0) | | | 12 (1.5) | 5 (1.3) | 7 (1.8) | |
| EF, % ($\bar{X}$ ± SD) | 60.2 ± 4.3 | 60.1 ± 4.5 | 60.4 ± 4.0 | 0.18 | 4 (0.4) | 60.4 ± 4.1 | 60.4 ± 4.2 | 60.4 ±4.0 | 0.90 |
| AR>moderate (*n*, %) | 110 (11.8) | 70 (13.4) | 40 (9.9) | 0.09 | 1 (0.1) | 74 (9.5) | 34 (8.8) | 40 (10.3) | 0.46 |
| Hemodynamic instability (*n*, %) | 47 (5.1) | 31 (6.0) | 16 (4.1) | 0.18 | 0 (0.0) | 29 (3.7) | 13 (3.4) | 16 (4.2) | 0.58 |
| Tamponade | 10 (1.1) | 4 (0.8) | 6 (1.5) | 0.30 | | 6 (0.8) | 3 (0.7) | 4 (1.0) | 0.70 |
| Entry tear (*n*, %) | | | | 0.009 | 0 (0.0) | | | | 0.68 |
| aAO | 608 (65.4) | 363 (69.4) | 245 (60.3) | | | 483 (62.2) | 243 (62.6) | 240 (61.9) | |
| Arch | 260 (28.0) | 126 (24.1) | 134 (33.0) | | | 236 (30.4) | 114 (29.4) | 122 (31.4) | |
| DTA | 61 (6.6) | 34 (6.5) | 27 (6.7) | | | 57 (7.3) | 31 (8.0) | 26 (6.7) | |
| Extent (*n*, %) | | | | 0.14* | 0 (0.0) | | | | 0.29 |
| To arch | 60 (6.5) | 41 (7.8) | 19 (4.7) | | | 46 (5.9) | 29 (7.5) | 17 (4.4) | |
| To DTA | 5 (0.5) | 3 (0.6) | 2 (0.5) | | | 4 (0.5) | 2 (0.5) | 2 (0.5) | |
| To distal AA | 864 (93.0) | 479 (91.6) | 385 (94.8) | | | 726 (93.6) | 357 (92.0) | 369 (95.1) | |
| IA-FL (*n*, %) | 22 (2.4) | 13 (2.5) | 9 (2.2) | 0.79 | 0 (0.0) | 19 (2.4) | 10 (2.6) | 9 (2.3) | 1.00 |
| IAS (*n*, %) | 23 (2.5) | 15 (2.9) | 8 (2.0) | 0.37 | 0 (0.0) | 15 (1.9) | 8 (2.1) | 7 (1.8) | 1.00 |
| Coronary malperfusion (*n*, %) | 26 (2.8) | 19 (3.6) | 7 (1.7) | 0.07 | 0 (0.0) | 13 (1.7) | 6 (1.5) | 7 (1.8) | 1.00 |
| Cerebral malperfusion (*n*, %) | | | | 0.004* | 0 (0.0) | | | | 0.80 |
| No | 882 (94.9) | 487 (93.1) | 395 (97.3) | | | 757 (97.6) | 380 (97.9) | 377 (97.2) | |
| Unilateral | 45 (4.8) | 35 (6.7) | 10 (2.5) | | | 17 (2.2) | 7 (1.8) | 10 (2.6) | |
| Bilateral | 2 (0.2) | 1 (0.2) | 1 (0.2) | | | 2 (0.3) | 1 (0.3) | 1 (0.3) | |
| SMA-malperfusion (*n*, %) | | | | 0.85* | 0 (0.0) | | | | 0.97 |

*(Continued)*

**TABLE 1** | Continued

| Variable | Unmatched | | | | Missing | Matched | | | |
|---|---|---|---|---|---|---|---|---|---|
| | Overall $n = 929$ | DAC $n = 523$ | SAC $n = 406$ | *P* | | Overall $n = 776$ | DAC $n = 388$ | SAC $n = 388$ | *P* |
| No | 777 (83.6) | 434 (83.0) | 343 (84.5) | | | 659 (84.9) | 331 (85.3) | 328 (84.5) | |
| Dynamic | 131 (14.1) | 78 (14.9) | 53 (13.1) | | | 98 (12.6) | 48 (12.4) | 50 (12.9) | |
| Static | 19 (2.0) | 10 (1.9) | 9 (2.2) | | | 18 (2.3) | 9 (2.3) | 9 (2.3) | |
| Mix | 2 (0.2) | 1 (0.2) | 1 (0.2) | | | 1 (0.1) | 0 (0.0) | 1 (0.3) | |
| Renal malperfusion | 62 (6.7) | 32 (6.1) | 30 (7.4) | 0.44 | | 59 (7.6) | 32 (8.2) | 27 (7.0) | 0.50 |
| Left lower limb malperfusion (*n*, %) | | | | 0.15* | 0 (0.0) | | | | 0.99 |
| No | 876 (94.3) | 498 (95.2) | 378 (93.1) | | | 730 (94.1) | 366 (94.3) | 364 (93.8) | |
| Dynamic | 51 (5.5) | 25 (4.8) | 26 (6.4) | | | 46 (5.9) | 22 (5.7) | 24 (6.2) | |
| Static | 2 (0.2) | 0 (0.0) | 2 (0.5) | | | 0 | 0 (0.0) | 0 (0.0) | |
| Right lower limb malperfusion (*n*, %) | | | | 0.61 | 0 (0.0) | | | | 0.78 |
| No | 863 (92.9) | 489 (93.5) | 374 (92.1) | | | 722 (93.0) | 362 (93.3) | 360 (92.8) | |
| Dynamic | 41 (4.4) | 20 (3.8) | 21 (5.2) | | | 38 (4.9) | 19 (4.9) | 19 (4.9) | |
| Static | 25 (2.7) | 14 (2.7) | 11 (2.7) | | | 16 (2.1) | 7 (1.8) | 9 (2.3) | |

*DAC, dual arterial cannulation; SAC, axillary artery cannulation; BMI, body mass index; HT, hypertension; CAD, coronary artery disease; AF, atrial fibrillation; DM, diabetes mellitus; CRI, chronic renal insufficiency; Scr, serum creatinine; TEVAR, thoracic endovascular aortic repair; AVR, aortic valve replacement; AR, aortic regurgitation; aAO, ascending aorta; DTA, descending thoracic aorta; AA, abdominal aorta; IA-FL, innominate artery originating from false lumen; IAS, innominate artery stenosis; and SMA, superior mesenteric artery. *Fisher's exact test was used.*

axillary conduit owing to insufficient flow volume. Venous return was achieved *via* a two-staged cannula placed in the right atrium or cannulas in the vena cava as appropriate. Indication and technique of performing TAR combined with FET (CRONUS; MicroPort, Shanghai, China) in our institution were similar to those described by Sun et al. (5) (More detailed information about indication and technique was available in **Supplementary Material** Expanded Methods). Briefly, we used a 4-branch prosthetic graft to replace the arch and a stented graft that is deployed anterogradely into a descending aorta to isolate the false lumen. During FET deployment and distal arch anastomosis, hypothermia circulatory arrest (HCA) and unilateral selective cerebral perfusion were applied. The target nasopharyngeal temperature during HCA was 18–25°C in different periods.

## Statistical Analysis

Data were presented as mean and standard deviation for a continuous data conforming to the normal distribution and as number (%) for categorical data. The mean of two continuous normally distributed variables was compared by independent samples student *t*-test. Comparison of categoric variables between groups was analyzed by the likelihood ratio of Chi-square test or Fisher's exact test. The continuous variable that did not conform to a normal distribution was demonstrated as the median and interquartile range (IQR) and were compared by Wilcoxon signed-rank test. The missing quantitative data were filled with mean and the qualitative data were filled with maximum frequency.

Propensity score matching was applied to achieve a balanced exposure between groups at baseline (i.e., minimal confounding). The probability of each patient having a dual arterial cannulation (i.e., the propensity score) was calculated using a logistic regression model. Covariates included age, gender, preoperative comorbidities, and pathologic features of dissection were adjusted (see **Supplementary Table I**). Patients were then matched one-to-one using the Nearest-neighbor matching and caliper width of 0.1 of the standard deviation of the logit of the propensity score. After propensity score matching, a comparison of continuous data conforming to normal distribution between groups was analyzed by paired *t*-test. Paired Chi-square test was used to compare multiple categorical variables between the two groups, statistics and the *P* value of the symmetric test were adopted. The McNemar test was used to compare binary variables between the two groups. To investigate the influence of cannulation strategy on primary outcomes and to avoid a large deviation result, three multivariate logistic regression models adjusting to different confounders were constructed. Confounders were determined according to our clinical experience and previous studies (6, 7). Stratified analysis was conducted to identify whether a dual arterial cannulation had an advantage over a single axillary artery cannulation for a particular population. Statistical significance was denoted by *P* values $< 0.05$. The statistical analyses were conducted by SAS (version 9.4, SAS Institute Inc., Cary, North Carolina, America).

**TABLE 2** | Operative characteristics.

| Variable | Unmatched | | | *P* | Matched | | | *P* |
|---|---|---|---|---|---|---|---|---|
| | Overall *n* = 929 | DAC *n* = 523 | SAC *n* = 406 | | Overall *n* = 776 | DAC *n* = 388 | SAC *n* = 388 | |
| Aortic root surgery (*n*, %) | | | | 0.019 | | | | 0.07 |
| Supracoronary aortic replacement | 667 (71.8) | 377 (72.1) | 290 (71.4) | | 564 (72.7) | 290 (74.7) | 274 (70.6) | |
| Bentall | 241 (25.9) | 136 (26.0) | 105 (25.9) | | 193 (24.9) | 90 (23.2) | 103 (26.5) | |
| David | 9 (1.0) | 1 (0.2) | 8 (2.0) | | 8 (1.0) | 0 (0.0) | 8 (2.1) | |
| AVR | 12 (2.3) | 9 (1.7) | 3 (0.7) | | | 8 (2.1) | 3 (0.8) | |
| CABG (*n*, %) | 113 (12.2) | 66 (12.6) | 47 (11.6) | 0.63 | 83 (10.7) | 38 (9.8) | 45 (11.6) | 0.41 |
| Femoral artery bypass (*n*, %) | 32 (3.4) | 22 (4.2) | 9 (2.2) | 0.35 | 30 (3.9) | 21 (5.4) | 9 (2.3) | 0.025 |
| Carotid artery bypass (*n*, %) | 15 (1.6) | 10 (1.9) | 5 (1.2) | 0.42 | 13 (1.7) | 8 (2.1) | 5 (1.3) | 0.40 |
| CPB duration, min ($\bar{X}$ ± SD) | 195.1 ± 68.1 | 204.8 ± 62.7 | 182.7 ± 72.7 | <0.001 | 192.6 ± 70.0 | 202.2 ± 64.6 | 183.0 ± 73.9 | <0.001 |
| X-clamp duration, min ($\bar{X}$ ± SD) | 108.3 ± 33.8 | 112.9 ± 31.9 | 102.4 ± 35.3 | <0.001 | 106.6 ± 33.2 | 110.7 ± 30.3 | 102.4 ± 35.5 | <0.001 |
| HCA duration, min ($\bar{X}$ ± SD) | 18.7 ± 6.8 | 18.8 ± 8.0 | 18.6 ± 4.8 | 0.51 | 18.8 ± 6.6 | 19.13 ± 8.0 | 18.5 ± 4.7 | 0.29 |
| SCP duration, min ($\bar{X}$ ± SD) | 27.1 ± 8.5 | 29.5 ± 8.7 | 23.9 ± 7.0 | <0.001 | 26.8 ± 8.5 | 29.7 ± 8.9 | 23.9 ± 6.9 | <0.001 |
| Nasopharyngeal temperature, °C ($\bar{X}$ ± SD) | 22.0 ± 3.6 | 21.6 ± 3.8 | 22.4 ± 3.2 | 0.001 | 21.9 ± 3.5 | 21.5 ± 3.7 | 22.4 ± 3.2 | <0.001 |
| Rectal temperature, °C ($\bar{X}$ ± SD) | 24.9 ± 4.0 | 24.0 ± 3.9 | 26.2 ± 3.8 | <0.001 | 25.0 ± 4.0 | 23.9 ± 3.8 | 26.1 ± 3.9 | <0.001 |

*DAC, dual arterial cannulation; SAC, axillary artery cannulation; AVR, aortic valve replacement; CABG, coronary artery bypass grafting; CPB, cardiopulmonary bypass; HCA, hypothermic circulatory arrest; and SCP, selective cerebral perfusion.*

**TABLE 3** | Perioperative outcome characteristics.

| Variable | Unmatched | | | *P* | Matched | | | *P* |
|---|---|---|---|---|---|---|---|---|
| | Overall *n* = 929 | DAC *n* = 523 | SAC *n* = 406 | | Overall *n* = 776 | DAC *n* = 388 | SAC *n* = 388 | |
| MV duration, hour (median, IQR) | 22.0 (14.0–56.0) | 24.0 (14.0–64.0) | 20.0 (14.0–45.0) | 0.019* | 22.0 (14.0–50.5) | 24.0 (14.0–61.0) | 20.0 (14.0–44.5) | 0.038* |
| ICU stay, day (median, IQR) | 3.0 (2.0–6.0) | 4.0 (2.0–6.0) | 3.0 (2.0–5.0) | <0.001* | 3.0 (2.0–6.0) | 4.0 (2.0–6.0) | 3.0 (2.0–5.0) | 0.002* |
| Operative mortality (*n*, %) | 57 (6.1) | 35 (6.7) | 22 (5.4) | 0.42 | 42 (5.4) | 21 (5.4) | 21 (5.4) | 1.00 |
| PMI (*n*, %) | 4 (0.4) | 3 (0.6) | 1 (0.2) | 0.64† | 3 (0.4) | 2 (0.5) | 1 (0.3) | 1.00 |
| Stroke (*n*, %) | 57 (6.1) | 35 (6.7) | 22 (5.4) | 0.42 | 45 (5.8) | 25 (6.4) | 20 (5.2) | 0.44 |
| Spinal cord injury (*n*, %) | 49 (5.3) | 26 (5.0) | 23 (5.7) | 0.64 | 43 (5.5) | 21 (5.4) | 22 (5.7) | 1.00 |
| Reoperation for bleeding (*n*, %) | 41 (4.4) | 21 (4.0) | 20 (4.9) | 0.50 | 38 (4.9) | 18 (4.6) | 20 (5.2) | 0.87 |
| IABP (*n*, %) | 3 (0.3) | 1 (0.2) | 2 (0.5) | 0.58† | 3 (0.4) | 1 (0.3) | 2 (0.5) | 1.00 |
| ECMO (*n*, %) | 6 (0.6) | 1 (0.2) | 5 (1.2) | 0.09† | 6 (0.8) | 1 (0.3) | 5 (1.3) | 0.22 |
| CRRT (*n*, %) | 111 (11.9) | 72 (13.8) | 39 (9.6) | 0.05 | 86 (11.1) | 49 (12.6) | 37 (9.5) | 0.17 |
| Tracheotomy (*n*, %) | 24 (2.6) | 15 (2.9) | 9 (2.2) | 0.53 | 21 (2.7) | 12 (3.1) | 9 (2.3) | 0.66 |
| Intestinal ischemia (*n*, %) | 12 (1.3) | 8 (1.5) | 4 (1.0) | 0.46 | 9 (1.6) | 5 (1.3) | 4 (1.0) | 1.00 |

*DAC, dual arterial cannulation; SAC, axillary artery cannulation; MV, mechanical ventilation; IQR, Interquartile Range; ICU, intensive care unit; PMI, perioperative myocardial infarction; IABP, intra-aortic balloon pump implantation; ECMO, extracorporeal membrane oxygenation; and CRRT, continuous renal replacement therapy. *Wilcoxon signed rank test was used. †Fisher's exact test was used.*

# RESULTS

## Baseline Characteristics

Between January 2010 and December 2019, a total of 1,119 patients suffering from ATAAD were admitted emergently for undergoing TAR and FET, whereas 185 met the criteria for exclusion (**Supplementary Figure I**). Of this total, 929 patients comprised the interest cohort.

The mean age of the patient was 46.8 ± 10.1years, with a male preponderance (81.5%). A total of 523 patients (56.3%) accepted dual arterial cannulation (DAC group), and 406 patients (43.7%) received single axillary artery cannulation (SAC group). The preoperative serum creatinine level was significantly higher in the DAC group. Entry tear locating in ascending aorta was more common in the DAC group (69.4 vs. 60.3%, $P = 0.009$), on the other hand, the patients in the SAC group were more likely to have entry tear in the arch (24.1 vs. 33.0%, $P = 0.009$). The proportion of unilateral cerebral malperfusion was significantly higher in the DAC group (6.7 vs. 2.5%, $P = 0.004$). Other preoperative features were similarly distributed between the two groups. The baseline characteristics were shown in **Table 1**. For the whole cohort, 667 (71.8%) patients received a supracoronary aortic replacement. Bentall procedure, David procedure, and aortic valve replacement were carried out in 241 (25.9%), 9 (1.0%), and 12 (2.3%) patients, respectively. A total of 113 (12.2%) patients underwent a coronary artery bypass grafting for coronary artery disease or coronary artery involvement. Femoral and carotid artery bypass operations were implemented to rescue severely dissected vessels from occlusion caused by a thrombus compression. These bypass operations were performed in 32 (3.4%) and 15 (1.6%) patients. A similar proportion of concomitant procedures was found in the two groups. For patients undergoing dual arterial cannulation, CPB duration, X-clamp duration, and SCP, duration were all longer than those in the SAC group (204.8 ± 62.7 vs. 182.7 ± 72.6 min, 112.9 ± 31.9 vs. 102.4 ± 35.3 min, 29.5 ± 8.7 vs. 23.9 ± 7.0 min, $P < 0.001$). The nasopharyngeal temperature in the DAC group was significantly lower than in the SAC group (21.6 ± 3.8 vs. 22.4 ± 3.2°C, $P = 0.004$). Operative characteristics were demonstrated in **Table 2**. Altogether, 388 pairs of patients were matched using a propensity score matching. It was demonstrated that well-balanced absolute standardized differences between the two groups were achieved regarding the baseline characteristics (**Supplementary Table II**). After matching, there was no significant difference in terms of baseline characteristics between the 2 groups, although CPB duration, X-clamp duration, SCP duration, and nasopharyngeal temperature were still significantly different.

## Perioperative Outcomes

In the whole cohort, 57 patients (6.1%) died, and the main presumed causes of death were heart-related circulatory failure, acidosis induced by visceral malperfusion, and stroke. Stroke and spinal cord injury occurred in 57 (6.1%) and 49 (5.3%) patients, respectively. In total, 111 (11.9%) patients had acute renal failure and required CRRT. Operative mortality was similar between the 2 groups (6.7 vs. 5.4%, $P = 0.42$ before matching; 5.4 vs. 5.4%, $P = 1$ after matching). Unadjusted and adjusted risks of stroke were similar across the initial cannulation sites (6.7 vs. 5.4%, $P = 0.42$ before matching; 6.4 vs. 5.2%, $P = 0.44$ after matching). Spinal cord injury was also distributed similarly in the two groups (5 vs. 5.7%, $P = 0.64$ before matching; 5.4 vs. 5.7%, $P = 1$ after matching). A trend that CRRT was more frequent in the DAC group was observed (13.8 vs. 9.6%, $P = 0.05$), but the trend disappeared after matching (12.6 vs. 9.5%, $P = 0.17$). The incidences of other complications were similar between the 2 groups whether before or after matching. The perioperative outcomes were listed in **Table 3**.

## Multivariate Logistic Regression Analysis and Stratification Analysis

Dual arterial cannulation was not an independent protective factor of operative mortality (odds ratio [OR] 1.01, 95% confidence interval [CI] 0.55–1.86), stroke (OR 1.17, 95% CI 0.65–2.11), spinal cord injury (OR 1.17, 95% CI 0.65–2.11), and acute renal failure requiring CRRT (OR 1.24, 95% CI 0.78–1.97) after adjusting for confounding factors by multivariable logistic regression analysis (see detailed results of three models in **Table 4**). After stratification according to BMI, dual arterial cannulation was associated with a significantly higher risk of CRRT in patients with a body mass index (BMI) of ≤ 26 (OR, 1.98; 95% CI 1.06–3.7). In other subgroups of entry tear location, innominate artery originating from false lumen, superior mesenteric artery malperfusion, and innominate artery stenosis, and dual arterial cannulation had no significant advantage over a single axillary artery cannulation on the primary outcomes. The incidence of stroke, spinal cord injury, and CRRT in the subgroup of IAS was low or even 0, making stratification results meaningless so that subgroup analysis of IAS was conducted only for operative mortality. The results of subgroup analysis were demonstrated in **Figures 1–4**.

**TABLE 4** | Multivariable analyses of operative mortality, stroke, spinal cord injury, and acute renal failure requiring CRRT for dual arterial cannulation vs. single axillary artery cannulation.

| | Odds ratio (95% CI) | *P* value | Reference |
|---|---|---|---|
| Operative mortality | | | Axillary cannulation |
| Model 1 | 1.06 (0.58, 1.92) | 0.85 | |
| Model 2 | 1.04 (0.57, 1.9) | 0.89 | |
| Model 3 | 1.01 (0.55, 1.86) | 0.98 | |
| Stroke | | | Axillary cannulation |
| Model 1 | 1.11 (0.62, 1.96) | 0.73 | |
| Model 2 | 1.12 (0.63, 1.99) | 0.70 | |
| Model 3 | 1.17 (0.65, 2.11) | 0.60 | |
| Spinal cord injury | | | Axillary cannulation |
| Model 1 | 0.83 (0.45, 1.5) | 0.53 | |
| Model 2 | 0.85 (0.46, 1.54) | 0.59 | |
| Model 3 | 1.17 (0.65, 2.11) | 0.60 | |
| ARF-CRRT | | | Axillary cannulation |
| Model 1 | 1.17 (0.75, 1.81) | 0.49 | |
| Model 2 | 1.18 (0.76, 1.84) | 0.46 | |
| Model 3 | 1.24 (0.78, 1.97) | 0.36 | |

*OR, odds ratio; CI, confident interval. Model 1: adjusted for age/CAD/previous stroke/coronary malperfusion/cerebral malperfusion/superior mesenteric artery malperfusion/hemodynamic instability/CPB duration/preoperative serum creatinine. Model 2: adjusted for age/BMI /CAD/EF/previous stroke/chronic renal insufficiency/ aortic regurgitation>moderate/coronary malperfusion/ cerebral malperfusion/superior mesenteric artery malperfusion/hemodynamic instability/CPB duration/preoperative serum creatinine. Model 3: adjusted for age/BMI /CAD/EF/previous stroke/chronic renal insufficiency/ aortic regurgitation>moderate/coronary malperfusion/ cerebral malperfusion/superior mesenteric artery malperfusion/hemodynamic instability/CPB duration/preoperative serum creatinine/left lower limb malperfusion/right lower limb malperfusion.*

## DISCUSSION

The present study is important because it compares two cannulation strategies in the context of varying complexity of acute type A aortic dissection. The main findings of our study can be summarized as follows:

1) Regarding pathological features of dissection, single axillary cannulation was comparable with dual arterial cannulation for complex arch repair in the acute type A aortic dissection.

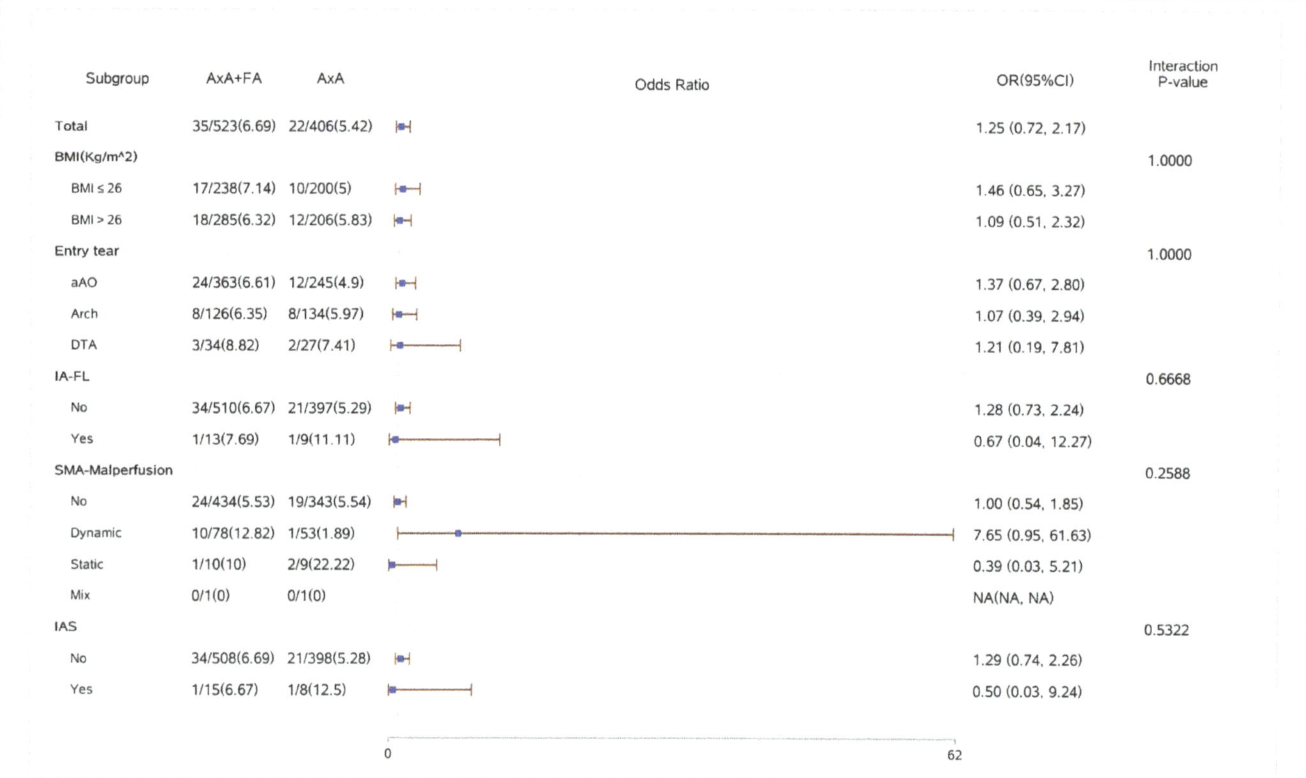


**FIGURE 1 |** Forest plot of dual arterial cannulation vs. axillary artery cannulation regarding operative mortality by subgroups. AXA+FA, axillary artery cannulation+femoral artery cannulation; AXA, axillary artery cannulation; IA-FL, innominate artery originating from false lumen; SMA, superior mesenteric artery; and IAS, innominate artery stenosis.

2) Based on antegrade perfusion, adding femoral artery cannulation did not result in an elevated rate of stroke caused by a retrograde blood flow.

Total arch replacement (TAR) combined with FET could provide a stable distal anastomosis and ideal remodeling of the downstream aorta, therefore, it was appropriate for patients with extensive dissection, presenting with satisfactory early and long-term results (5, 6, 8). Overall, compared with recent studies (6, 7), we had a lower operative mortality and a comparable incidence of main complications in the present study. The SCP time of the single axillary group was 5 min faster than that of the dual arterial group, in fact, the dual cannulation group mainly consisted of the patients who received operation in the earlier stage, and the single axillary cannulation group mainly consisted of the patients in the later stage. We became more skillful and the SCP time was shorter in the later stage. A higher incidence of spinal cord injury was found in our study. The FET products we used had only two length specifications: 100 mm and 120 mm. In most cases, we preferred a 120 mm FET in order to achieve a better remodeling of the distal aorta. The FET depth, which varied with body height, ranged from T5-T8 vertebral body. It was well-discussed that an intercostal artery originating from false lumen is a risk factor of spinal cord injury besides application of FET. So, we speculated that longer FETs for patients who were at risk of SCI were responsible for the high incidence of SCI in our cohort.

Restoring organ perfusion was critical in the early stage of CPB because pulsatile blood flow attenuated and even disappeared. The arterial cannulation site was an important issue of the whole procedure. Many types of research (9–12) were conducted to discover the optimal cannulation strategy, drawing an identical or conflicting conclusion. Axillary artery cannulation providing antegrade perfusion was advocated by more surgeons. The advantages and limitations of axillary artery cannulation vs. femoral artery cannulation were well-discussed in previous studies (13, 14). Some investigators attempted to apply a dual arterial cannulation to overcome their respective drawbacks (15, 16). It was considered reasonable that morphologic variability of dissection might interplay with cannulation and affect outcomes (17). That is why the cannulation site would possibly make a difference in clinical outcomes, although it worked for a short period of time (usually less than 1 h) from the establishment of CPB to the initiation of hypothermic circulatory arrest. But, this point was seldom taken into full consideration when the cannulation strategy was investigated in previous studies. In our study, we adjusted the preoperative comorbidities and special pathological features of aortic dissection by propensity-score matching. Judging from the statistical results, single axillary artery cannulation was competent in a complex aortic dissection regarding primary outcomes. According to the analysis of some investigators (18–20), persistent false lumen perfusion and true lumen collapse after initiation of CPB might lead to an

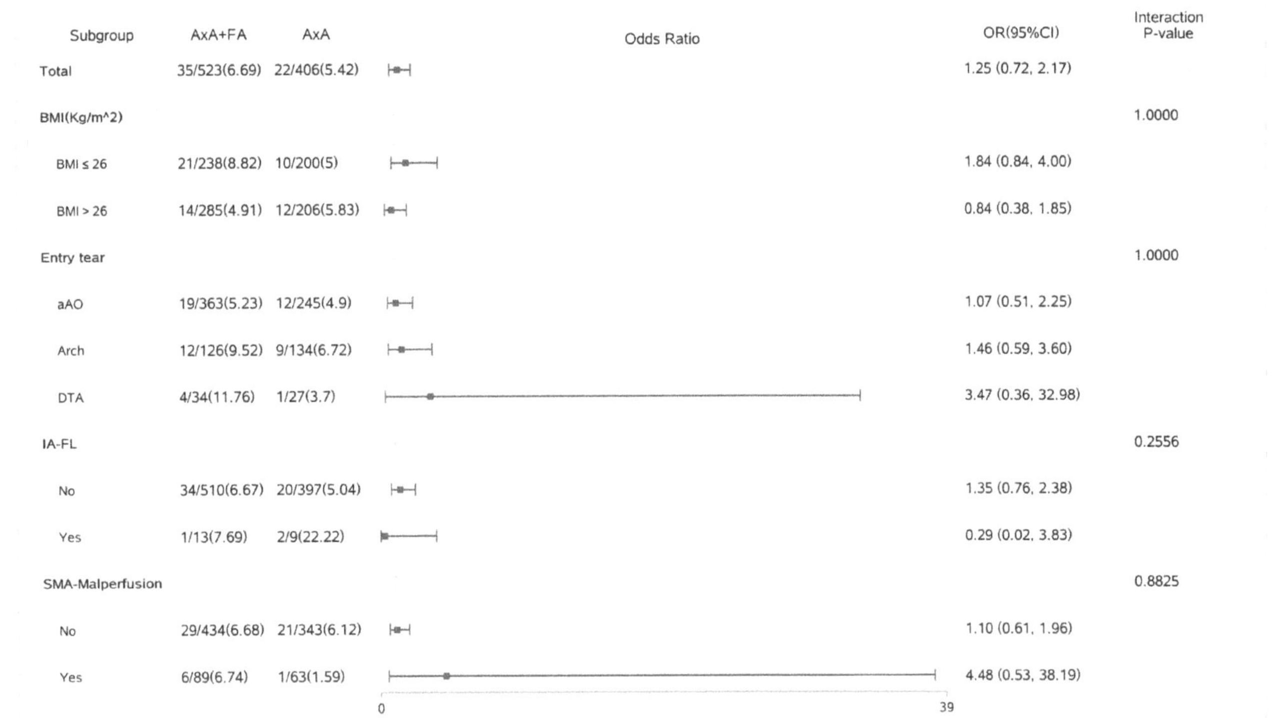


**FIGURE 2 |** Forest plot of dual arterial cannulation vs. axillary artery cannulation regarding stroke by subgroups. AXA+FA, axillary artery cannulation+femoral artery cannulation; AXA, axillary artery cannulation; IA-FL, innominate artery originating from false lumen; and SMA, superior mesenteric artery.

exacerbation of pre-existing malperfusion or a newly emerging malperfusion. Theoretically, a persistent false lumen perfusion occurred more frequently in patients using a retrograde blood flow through femoral artery cannulation (18, 19); and if entry tear is located farther distally (in or beyond the transverse arch) or an innominate artery is originated from false lumen, the same phenomenon might occur when axillary artery cannulation was applied. As Orihashi et al. (18) reported, false lumen perfusion was detected in 8.5% of cases while axillary artery cannulation was used. Lin and coworkers (15) reported that dual arterial cannulation had significant advantages on hospital mortality, stroke, and malperfusion-related complications over a single arterial cannulation. In their single arterial cannulation group, femoral artery cannulation was predominant so that the gap in results might be exaggerated. In our cohort, either operative mortality or incidence of main complications was similar between the two groups. When the innominate artery was involved, axillary artery cannulation was also safe, this finding was similar to previous studies (21, 22). Regarding malperfusion-related complications, such as acute renal failure and intestinal ischemia, there was still no significant difference. The statistical results of the three models were consistent no matter how many variables were adjusted. In stratification analysis, for patients with innominate artery originating from the false lumen and distal entry tear, the single axillary artery cannulation group did not have disadvantages on primary outcomes. On the other hand, there were still some studies showing comparable results of single femoral artery cannulation without a raised risk of malperfusion-related complications (13, 14). According to these findings, it can be hypothesized that a persistent false lumen perfusion might be a random effect and is not as common as Orihashi et.al reported (18). As Rosinski proposed (9): "outcomes are largely determined according to patient presentation rather than cannulation site". To prevent over-interpretation of the results, a detailed monitoring and fluid dynamics analysis were needed to explain the mechanism.

Indeed, whether using additional cannulation should base on intraoperative findings. Firstly, if high-flow resistance occurred when a single axillary artery was used, an extra femoral artery cannulation was necessary (9, 23). In fact, we seldom encountered insufficient flow volume *via* single axillary artery cannulation because patients in our cohort had a relatively small body mass index. Even single axillary artery cannulation was competent in 8 patients with innominate artery stenosis. Secondly, if malperfusion was detected after initiation of CPB, shifting or adding cannulation should be considered (17–19). Peripheral arterial blood pressure and near-infrared spectroscopy were available in most institutes. Transesophageal echocardiography and orbital Doppler could be used to detect intraoperative superior mesenteric artery and cerebral malperfusion (18). Even though it is not easy to implement multiple monitoring methods

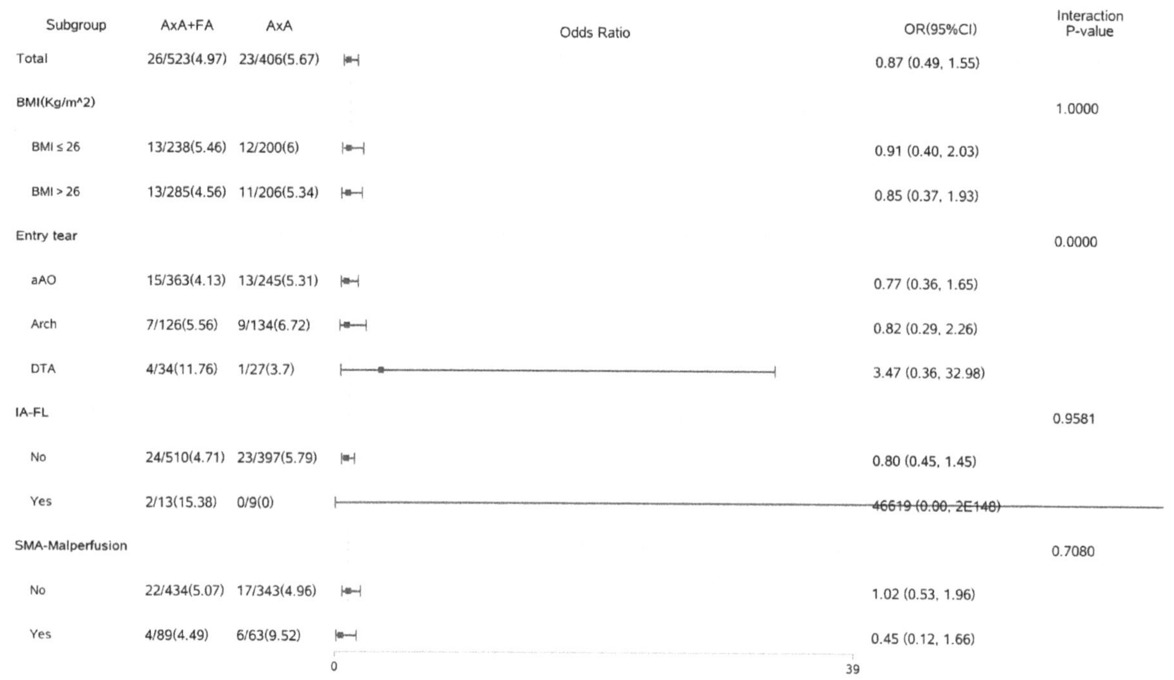


**FIGURE 3 |** Forest plot of dual arterial cannulation vs. axillary artery cannulation regarding spinal cord injury by subgroups. AXA+FA, axillary artery cannulation+femoral artery cannulation; AXA, axillary artery cannulation; IA-FL, innominate artery originating from false lumen; and SMA, superior mesenteric artery.

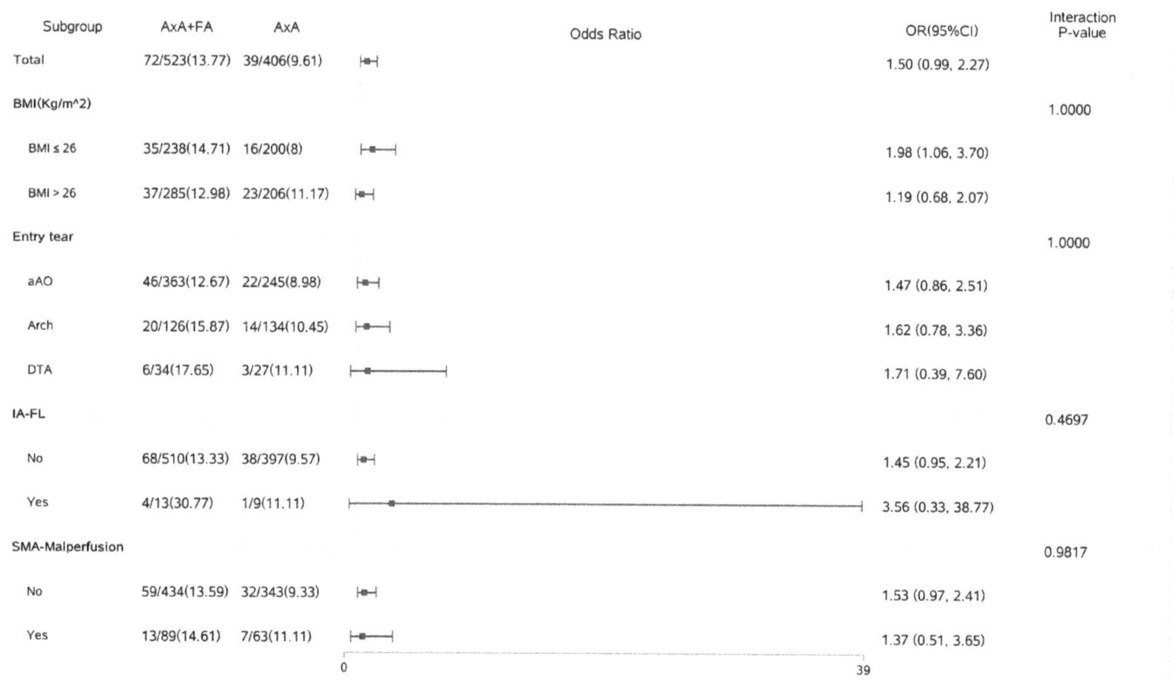


**FIGURE 4 |** Forest plot of dual arterial cannulation vs. axillary artery cannulation regarding acute renal failure requiring dialysis by subgroups. AXA+FA, axillary artery cannulation+femoral artery cannulation; AXA, axillary artery cannulation; IA-FL, innominate artery originating from false lumen; and SMA, superior mesenteric artery.

simultaneously, we still believe that an accurate monitoring can avoid strategic blindness.

This study has some important limitations. Firstly, it is a retrospective study and selection bias might exist although a propensity-score matching partially made up for the deficiency. Secondly, we did not use a direct intraoperative surveillance to evaluate malperfusion during CPB. Third, cases with adverse events were very few in subgroups and statistical analysis was of limited significance.

## CONCLUSION

Single axillary artery cannulation was competent in most cases, presenting with a satisfactory result as dual arterial cannulation. Adding femoral artery cannulation was necessary when the sufficient flow volume could not be achieved by axillary artery cannulation or lower limb malperfusion existed. Under antegrade blood flow, femoral artery cannulation would not increase the stroke risk.

## ETHICS STATEMENT

The studies involving human participants were reviewed and approved by The Ethics Committee of Fuwai Hospital. Written informed consent for participation was not required for this study in accordance with the national legislation and the institutional requirements.

## AUTHOR CONTRIBUTIONS

YC was responsible for the conceptualization, data curation, statistical analysis, and writing—original draft. HL was responsible for the statistical analysis. XQ was responsible for the conceptualization, methodology, investigation, and funding acquisition. HG, CY, XS, BW, QM, YW, and YS were responsible for the investigation. All authors contributed to the article and approved the submitted version.

## ACKNOWLEDGMENTS

We thank Yuan-yuan Feng and Yanyan Zhao for their help with the statistical analysis.

## REFERENCES

1. Malaisrie SC, Szeto WY, Halas M, Girardi LN, Coselli JS, Sundt TM, et al. AATS Clinical Practice Standards Committee: Adult Cardiac Surgery. 2021 The American Association for Thoracic Surgery expert consensus document: Surgical treatment of acute type A aortic dissection. *J Thorac Cardiovasc Surg.* (2021) 162:735–58. doi: 10.1016/j.jtcvs.2021.04.053
2. Slonim SM, Miller DC, Mitchell RS, et al. Percutaneous balloon fenestration and stenting for life-threatening ischemic complications in patients with acute aortic dissection. *J Thorac Cardiovasc Surg.* (1999) 117:1118–26. doi: 10.1016/S0022-5223(99)70248-5
3. Deeb GM, Patel HJ, Williams DM. Treatment for malperfusion syndrome in acute type A and B aortic dissection: a long-term analysis. *J Thorac Cardiovasc Surg.* (2010) 140:S98–S100. doi: 10.1016/j.jtcvs.2010.07.036
4. Patel HJ, Williams DM, Dasika NL, et al. Operative delay for peripheral malperfusion syndrome in acute type A aortic dissection: a long-term analysis. *J Thorac Cardiovasc Surg.* (2008) 135:1288–95. doi: 10.1016/j.jtcvs.2008.01.026
5. Sun L, Qi R, Zhu J, Liu Y, Zheng J. Total arch replacement combined with stented elephant trunk implantation: a new "standard" therapy for type a dissection involving repair of the aortic arch? *Circulation.* (2011) 123:971–8. doi: 10.1161/CIRCULATIONAHA.110.015081
6. Poon SS, Tian DH, Yan T, Harrington D, Nawaytou O, Kuduvalli M, et al. International Aortic Arch Surgery Study Group. Frozen elephant trunk does not increase incidence of paraplegia in patients with acute type A aortic dissection. *J Thorac Cardiovasc Surg.* (2020) 159:1189–96. doi: 10.1016/j.jtcvs.2019.03.097
7. Rosinski BF, Idrees JJ, Roselli EE, Germano E, Pasadyn SR, Lowry AM, et al. Cannulation strategies in acute type A dissection repair: a systematic axillary artery approach. *J Thorac Cardiovasc Surg.* (2019) 158:647–59. doi: 10.1016/j.jtcvs.2018.11.137
8. Chen Y, Ma WG, Zhi AH, Lu L, Zheng J, Zhang W, et al. Fate of distal aorta after frozen elephant trunk and total arch replacement for type A aortic dissection in Marfan syndrome. *J Thorac Cardiovasc Surg.* (2019) 157:835–49. doi: 10.1016/j.jtcvs.2018.07.096
9. Stamou SC, Gartner D, Kouchoukos NT, Lobdell KW, Khabbaz K, Murphy E, et al. Axillary versus femoral arterial cannulation during repair of type A aortic dissection? *AORTA.* (2016) 4:115–23. doi: 10.12945/j.aorta.2016.16.007
10. Kamiya H, Kallenbach K, Halmer D, Özsöz M, Ilg K, Lichtenberg A, et al. Comparison of ascending aorta versus femoral artery cannulation for acute aortic dissection type A. *Circulation.* (2009) 120:S282–6. doi: 10.1161/CIRCULATIONAHA.108.844480
11. Peterson MD, Mazine A, El-Hamamsy I, Manlhiot C, Ouzounian M, MacArthur RG, et al. Knowledge, attitudes, and practice preferences of Canadian cardiac surgeons toward the management of acute type A aortic dissection. *J Thorac Cardiovasc Surg.* (2015) 150:e821–5. doi: 10.1016/j.jtcvs.2015.07.026
12. Etz CD, von Aspern K, da Rocha ESJ, Girrbach FF, Leontyev S, Luehr M, et al. Impact of perfusion strategy on outcome after repair for acute type A aortic dissection. *Ann Thorac Surg.* (2014) 97:78–85. doi: 10.1016/j.athoracsur.2013.07.034
13. Gulbins H, Pritisanac A, Ennker J. Axillary versus femoral cannulation for aortic surgery: enough evidence for a general recommendation? *Ann Thorac Surg.* (2007) 83:1219–24. doi: 10.1016/j.athoracsur.2006.10.068
14. Parikh N, Trimarchi S, Gleason TG, Kamman AV, di Eusanio M, Myrmel T, et al. Changes in operative strategy for patients enrolled in the International Registry of Acute Aortic Dissection interventional cohort program. *J Thorac Cardiovasc Surg.* (2017) 153:74–9. doi: 10.1016/j.jtcvs.2016.12.029
15. Lin CY, Tseng CN, Lee HA, Ho HT, Tsai FC. Double arterial cannulation strategy for acute type A aortic dissection repair: A 10-year single-institution experience. *PLoS ONE.* (2019) 14:e0211900. doi: 10.1371/journal.pone.0211900
16. Huang LC, Xu QC, Chen DZ Dai XF, Chen LW. Combined femoral and axillary perfusion strategy for Stanford type a aortic dissection repair. *J Cardiothorac Surg.* (2020) 15:326. doi: 10.1186/s13019-020-01371-0
17. Orihashi K, Sueda T, Okada K, Imai K. Detection and monitoring of complications associated with femoral or axillary arterial cannulation for surgical repair of aortic dissection. *J Cardiothor Vasc Anesth.* (2006) 20:20–5. doi: 10.1053/j.jvca.2005.11.010
18. Orihashi K. Malperfusion in acute type A aortic dissection: unsolved problem. *Ann Thorac Surg.* (2013) 95:1570–6. doi: 10.1016/j.athoracsur.2013.02.025
19. Shiiya N, Matsuzaki K, Kunihara T, Murashita T, Matsui Y. Management of vital organ malperfusion in acute aortic dissection: proposal of a mechanism-specific approach. *Gen Thorac Cardiovasc Surg.* (2007) 55:85–90. doi: 10.1007/s11748-006-0080-8
20. Orihashi K, Sueda T, Okada K, Imai K. Perioperative diagnosis of mesenteric ischemia in acute aortic dissection by transesophageal echocardiography. *Eur*

*J Cardiothorac Surg.* (2005) 28:871–6. doi: 10.1016/j.ejcts.2005.09.017
21. Rylski B, Czerny M, Beyersdorf F, Kari FA, Siepe M, Adachi H, et al. Is right axillary artery cannulation safe in type A aortic dissection with involvement of the innominate artery? *J Thorac Cardiovasc Surg.* (2016) 152:801–7. doi: 10.1016/j.jtcvs.2016.04.092
22. Ohira S, Malekan R, Kai M, Goldberg JB, Spencer PJ, Lansman SL, et al. Direct axillary artery cannulation for type A dissection and impact of dissected innominate artery. *Ann Thorac Surg.* (2021) 27:S0003-4975(21)00905-X. doi: 10.1016/j.athoracsur.2021.05.008
23. Minatoya K, Ogino H, Matsuda H, Sasaki H. Rapid and safe establishment of cardiopulmonary bypass in repair of acute aortic dissection: improved results with double cannulation. *Interact Cardiovasc Thorac Surg.* (2008) 7:951–3. doi: 10.1510/icvts.2007.171546

22

# Long Term Outcome of Postoperative Atrial Fibrillation After Cardiac Surgery—A Propensity Score-Matched Cohort Analysis

*Jung-Chi Hsu*[1,2], *Chen-Yu Huang*[2,3], *Shu-Lin Chuang*[4,5], *Hsu-Yu Yu*[6], *Yih-Sharng Chen*[6], *Chih-Hsien Wang*[6*] and *Lian-Yu Lin*[2,7,8*]

[1] Division of Cardiology, Department of Internal Medicine, Camillian Saint Mary's Hospital Luodong, Yilan, Taiwan, [2] Division of Cardiology, Department of Internal Medicine, National Taiwan University Hospital, Taipei, Taiwan, [3] Division of Cardiology, Department of Internal Medicine, Taoyuan General Hospital, Ministry of Health and Welfare, Taoyuan, Taiwan, [4] Department of Medical Research, National Taiwan University Hospital, Taipei, Taiwan, [5] Graduate Institute of Epidemiology and Preventive Medicine, College of Public Health, National Taiwan University, Taipei, Taiwan, [6] Division of Cardiovascular Surgery, Department of Surgery, National Taiwan University Hospital and College of Medicine, National Taiwan University, Taipei, Taiwan, [7] Department of Internal Medicine, College of Medicine, National Taiwan University, Taipei, Taiwan, [8] Division of Electrophysiology, Cardiovascular Center, National Taiwan University Hospital, Taipei, Taiwan

***Correspondence:**
Lian-Yu Lin
lianyulin94@gmail.com
Chih-Hsien Wang
wchemail.us@gmail.com

**Background:** Postoperative atrial fibrillation (POAF) results in a longer hospital stay and excess mortality. However, whether POAF would increase stroke rate has been debated for years. When and how long should anticoagulation be used to prevent stroke are unknown. In the study, we planned to investigate the clinical demographics and long-term outcomes of POAF after cardiac surgery in a single-center cohort.

**Methods:** The cohort study used a database from National Taiwan University Hospital, a single tertiary medical center in Taiwan, between 2007 and 2017, to identify patients with prior normal sinus rhythm developing POAF after cardiac surgery. Patients without POAF after cardiac surgery were used as controls. Propensity score matching with 1:1 ratio and Cox regression models were employed to estimate the risk of transient ischemic accident (TIA) or ischemic stroke.

**Results:** From 2007 to 2017, a total of 8,374 patients received open-heart surgery, in which 1,585 patients with a history of AF were excluded. The overall incidence of TIA/ischemic stroke was 3.9% in a median 9.2-years of follow-up. After propensity matching, 1,965 matched paired subjects were included for analysis. Postoperative atrial fibrillation was associated with an increased risk of future AF [Hazard ratio (HR) 1.40, 95% confidence interval (95%CI) = 1.09–1.79, $p = 0.008$] and heart failure (HF) hospitalization (HR 1.58, 95%CI 1.23–2.04, $p < 0.001$); however, POAF did not significantly correlate with the risk of TIA/ischemic stroke (HR 1.17, 95%CI 0.85–1.60, $p = 0.043$). Kaplan-Meier analysis showed that POAF was a significant predictor for future AF, HF hospitalization, and overall mortality, but not for TIA/ischemic stroke.

**Conclusion:** In the Asian population, POAF after cardiac surgery increased the risk of future AF, HF, and overall mortality, but was not associated with future TIA/ischemic stroke.

**Keywords: postoperative atrial fibrillation, open heart surgery, coronary artery bypass grafting, stroke, atrial fibrillation**

## INTRODUCTION

Atrial fibrillation (AF) is the most common perioperative arrhythmia, with an incidence of 3% in major non-cardiac surgery. The incidence was estimated to be 11–40% in patients receiving coronary artery bypass grafting (CABG) and even higher (>50%) after valvular surgery (1, 2). New-onset AF during the perioperative period could be provoked by physiological stress and sepsis and were considered to be associated with both short and long-term risks of stroke (3). Nevertheless, cardiac operations-associated AF, so-called Postoperative atrial fibrillation (POAF), appears to be a consequence of direct response of pericardial inflammation and is often believed to be self-limiting and probably has little impact on long-term outcome since the majority of patients return to normal sinus rhythm within a few weeks after surgery (4). Even though some studies have shown that new-onset POAF following CABG was associated with a significantly higher risk of short and long-term mortality, the long-term stroke risk remained controversial (5, 6). Some reported no association (7, 8), while some advocated increased risk of stroke after cardiac surgery (9–11).

Despite lack of strong evidence, the consensus of AHA/ACC/HRS guidelines recommended anticoagulation therapy for patients with prolonged duration of POAF (>48 h) and concomitant multiple stroke risk factors (12). The 2017 EACTS guidelines also recommended giving anticoagulation therapy to patients who developed POAF after cardiac surgery to avoid early stroke (13).

Since POAF is usually transient, when the sinus rhythm restores, whether the long-term stroke risk increases is still not known. In this study, we plan to investigate the long-term outcomes of the patients with POAF after cardiac surgery.

## METHODS

### Data Collection

The study database was from National Taiwan University Hospital integrated Medical Database (NTUH-iMD) which was composed of detailed medical and procedural information from a tertiary medical center in Taiwan. Atrial fibrillation and its occurrence time were identified by the diagnosis of electronic health records and the electrocardiograms. Comorbidities including hypertension (HTN), diabetes mellitus (DM), hyperlipidemia, heart failure (HF), coronary artery disease (CAD), myocardial infarction (MI), chronic obstructive pulmonary disease (COPD), peripheral arterial occlusive disease (PAOD), chronic kidney disease (CKD) were also coded from the records. Prescription information were categorized into antiarrhythmic agents, beta-blockers, angiotensin-converting enzyme inhibitors (ACEI), angiotensin receptor blockers (ARB), mineralocorticoid-receptor antagonists (MRA), and anticoagulants including direct oral anticoagulants (DOAC) and warfarin. The open heart procedures included CABG, valvuloplasty, and valve replacement. The echocardiographic data and outcomes including TIA, ischemic stroke, HF hospitalization, and mortality were also obtained from the electronic health records. The study was approved by the Institutional Review Board (IRB) of National Taiwan University Hospital.

### Patient Selection

In this study, all patients above 18 years of age undergoing first-time open-heart surgery at the National Taiwan University Hospital from February 1, 2007, to February 30, 2017 were included for analysis. Patients with previous documented AF, who received anticoagulant therapy within 6 months before the open-heart surgery or during the follow-up period, could not survive the open-heart procedures, could not receive regular follow-up at the out-patient clinics were all excluded. The definition of POAF was new-onset AF, which sustained for over 30 s, detected by either continuous telemetry in the intensive care unit, standard 12-lead electrocardiogram, or implanted devices. Future AF was defined as documented AF 1 month after surgery or discharge. All medical records were followed until their last clinical visit, repeat cardiac surgery, or death. The index date of outcomes was defined as the date of diagnosis.

### Statistical Analysis

Continuous variables were denoted as mean (SD) while categorical variables were presented as numbers and percentages. Baseline demographics between groups were compared by using Student's $t$-test for continuous variables and Chi-square test for categorical variables.

Missing data for variables of interest were handled by multiple imputations with chained equations before propensity score matching. Propensity score matching was used to adjust for potentially confounding variables. We calculated the propensity scores by hierarchical logistic regression. Covariates included in the logistic model were age, gender, HTN, DM, hyperlipidemia, COPD, CHF, CAD, CKD, CHA2DS2-VASc score, echocardiography parameters, and medications. Considering the statistical power and distribution of sample size, patients with POAF were matched 1:1 to non-POAF patients, using the nearest neighbor method without replacement and with caliper 0.2 which was statically optimal width (14, 15). The matching result was estimated by calculating the absolute standard differences of baseline characteristics between patients with POAF and non-POAF. A value of <10% was considered well-matched. A Cox proportional hazard model was used to estimate the association between POAF and outcomes. Results were expressed as hazard ratios (HRs) with 95% confidence intervals (CIs). Factors that were statistically significant in univariate analysis would be put into multivariate analysis. Survival analyses were illustrated by the Kaplan-Meier curve. A two-tailed $p$-value of $<0.05$ was considered statistically significant. All statistical analyses were performed using SPSS V.25.0 (SPSS, Inc., Chicago, Illinois) and R software (R software version 3.3.3).

## RESULTS

### Baseline Characteristics

A total of 8,374 patients received cardiac surgery between 2007 and 2017, of which 1,585 patients were excluded because of pre-existing AF. After excluding patients with anticoagulant, a

**TABLE 1** | Basic characteristics of enrolled patients before and after propensity score matching.

| | Pre-Match | | | | Post-Match | | | |
|---|---|---|---|---|---|---|---|---|
| | POAF (*N* = 2,015) | Non-POAF (*N* = 4,252) | Std. Diff. | *p*-Value | POAF (*N* = 1,965) | Non-POAF (*N* = 1,965) | Std. Diff. | *p*-Value |
| Age | 65.2 ± 13.6 | 60.5 ± 13.5 | 0.35 | **<0.001** | 65.0 ± 13.6 | 64.5 ± 13.8 | 0.03 | 0.339 |
| Gender (male) | 1,502 (74.5%) | 3,318 (78.0%) | −0.08 | **0.002** | 1,469 (74.8%) | 1,501 (73.4%) | −0.04 | 0.235 |
| Hypertension | 1,349 (66.9%) | 2,959 (69.6%) | −0.06 | 0.035 | 1,319 (67.1%) | 1,349 (67.7%) | −0.03 | 0.305 |
| Type 2 DM | 891 (44.2%) | 1,854 (43.6%) | 0.01 | 0.647 | 871 (44.3%) | 894 (45.5%) | 0.02 | 0.461 |
| Hyperlipidemia | 886 (44.0%) | 2,636 (62.0%) | −0.36 | **<0.001** | 878 (44.6%) | 903 (46.0%) | −0.03 | 0.423 |
| COPD | 205 (10.2%) | 375 (8.8%) | 0.08 | **0.037** | 199 (10.1%) | 210 (10.7%) | −0.02 | 0.566 |
| CHF | 541 (26.8%) | 608 (14.3%) | 0.28 | **<0.001** | 512 (26.1%) | 465 (23.7%) | 0.05 | 0.083 |
| CAD | 1,635 (81.1%) | 3,731 (87.7%) | −0.17 | **<0.001** | 1,607 (81.8%) | 1,616 (82.2%) | −0.01 | 0.709 |
| CKD | 542 (26.9%) | 744 (17.5%) | 0.19 | **<0.001** | 500 (25.4%) | 496 (25.2%) | 0.01 | 0.883 |
| CHA2DS2-VASc score | 2.64 ± 1.60 | 2.15 ± 1.49 | 0.31 | **<0.001** | 2.61 ± 1.59 | 2.56 ± 1.59 | 0.03 | 0.321 |
| UCG | | | | | | | | |
| LVEF (%) | 54.00 ± 12.38 | 59.62 ± 12.38 | −0.11 | **<0.001** | 43.23 ± 13.05 | 48.42 ± 12.17 | −0.03 | **<0.001** |
| LV mass (g) | 231.94 ± 84.13 | 209.50 ± 70.96 | −0.11 | **<0.001** | 230.33 ± 82.02 | 217.48 ± 77.94 | −0.03 | **<0.001** |
| LA size (mm) | 3.89 ± 0.73 | 3.64 ± 0.67 | −0.08 | **<0.001** | 3.88 ± 0.73 | 3.73 ± 0.72 | −0.02 | **<0.001** |
| E | 89.69 ± 34.61 | 81.37 ± 29.53 | −0.07 | **<0.001** | 89.17 ± 34.33 | 85.61 ± 31.97 | −0.02 | **0.001** |
| A | 85.27 ± 29.67 | 81.37 ± 29.53 | 0.02 | 0.502 | 85.45 ± 29.78 | 86.02 ± 26.50 | 0.02 | 0.636 |
| E/A | 1.14 ± 0.62 | 1.01 ± 0.50 | 0.02 | **<0.001** | 1.13 ± 0.62 | 1.06 ± 0.57 | 0.02 | **0.003** |
| DT | 0.27 ± 2.44 | 0.26 ± 2.93 | −0.04 | 0.934 | 0.27 ± 2.48 | 0.32 ± 4.27 | 0.01 | 0.711 |
| Medication | | | | | | | | |
| Anti-arrhythmic agents | 20 (1.0%) | 16 (0.4%) | 0.06 | **0.003** | 15 (0.8%) | 13 (0.7%) | 0.01 | 0.704 |
| Beta-blocker | 903 (44.8%) | 2,646 (62.2%) | −0.35 | **<0.001** | 893 (45.4%) | 933 (47.5%) | −0.04 | 0.201 |
| ACEI | 121 (6.0%) | 385 (9.1%) | −0.13 | **<0.001** | 120 (6.1%) | 123 (6.3%) | −0.01 | 0.843 |
| ARB | 618 (30.7%) | 1,744 (41.0%) | −0.22 | **<0.001** | 611 (31.1%) | 637 (32.4%) | −0.03 | 0.373 |
| MRA | 228 (11.3%) | 290 (6.8%) | 0.14 | **<0.001** | 214 (10.9%) | 211 (10.7%) | 0.05 | 0.878 |
| Outcome | | | | | | | | |
| Future AF | 267 (13.1%) | 343 (8.1%) | | **<0.001** | 261(13.3%) | 169 (8.6%) | | **<0.001** |
| TIA/Stroke | 82 (4.1%) | 164 (3.9%) | | 0.686 | 77 (3.9%) | 75 (3.8%) | | 0.869 |
| HF hospitalization | 146 (7.3%) | 208 (4.9%) | | **<0.001** | 144 (7.3%) | 103 (5.2%) | | **0.007** |
| Mortality | 19 (0.9%) | 9 (0.2%) | | **<0.001** | 18 (0.9%) | 5 (032%) | | **0.010** |

*Absolute standard differences are defined as the difference in means, proportions, or ranks divided by the mutual standard deviation. DM, diabetes mellitus; COPD, chronic obstructive pulmonary disease; CHF, congestive heart failure; CAD, coronary artery disease; CKD, chronic kidney disease; TIA, transient ischemia accident; LVEF, left ventricular ejection fraction; LV mass, left ventricular mass; LA size, left atrium size; ACEI, angiotensin-converting enzyme inhibitors; ARB, angiotensin receptor blockers; MRA, mineralocorticoid-receptor antagonists; AF, atrial fibrillation; HF hospitalization, heart failure hospitalization.*

total of 6,267 patients was enrolled to this cohort. As shown in **Table 1**, before propensity matching, patients with POAF were elder (65.2 ± 13.6 vs. 60.5 ± 13.5, $p < 0.001$), more often female (25.5 vs. 22.0%, $p = 0.002$), had fewer comorbidities including HTN (66.9 vs. 69.6%, $p = 0.035$), hyperlipidemia (44.0 vs. 62.0%, $p < 0.001$), and CAD (81.1 vs. 87.7%, $p < 0.001$). The prevalence of other comorbidities such as COPD (10.2 vs. 8.8%, $p = 0.037$), CHF (26.8 vs. 14.3%, $p < 0.001$), CKD (26.9 vs. 17.5%, $p < 0.001$), together with the average CHA2DS2-VASc score (2.64 ± 1.60 vs. 2.15 ± 1.49, $p < 0.001$) were significantly higher in POAF group. The echocardiographic parameters including left ventricular ejection fraction (LVEF) (54.00 ± 12.38 vs. 59.62 ± 12.38, $p < 0.001$) was lower while the left ventricular mass (LVM) (231.94 ± 84.13 vs. 209.50 ± 70.96, $p < 0.001$) and the left atrial size (3.89 ± 0.73 vs. 3.64 ± 0.67 mm, $p < 0.001$) were larger in patients with POAF. The chances of taking MRA (11.3 vs. 6.8%, $p < 0.001$) and anti-arrhythmic agents (1.0 vs. 0.4%, $p < 0.001$) were higher in patients with POAF while less patients in the POAF group taking beta-blockers (44.8 vs. 62.2%, $p < 0.001$) and ACEI/ARBs (ACEIs 6.0 vs. 9.1%, $p < 0.001$; ARBs 30.7 vs. 41.0%, $p < 0.001$). After propensity matching, 1,965 paired matched patients were included for analysis. As demonstrated in **Table 1**, all of the absolute standard differences of the demographic and clinical characteristics between groups were within 10% and the *p*-value of the overall balance test (Hansen&Bowers) was 0.962, which was suggestive of well-matched. After PS matching, only echocardiographic parameters remained significantly different between groups. Multiple regression would be further applied to adjust all these confounders.

**TABLE 2 |** Univariate and multivariate Cox regression models in patients with postoperative atrial fibrillation in matched cohort.

| | Future atrial fibrillation | | | | TIA/Ischemic stroke | | | | Heart failure hospitalization | | | | Mortality | | | |
|---|---|---|---|---|---|---|---|---|---|---|---|---|---|---|---|---|
| | Univariate | | Multivariate | | Univariate | | Multivariate | | Univariate | | Multivariate | | Univariate | | Multivariate | |
| **Parameters** | **HR (95%CI)** | ***p*-Value** | **HR (95%CI)** | ***p*-Value** | **HR (95%CI)** | ***p*-Value** | **HR (95%CI)** | ***p*-Value** | **HR (95%CI)** | ***p*-Value** | **HR (95%CI)** | ***p*-Value** | **HR (95%CI)** | ***p*-Value** | **HR (95%CI)** | ***p*-Value** |
| POAF | 1.792 (1.476–2.176) | **<0.001** | 1.401 (1.092–1.798) | **0.008** | 1.166 (0.849–1.603) | 0.343 | | | 1.581 (1.227–2.036) | **<0.001** | 1.819 (1.292–2.563) | **0.001** | 3.732 (1.385–10.055) | **0.009** | 2.851 (0.923–8.806) | 0.069 |
| CHA2DS2-VASc score | 1.419 (1.336–1.508) | **<0.001** | 1.182 (1.182–1.397) | **<0.001** | 1.651 (1.498–1.819) | **<0.001** | 1.630 (1.422–1.867) | **<0.001** | 1.143 (1.056–1.238) | **<0.001** | 0.944 (0.843–1.058) | 0.324 | 0.909 (0.691–1.196) | 0.497 | | |
| Hyperlipidemia | 0.936 (0.772–1.134) | 0.936 | | | 1.443 (1.038–2.007) | **0.029** | 1.675 (1.077–2.605) | **0.022** | 0.994 (0.734–1.214) | 0.651 | | | 0.767 (0.334–1.764) | 0.532 | | |
| COPD | 1.848 (1.451–2.354) | **<0.001** | 1.067 (0.750–1.519) | 0.719 | 1.226 (0.766–1.963) | 0.395 | | | 1.647 (1.186–2.289) | **0.003** | 1.515 (0.968–2.370) | 0.069 | 0.793 (0.186–3.383) | 0.754 | | |
| CKD | 2.481 (2.048–3.005) | **<0.001** | 2.076 (1.602–2.689) | **<0.001** | 2.400 (1.741–3.309) | **<0.001** | 1.557 (1.009–2.403) | **0.046** | 3.078 (2.395–3.946) | **<0.001** | 2.756 (1.940–3.914) | **<0.001** | 3.290 (1.451–7.460) | **0.004** | 2.950 (1.138–7.649) | **0.026** |
| LVEF | 0.982 (0.974–0.990) | **<0.001** | 0.987 (0.978–0.995) | **0.002** | 0.994 (0.980–1.009) | 0.441 | | | 0.975 (0.964–0.985) | **<0.001** | 0.980 (0.969–0.991) | **<0.001** | 0.962 (0.934–0.990) | **0.008** | 0.967 (0.939–0.996) | **0.025** |
| LV mass | 1.001 (0.999–1.002) | 0.280 | | | 1.002 (1.000–1.005) | **0.036** | 1.003 (1.000–1.005) | **0.019** | 1.002 (1.000–1.004) | **0.032** | 1.000 (0.998–1.002) | 0.966 | 0.998 (0.992–1.005) | 0.582 | | |
| LA size | 1.335 (1.137–1.568) | **<0.001** | 1.164 (0.980–1.382) | 0.083 | 0.984 (0.737–1.315) | 0.915 | | | 1.076 (0.857–1.351) | 0.528 | | | 0.477 (0.223–1.024) | 0.057 | | |
| Beta-blocker use | 0.979 (0.806–1.190) | 0.832 | | | 0.814 (0.591–1.120) | 0.814 | | | 1.088 (0.842–1.405) | 0.518 | | | 0.569 (0.242–1.336) | 0.195 | | |
| ACEI/ARB use | 0.943 (0.778–1.141) | 0.545 | | | 1.133 (0.822–1.561) | 0.446 | | | 0.877 (0.681–1.128) | 0.877 | | | 0.579 (0.234–1.434) | 0.238 | | |

*HR, hazard ratio, with 95% confidence interval (CI), $p < 0.05$ statistically significant.*

*COPD, chronic obstructive pulmonary disease; CKD, chronic kidney disease; LVEF, left ventricular ejection fraction; LV mass, left ventricular mass; LA size, left atrium size; ACEI, angiotensin-converting enzyme inhibitors; ARB, angiotensin receptor blockers.*

## Outcomes

In the matched cohort, the overall TIA/ischemic stroke rate was 3.9% in the POAF group and 3.8% in the control group during a median of 9.2-year follow-up. The incidence of future AF was higher in patients with POAF (13.1 vs. 8.1%, $p < 0.001$). Other outcomes including the rates of CHF hospitalization (7.3 vs. 4.9%, $p < 0.001$), and overall mortality (0.9 vs. 0.2%, $p < 0.001$) were significantly higher in patients with POAF. Univariate cox regression analysis revealed that POAF, CHA2DS2-VASc score, COPD, CKD, poorer LVEF, larger LA size were significant predictors for future AF. Multivariate analysis showed that POAF (HR 1.33, 95%CI 1.04–1.71, $p = 0.025$), CHA2DS2-VASc score (HR 1.18, 95%CI 1.18–1.39, $p < 0.001$), CKD (HR 2.08, 95%CI 1.60–2.69), poorer LVEF (HR 0.98, 95%CI 0.97–0.99, $p < 0.001$), and larger LA size (HR 1.34, 95%CI 1.14–1.57, $p = 0.001$) were predictors for future AF (**Table 2**). For TIA/ischemic stroke, univariate, and multivariate analysis showed that CHA2DS2-VASc score (HR 1.63, 95%CI 1.42–1.87), hyperlipidemia (HR 1.68, 95%CI 1.08–2.61), CKD (HR 1.56, 95%CI 1.01–2.40), and higher LV mass were significantly associated with TIA/ischemic stroke (HR 1.003, 95%CI 1.000–1.006, $p = 0.027$). Of noted, POAF was not significantly

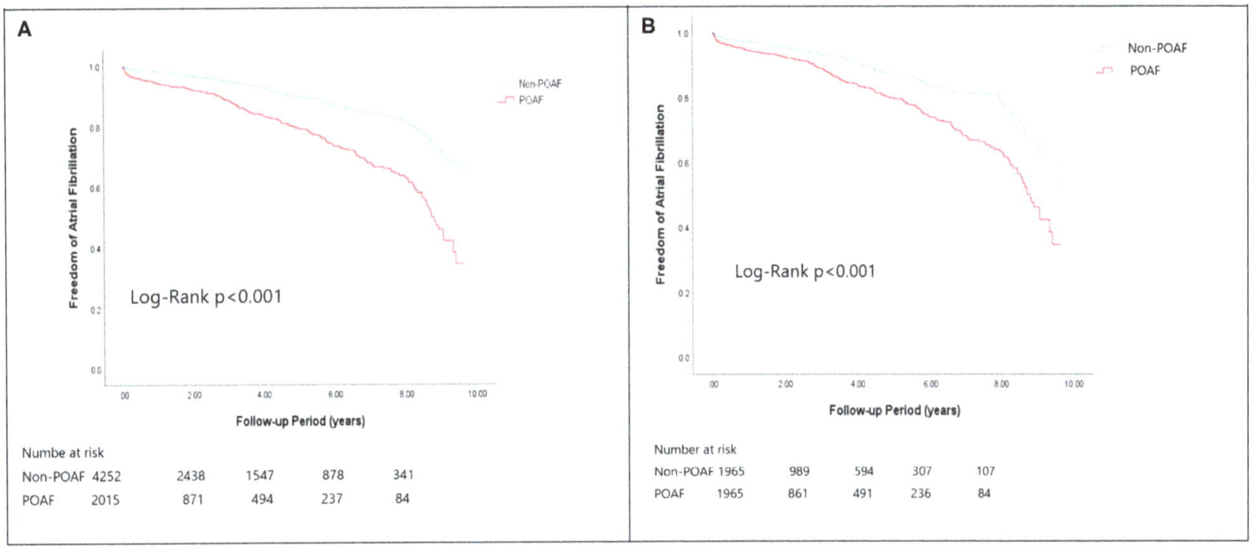


**FIGURE 1** | The Kaplan-Meier curve of **(A)** atrial fibrillation (crude) and **(B)** atrial fibrillation (matched).

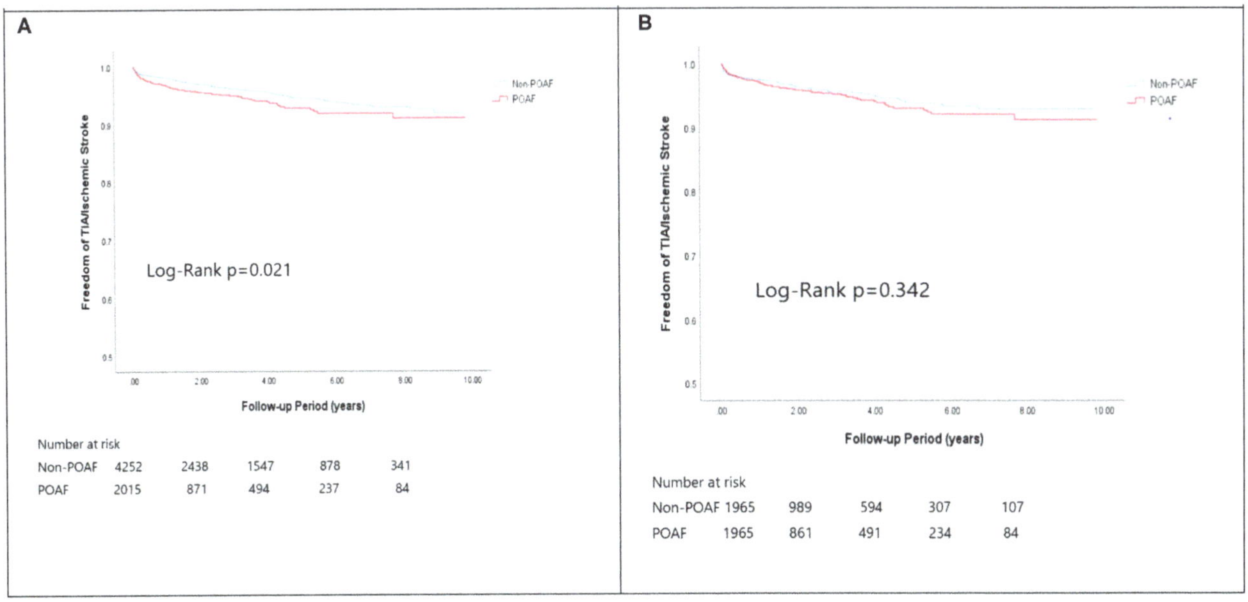


**FIGURE 2** | The Kaplan-Meier curve of **(A)** TIA/Ischemic stroke (crude) and **(B)** The Kaplan-Meier curve of atrial fibrillation (matched).

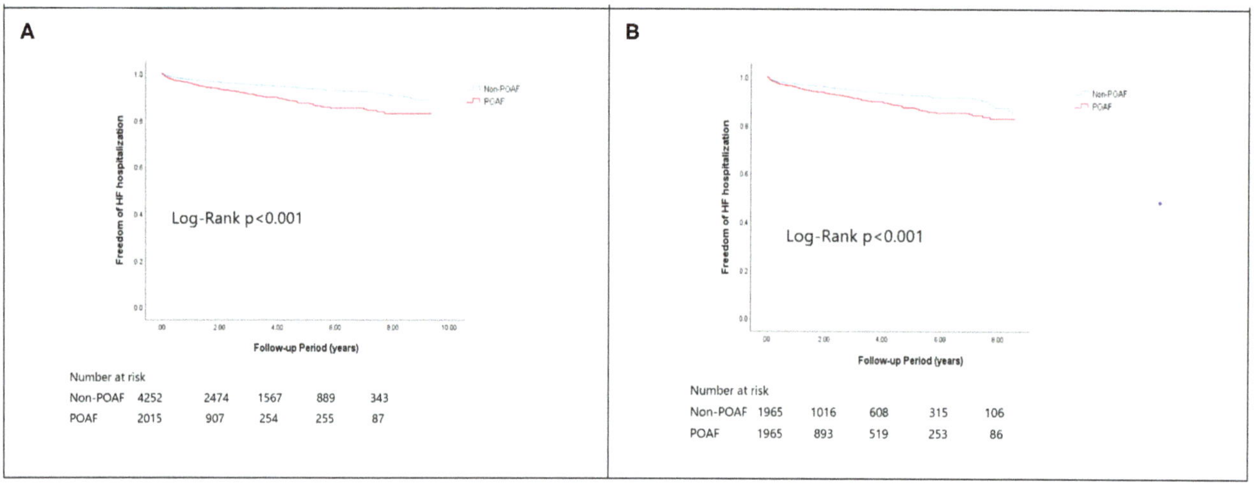


**FIGURE 3 |** The Kaplan-Meier curve of **(A)** HF hospitalization (crude) and **(B)** HF hospitalization (matched).

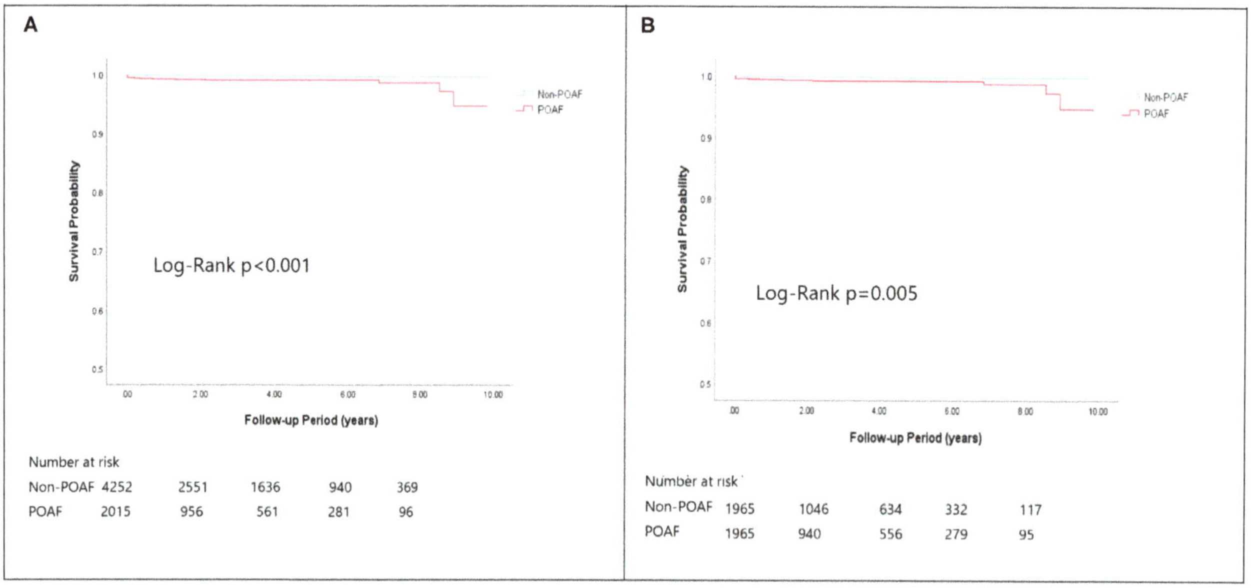


**FIGURE 4 |** The Kaplan-Meier curve of **(A)** overall mortality (crude) and **(B)** overall mortality (matched).

associated with future TIA/ischemic stroke (HR 1.17, 95%CI 0.85–1.60, $p = 0.343$). For HF hospitalization, univariate analysis showed that POAF (HR 1.58, 95%CI 1.23–2.04, $p < 0.001$), CHA2DS2-VASc score (HR 1.14, 95%CI 1.06–1.24), COPD (HR 1.52, 95%CI 0.97–2.37), CKD (HR 3.08, 95%CI 2.39–3.95), poorer LVEF (HR 0.98, 95%CI 0.96–0.99, $p < 0.001$), and higher LV mass (HR 1.002, 95%CI 1.000–1.004, $p = 0.039$) were associated with HF hospitalization, in which POAF (HR 1.82, 95%CI 1.29–2.56, $p = 0.001$), CKD (HR 2.76, 95%CI 1.94–3.91), and poorer LVEF (HR 0.98, 95%CI 0.97–0.99, $p < 0.001$) were predictors in multivariate analysis. As for overall mortality, univariate analysis revealed that POAF (HR 3.73, 95%CI 1.39–10.06, $p = 0.009$), CKD (HR 3.29, 95%CI 1.45–7.46), and poorer LVEF (HR 0.96, 95%CI 0.93–0.99, $p = 0.008$) were significant predictors, but after adjustment, only CKD (HR 2.95, 95%CI 1.14–7.65) and poorer LVEF (HR 0.967, 95%CI 0.939–0.996, $p = 0.025$) remained significant. Kaplan-Meier analysis showed that the chance of future AF was significantly higher in patients with POAF both before (Log-rank $p < 0.001$) (**Figure 1A**) and after (**Figure 1B**) propensity matching (Log-rank $p < 0.001$), while the risk of future TIA/ischemic stroke was significantly higher in patients with POAF before matching (Log-rank $p = 0.021$) (**Figure 2A**) but became non-significant after matching (Log-rank $p = 0.342$) (**Figure 2B**). Kaplan-Meier analysis also demonstrated that patients with POAF had higher chances of HF hospitalization and mortality both before and after matching (all Log-rank $p < 0.001$) (**Figures 3, 4**).

## DISCUSSION

In this study, we investigated the development of future AF and TIA/ischemic stroke after cardiac surgery during a long-term follow-up. We found that POAF increased the risk of future AF, HF hospitalization, and overall mortality, but was not associated with TIA/ischemic stroke.

In a large cohort study, the rate of new-onset perioperative AF during index hospitalization was 1.43% and the cumulative 1-year ischemic stroke rate was 1.47% after non-cardiac surgery and 0.99% after cardiac surgery. Perioperative AF was found to be significantly correlated with ischemic stroke, with a HR of 2.0 and 1.3 in non-cardiac and cardiac surgery, respectively (3). A very recent study reported a significantly increased risk of stroke, MI, and death at 1 year in patients with POAF following non-cardiac surgery (16). In cardiac surgery, another large cohort study revealed that the incidence of post-CABG AF was around 30%, which was much higher than non-cardiac surgery and the incidence varied little over time (9' 17–19). Post-CABG AF occurs most commonly 24–72 h after surgery, with a peak incidence on the second postoperative day. The onset is typically within 6 days after operation with 15–20% of episodes spontaneously converting to sinus rhythm within several hours (19, 20). It seems that although POAF is easier to develop in cardiac surgery but it carries a higher risk of stroke in non-cardiac surgery. One reason leading to this discrepancy might be attributed to different underlying pathophysiologies. For cardiac surgery, POAF tends to be triggered by direct irritation of the atrial tissues while in non-cardiac surgery, intrinsic atriopathy might be the leading cause and thus result in higher stroke risk. As a whole, the mechanisms of POAF are complex, including atrial ischemia, inflammation, hypoxia, acidosis, oxidative stress, electrolyte abnormalities, and intra-atrial conduction delay and dispersion of refractoriness of the atrial tissue (21). Interestingly, a small study showed that pulmonary vein isolation does not decrease the incidence of POAF or its clinical impact, suggestive of non-pulmonary vein mechanisms (22). In our study, the incidence of POAF was 32.1% which was compatible with previous studies.

Our study showed that patients with POAF were elder, had a higher prevalence of CKD, higher CHA2DS2-VASc score, and poorer echocardiographic profile, all of which are compatible with previous studies (23–26). Also noted, patients in POAF group were less frequently taking ACEI/ARBs and beta-blockers, both medications were proved to be able to prevent the development of POAF (27, 28).

Patients with secondary AF following clinical events such as surgery, infection, acute MI, or thyrotoxicosis, were found to carry higher long-term risks of stroke and mortality (19). Postoperative atrial fibrillation is a secondary AF, but it should be considered as an independent entity. Previous studies have shown that patients with POAF have taken a 3- to 8-time risk of developing future AF and have higher risks of cerebrovascular events and cardiovascular mortality (10, 11). However a cohort study demonstrated that AF developing late after operation, rather than POAF, is independently associated with long-term mortality (29). Another study also showed that patients with new-onset POAF after CABG had a lower long-term thromboembolic risk than those who had non-valvular AF (30). These findings are in accord with ours that POAF is not a predictor for future TIA/ischemic stroke. Since most studies focused on the early risk of ischemic stroke after cardiac surgery, our study is unique because it provided the first Asian long-term and large sample cohort data.

Given that POAF might not be associated with long-term prognosis, patients with POAF might be prone to late AF. Nevertheless, the long-term data for late AF in POAF patients remains sparse. Some studies have reported that one- to two-thirds of patients had late AF after CABG when closely monitoring (31–33). The incidence of late AF in our study was 15.9%, which was much lower than previous reports. The reasons are not unclear but might probably be related to differences in patients' characteristics or AF detection methods. The current guideline recommends anticoagulation therapy for patients with POAF for at least 4 weeks, but when to discontinue anticoagulants is still uncertain. Since the CHA2DS2-VASc score itself represented the risk factors for AF incidence, the mean CHA2DS2-VASc score in our patients receiving open heart surgery was above score 2 in both POAF and non-POAF group, suggesting that all patients should be aware of AF occurrence. Furthermore, the average of CHA2DS2-VASc score was 2.6 in our POAF group, which reached the criteria for anticoagulation therapy once late AF developed. As a result, for patients with POAF who are at high risk for late AF, physicians should carefully monitor those patients to start anticoagulation therapy at the right time.

## LIMITATION

The study has some limitations. First, this is a retrospective analysis from an integrated database from a single medical tertiary center in Taiwan. Second, AF was identified by diagnostic code, electrocardiogram, and medical history, not by long-term recorder, some patients with AF might be underdiagnosed.

## CONCLUSION

In conclusion, in this large Asian cohort, POAF after cardiac surgery increased the risk of future AF, HF, and overall mortality, but was not associated with future TIA/ischemic stroke.

## ETHICS STATEMENT

The study was approved by the Institutional Review Board (IRB) of National Taiwan University Hospital.

## AUTHOR CONTRIBUTIONS

L-YL, contributed to the conception, design, acquisition of the work, and critically revised the manuscript. C-YH, J-CH, and S-LC contributed to the analysis, or interpretation of data for the work. J-CH drafted the manuscript. All authors gave final approval and agree to be accountable for all aspects of work ensuring integrity and accuracy.

## ACKNOWLEDGMENTS

The authors would like to express their thanks to the staff of the Department of Medical Research for providing clinical data from National Taiwan University Hospital-integrated Medical Database (NTUH-iMD).

## REFERENCES

1. Bhave PD, Goldman LE, Vittinghoff E, Maselli J, Auerbach A. Incidence, predictors, and outcomes associated with postoperative atrial fibrillation after major noncardiac surgery. *Am Heart J.* (2012) 164:918–24. doi: 10.1016/j.ahj.2012.09.004
2. Ommen SR, Odell JA, Stanton MS. Atrial arrhythmias after cardiothoracic surgery. *N Engl J Med.* (1997) 336:1429–34. doi: 10.1056/NEJM199705153362006
3. Gialdini G, Nearing K, Bhave PD, Bonuccelli U, Iadecola C, Healey JS, et al. Perioperative atrial fibrillation and the long-term risk of ischemic stroke. *JAMA.* (2014) 312:616–22. doi: 10.1001/jama.2014.9143
4. Tanawuttiwat T, O'Neill BP, Cohen MG, Chinthakanan O, Heldman AW, Martinez CA, et al. New-onset atrial fibrillation after aortic valve replacement: comparison of transfemoral, transapical, transaortic, and surgical approaches. *J Am Coll Cardiol.* (2014) 63:1510–9. doi: 10.1016/j.jacc.2013.11.046
5. El-Chami MF, Kilgo P, Thourani V, Lattouf OM, Delurgio DB, Guyton RA, et al. New-onset atrial fibrillation predicts long-term mortality after coronary artery bypass graft. *J Am Coll Cardiol.* (2010) 55:1370–6. doi: 10.1016/j.jacc.2009.10.058
6. Phan K, Ha HS, Phan S, Medi C, Thomas SP, Yan TD. New-onset atrial fibrillation following coronary bypass surgery predicts long-term mortality: a systematic review and meta-analysis. *Eur J Cardiothorac Surg.* (2015) 48:817–24. doi: 10.1093/ejcts/ezu551
7. Rubin DA, Nieminski KE, Reed GE, Herman MV. Predictors, prevention, and long-term prognosis of atrial fibrillation after coronary artery bypass graft operations. *J Thorac Cardiovasc Surg.* (1987) 94:331–5.
8. Weidinger F, Schachner T, Bonaros N, Hofauer B, Lehr EJ, Vesely M, et al. Predictors and consequences of postoperative atrial fibrillation following robotic totally endoscopic coronary bypass surgery. *Eur J Cardiothorac Surg.* (2014) 45:318–22. doi: 10.1093/ejcts/ezt282
9. Horwich P, Buth KJ, Légaré JF. New onset postoperative atrial fibrillation is associated with a long-term risk for stroke and death following cardiac surgery. *J Card Surg.* (2013) 28:8–13. doi: 10.1111/jocs.12033
10. Ahlsson A, Fengsrud E, Bodin L, Englund A. Postoperative atrial fibrillation in patients undergoing aortocoronary bypass surgery carries an eightfold risk of future atrial fibrillation and a doubled cardiovascular mortality. *Eur J Cardiothorac Surg.* (2010) 37:1353–9. doi: 10.1016/j.ejcts.2009.12.033
11. Thorén E, Wernroth ML, Christersson C, Grinnemo KH, Jidéus L, Ståhle E. Compared with matched controls, patients with postoperative atrial fibrillation (POAF) have increased long-term AF after CABG, and POAF is further associated with increased ischemic stroke, heart failure and mortality even after adjustment for AF. *Clin Res Cardiol.* (2020) 109:1232–42. doi: 10.1007/s00392-020-01614-z
12. Jagadish PS, Kirolos I, Khare S, Rawal A, Lin V, Khouzam RN. Post-operative atrial fibrillation: should we anticoagulate? *Ann Transl Med.* (2019) 7:407. doi: 10.21037/atm.2019.07.10
13. Sousa-Uva M, Head SJ, Milojevic M, Collet JP, Landoni G, Castella M, et al. 2017 EACTS Guidelines on perioperative medication in adult cardiac surgery. *Eur J Cardiothorac Surg.* (2018) 53:5–33. doi: 10.1093/ejcts/ezx314
14. Austin PC. Optimal caliper widths for propensity-score matching when estimating differences in means and differences in proportions in observational studies. *Pharm Stat.* (2011) 10:150–61. doi: 10.1002/pst.433
15. Heinze G, Jüni P. An overview of the objectives of and the approaches to propensity score analyses. *Eur Heart J.* (2011) 32:1704–8. doi: 10.1093/eurheartj/ehr031
16. Conen D, Alonso-Coello P, Douketis J, Chan MTV, Kurz A, Sigamani A, et al. Risk of stroke and other adverse outcomes in patients with perioperative atrial fibrillation 1 year after non-cardiac surgery. *Eur Heart J.* (2020) 41:645–51. doi: 10.1093/eurheartj/ehz431
17. Almassi GH, Schowalter T, Nicolosi AC, Aggarwal A, Moritz TE, Henderson WG, et al. Atrial fibrillation after cardiac surgery: a major morbid event? *Ann Surg.* (1997) 226:501–11. doi: 10.1097/00000658-199710000-00011
18. Villareal RP, Hariharan R, Liu BC, Kar B, Lee VV, Elayda M, et al. Postoperative atrial fibrillation and mortality after coronary artery bypass surgery. *J Am Coll Cardiol.* (2004) 43:742–8. doi: 10.1016/j.jacc.2003.11.023
19. Filardo G, Damiano RJ Jr, Ailawadi G, Thourani VH, Pollock BD, Sass DM, et al. Epidemiology of new-onset atrial fibrillation following coronary artery bypass graft surgery. *Heart.* (2018) 104:985–92. doi: 10.1136/heartjnl-2017-312150
20. Westaby S. Atrial fibrillation after cardiac surgery: benign or deserving of prophylaxis. *J Atr Fibrillation.* (2010) 3:337. doi: 10.4022/jafib.337
21. Pires LA, Wagshal AB, Lancey R, Huang SK. Arrhythmias and conduction disturbances after coronary artery bypass graft surgery: epidemiology, management, and prognosis. *Am Heart J.* (1995) 129:799–808. doi: 10.1016/0002-8703(95)90332-1
22. Kiaii B, Fox S, Chase L, Fernandes M, Stitt LW, Guo R, et al. Postoperative atrial fibrillation is not pulmonary vein dependent: Results from a randomized trial. *Heart Rhythm.* (2015) 12:699–705. doi: 10.1016/j.hrthm.2015.01.014
23. Zaman AG, Archbold RA, Helft G, Paul EA, Curzen NP, Mills PG. Atrial fibrillation after coronary artery bypass surgery: a model for preoperative risk stratification. *Circulation.* (2000) 101:1403–8. doi: 10.1161/01.cir.101.12.1403
24. Chua SK, Shyu KG, Lu MJ, Lien LM, Lin CH, Chao HH, et al. Clinical utility of CHADS2 and CHA2DS2-VASc scoring systems for predicting postoperative atrial fibrillation after cardiac surgery. *J Thorac Cardiovasc Surg.* (2013) 146:919–26. doi: 10.1016/j.jtcvs.2013.03.040
25. Chua SK, Shyu KG, Lu MJ, Hung HF, Cheng JJ, Chiu CZ, et al. Renal dysfunction and the risk of postoperative atrial fibrillation after cardiac surgery: role beyond the CHA2DS2-VASc score. *Europace.* (2015) 17:1363–70. doi: 10.1093/europace/euu360
26. Her AY, Kim JY, Kim YH, Choi EY, Min PK, Yoon YW, et al. Left atrial strain assessed by speckle tracking imaging is related to new-onset atrial fibrillation after coronary artery bypass grafting. *Can J Cardiol.* (2013) 29:377–83. doi: 10.1016/j.cjca.2012.06.006
27. Celik T, Iyisoy A, Jata B, Celik M, Gunay C, Isik E. Beta blockers for the prevention of atrial fibrillation after coronary artery bypass surgery: carvedilol versus metoprolol. *Int J Cardiol.* (2009) 135:393–6. doi: 10.1016/j.ijcard.2007.12.026
28. Chen S, Acou WJ, Kiuchi MG, Meyer C, Sommer P, Martinek M, et al. Association of preoperative renin-angiotensin system inhibitors with prevention of postoperative atrial fibrillation and adverse events: a systematic review and meta-analysis. *JAMA Netw Open.* (2019) 2:e194934. doi: 10.1001/jamanetworkopen.2019.4934
29. Melduni RM, Schaff HV, Bailey KR, Cha SS, Ammash NM, Seward JB, et al. Implications of new-onset atrial fibrillation after cardiac surgery on long-term prognosis: a community-based study. *Am Heart J.* (2015) 170:659–68. doi: 10.1016/j.ahj.2015.06.015
30. Butt JH, Xian Y, Peterson ED, Olsen PS, Rørth R, Gundlund A, et al. Long-term thromboembolic risk in patients with postoperative atrial fibrillation after coronary artery bypass graft surgery and patients with nonvalvular atrial fibrillation. *JAMA Cardiol.* (2018) 3:417–24. doi: 10.1001/jamacardio.2018.0405
31. Lubitz SA, Yin X, Rienstra M, Schnabel RB, Walkey AJ, Magnani JW, et al. Long-term outcomes of secondary atrial fibrillation in the community: the Framingham Heart Study. *Circulation.* (2015) 131:1648–55. doi: 10.1161/CIRCULATIONAHA.114.014058

32. Lowres N, Mulcahy G, Jin K, Gallagher R, Neubeck L, Freedman B. Incidence of postoperative atrial fibrillation recurrence in patients discharged in sinus rhythm after cardiac surgery: a systematic review and meta-analysis. *Interact Cardiovasc Thorac Surg.* (2018) 26:504–11. doi: 10.1093/icvts/ivx348

33. El-Chami MF, Merchant FM, Smith P, Levy M, Nelms AG, Merlino J, et al. Management of new-onset postoperative atrial fibrillation utilizing insertable cardiac Monitor Technology to Observe Recurrence of AF (MONITOR-AF). *Pacing Clin Electrophysiol.* (2016). 39:1083–9. doi: 10.1111/pace.12949

# 23

# Relationship Between First 24-h Mean Body Temperature and Clinical Outcomes of Post-cardiac Surgery Patients

*Fei Xu , Cheng Zhang , Chao Liu , Siwei Bi and Jun Gu*[3*]

[1] Department of Anesthesiology, The Affiliated Hospital, School of Medicine, Chengdu Women's & Children's Central Hospital, UESTC, Chengdu, China, [2] West China of Medical School, Sichuan University, Chengdu, China, [3] Department of Cardiovascular Surgery, West China Hospital, Sichuan University, Chengdu, China

***Correspondence:**
Jun Gu
gujun@wchscu.cn

**Background:** This study was aimed to investigate the relationship between first 24-h mean body temperature and clinical outcomes of post cardiac surgery patients admitted to intensive care unit (ICU) in a large public clinical database.

**Methods:** This is a retrospectively observational research of MIMIC III dataset, a total of 6,122 patients included. Patients were divided into 3 groups according to the distribution of body temperature. Multivariate cox analysis and logistic regression analysis were used to investigate the association between abnormal temperature, and clinical outcomes.

**Results:** Hypothermia (<36°C) significantly associated with increasing in-hospital mortality (HR 1.665, 95%CI 1.218–2.276; $p = 0.001$), 1-year mortality (HR 1.537, 95% CI 1.205–1.961; $p = 0.001$), 28-day mortality (HR 1.518, 95% CI 1.14–2.021; $p = 0.004$), and 90-day mortality (HR 1.491, 95% CI 1.144–1.943; $p = 0.003$). No statistical differences were observed between short-term or long-term mortality and hyperthermia (>38°C). Hyperthermia was related to the extended length of ICU stay ($p < 0.001$), and hospital stay ($p < 0.001$).

**Conclusion:** Hypothermia within 24h after ICU admission was associated with the increased mortality of post cardiac surgery patients. Enhanced monitoring of body temperature within 24h after cardiac surgery should be taken into account for improving clinical outcomes.

**Keywords: hypothermia, hyperthermia, clinical outcome, post-cardiac surgery, intensive care unit**

## INTRODUCTION

The management of body temperature (BT) was very important to the recovery of postoperative patients, especially for critically ill patients who have relatively severe physical conditions. Almost 57.1% patients were exposed to hypothermia (BT < 36.0°C) among the patients admitted to intensive care unit (ICU) after operation (1) which claimed to be associated with mortality (2). Postoperative hyperthermia might be relevant to adverse clinical outcomes (3), and infection (4) in critically ill patients. Previous studies had indicated general anesthesia and surgical influence disturbed normal temperature regulation mechanism (5). Without preventative actions, influence of abnormal body temperature could be exaggerated with serious consequences.

As a special operation type, cardiac surgery had a great impact on circulation and physiology, and also brought enormous challenges to reduce mortality. Hypothermia and hyperthermia might occur after cardiac surgery attributed to long-term anesthesia and surgery exposure, the failure of the temperature maintenance, special hypothermia treatment and inflammatory response, and so on. Hyperthermia after cardiovascular surgery with cardiopulmonary bypass (CPB) could cause cognitive decline (3, 6). Grocott and colleagues revealed that postoperative high fever was associated with cognitive impairment at 6 weeks after coronary artery bypass grafting (6). Besides, there was study reporting that hypothermia effectively promoted endotoxin release through ischemic intestinal mucosa and had bad effects on brain tissue (7). Abnormal body temperature is disadvantageous to the prognosis of patients.

There were few studies explored the relationship between body temperature and adverse outcomes of patients after cardiac surgery, and no unified conclusion was obtained. Body temperature at single point in time raised bias risk inevitably (8), and could not fully reflect the overall effect of early postoperative body temperature. The object of this study was to investigate the association between first 24-h mean body temperature and clinical outcomes of post cardiac surgery patients admitted to ICU in a large public clinical database.

## MATERIALS AND METHODS

### Data Source

The study is a retrospective study with data collected from Medical Information Mart for Intensive Care-III (MIMIC-III) database (9, 10). This is a large intensive care database open to the public including more than 40,000 patients admitted to ICU from Beth Israel Deaconess Medical Center (Boston, Massachusetts, USA) between 2001 and 2012. Beth Israel Deaconess Medical Center and the Beth Israel Deacon Medical Center's institutional review board approved the application of the database (approval code 40043439) and personal informed consent was abandoned.

### Study Population

Patients with cardiac surgery were identified using current procedural terminology numbered from 33,010 to 37,799. 18 to 89 years old patients were enrolled into the study. If patients were admitted to hospital or ICU multiple times, only the first record was analyzed. Patients stayed ICU <24h were excluded. Based on the attribution of temperature and existing research (11), Patients were divided into 3 groups: hypothermia group (BT < 36.0°C), normal group (36.0°C ≤ BT ≤ 38.3°C), hyperthermia group (BT > 38.3°C).

### Data Collection and Definitions

The data was extracted from database by using structure query language (PostgreSQL, version 9.4.6, www.postgresql.org),and the codes in MIMIC Code Repository (https://github.com/MIT-LCP/mimic-website). Variables of this study included demographics, comorbidities, scoring systems, laboratory tests, and vital signs. Calculate the average of vital signs and laboratory tests with multiple results within 24h after ICU admission. Data analysis excluded variables with missing values exceeding 30% to avoid potential bias. Multiple imputation method was used to process variables with missing values <30%.

### Outcomes

The primary outcomes were in-hospital and 1-year mortality. The secondary outcomes included survival time, 28-day mortality, 90-day mortality, length of hospital stay and ICU stay, the intervention of continuous renal replacement therapy (CRRT) within 24h admitted to ICU, the incidence of acute kidney injury (AKI) within 7 days after ICU admission. The diagnosis of AKI was confirmed following the Kidney Disease: improving global outcomes (KDIGO) guideline (12).

### Statistical Analysis

Most continuous variables in this research were checked to be non-normally distributed and described as medians with interquartile ranges (IQRs), the rest were reported as mean ± standard deviation. Categorical variables were described as

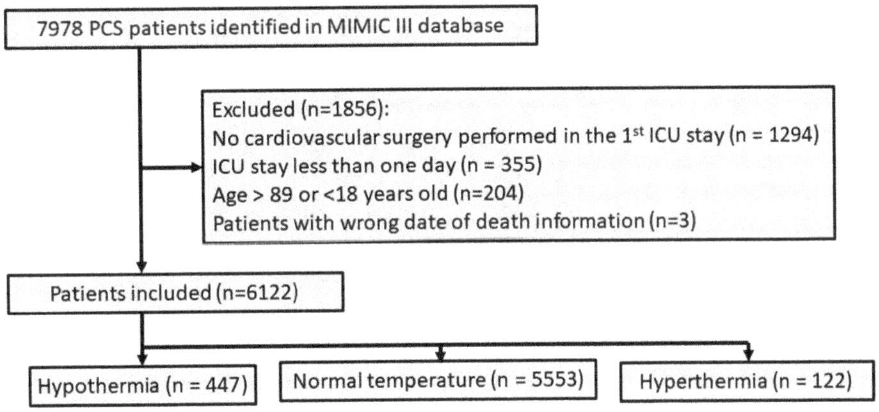


**FIGURE 1** | Flowchart of study cohort selection.

**TABLE 1** | Clinical and laboratory baseline characteristics of the overall cohort.

| Characteristics | Over all ($n$ = 6,122) | Low temperature group ($n$ = 447) | Normal temperature group ($n$ = 5,553) | High temperature group ($n$ = 122) | $p$-value |
|---|---|---|---|---|---|
| Temperature, median [IQR] | 36.81 [36.43, 37.24] | 35.8 [35.56, 35.9] | 36.86 [36.52, 37.25] | 38.58 [38.43, 38.71] | <0.001 |
| Age, median [IQR] | 66 [55, 76] | 68.0 [59.0, 78.0] | 66.0 [55.0, 76.0] | 54.0 [40.0, 66.0] | <0.001 |
| BMI, median [IQR] | 27.84 [24.39, 31.84] | 27.14 [24.21, 31.18] | 27.83 [24.37, 31.79] | 30.78 [26.7, 35.91] | <0.001 |
| Male gender, n (%) | 3,704 (60.503) | 259 (57.942) | 3,364 (60.580) | 81 (66.393) | 0.222 |
| Admission type, $n$ (%) | | | | | |
| Elective | 1,535 (25.074) | 100 (22.371) | 1,429 (25.734) | 6 (4.918) | <0.001 |
| Emergency | 4,487 (73.293) | 342 (76.510) | 4,031 (72.591) | 114 (93.443) | |
| Urgent | 100 (1.633) | 5 (1.119) | 93 (1.675) | 2 (1.639) | |
| **Comorbidity, $n$ (%)** | | | | | |
| Drug abuse, $n$ (%) | 208 (3.398) | 14 (3.132) | 186 (3.350) | 8 (6.557) | 0.146 |
| Alcohol abuse, $n$ (%) | 474 (7.743) | 44 (9.843) | 414 (7.455) | 16 (13.115) | 0.016 |
| Deficiency anemias, $n$ (%) | 1 340 (21.888) | 94 (21.029) | 1 209 (21.772) | 37 (30.328) | 0.070 |
| Rheumatoid arthritis, $n$ (%) | 182 (2.973) | 13 (2.908) | 165 (2.971) | 4 (3.279) | 0.977 |
| Metastatic cancer, $n$ (%) | 214 (3.496) | 12 (2.685) | 199 (3.584) | 3 (2.459) | 0.500 |
| Liver disease, $n$ (%) | 463 (7.563) | 52 (11.633) | 408 (7.347) | 3 (2.459) | <0.001 |
| Renal failure, $n$ (%) | 869 (14.195) | 81 (18.121) | 769 (13.848) | 19 (15.574) | 0.041 |
| Diabetes uncomplicated, $n$ (%) | 1,448 (23.652) | 97 (21.700) | 1,324 (23.843) | 27 (22.131) | 0.546 |
| Hypertension, $n$ (%) | 758 (12.382) | 66 (14.765) | 680 (12.246) | 12 (9.836) | 0.206 |
| Peripheral vascular, $n$ (%) | 794 (12.970) | 73 (16.331) | 709 (12.768) | 12 (9.836) | 0.057 |
| Pulmonary circulation, $n$ (%) | 258 (4.214) | 28 (6.264) | 224 (4.034) | 6 (4.918) | 0.072 |
| Valvular disease, $n$ (%) | 254 (4.149) | 17 (3.803) | 233 (4.196) | 4 (3.279) | 0.820 |
| Cardiac arrhythmias, $n$ (%) | 911 (14.881) | 87 (19.463) | 805 (14.497) | 19 (15.574) | 0.017 |
| **Laboratory tests within 24h after ICU** | | | | | |
| $F$ calcium mean, median [IQR] | 1.13 [1.08, 1.18] | 1.11 [1.06, 1.16] | 1.13 [1.08, 1.18] | 1.1[1.02, 1.14] | <0.001 |
| $T$ calcium mean, median [IQR] | 8.1 [7.65, 8.6] | 8.15 [7.7, 8.7] | 8.1 [7.65, 8.6] | 7.8 [7.2, 8.4] | <0.001 |
| WBC mean, median [IQR] | 11.93 [8.9, 15.55] | 11.4 [7.84, 14.47] | 11.97 [9.0, 15.6] | 13.2 [8.43, 17.1] | 0.004 |
| BUN mean, median [IQR] | 18.33 [13.0, 29.4] | 23.5 [15.5, 42.0] | 18.0 [13.0, 28.0] | 22.5 [14.5, 38.0] | <0.001 |
| PT mean, median [IQR] | 14.65 [13.6, 16.2] | 15.2 [13.8, 18.05] | 14.6 [13.55, 16.1] | 14.83 [13.6, 16.6] | <0.001 |
| INR mean, median [IQR] | 1.3 [1.2, 1.5] | 1.35 [1.2, 1.75] | 1.3 [1.2, 1.5] | 1.33 [1.2, 1.6] | <0.001 |
| PTT mean, median [IQR] | 33.3 [28.65, 41.6] | 37.4 [30.7, 49.5] | 33.0 [28.55, 41.1] | 33.0 [28.05, 40.07] | <0.001 |
| $K^+$ mean, median [IQR] | 4.19[3.87,4.5] | 4.22[3.87,4.56] | 4.19[3.88,4.5] | 4.04[3.7,4.4] | 0.004 |
| Platelet mean, median [IQR] | 175.33 [130.33, 233.33] | 161.67 [111.33, 217.0] | 176.0 [132.0, 234.0] | 199.5 [134.0, 269.0] | <0.001 |
| Lactate mean, median [IQR] | 1.93 [1.4, 2.7] | 2.3 [1.52, 3.4] | 1.9 [1.4, 2.6] | 2.0 [1.25, 3.07] | <0.001 |
| Hemoglobin mean, median [IQR] | 10.15 [9.15, 11.4] | 10.09 [9.1, 11.2] | 10.15 [9.15, 11.4] | 10.35 [9.28, 12.3] | 0.080 |
| Hematocrit mean, median [IQR] | 30.0 [27.3, 33.58] | 29.88 [27.0, 33.45] | 30.0 [27.3, 33.57] | 30.8 [27.82, 36.0] | 0.261 |
| Glucose mean, median [IQR] | 130.57 [116.0, 150.89] | 133.0 [117.0, 159.25] | 130.17 [116.0, 150.0] | 139.25 [118.67, 165.33] | <0.001 |
| Creatinine mean, median [IQR] | 0.95 [0.72, 1.37] | 1.05 [0.8, 2.0] | 0.93 [0.7, 1.33] | 1.08 [0.85, 2.13] | <0.001 |
| **Vital sign** | | | | | |
| $Spo_2$ mean, median [IQR] | 97.77 [96.52, 98.81] | 97.85 [96.39, 98.96] | 97.77 [96.56, 98.81] | 96.96 [95.33, 98.39] | <0.001 |
| Respirate mean, median [IQR] | 18.12 [16.08, 21.17] | 17.78 [15.92, 20.85] | 18.08 [16.07, 21.03] | 23.03 [19.81, 26.62] | <0.001 |
| Mean bp mean, median [IQR] | 75.11 [70.17, 81.36] | 74.61 [69.46, 80.39] | 75.16 [70.24, 81.38] | 74.96 [69.63, 83.87] | 0.121 |
| Dias bp mean, median [IQR] | 58.39 [53.15, 64.3] | 58.11 [52.44, 63.88] | 58.41 [53.18, 64.29] | 58.96 [54.1, 66.07] | 0.276 |
| Sys bp mean, median [IQR] | 112.86 [105.52, 122.26] | 111.13 [102.96, 118.56] | 112.97 [105.71, 122.54] | 113.15 [104.58, 125.96] | <0.001 |
| Heart rate mean, median [IQR] | 85.83 [77.53, 96.52] | 80.97 [71.7, 90.64] | 86.0 [77.9, 96.5] | 105.52 [92.33, 117.19] | <0.001 |

*(Continued)*

**TABLE 1** | Continued

| Characteristics | Over all ($n$ = 6,122) | Low temperature group ($n$ = 447) | Normal temperature group ($n$ = 5,553) | High temperature group ($n$ = 122) | $p$-value |
|---|---|---|---|---|---|
| **Score system** | | | | | |
| SPAS ii, median [IQR] | 38 [30, 48] | 44.0 [34.0, 56.0] | 37.0 [30.0, 47.0] | 43.0 [33.0, 55.0] | <0.001 |
| SOFA, median [IQR] | 5 [3, 8] | 6.0 [4.0, 9.0] | 5.0 [3.0, 7.0] | 7.0 [5.0, 10.0] | <0.001 |
| **Outcome** | | | | | |
| Hospital interval, median [IQR] | 9.91 [6.07, 17.69] | 10.0 [5.94, 19.09] | 9.85 [6.06, 17.27] | 17.91 [10.14, 30.06] | <0.001 |
| ICU interval, median [IQR] | 3.34 [1.86, 8.14] | 3.86 [2.03, 9.15] | 3.28 [1.83, 7.86] | 9.99 [4.51, 17.22] | <0.001 |
| Survival time, median [IQR] | 11.15 [6.26, 27.17] | 12.12 [6.03, 31.47] | 11.01 [6.25, 26.75] | 20.03 [10.34, 33.56] | <0.001 |
| AKI 7-day, n (%) | 4,563 (74.534) | 360 (80.537) | 4,094 (73.726) | 109 (89.344) | <0.001 |
| CRRT, n (%) | 299 (4.884) | 38 (8.501) | 252 (4.538) | 9 (7.377) | <0.001 |
| Death in hospital, n (%) | 925 (15.109) | 133 (29.754) | 763 (13.740) | 29 (23.770) | <0.001 |
| Death 28-day, n (%) | 1,114 (18.197) | 153 (34.228) | 925 (16.658) | 36 (29.508) | <0.001 |
| Death 90-day, n (%) | 1,301 (21.251) | 174 (38.926) | 1,089 (19.611) | 38 (31.148) | <0.001 |
| Death1-year, n (%) | 1,606 (26.233) | 201 (44.966) | 1,362 (24.527) | 43 (35.246) | <0.001 |

*BMI, body mass index; F calcium, free calcium; T calcium, total calcium; WBC, white blood cell count; BUN, Blood urea nitrogen; PT, prothrombin time; INR, international normalized ratio; PTT, partial thromboplastin time; SOFA, sequential organ failure assessment; SPAS, simplified acute physiology score; AKI, acute kidney injury; CRRT, continuous renal replacement therapy; ICU, the intensive care unit; SPO2, pulse oxygen saturation; BT, body temperature; Data are represented as median (interquartile range) or n (%), mean (SD, Standard Deviation).*

number and rate. Comparisons were performed with Kruskal-Wallis test or Mann-Whitney U or Welch's $t$ test for continuous variables and chi-square or Fisher's exact tests for categorical variables. Propensity score matching (PSM) (13) was performed to adjust the imbalance of baseline between different groups. All selected variables were analyzed by univariate analysis firstly. Multivariate cox analysis or multivariate logistic regression analysis were performed to investigate relationships between abnormal temperature and clinical outcomes through adjusting confounding factors post-matched which had been analyzed in univariate analysis models with $P < 0.05$. Kaplan-Meier survival curves of 1 year mortality in different groups were constructed and compared by the log-rank test.

Data cleaning, statistical analyses and illustrations were conducted by using SPSS software version 24.0 (IBM Corporation, Armonk, NY, USA) and R software (version 4.0.3) consisted of "tableone" (14), "ggplot2" (15), "survival" (16), "survminer" (17), "lubridate" (18), "tidyverse" (19). $P < 0.05$ was considered statistically significant.

## RESULT

### Baseline Characteristics

There were 6,122 patients concluded in our study (**Figure 1**), 447 patients (7.3%) belonged to hypothermia, 122 patients (2.0%) belonged to hyperthermia, 5,553 patients (90.7%) belonged to normal group. Clinical and laboratory test baseline characteristics of the populations were reported in **Table 1**. The association between body temperature and in-hospital mortality was described in **Figure 2A** (95% CI −0.043, −0.016, $p < 0.001$). The relationship between body temperature and 1-year mortality was shown in **Figure 2B** (95% CI −0.065, −0.032, $p < 0.001$). There were statistical differences between body temperature distribution of first 24- h after ICU admission and long-term mortality, that was described in **Figure 3** (log-rank $p < 0.001$).

### Hypothermia

The comparison between hypothermia and normal group was performed before (**Supplemental Table 1**) and after (**Supplemental Table 2**, **Table 2**) PSM. There were no significant differences in hospital interval, ICU interval and survival time (**Table 2**) across univariate analysis. After adjusting potential confounding factors, the results of multivariate cox analysis and multivariate logistic regression analysis were that in-hospital mortality (HR 1.665, 95% CI 1.218–2.276; $p$ = 0.001) and 1-year mortality (HR 1.537, 95% CI 1.205–1.961; $p$ = 0.001) significantly increased in hypothermia group. There were higher 28-day mortality (HR 1.518, 95% CI 1.14–2.021; $p$ = 0.004) and 90-day mortality (HR 1.491, 95% CI 1.144–1.943; $p$ = 0.003) compared to normal group. The incidence of AKI within 7-day and intervention of CRRT within the first day after ICU admission were both showed no significant differences between 2 groups (**Table 3**).

### Hyperthermia

The comparison between hyperthermia and normal group was conducted before (**Supplemental Table 3**) and after (**Supplemental Table 4**, **Table 4**) PSM. The length of hospital stay and ICU stay were longer in hyperthermia group than normal group, respectively ($p < 0.001$,**Table 4**) across univariate analysis. After adjustment for potential confounding factors, there were no statistical differences in in-hospital mortality, 28-day mortality, 90-day mortality, 1-year mortality, the incidence of AKI within 7-day or the intervention of CRRT within the first day after ICU admission between hyperthermia group and normal group across multivariate analysis (**Table 5**).

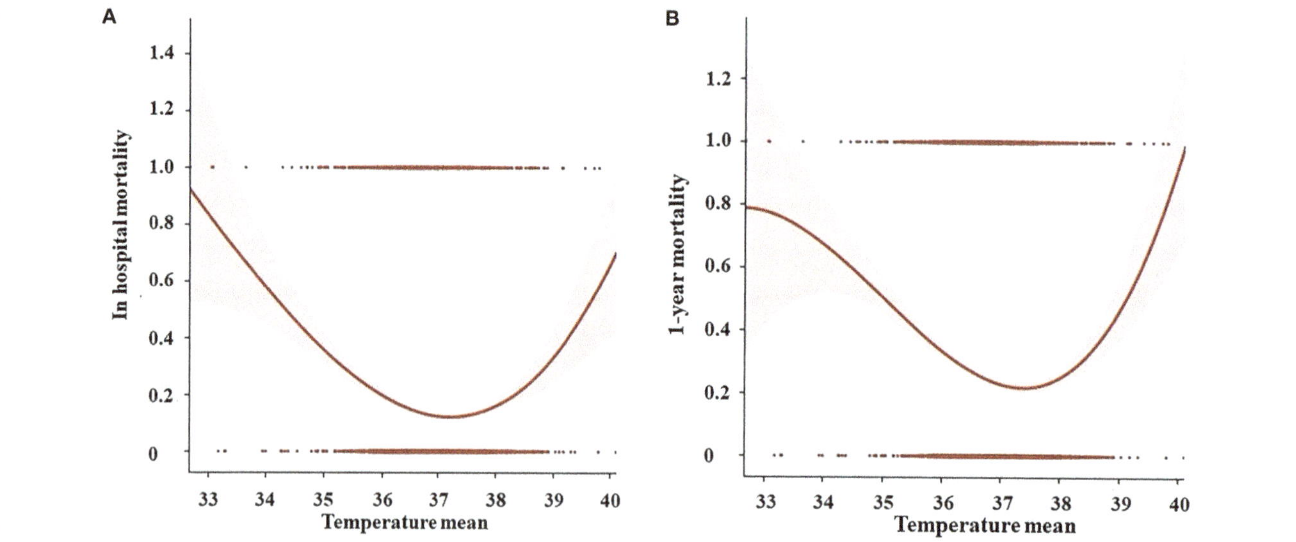


**FIGURE 2** | The relationship between **(A)** body temperature and in-hospital mortality; **(B)** body temperature and 1-year mortality by Polynomial regression.

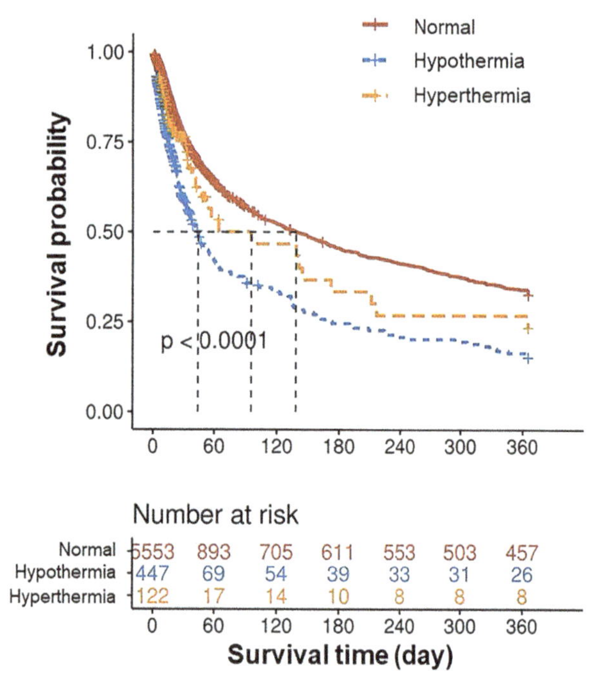


**FIGURE 3** | Kaplan-Meier curves of 1-year mortality by temperature category.

## DISCUSSION

This study demonstrated hypothermia within first 24-h after ICU admission was significantly associated with the increased short-term mortality and long-term mortality of post-cardiac surgery patients. Otherwise, no statistical associations were observed between hyperthermia and mortality. Hyperthermia was related to the prolonged length of hospital stay and ICU stay. Incidence of acute renal injury and intervention of continuous renal replacement therapy were not associated with hypothermia or hyperthermia.

Previous study considered body temperature could be used to assess prognostic risk independently. Hypothermia increased one-year mortality and seemed more harmful than hyperthermia (20). This is in line with our results. The reason may be relative to the great physiological changes produced by hypothermia (such as left shift of oxygenation curve, decline of coagulation function and arrhythmia and so on), which may lead to aggravate tissue hypoxia, aggravation of multiple organ functions (21), and failure of fluid resuscitation (22). For patients who were diagnosed sepsis within 24h, hypothermia (< 36.0°C) could increase 28-day mortality and 1-year mortality (23). Besides, hypothermia was also associated with the mortality of none-elderly sepsis patients (11). Moreover, patients whose bladder core temperature were <36°C after ICU admission associated with worse outcomes after coronary artery bypass grafting (CABG) under CPB (5). The results of these researches are consistent with ours. Contrary to our study, Jiwook Kim's study suggested hypothermia or hyperthermia were not interrelated with long-term mortality of severe surgery patients except cardiovascular surgery patients (24). This can be explained by the inconsistence at the key time of temperature. Owing to enlarge sample size in our study, association between the distribution of body temperature and long-term mortality was significant. Relative research confirmed that changes in body temperature could easily induce acute and further cardiovascular outcomes (25). Thus, temperature monitoring of critically ill patients is extremely necessary. Emphasizing the importance of temperature monitoring within first 24-h after ICU admission is a new sight to improve the clinical outcomes of post-cardiac surgery patients.

**TABLE 2** | Post-PSM matched between hypothermia and normal group.

| | Over all ($n = 894$) | Normal ($n = 447$) | Hypothermia ($n = 447$) | *p*-value |
|---|---|---|---|---|
| **Laboratory tests within 24h after ICU** | | | | |
| *F* calcium mean, median [IQR] | 1.12 [1.07, 1.18] | 1.13 [1.09, 1.19] | 1.11 [1.06, 1.16] | <0.001 |
| *T* calcium mean, median [IQR] | 8.1 [7.67, 8.7] | 8.1 [7.65, 8.6] | 8.15 [7.7, 8.7] | 0.281 |
| WBC mean, median [IQR] | 11.47 [8.37, 15.05] | 11.57 [8.8, 15.4] | 11.4 [7.84, 14.47] | 0.068 |
| BUN mean, median [IQR] | 20.0 [14.5, 35.25] | 18.5 [14.0, 30.67] | 23.5 [15.5, 42.0] | <0.001 |
| PT mean, median [IQR] | 14.97 [13.8, 17.1] | 14.7 [13.8, 16.4] | 15.2 [13.8, 18.05] | 0.003 |
| INR mean, median [IQR] | 1.35 [1.2, 1.6] | 1.3 [1.2, 1.5] | 1.35 [1.2, 1.75] | 0.006 |
| PTT mean, median [IQR] | 35.3 [29.75, 44.9] | 33.8 [29.1, 41.9] | 37.4 [30.7, 49.5] | <0.001 |
| $K^+$ mean, median [IQR] | 4.2 [3.87, 4.53] | 4.2 [3.89, 4.51] | 4.22 [3.87, 4.56] | 0.649 |
| Platelet mean, median [IQR] | 166.0 [121.0, 223.0] | 169.0 [130.0, 226.33] | 161.67 [111.33, 217.0] | 0.018 |
| Lactate mean, median [IQR] | 2.1 [1.45, 3.09] | 2.0 [1.4, 2.8] | 2.3 [1.52, 3.4] | <0.001 |
| Hemoglobin mean median [IQR] | 10.04 [9.07, 11.28] | 10.0 [9.07, 11.37] | 10.09 [9.1, 11.2] | 0.789 |
| Hematocrit mean median [IQR] | 29.8 [27.2, 33.46] | 29.52 [27.32, 33.43] | 29.88 [27.0, 33.45] | 0.886 |
| Glucose mean median [IQR] | 132.6 [116.29, 153.0] | 131.7 [115.62, 150.0] | 133.0 [117.0, 159.25] | 0.166 |
| Creatinine mean median [IQR] | 1.0 [0.75, 1.6] | 0.95 [0.73, 1.4] | 1.05 [0.8, 2.0] | <0.001 |
| **Score system** | | | | |
| SPAS ii, median [IQR] | 41 [32, 53] | 38.0 [31.0, 49.0] | 44.0 [34.0, 56.0] | <0.001 |
| SOFA, median [IQR] | 6 [4, 8] | 5.0 [3.0, 8.0] | 6.0 [4.0, 9.0] | <0.001 |
| **Vital sign** | | | | |
| $Spo_2$ mean, median [IQR] | 97.79 [96.46, 98.95] | 97.78 [96.56, 98.9] | 97.85 [96.39, 98.96] | 0.859 |
| Temperature mean, median [IQR] | 35.99 [35.8, 36.86] | 36.86 [36.52, 37.2] | 35.8 [35.56, 35.9] | <0.001 |
| Respirate mean, median [IQR] | 17.88 [15.97, 20.93] | 18.05 [16.07, 20.95] | 17.78 [15.92, 20.85] | 0.359 |
| Mean bp mean, median [IQR] | 74.71 [69.71, 80.35] | 74.84 [70.1, 80.23] | 74.61 [69.46, 80.39] | 0.592 |
| Dias bp mean, median [IQR] | 57.91 [52.33, 63.58] | 57.55 [52.19, 63.19] | 58.11 [52.44, 63.88] | 0.530 |
| Sys bp mean, median [IQR] | 112.11 [104.14, 120.28] | 113.08 [105.27, 122.84] | 111.13 [102.96, 118.56] | <0.001 |
| Heart rate mean, mean (SD) | 83.53 [74.5, 93.04] | 86.21 [78.3, 95.29] | 80.97 [71.7, 90.64] | <0.001 |
| **Outcomes** | | | | |
| Hospital interval, median [IQR] | 9.97 [6.03, 17.97] | 9.9 [6.33, 17.04] | 10.0 [5.94, 19.09] | 0.873 |
| ICU interval, median [IQR] | 3.77 [2.0, 8.7] | 3.47 [1.98, 8.11] | 3.86 [2.03, 9.15] | 0.621 |
| Survival time, median [IQR] | 11.8 [6.31, 30.0] | 11.7 [6.97, 29.29] | 12.12 [6.03, 31.47] | 0.341 |
| Death in hospital, *n* (%) | 205 (22.931) | 72 (16.107) | 133 (29.754) | <0.001 |
| CRRT, *n* (%) | 59 (6.600) | 21 (4.698) | 38 (8.501) | 0.022 |
| AKI 7-day, *n* (%) | 689 (77.069) | 329 (73.602) | 360 (80.537) | 0.014 |
| Death 28-day, *n* (%) | 241 (26.957) | 88 (19.687) | 153 (34.228) | < 0.001 |
| Death 90-day, *n* (%) | 280 (31.320) | 106 (23.714) | 174 (38.926) | < 0.001 |
| Death 1-year, *n* (%) | 329 (36.801) | 128 (28.635) | 201 (44.966) | <0.001 |

*F calcium, free calcium; T calcium, total calcium; WBC, white blood cell count; BUN, Blood urea nitrogen; PT, prothrombin time; INR, international normalized ratio; PTT, partial thromboplastin time; SOFA, sequential organ failure assessment; SPAS, simplified acute physiology score; AKI, acute kidney injury; CRRT, continuous renal replacement therapy; ICU, the intensive care unit; SPO2, pulse oxygen saturation; BT, body temperature; Data are represented as median (interquartile range) or n (%), mean (SD, Standard Deviation).*

The effects of hyperthermia and hypothermia on human body were complicated (26, 27). Hyperthermia was likely a powerful factor in strengthening immunity to remove subsequent pathogen by itself (28). Infection (29) and systemic inflammatory response syndrome (SIRS) caused by CPB (30) both lead to hyperthermia after cardiac surgery (31). Recent study claimed that hyperthermia in first 24h can be used to diagnose inflammatory response and possible outcomes after CPB, in this study in-hospital mortality was not significantly different comparing SIRS with no SIRS patients, while length of ICU stay was longer in SIRS patients (30). Besides, earlier studies suggested hyperthermia was beneficial for some outcomes (23, 32) and did not improve 1-year mortality of post-cardiac surgery patients (24). In line with our research, relationship between hyperthermia and mortality was not statistically significant, but hyperthermia was related to the prolonged length of ICU and hospital stay.

The strength of our study is focusing on the impact of overall body temperature changes within 24h after cardiac surgery on clinical outcomes rather than emphasizing the

**TABLE 3 |** Multivariable cox regression and logistic regression analysis for hypothermia.

| | <36.0°C (Pre-matched) | | | <36.0°C (Post-matched) | | |
|---|---|---|---|---|---|---|
| | HR/OR | 95%CI | *P*-value | HR/OR | 95%CI | *p*-value |
| Death in-hospital | 1.475 | 1.204–1.806 | <001 | 1.665 | 1.218 – 2.276 | 0.001 |
| Death 1-year | 1.409 | 1.199–1.655 | <001 | 1.537 | 1.205–1.961 | 0.001 |
| Death 28-day | 1.387 | 1.15–1.674 | 0.001 | 1.518 | 1.14–2.021 | 0.004 |
| Death 90-day | 1.389 | 1.166–1.656 | <001 | 1.491 | 1.144–1.943 | 0.003 |
| AKI 7-day | 0.871 | 0.521–1.417 | 0.588 | 1.094 | 0.762–1.573 | 0.627 |
| CRRT | 1.004 | 0.764–1.329 | 0.976 | 1.021 | 0.457–2.31 | 0.959 |

*AKI, acute kidney injury; CRRT, continuous renal replacement therapy; HR, hazard ratio; OR, odds ratio.*

**TABLE 4 |** Post-PSM matched between hyperthermia and normal group.

| | Over all ($n$ = 244) | Normal ($n$ = 122) | Hyperthermia($n$ = 122) | *p*-value |
|---|---|---|---|---|
| **Laboratory tests within 24h after ICU** | | | | |
| *F* calcium mean, median [IQR] | 1.11 [1.06, 1.15] | 1.12[1.08, 1.16] | 1.1 [1.02, 1.14] | 0.002 |
| *T* calcium mean, median [IQR] | 8.03 [7.4, 8.5] | 8.2 [7.7, 8.55] | 7.8 [7.2, 8.4] | 0.003 |
| WBC mean, median [IQR] | 12.43 [8.77, 16.73] | 11.85 [8.8, 16.05] | 13.2 [8.43, 17.1] | 0.617 |
| BUN mean, median [IQR] | 18.67 [13.0, 33.0] | 17.0 [12.0, 24.67] | 22.5 [14.5, 38.0] | 0.005 |
| PT mean, median [IQR] | 14.57 [13.6, 16.4] | 14.3 [13.4, 15.9] | 14.83 [13.6, 16.6] | 0.122 |
| INR mean, median [IQR] | 1.3 [1.2, 1.55] | 1.3 [1.2, 1.5] | 1.33 [1.2, 1.6] | 0.113 |
| PTT mean, median [IQR] | 32.1 [27.9, 38.36] | 30.7 [27.7, 37.65] | 33.0 [28.05, 40.07] | 0.104 |
| $K^+$ mean, median [IQR] | 4.11 [3.75, 4.4] | 4.14 [3.81, 4.41] | 4.04 [3.7, 4.4] | 0.146 |
| Platelet mean, median [IQR] | 202.5 [140.5, 267.0] | 206.8 [147.0, 263.0] | 199.5 [134.0, 269.0] | 0.565 |
| Lactate mean, median [IQR] | 1.9[1.37, 2.68] | 1.85 [1.4, 2.4] | 2.0 [1.25, 3.07] | 0.626 |
| Hemoglobin mean, median [IQR] | 10.5 [9.37, 12.3] | 10.6 [9.5, 12.5] | 10.35 [9.28, 12.3] | 0.544 |
| Hematocrit mean, median [IQR] | 31.0 [27.62, 35.3] | 31.1 [27.53, 35.03] | 30.8 [27.82, 36.0] | 0.657 |
| Glucose mean, median [IQR] | 136.2 [117.88, 157.75] | 131.0 [117.25, 149.2] | 139.25 [118.67, 165.33] | 0.044 |
| Creatinine mean, median [IQR] | 1.0 [0.8, 1.65] | 0.95 [0.7, 1.2] | 1.08 [0.85, 2.13] | 0.005 |
| **Score system** | | | | |
| SPAS ii, median [IQR] | 37 [29, 49] | 34.0 [25.0, 42.0] | 43.0 [33.0, 55.0] | <0.001 |
| SOFA, median [IQR] | 6 [4, 9] | 5.0 [2.0, 7.0] | 7.0 [5.0, 10.0] | <0.001 |
| **Vital sign** | | | | |
| $SpO_2$ mean, median [IQR] | 97.59 [96.04, 98.9] | 97.92 [96.7, 99.18] | 96.96 [95.33, 98.39] | <0.001 |
| Temperature mean, median [IQR] | 38.31 [37.0, 38.58] | 36.99 [36.64, 37.44] | 38.58 [38.43, 38.71] | <0.001 |
| Resp rate mean, median [IQR] | 20.42 [17.3, 24.38] | 17.82 [15.97, 21.29] | 23.03 [19.81, 26.62] | <0.001 |
| Mean bp mean, median [IQR] | 76.14 [70.0, 84.69] | 77.1 [70.58, 87.36] | 74.96 [69.63, 83.87] | 0.092 |
| Dias bp mean, median [IQR] | 59.91 [54.68, 67.32] | 61.45 [55.07, 68.72] | 58.96 [54.1, 66.07] | 0.155 |
| Sys bp mean, median [IQR] | 114.83 [105.94, 125.07] | 114.94 [108.25, 125.07] | 113.15 [104.58, 125.96] | 0.279 |
| Heart rate mean, mean (SD) | 97.326 (17.954) | 90.644 (15.142) | 104.008 (18.059) | <0.001 |
| **Outcomes** | | | | |
| Hospital interval, median [IQR] | 14.18 [7.76, 24.93] | 10.84 [6.25, 20.44] | 17.91 [10.14, 30.06] | <0.001 |
| ICU interval, median [IQR] | 6.29 [2.58, 13.2] | 3.74 [2.04, 9.01] | 9.99 [4.51, 17.22] | <0.001 |
| Survival time, median [IQR] | 15.7 [7.9, 30.67] | 12.25 [6.31, 24.2] | 20.03 [10.34, 33.56] | 0.001 |
| CRRT, *n* (%) | 14 (5.738) | 5 (4.098) | 9 (7.377) | 0.271 |
| AKI 7-day, *n* (%) | 193 (79.098) | 84 (68.852) | 109 (89.344) | <0.001 |
| Death in hospital, *n* (%) | 46 (18.852) | 17 (13.934) | 29 (23.770) | 0.050 |
| Death 28-day, *n* (%) | 55 (22.541) | 19 (15.574) | 36 (29.508) | 0.009 |
| Death 90-day, *n* (%) | 62 (25.410) | 24 (19.672) | 38 (31.148) | 0.040 |
| Death 1-year, *n* (%) | 67 (27.459) | 24 (19.672) | 43 (35.246) | 0.006 |

*F calcium,free calcium; T calcium, total calcium; WBC, white blood cell count; BUN, Blood urea nitrogen; PT, prothrombin time; INR, international normalized ratio; PTT, partial thromboplastin time; SOFA, sequential organ failure assessment; SPAS, simplified acute physiology score; AKI, acute kidney injury; CRRT, continuous renal replacement therapy; ICU, the intensive care unit; SPO2, pulse oxygen saturation; BT, body temperature; Data are represented as median (interquartile range) or n (%), mean (SD, Standard Deviation).*

**TABLE 5** | Multivariable cox regression and logistic regression analysis for hyperthermia.

| | >38.3°C (Pre-matched) | | | >38.3°C (Post-matched) | | |
|---|---|---|---|---|---|---|
| | **HR/OR** | **95%CI** | ***P*-value** | **HR/OR** | **95%CI** | ***P*-value** |
| Death in-hospital | 1.001 | 0.686–1.46 | 0.995 | 1.061 | 0.492–2.29 | 0.88 |
| Death 1-year | 1.069 | 0.785–1.456 | 0.672 | 1.049 | 0.567–1.94 | 0.878 |
| Death 28-day | 1.068 | 0.761–1.499 | 0.704 | 1.126 | 0.561–2.259 | 0.739 |
| Death 90-day | 1.033 | 0.743–1.436 | 0.846 | 0.917 | 0.484–1.74 | 0.791 |
| AKI 7-day | 1.573 | 0.869–3.061 | 0.155 | 2.329 | 0.938–6.058 | 0.073 |
| CRRT | 0.684 | 0.251–1.644 | 0.427 | 3.909 | 0.656–34.76 | 0.164 |

*AKI, acute kidney injury; CRRT, continuous renal replacement therapy; HR, hazard ratio; OR, odds ratio.*

adverse results associated with a single time point. This study may be of beneficial in alleviating the adverse outcomes of hypothermia in post-cardiac surgery patients. Our study also has some limitations. Firstly, number of hyperthermia samples is relatively small, enlarging sample size and multicenter database are necessary for verification in future. Secondly, method and site of body temperature measurement were not clarified in MIMIC-III database which could cause bias to results, more researches deserve to carry out to clarify details. Thirdly, this is a retrospective single center study, results should be explained with caution in other populations and regions.

## CONCLUSION

This retrospective observational study confirmed hypothermia within 24-h after ICU admission was associated with the elevated mortality of post-cardiac surgery patients while hyperthermia was not. The importance of temperature monitoring is worthy of attention to improve clinical outcomes after cardiac surgery in clinical treatment.

## ETHICS STATEMENT

Ethical review and approval was not required for the study on human participants in accordance with the local legislation and institutional requirements. Written informed consent for participation was not required for this study in accordance with the national legislation and the institutional requirements.

## AUTHOR CONTRIBUTIONS

FX, CL, and SB gathered and processed the data. CL and CZ prepared the results. FX and SB contributed in writing the manuscript. JG put forward the idea and revised the manuscript. All authors have read and approved the final manuscript.

## REFERENCES


1. Kongsayreepong S, Chaibundit C, Chadpaibool J, Komoltri C, Suraseranivongse S, Suwannanonda P, et al. Predictor of core hypothermia and the surgical intensive care unit. *Anesth Analg.* (2003) 96:826–33. doi: 10.1213/01.ANE.0000048822.27698.28
2. Karalapillai D, Story DA, Calzavacca P, Licari E, Liu YL, Hart GK. Inadvertent hypothermia and mortality in postoperative intensive care patients: retrospective audit of 5050 patients. *Anesthesia.* (2009) 64:968–72. doi: 10.1111/j.1365-2044.2009.05989.x
3. Grocott HP, Mackensen GB, Grigore AM, Mathew J, Reves JG, Phillips-Bute B, et al. Postoperative hyperthermia is associated with cognitive dysfunction after coronary artery bypass graft surgery. *Stroke.* (2002) 33:537–41. doi: 10.1161/hs0202.102600
4. Vermeulen H, Storm-Versloot MN, Goossens A, Speelman P, Legemate DA. Diagnostic accuracy of routine postoperative body temperature measurements. *Clin Infect Dis.* (2005) 40:1404–10. doi: 10.1086/429621
5. Insler SR, O'Connor MS, Leventhal MJ, Nelson DR, Starr NJ. Association between postoperative hypothermia and adverse outcome after coronary artery bypass surgery. *Ann Thorac Surg.* (2000) 70:175–81. doi: 10.1016/S0003-4975(00)01415-6
6. Nathan HJ, Wells GA, Munson JL, Wozny D. Neuroprotective effect of mild hypothermia in patients undergoing coronary artery surgery with cardiopulmonary bypass: a randomized trial. *Circulation.* (2001) 104:I85–91. doi: 10.1161/hc37t1.094710
7. Gercekoglu H, Tarim O, Agar I, Korukcu A, Karabulut H, Soydemir H, et al. Effects of hypothermia on blood endogenous endotoxin levels during cardiopulmonary bypass. *J Card Surg.* (1997) 12:223–7. doi: 10.1111/j.1540-8191.1997.tb00129.x
8. Shen Y, Lou Y, Zhu S. Hyperthermia is a predictor of high mortality in patients with sepsis. *Crit Care.* (2020) 24:543. doi: 10.1186/s13054-020-03263-0
9. Goldberger AL, Amaral LA, Glass L, Hausdorff JM, Ivanov PC, Mark RG, et al. PhysioBank, PhysioToolkit, and PhysioNet: components of a new research resource for complex physiologic signals. *Circulation.* (2000) 101:E215–20. doi: 10.1161/01.CIR.101.23.e215
10. Johnson AE, Pollard TJ, Shen L, Lehman LW, Feng M, Ghassemi M, et al. MIMIC-III, a freely accessible critical care database. *Sci Data.* (2016) 3:160035. doi: 10.1038/sdata.2016.35
11. Shimazui T, Nakada TA, Walley KR, Oshima T, Abe T, Ogura H, et al. Significance of body temperature in elderly patients with sepsis. *Crit Care.* (2020) 24:387. doi: 10.1186/s13054-020-02976-6
12. Levin A, Stevens PE, Bilous RW, Coresh J, Winearls CG. Kidney disease: Improving global outcomes (KDIGO) CKD work group. KDIGO 2012 clinical practice guideline for the evaluation and management of chronic kidney disease. *Kidney Int.* (2013) Supplements 3:1–150. doi: 10.1038/kisup.2012.73
13. McCaffrey DF, Griffin BA, Almirall D, Slaughter ME, Ramchand R, Burgette LF. A tutorial on propensity score estimation for multiple treatments using generalized boosted models. *Stat Med.* (2013) 32:3388–414. doi: 10.1002/sim.5753
14. Yoshida K, Bohn J and Yoshida MK. *Package 'tableone'.* Vienna: R Foundation for Statistical Computing (2019).
15. Ginestet C. ggplot2. Elegant graphics for data analysis. *J R Stat Soc.* (2011) 174:245–6. doi: 10.1111/j.1467-985X.2010.00676_9.x
16. Therneau T. A package for survival analysis. *Package R.* (2012) 2:37–2.

17. Kassambara A, Kosinski M, Biecek P. *Survminer. Drawing Survival Curves using 'ggplot2'.* (2016).
18. Grolemund G, Wickham H. Dates and times made easy with lubridate. *J StatSoftw.* (2011) 40:1–25. doi: 10.18637/jss.v040.i03
19. Wickham H, Averick M, Bryan J, Chang W, Yutani H. Welcome to the tidyverse. *J Open Source Softw.* (2019) 4:1686. doi: 10.21105/joss.01686
20. Erkens R, Wernly B, Masyuk M, Muessig JM, Franz M, Schulze PC, et al. Admission body temperature in critically ill patients as an independent risk predictor for overall outcome. *Med Princ Pract.* (2020) 29:389–95. doi: 10.1159/000505126
21. Martini WZ. The effects of hypothermia on fibrinogen metabolism and coagulation function in swine. *Metabolism.* (2007) 56:214–21. doi: 10.1016/j.metabol.2006.09.015
22. Leisman DE, Doerfler ME, Schneider SM, Masick KD, D'Amore JA, D'Angelo JK. Predictors, prevalence, and outcomes of early crystalloid responsiveness among initially hypotensive patients with sepsis and septic shock. *Crit Care Med.* (2018) 46:189–98. doi: 10.1097/CCM.0000000000002834
23. Drewry AM, Fuller BM, Skrupky LP, Hotchkiss RS. The presence of hypothermia within 24 hours of sepsis diagnosis predicts persistent lymphopenia. *Crit Care Med.* (2015) 43:1165–9. doi: 10.1097/CCM.0000000000000940
24. Kim J, Oh TK, Lee J, Kim S, Song IA. Association of immediate postoperative temperature in the surgical intensive care unit with 1-year mortality: retrospective analysis using digital axillary thermometers. *Acute Crit Care.* (2019) 34:53–9. doi: 10.4266/acc.2019.00255
25. Kawashima C, Matsuzawa Y, Akiyama E, Konishi M, Suzuki H, Hashiba K, et al. Prolonged fever after st-segment elevation myocardial infarction and long-term cardiac outcomes. *J Am Heart Assoc.* (2017) 6:e005463. doi: 10.1161/JAHA.116.005463
26. Launey Y, Nesseler N, Malledant Y, Seguin P. Clinical review: fever in septic ICU patients–friend or foe? *Crit Care.* (2011) 15:222. doi: 10.1186/cc10097
27. Annane D. Body temperature in sepsis: a hot topic. *Lancet Respir Med.* (2018) 6:162–3. doi: 10.1016/S2213-2600(18)30003-1
28. Evans SS, Repasky EA, Fisher DT. Fever and the thermal regulation of immunity: the immune system feels the heat. *Nat Rev Immunol.* (2015) 15:335–49. doi: 10.1038/nri3843
29. Sessler DI. Temperature monitoring and perioperative thermoregulation. *Anesthesiology.* (2008) 109:318–38. doi: 10.1097/ALN.0b013e31817f6d76
30. Squiccimarro E, Labriola C, Malvindi PG, Margari V, Guida P, Visicchio G, et al. Prevalence and clinical impact of systemic inflammatory reaction after cardiac surgery. *J Cardiothorac Vasc Anesth.* (2019) 33:1682–90. doi: 10.1053/j.jvca.2019.01.043
31. Zakkar M, Guida G, Suleiman MS, Angelini GD. Cardiopulmonary bypass and oxidative stress. *Oxid Med Cell Longev.* (2015) 2015:189863. doi: 10.1155/2015/189863
32. Rumbus Z, Matics R, Hegyi P, Zsiboras C, Szabo I, Illes A, et al. Fever is associated with reduced, hypothermia with increased mortality in septic patients: a meta-analysis of clinical trials. *PLoONE.* (2017) 12:e0170152. doi: 10.1371/journal.pone.0170152

24

# 1-Year Outcomes of a Multicenter Randomized Controlled Trial of the Ankura II Thoracic Endoprosthesis for the Endovascular Treatment of Stanford Type B Aortic Dissections

*Chang Shu[1,2*†], Hao He[1†], Weiguo Fu[3], Wei Guo[4], Ming Li[1,5], Erping Xi[6], Shuguang Guo[7], Xueming Chen[8], Zhanxiang Xiao[9], Shiqiang Yu[10], Jianhua Huang[11], Xiangchen Dai[12], Zhiwei Wang[13], Wei Li[14], Qingshan Zheng[15], Quanming Li[1], Lunchang Wang[1], Xin Li[1], Junwei Wang[1] and Feng Gu[1]*

*[1] Department of Vascular Surgery, Second Xiangya Hospital, Central South University, Changsha, China, [2] Department of Vascular Surgery, Fuwai Hospital, Chinese Academy of Medical Science & Peking Union Medical College, Beijing, China, [3] Department of Vascular Surgery, Institute of Vascular Surgery, Zhongshan Hospital, Fudan University, Shanghai, China, [4] Department of Vascular and Endovascular Surgery, Chinese PLA General Hospital, Beijing, China, [5] Department of Vascular Surgery, The First Affiliated Hospital of Medical School of Zhejiang University, Hangzhou, China, [6] Department of Vascular Surgery, Wuhan General Hospital of Guangzhou Military Region, Wuhan, China, [7] Department of Vascular Surgery, Kunming General Hospital of Chengdu Military Region, Kunming, China, [8] Department of Vascular Surgery, Beijing Friendship Hospital, Capital Medical University, Beijing, China, [9] Department of Vascular Surgery, Hainan Provincial People's Hospital, Haikou, China, [10] Department of Vascular Surgery, The First Affiliated Hospital of the Fourth Military Medical University, Xi'an, China, [11] Department of Vascular Surgery, Xiangya Hospital, Central South University, Changsha, China, [12] Department of Vascular Surgery, General Hospital of Tianjin Medical University, Tianjin, China, [13] Department of Vascular Surgery, Wuhan University People's Hospital, Wuhan, China, [14] Medical Research and Statistics Center, Fuwai Hospital, Chinese Academy of Medical Sciences, Beijing, China, [15] Drug Clinical Research Center, Shanghai University of Traditional Chinese Medicine, Shanghai, China*

***Correspondence:**
*Chang Shu*
*shuchang@csu.edu.cn*

*†These authors have contributed equally to this work*

**Background:** The Ankura II Thoracic Stent Graft System (Lifetech, Shenzhen, China) is an evolution of the Ankura stent graft. This study reports one-year outcomes of the Ankura II Thoracic Stent Graft System for endovascular treatment of Stanford type B aortic dissections.

**Methods:** The Ankura II Thoracic Aortic Endovascular Trial was a randomized, single-blinded, clinical trial conducted at 12 Chinese institutes. The enrolled patients diagnosed with Stanford type B aortic dissections (TBADs) were randomly assigned to the Ankura group or Ankura II group. Standard follow-up examinations were performed at 1, 6, and 12 months. Safety and efficacy data were analyzed.

**Results:** 132 patients with TBADs were enrolled. The outcomes for the primary safety end points revealed that the Ankura II stent graft was statistically non-inferior compared to the Ankura stent graft. The 1-month device-related major adverse events (1.6 vs. 0%; $p = 0.48$), 1-month all-cause mortality (1.7 vs. 4.5%; $p = 0.621$), 12-month survival rate (95.2 ± 2.7% vs. 94.1 ± 2.9%; $p = 0.769$), and major adverse event (MAE) rate (5.1 vs. 4.7% at 1 month; $p = 0.73$ and 5.8 vs. 8.9% at 12 months; $p = 0.718$) of Ankura II group are all comparable to Ankura group. The two groups showed similar primary effectiveness and true lumen expansion effect, and false lumen remodeling was improved in Ankura II group (−100.0 vs. −48.5%; $p = 0.08$).

**Conclusions:** The one-year outcomes from this prospective, randomized, multicenter study demonstrate that Ankura II stent graft shows comparable results to Ankura for treating TBADs, resulting in low mortality rates, MAEs and reintervention rates.

**Clinical Trial Registration:** ChiCTR-TRC-12002844.

**Keywords: Ankura II, RCT, thoracic endovascular aortic repair, type B aortic dissection, stent – evolution**

## INTRODUCTION

The thoracic endovascular aortic repair (TEVAR) has been well-studied and demonstrated it can improve the early treatment outcomes of thoracic lesions compared to conventional best medical therapy (BMT) and open surgery (1, 2). The several pioneering thoracic stent graft clinical trials established TEVAR combined with BMT as a safe and effective strategy for treating Stanford type B aortic dissection (TBADs), especially for high risk and complicated patients (3–5). Recently, TEVAR was extended to manage stable uncomplicated type B dissection due to the potential role of remodeling dissected aorta and preventing late expansion and malperfusion (6, 7). The booming of TEVAR really changes the treatment therapy of thoracic lesions.

However, the current commercialized stent graft design still faces some anatomic challenge, since the diameter of thoracic aorta is decreasing from proximal end to distal end (8). The size mismatch between the distal end of the stent graft and the remarkably small diameter of a compressed distal true lumen (TL) may contribute to the distal endoleak or stent graft-induced new entry (SINE) (9, 10). Moreover, the relative short stent can cause incomplete false lumen (FL) thrombosis of the aorta, thus affecting vessel remodeling (11). Recent studies have shown that the degree of FL thrombosis and aortic remodeling are associated with better long-term outcomes of TEVAR (12, 13).

Given the challenge as we mentioned above, the Ankura II Thoracic Stent Graft System (Lifetech, Shenzhen, China), an evolution of the Ankura stent graft, is designed. Compared to first generation product, The Ankura II stent graft is available in straight or tapered configurations. And the new shape provides flexibility and conformability in the stent graft, exerting radial force to enhance seal and fixation. The old system has already showed early evidence of a safe, effective, and durable endoprosthesis for the treatment of descending aortic aneurysms (14). Yet no study has been done for the Ankura II system. Since the new system has many theoretical advantages and available to more patients, we conduct this non-inferiority study. Our goal is to present characteristics and early outcomes of this novel endovascular stent graft, Ankura II Thoracic Stent Graft System, for the treatment of TBADs. Our early data from multicenter in China reveals the safety and efficacy of the Ankura II stent graft in the treatment of TBADs and better aortic remodeling compared to Ankura stent graft.

## MATERIALS AND METHODS

### Enrollment

The Ankura II Thoracic Aortic Endovascular Trial was a prospective, randomized, multicenter study designed to evaluate the safety and efficacy of the Ankura II Graft System for the treatment of thoracic lesion (Clinical trial registration number: ChiCTR-TRC-12002844). The study was approved by the Institutional Review Board of each participating institution. All participates were well-informed the potential benefit and risk and signed the consent. The trial enrolled 134 patients (two patients withdrew consent before surgery) with TBADs and 10 patients with aortic aneurysm from 12 institutions in China between November 2012 and December 2016. Since the sample size of aneurysmal patients was too small, only patients with TBADs were analyzed in this article to ensure homogeneous results. Data from aneurysmal patients can be provided to readers with reasonable require. The block randomization method was adopted, with a block size of four. The random envelopes were used. Patients were randomly assigned to the Ankura II group or Ankura group in a 1:1 ratio. The anatomic and medical inclusion and exclusion criteria were described in **Table 1**. All the anatomic enrollment criteria were assessed by independent clinical research associates and attending physicians together.

**TABLE 1** | Anatomic and medical inclusion and exclusion criteria.

| |
|---|
| ***Inclusion criteria*** |
| Age ≥18-years-old; |
| Diagnosed with Stanford type B aortic dissection, landing zone ≥20 mm distance to the left subclavian artery (or the landing zone ≥20 mm distance to the left common cervical artery and the left vertebral artery is non-superior); |
| Patent femoral and iliac arteries or can tolerate a vascular conduit allowing endovascular access to dissection area via a delivery system; |
| • Life expectancy ≥1 year. |
| ***Exclusion criteria*** |
| Pregnant or breastfeeding women; |
| Medical history of aortic surgery (open or endovascular); |
| History of cardiac or cerebral infarction within 3 months; |
| Diagnosed with connective tissue disease or active systemic infection; |
| Severe coagulation dysfunction; |
| Potential genetic deficiencies and congenital diseases; |
| Trauma patients or patients using illicit drugs. |

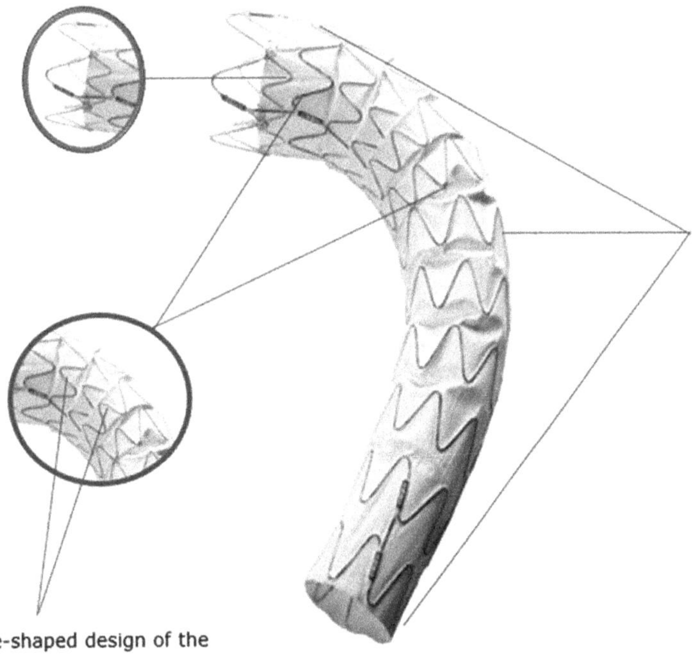


**FIGURE 1** | Overall observation of the Ankura II stent graft.

## Device Description

The Ankura II Thoracic Stent Graft System is a modular device comprising of a self-expanding metal stent dual-layer hot oxygen fusion polytetrafluoroethylene membrane with a bare proximal stent and covered distal stent. Based on the original Ankura stent graft, Ankura II includes some new improvements as shown in **Figure 1**. No suture was found on the main body to avoid pinhole leakage, thus providing better biocompatibility and durability. The sinusoidal shape and placement of the self-expanding nitinol springs also provide flexibility and conformability in the stent graft, exerting radial force to enhance seal and fixation. The Ankura II stent graft is available in straight or tapered configurations (6-mm, 8-mm or 10-mm taper) and is offered in diameters ranging from 24 to 42 mm and covered lengths ranging from 60 to 200 mm. The detailed deployment process is described in the **Supplementary data**. The consistency of treatment was tested after the deployment process.

## End Points and Definitions

The primary safety end point was device-related major adverse events (MAEs) rate at 1 month, which includes stent could not open successfully; stent thrombosis, migration, collapse, and fracture, accidental blockage of other branches of blood vessels, and stent-related endoleaks.

The secondary safety end points were all-cause mortality rates and MAEs rates at 1, 6, and 12 months after surgery. The definitions of MAEs were as follows: cardiovascular events [heart failure, myocardial infarction, cardiac tamponade, retrograde type A aortic dissection (RTAD), rupture of dissection and ischemia of left subclavian artery (LSA)], neurological events (stroke, paraplegia, and coma), acute kidney failure, respiratory failure needs non-invasive or invasive respiratory support, and death. The primary effectiveness end points were clinically successful treatments, which were defined as the absence of any type I or type III endoleaks. The FL thrombosis rates and diameter and area changes in the FL and TL were also compared at 1, 6, and 12 months after surgery.

Endoleaks were defined according to the well-established type I to IV nomenclature (15). Migration was defined as >10 mm proximal or distal movement of the stent graft relative to fixed anatomic landmarks.

## Data Management and Statistical Analysis

The standard follow-up protocol for the study included physical examination and computed tomography angiography (CTA) at 1, 6, and 12 months after surgery. We reported our data based on either intention-to-treat analysis (ITT) or per-protocol (PP) analysis. Due to the missing data, we cannot perform full set ITT analysis. For those who had missing category data, we consider the data from previous time follow-up as this time follow-up.

All data analysis and reports of aortic dissection followed the Society for Vascular Surgery and Society of Thoracic Surgeons' reporting standards (3). All imaging studies were performed at the participating sites and reviewed by the core laboratory, which was in second Xiangya hospital, Changsha, Hunan, China. To assess the change and remodeling of the aortic lumen

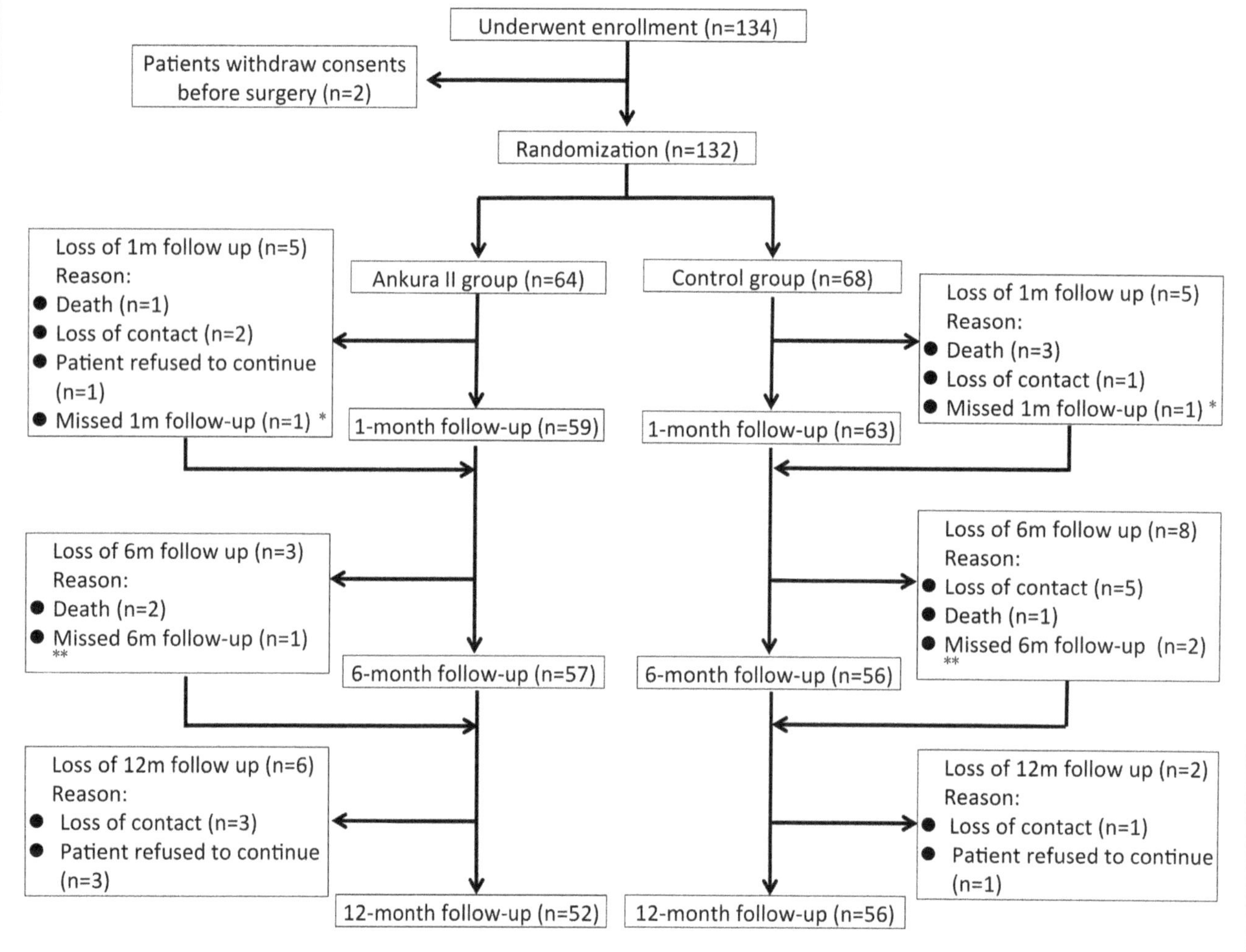


**FIGURE 2 |** Illustration of the study cohort and the follow-up process. *Ankura II group Patient No. 11 and Ankura group Patient No. 129 missed the 1-month follow-up but finished the 6- and 12-month follow-ups. **Ankura II group Patient No. 117 and Ankura group Patient No. 50 and No. 120 missed the 6-month follow-up but finished the 12-month follow-up.

during follow-up, three different representative aortic planes were selected. Plane 1 was the aorta plane with the maximal diameter. Plane 2 was the aorta plane where the TL was most constricted by the FL. Plane 3 was the aorta plane of the distal end of the stent.

All deaths and MAEs were reported by the participating site and adjudicated by the clinical events committee to determine whether they were secondary to failure of the device, related to the procedure, or both.

The normally distributed continuous variables were expressed as mean ± standard deviation and other continuous variables were presented as median (interquartile range). Categorical variables were expressed as proportions (percentage). The two-sided Student's *t*-test and Mann-Whitney *U* test are used to compare continuous variables. And Chi-square test or Fisher's exact probabilities were used to compare category variables. The cumulative survival estimates were generated by using the Kaplan-Meier non-parametric method and compared using the log-rank test. The primary safety end point, the device-related MAEs rates at 1 month, was submitted to a non-inferiority comparison with a null hypothesis that $Rate_{AnkuraII}$-$Rate_{Ankura}$ $\leq$-.1. (The rate refers the risk of the MAEs)

The sample size calculation was based on power analysis. According to a previous report, the incidence of device-related MAEs was.05 in the control group at the 1-month follow-up (16–18). Based on statistical requirements (unilateral $\alpha$ =0.05, $\beta$ = 0.20, non-inferiority margin $\delta$ = 0.1), 118 cases were required after calculation. Considering that the 1-month follow-up rate should not be lower than 90%, the total sample size required was 130 cases. In the trial, 132 dissecting patients were enrolled to ensure statistical power.

## RESULTS

### Follow-Up Process and Results

134 patients with TBADs were enrolled in the study, two of which withdrew consent before surgery. The study cohort and follow-up process are described in **Figure 2**. A total of 108 (81.8%) patients

**TABLE 2** | Demographics of the enrolled subjects.

| | Ankura II %(n/N) | Ankura %(n/N) | *P*-value |
|---|---|---|---|
| Age (year) | 56.4 ± 10.5 | 55.8 ± 11.7 | 0.85 |
| Height (cm) | 167.0 ± 8.2 | 166.9 ± 7.4 | 0.79 |
| Weight (kg) | 68.7 ± 12.3 | 66.8 ± 11.4 | 0.22 |
| Male | 81.3% (52/64) | 83.8% (57/68) | 0.70 |
| Smoking | 42.2% (27/64) | 44.1% (30/68) | 0.82 |
| Cardiovascular history | 65.6% (42/64) | 64.7% (44/68) | 0.91 |
| Hypertension | 64.1% (41/64) | 61.8% (42/68) | 0.78 |
| Coronary artery disease | 1.6% (1/64) | 2.9% (2/68) | 0.96 |
| PCI | 1.6% (1/64) | 1.5% (1/68) | 0.50 |
| Medical treatment | 65.6% (42/64) | 64.7% (44/68) | 0.91 |
| Cerebral infarction History | 3.1% (2/64) | 1.5% (1/68) | 0.96 |
| Diabetes | 6.3% (4/64) | 4.4% (3/68) | 0.93 |
| COPD | 1.6% (1/64) | 0% (0/68) | 0.48 |
| Chronic renal failure | 0% (0/64) | 0% (0/68) | |
| Back pain | 67.2% (43/64) | 73.5% (50/68) | 0.70 |
| Chest pain | 15.6% (10/64) | 8.8% (6/68) | 0.23 |
| Abdominal pain | 28.1% (18/64) | 22.1% (15/68) | 0.69 |
| Asymptomatic | 7.8% (5/64) | 8.8% (6/68) | 0.83 |
| **High-rsik TBADs** | | | |
| Aorta diameter >40 or false lumen diameter >22 mm | 79.7% (51/64) | 66.2% (45/68) | 0.08 |
| Refractory pain | 76.6% (49/64) | 70.6% (48/68) | 0.44 |
| **Complicated TBADs** | | | |
| Ischemia of branch arteries | 9.4% (6/64) | 11.8% (8/68) | 0.66 |
| HR with medicine (bpm) | 74.2 ± 10.5 | 74.5 ± 11.5 | 0.88 |
| BP with medicine (mmHg) | 127.0 ± 19.2/78.2 ± 12.0 | 126.4 ± 16.1/74.5 ± 9.4 | 0.85/0.050 |

*Bpm, beats per minute; BP, blood pressure, systolic/diastolic; COPD, Chronic obstructive pulmonary disease; HR, heart rate; PCI, Percutaneous coronary intervention; TBAD, Stanford type B aortic dissection.*

completed the 12-month follow-up, 7 patients (5.2%) died during the follow-up, and 17 (12.9%) patients were lost to follow-up. Of the patients who were lost to follow-up, 12 were unfortunately lost to contact, and five patients refused to continue in the study. Overall, 132 patients were included in ITT analysis and 108 patients were included in PP analysis.

## Demographics of the Enrolled Subjects

The demographics and risk factors showed no significant differences between the Ankura II and Ankura group (**Table 2**). Based on the definition of high-risk and complicated TBADs from Society for Vascular Surgery in 2020, we clarified the type of TBADs in both group by the data we had. The high risk of TABDs is defined as having an aorta diameter >40 mm or false lumen diameter >22 mm. The complicated TABDs is defined as existing ischemia of branch arteries. 66.2% of patients in Ankura group are high risk patients and 79.7% of patients in Ankura II group are high risk patients ($p = 0.120$). 11.8% of patients in Ankura group are complicated patients and 9.4% of patients in Ankura II group are complicated TABDs patients ($p = 0.656$). Besides, the rates of persistence of pain despite adequate blood pressure control and pain medications was 77.4% in Ankura group vs. 83.1% in Ankura II group ($p = 0.499$).

## Baseline Anatomical Features of Aortic Lesions

Comparable baseline anatomical features, including important anatomical factors such as ischemia of branch arteries, primary entry tear site, landing zone situation, and TL and FL diameter, were found between the Ankura II and Ankura group, Detailed information is listed in the **Supplementary data** and **Supplementary Table 1**.

## Surgical Procedures

The detailed results of the surgical procedures, including the deployment of stents, anesthesia methods, total surgery time, time for stent deployment, contrast agent volume and digital subtraction angiography (DSA) time, are described and compared (**Supplementary data** and **Supplementary Table 2**). No significant difference was found between the two groups.

## Device-Related Major Adverse Events, Mortality, and MAEs

Migration, collapse, fracture, or thrombosis of the stent was not found in either group during the 12-month follow-up, only one stent-related endoleaks (Type IV) occurred in the Ankura II group (**Table 3**). The incidence of 1-month device-related MAEs was 1.6% in the Ankura II group and 0% in the Ankura group.

**TABLE 3 |** Device-related major adverse events, mortality, and major adverse events.

| | 1 month (ITT analysis) | | | 12 months (PP analysis) | | |
|---|---|---|---|---|---|---|
| | **Ankura II (n/N)** | **Ankura (n/N)** | ***P*-value** | **Ankura II (n/N)** | **Ankura (n/N)** | ***P*-value** |
| Device-related MAEs | 1.6% (1/64) | 0% (0/68) | 0.48 | - | - | - |
| Stent migration | 0% (0/64) | 0% (0/68) | - | 0% (0/52) | 0% (0/56) | - |
| Stent collapse | 0% (0/64) | 0% (0/68) | - | 0% (0/52) | 0% (0/56) | - |
| Stent fracture | 0% (0/64) | 0% (0/68) | - | 0% (0/52) | 0% (0/56) | - |
| Stent thrombosis | 0% (0/64) | 0% (0/68) | - | 0% (0/52) | 0% (0/56) | - |
| Stent-related endoleaks (IV) | 1.6% (1/64) | 0% (0/68) | .48 | 1.9% (1/52) | 0% (0/56) | 0.48 |
| Device-related re-intervention | 0% (0/64) | 0% (0/68) | - | 0% (0/52) | 0% (0/56) | - |
| 1-month all-cause mortality | 1.6% (1/64) | 4.4% (3/68) | 0.66 | - | - | - |
| 12-month survival | - | - | - | 95.2 ± 2.7% | 94.1 ± 2.9% | 0.77[a] |
| Major adverse events | 5.1% (3/64) | 4.7% (3/68) | .73 | 5.8% (3/52) | 8.9% (5/56) | 0.72 |
| **Cardiovascular events** | | | | | | |
| Heart failure | 1.6% (1/64) | 0% (0/68) | 0.48 | 1.9% (1/52) | 0% (0/56) | 0.48 |
| Cardiac tamponade | 0% (0/64) | 1.5% (1/68) | >0.99 | 0% (0/52) | 1.8% (1/56) | >0.99 |
| RTAD | 0% (0/64) | 1.5% (1/68) | >0.99 | 0% (0/52) | 1.8% (1/56) | >0.99 |
| Rupture of dissection | 0% (0/64) | 1.5% (1/68) | >0.99 | 0% (0/52) | 1.8% (1/56) | >0.99 |
| Ischemia of LSA | 0% (0/64) | 1.5% (1/68) | >0.99 | 0% (0/52) | 1.8% (1/56) | >0.99 |
| **Neurological events** | | | | | | |
| Stroke | 1.6% (1/64) | 0% (0/68) | 0.48 | 1.9% (1/52) | 3.6% (2/56) | >0.99 |
| Paraplegia | 1.6% (1/64) | 0% (0/68) | 0.48 | 1.9% (1/52) | 0% (0/56) | 0.48 |
| Coma | 1.6% (1/64) | 0% (0/68) | 0.48 | 1.9% (1/52) | 0% (0/56) | 0.48 |
| Acute kidney injury | 0% (0/64) | 0% (0/68) | - | 0% (0/52) | 0% (0/56) | - |
| Respiratory failure | 1.6% (1/64) | 0% (0/68) | 0.48 | 1.9% (1/52) | 0% (0/56) | 0.48 |
| Endoleaks | | | | | | |
| Endoleaks I | 3.1% (2/64) | 0% (0/68) | 0.23 | 1.9% (1/52) | 1.8% (1/56) | >0.99 |
| Endoleaks II | 1.6% (1/64) | 0% (0/68) | 0.48 | 0% (0/52) | 0% (0/56) | - |
| Endoleaks III | 0% (0/64) | 0% (0/68) | - | 0% (0/52) | 0% (0/56) | - |
| Re-intervention rates | 1.6% (1/64) | 0% (0/68) | 0.48 | 7.7% (4/52) | 7.1% (4/56) | >0.99 |

*LSA, left subclavian artery; MAE, major adverse events; RTAD, retrograde type A aortic dissection. [a]Log-rank test; ITT analysis, intention to treat analysis; PP analysis, per-protocol analysis.*

And the lower limit of the unilateral 95% CI between the Ankura II and Ankura group was -.055. According to the non-inferiority standard of -.1, the Ankura II stent system was non-inferior to the Ankura stent. No reintervention was required for device related MAEs in either group during the follow-up.

The 1-month all-cause mortality rate for the Ankura II group was 1.6% (1/64), that for the Ankura group was 4.4% (3/68). Considering the loss of follow-up, the 12-month cumulative survival (Ankura II 95.2 ± 2.7% vs. Ankura 94.1 ± 2.9%; $p = 0.769$) was compared instead of the mortality rate. No significant difference was found between the two groups (**Table 3**). The Kaplan-Meier survival analysis with the exact time of death for Ankura II and Ankura patients is presented in **Figure 3**.

One patient in the Ankura II group exhibited paraplegia immediately after surgery and stroke after 5 days. Considering the poor prognosis, his family discontinued all treatment, and the patient unfortunately died. And there were three patients in the Ankura group who died within 1 month. One patient died 1 day after surgery with acute shock possibly due to rupture. Another patient died of acute pericardial tamponade, and RTAD 2 days after surgery. The third patient suddenly died at home 17 days after surgery with unknown cause.

Within 12-month follow-up, there were another two deaths in the Ankura II group. One patient died of multiple organ failure 50 days after surgery, and another died suddenly at home 168 days after surgery with unknown cause. In the Ankura group, one patient suddenly died at home of an unknown cause 65 days after surgery.

The distribution of MAEs at 1 month (ITT analysis, Ankura II: 4.7% (3/64): Ankura: 4.4% (3/68), $p = 0.73$) and 12 months (PP analysis, Ankura II: 5.8% (3/52): Ankura: 8.9% (5/56), $p = 0.718$) is shown in **Table 3**. In the Ankura II group, the cardiovascular events included a 1.6% (1/64) heart failure rate with respiratory failure within 1 month. In the Ankura group, the cardiovascular events included the rupture of dissection (1.5%), ischemia of the LSA (1.5%) and RTAD with cardiac tamponade (1.5%) occurring within 1 month. Neurologic events in the Ankura II group included paraplegia complicated with a later stroke (1.5%) and transient coma (1.5%) within 1 month. In the Ankura group, two stroke events occurred within the 12-month follow-up.

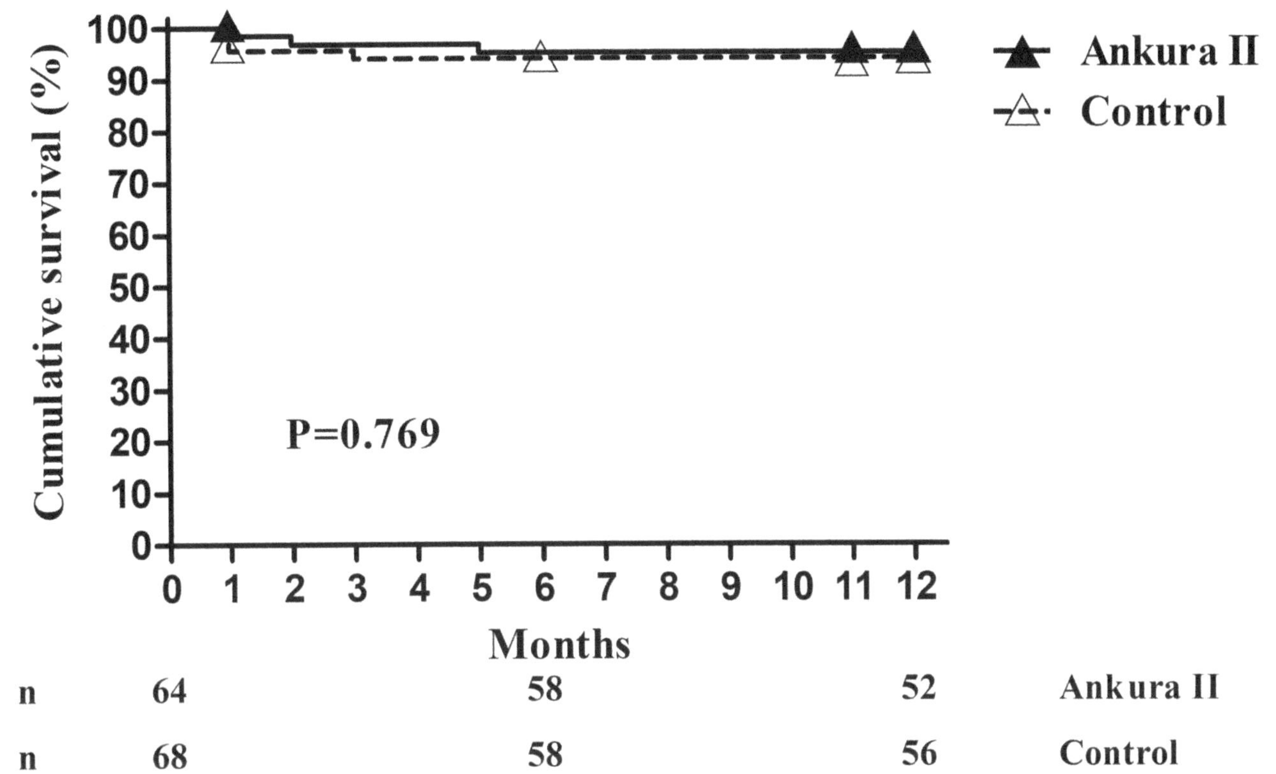


**FIGURE 3** | Kaplan-Meier survival analysis. The available number of patients between the Ankura II and Ankura groups was 64 and 68 at 0 months, 58 and 58 at 6 months, and 52 and 56 at 12 months, respectively.

The endoleaks rate was low for both groups. At 1 month, the type I endoleaks rate was 3.1% (2/64) in the Ankura II group and 0% in the Ankura group ($p$ = 0.232). At 12 months, the type I endoleaks rate was 1.9% (1/52) in the Ankura II group and 1.8% (1/56) in the Ankura group ($p$ = 1.000), medical treatment was continued. Additionally, one type II endoleaks occurred in the Ankura II group within 1 month but disappeared during the 12-month follow-up. No type III endoleaks occurred.

The reintervention rates for 1 month (1.6% vs. 0%: $p$=.48) and 12 months (7.7 vs. 7.1%: $p$ = 1.000) between the Ankura II and Ankura groups are also shown in **Table 3** and no dissection or aneurysm vascular-related intervention occurred in either group. Detailed reintervention events included one lumbar disc herniation, one renal cancer, one multiple organ failure and one adrenal adenoma in the Ankura II group and two strokes, one kidney stone and one lung cancer in the Ankura group.

## Stent Effectiveness and Remodeling of TL and FL in TBADs Patients

The 12-month follow-up was completed for 52 patients in Ankura II and 56 patients in Ankura group (**Table 4**). To evaluate the effectiveness of stents and compare the ability of stents to expand the TL and facilitate FL thrombosis in AD patients (51/52 and 55/56 patients in the Ankura II and Ankura group, respectively), the FL thrombosis rate was compared. Three different aorta planes were chosen, and the diameter and area of the TL and FL were measured before surgery and at the follow-up in dissection patients.

The two groups showed comparable clinical success rates- Ankura II: 51/52 (98.1%) vs. Ankura: 54/56 (96.4%), $p$ = 1.000. The complete thrombosis rate was significantly increased at 12 months compared with that at the 1-month follow-up in both groups. However, no significant difference in the thrombosis rate was found between the two groups.

The percentage change in the diameter and area 12 months after surgery was calculated before statistical analysis. In Plane 1 and Plane 2, the TL was expanded, and the FL diameter was decreased but without significant difference (**Table 4**). In Plane 3, Ankura II stents showed a possible advantage in facilitating thrombosis of the FL, with a decrease trend in diameter of −100.0% (−100.0 to −100.0%) (vs.−100.0% (−100.0% to −16.4%) for the Ankura; $p$ = 0.18) and a decrease trend in area of −100.0% (−100.0% to −67.5%) (vs. −48.5% (−100.0% to −3.6%) for the Ankura; $p$ = 0.08). The 12-month follow-up results demonstrated that the Ankura II and Ankura groups both performed well in expanding the TL and aortic remodeling was improved in patients treated with Ankura II.

## DISCUSSION

In the present trial, the Ankura II Thoracic Stent Graft System was safe and effective in treating TBADs. In terms of primary

**TABLE 4** | Effectiveness of Ankura II, remodeling of the aorta and percentage change in the TL and FL diameter and area in TBADs (PP analysis).

| | Ankura II (%) | Ankura (%) | *P*-value |
|---|---|---|---|
| Clinical successful treatment | 51/52 (98.1%) | 54/56 (96.4%) | >0.99 |
| **FL thrombosis rate** | | | |
| Partially, 1 month | 27 (45.8%) | 27 (43.5%) | 0.81 |
| Completely, 1 month | 32 (54.2%) | 35 (56.5%) | |
| Partially, 12 months | 20 (39.2%) | 15 (26.8%) | 0.15 |
| Completely, 12 months | 31 (60.8%) | 41 (73.2%) | |
| **12-month follow-up** | | | |
| **Plane 1** | | | |
| Diameter of TL | 36.4 (8.1–102.5) | 48.2 (23.4–111.0) | 0.18 |
| Diameter of FL | −100.0 (−100.0 to −100.0) | −100.0 (−100.0 to −99.8) | 0.76 |
| Area of TL | 153.7 ± 69.9 | 36.4 (8.1–102.5) | 0.23 |
| Area of FL | −100.0 (−100.0 to −100.0) | −100.0 (−100.0 to −100.0) | 0.17 |
| **Plane 2** | | | |
| Diameter of TL | 90.39 (8.6–332.3) | 89.9 (25.1–225.1) | 0.90 |
| Diameter of FL | −100.0 (−100.0 to −95.8) | −100.0 (−100.0–95.34) | 0.72 |
| Area of TL | 267.9 ± 79.1 | 170.2 ± 30.8 | 0.99 |
| Area of FL | −100.0 (−100.0 to −93.5) | −100.0 (−100.0 to −93.5) | 0.99 |
| **Plane 3** | | | |
| Diameter of TL | 56.8 (11.4–118.3) | 32.9 (1.4–121.0) | 00.35 |
| Diameter of FL | −100.0 (−100.0 to −100.0) | −100.0 (−100.0 to −16.4) | **0.18** |
| Area of TL | 128.7 ± 33.9 | 146.2 ± 49.8 | 0.82 |
| Area of FL | −100.0 (−100.0 to −67.5) | −48.5 (−100.0 to −3.6) | **0.08** |

*FL, false lumen; TL, true lumen. "-" stands for decrease in the diameter and area. PP analysis, per-protocol analysis. Plane 1 was the aorta plane with the maximal diameter. Plane 2 was the aorta plane where the TL was most constricted by the FL. Plane 3 was the aorta plane of the distal end of the stent.*

outcomes, no migration, collapse, fracture, or thrombosis of the stent occurred. Comparisons of the 1-month and 12-month MAEs showed no significant difference between Ankura and Ankura II. And comparison of 1-month and 12-month secondary outcomes further demonstrated that Ankura II had possible advantages in promoting FL thrombosis. Both groups had a low 1-month all-cause mortality rate (Ankura II 1.7 vs. Ankura 4.5%) and a high 12-month survival rate (Ankura II 94.2 ± 2.8 vs. Ankura 92.9 ± 3.1%) compared to other studies (7). Lower mortality rates are believed to result from multiple factors, including improvement in the stent design, good preoperative preparation and blood pressure control, and restricted inclusion criteria that excluded complicated cases.

Despite the benefits of TEVAR over conventional open repair, its adverse effects, reintervention rates and endoleaks events still raise concerns, particularly in situations with an unfavorable anatomy (9, 19). Notably results published by other centers suggest that the diameter mismatch between the stent and aortic lesions may be related to the occurrence of RTAD (10). In our trial, because of a smaller distal end diameter design compared to Ankura (27.7 ± 3.3 mm for Ankura II vs. 29.6 ± 3.1 mm for the Ankura; $p < 0.001$), the distal end of the stent in the Ankura II group complied better with the anatomy of the aorta. And follow-up results coincidentally showed that one RTAD and another dissection rupture occurred in the Ankura group. Furthermore, published results reveal that the rate of secondary intervention after elective TEVAR ranges from 0 to 32.3%, 1 month to 5 years, respectively (12, 20–22). Most were performed because of endoleaks or device-related complications. In our study, the reintervention rates for Ankura II group at 1 month is 1.7 and 7.7% after 12 months follow up.

Given the fact both endoleaks and reintervention rate are low in our study, we think it is most likely because of the improvements in the device design, thus resulting a better adherence between the graft and aorta, which also reminds surgeon to pay more attention to stent graft instructions when planning TEVAR to get a better adherence. But our follow up time is only 1 year, our data is far from sufficient to make any conclusions. the long-term reintervention rates and endoleaks are still required in following up and future studies are still warranted to prove the above conclusion.

Another interesting finding of current study is we found Ankura II stents could facilitate FL thrombosis better compared to the first-generation stent near the stent distal end area. As is all known, remodeling of the aorta after stent deployment, particularly FL thrombosis, is critical for stent stability and long-term outcomes (11). More importantly, the diameter of FL is negatively correlated with survival in patients undergoing endovascular therapy for chronic TBADs (12). Our trial showed the complete FL thrombosis rates at 12 months are 60.8 and 73.2% in the Ankura II and Ankura groups, respectively. Moreover, both groups had successful and satisfactory TL expansion rates and FL reducing rates. Ankura II stents also showed a possible advantage in facilitating FL thrombosis near the stent distal end area, with a decrease in the diameter (85.7 ± 4.4 vs. 66.9 ± 7.8%; $p = 0.048$) and a decrease in area (77.4 ±

7.9% (vs. 49.6 ± 10.1%). We speculate it is because of the tapered design of Ankura II and leading to better adhesion between the stent and aorta. And the availability of longer-length devices may also contribute to these more favorable outcomes (174.1 ± 19.2 mm for Ankura II vs. 165.6 ± 14.0 mm for the Ankura, $p = 0.003$). However, close postoperative surveillance by imaging with CTA or magnetic resonance angiography (MRA) remains extremely important for long-term results.

Several unavoidable limitations exist in this study. First, as a non-inferiority study, the non-inferiority margin (0.1) is a little wider compared to the incidence of MAEs (0.05), which makes the results underpower. Second, the follow up rate of current study is low (82.8% at 1 month) and thus have many missing data, making either ITT analysis or PP analysis have the type II or type I bias. And our total follow up time is limited (1 year), which is insufficient to make statistical conclusion. Finally, we haven't distinguished the complicated and uncomplicated TBAD during the patients recruiting process. Given the fact the complicated and uncomplicated TBAD behave differently in terms of MAE (23, 24), this is one major weakness of our study.

Overall, the 1-year outcomes from our prospective, randomized, multicenter study demonstrate that Ankura II shows comparable results to Ankura for treating TBADs and yields low mortality rates, MAEs and reintervention rates. Additionally, Ankura II shows a possible advantage in FL thrombosis. More data are warranted to evaluate the long-term effects of Ankura II and its performance in complicated cases.

## ETHICS STATEMENT

The studies involving human participants were reviewed and approved by Institutional Review Board of each participating institution. The patients/participants provided their written informed consent to participate in this study.

## AUTHOR CONTRIBUTIONS

CS and HH designed the study. HH, WF, WG, ML, EX, SG, XC, ZX, SY, JH, XD, ZW, WL, QZ, and FG collected the clinical data. HH, QL, LW, ML, XL, and JW analyzed and interpreted the data. HH and CS wrote the draft. CS, HH, WF, WG, ML, EX, SG, XC, ZX, SY, JH, XD, ZW, WL, QZ, QL, LW, ML, XL, JW, and FG edited the final version. CS guided all the process. All authors contributed to the article and approved the submitted version.

## REFERENCES


1. Shu C, He H, Li QM Li M, Jiang XH, Luo MY. Endovascular repair of complicated acute type-B aortic dissection with stentgraft: early and mid-term results. *Eur J Vasc Endovasc Surg.* (2011) 42:448–53. doi: 10.1016/j.ejvs.2011.05.013
2. Ehrlich MP, Dumfarth J, Schoder M, Gottardi R, Holfeld J, Juraszek A, et al. Midterm results after endovascular treatment of acute, complicated type B aortic dissection. *Ann Thorac Surg.* (2010) 90:1444–8. doi: 10.1016/j.athoracsur.2010.06.076
3. Lombardi JV, Hughes GC, Appoo JJ, Bavaria JE, Beck AW, Cambria RP, et al. Society for vascular surgery (SVS) and society of thoracic surgeons (STS) reporting standards for type B aortic dissections. *J Vasc Surg.* (2020) 71:723–47. doi: 10.1016/j.jvs.2019.11.013
4. Erbel R, Aboyans V, Boileau C, Bossone E, Bartolomeo RD, Eggebrecht H, et al. 2014 ESC Guidelines on the diagnosis and treatment of aortic diseases: document covering acute and chronic aortic diseases of the thoracic and abdominal aorta of the adult. The task force for the diagnosis and treatment of aortic diseases of the european society of cardiology (ESC). *Eur Heart J.* (2014) 35:2873–926. doi: 10.1093/eurheartj/ehu281
5. Tsai TT, Fattori R, Trimarchi S, Isselbacher E, Myrmel T, Evangelista A, et al. Long-term survival in patients presenting with type B acute aortic dissection: insights from the international registry of acute aortic dissection. *Circulation.* (2006) 114:2226–31. doi: 10.1161/CIRCULATIONAHA.106.622340
6. Stanley GA, Murphy EH, Knowles M, Ilves M, Jessen ME, Dimaio JM, et al. Volumetric analysis of type B aortic dissections treated with thoracic endovascular aortic repair. *J Vasc Surg.* (2011) 54:985–92. doi: 10.1016/j.jvs.2011.03.263
7. Nienaber CA, Kische S, Rousseau H, Eggebrecht H, Rehders TC, Kundt G, et al. Endovascular repair of type B aortic dissection: long-term results of the randomized investigation of stent grafts in aortic dissection trial. *Circ Cardiovasc Interv.* (2013) 6:407–16. doi: 10.1161/CIRCINTERVENTIONS.113.000463
8. Gu F, Randall EB, Whitesall S, Converso-Baran K, Carlson BE, Fink GD, et al. Potential role of intermittent functioning of baroreflexes in the etiology of hypertension in spontaneously hypertensive rats. *JCI Insight.* (2020) 5:139789. doi: 10.1172/jci.insight.139789
9. Luebke T, Brunkwall J. Outcome of patients with open and endovascular repair in acute complicated type B aortic dissection: a systematic review and meta-analysis of case series and comparative studies. *J Cardiovasc Surg (Torino).* (2010) 51:613–32.
10. Zhang S, Chen Y, Lu Q. Retrograde type A aortic dissection complicating endovascular therapy of type B aortic dissection and descending thoracic aneurysm disease. *Curr Opin Cardiol.* (2018) 33:581–6. doi: 10.1097/HCO.0000000000000567
11. Leshnower BG, Duwayri YM, Chen EP Li C, Zehner CA, Binongo JN, et al. Aortic remodeling after endovascular repair of complicated acute type B aortic dissection. *Ann Thorac Surg.* (2017) 103:1878–85. doi: 10.1016/j.athoracsur.2016.09.057
12. Mani K, Clough RE, Lyons OT, Bell RE, Carrell TW, Zayed HA, et al. Predictors of outcome after endovascular repair for chronic type B dissection. *Eur J Vasc Endovasc Surg.* (2012) 43:386–91. doi: 10.1016/j.ejvs.2012.01.016
13. Tolenaar JL, Kern JA, Jonker FH, Cherry KJ, Tracci MC, Angle JF, et al. Predictors of false lumen thrombosis in type B aortic dissection treated with TEVAR. *Ann Cardiothorac Surg.* (2014) 3:255–63. doi: 10.3978/j.issn.2225-319X.2014.05.17
14. Kratimenos T, Antonopoulos CN, Tomais D, Dedeilias P, Patris V, Samiotis I, et al. Repair of descending thoracic aortic aneurysms with Ankura Thoracic Stent Graft. *J Vasc Surg.* (2019) 69:996–1002. doi: 10.1016/j.jvs.2018.07.065
15. Fillinger MF, Greenberg RK, McKinsey JF, Chaikof EL, Society for vascular surgery *ad hoc* committee on TRS. Reporting standards for thoracic endovascular aortic repair (TEVAR). *J Vasc Surg.* (2010) 52:1022–33, 33. doi: 10.1016/j.jvs.2010.07.008
16. Li X, Li Q, Zhang W, Li M, He H, Luo M, et al. Early experience and technical aspects of physician-modified fenestration in thoracic endovascular aortic repair for aortic arch pathologies. *J Int Med Res.* (2020) 48:300060519870903. doi: 10.1177/0300060519870903
17. Wang T, Shu C, Li QM Li M, Li X, He H, et al. First experience with the double chimney technique in the treatment of aortic arch diseases. *J Vasc Surg.* (2017) 66:1018–27. doi: 10.1016/j.jvs.2017.02.035
18. Shu C, Fan B, Luo M, Li Q, Fang K, Li M, et al. Endovascular treatment for aortic arch pathologies: chimney, on-the-table fenestration, and *in-situ* fenestration techniques. *J Thorac Dis.* (2020) 12:1437–48. doi: 10.21037/jtd.2020.03.10
19. Desai ND, Burtch K, Moser W, Moeller P, Szeto WY, Pochettino A, et al. Long-term comparison of thoracic endovascular aortic repair (TEVAR) to open surgery for the treatment of thoracic aortic aneurysms. *J Thorac Cardiovasc*

*Surg.* (2012) 144:604–9. discussion 9–11. doi: 10.1016/j.jtcvs.2012.05.049

20. Yang KJ, Chi NH Yu HY, Chen YS, Wang SS, Wu IH. Outcome comparison between open and endovascular aortic repair for retrograde type a intramural hematoma with intimal tear in the descending thoracic aorta: a retrospective observational study. *Front Cardiovas Med.* (2021) 8:755214. doi: 10.3389/fcvm.2021.755214
21. Lee CJ, Rodriguez HE, Kibbe MR, Malaisrie SC, Eskandari MK. Secondary interventions after elective thoracic endovascular aortic repair for degenerative aneurysms. *J Vasc Surg.* (2013) 57:1269–74. doi: 10.1016/j.jvs.2012.10.124
22. Kamman AV, Jonker FH, Nauta FJ, Trimarchi S, Moll FL, van Herwaarden JA, et al. review of follow-up outcomes after elective endovascular repair of degenerative thoracic aortic aneurysms. *Vascular.* (2016) 24:208–16. doi: 10.1177/1708538115588648
23. Kamman AV, Yang B, Kim KM, Williams DM, Michael Deeb G, Patel HJ. Visceral malperfusion in aortic dissection: the michigan experience. *Semin Thorac Cardiovasc Surg.* (2017) 29:173–8. doi: 10.1053/j.semtcvs.2016.10.002
24. Criado FJ. Aortic dissection: a 250-year perspective. *Tex Heart Inst J.* (2011) 38:694–700.

# 25

# Comparative Evaluation of the Incidence of Postoperative Pulmonary Complications After Minimally Invasive Valve Surgery vs. Full Sternotomy

*Mohamed Abdulkadir Mohamed [1†], Shuai Ding [1†], Sayed Zulfiqar Ali Shah [2], Rui Li [2], Najib Isse Dirie [3], Cai Cheng [1*] and Xiang Wei [1*]*

*Division of Cardiothoracic and Vascular Surgery, Tongji Hospital, Tongji Medical College, Huazhong University of Science and Technology, Wuhan, China, [2] Department of Rehabilitation Medicine, Tongji Hospital, Tongji Medical College, Huazhong University of Science and Technology, Wuhan, China, [3] Division of Urology, Tongji Hospital, Tongji Medical College, Huazhong University of Science and Technology, Wuhan, China*

***Correspondence:**
*Cai Cheng*
*cai.cheng@hotmail.com*
*Xiang Wei*
*xiangwei@tjh.tjmu.edu.cn*

*† These authors have contributed equally to this work*

**Background:** Postoperative pulmonary complications remain a leading cause of increased morbidity, mortality, longer hospital stays, and increased costs after cardiac surgery; therefore, our study aims to analyze whether minimally invasive valve surgery (MIVS) for both aortic and mitral valves can improve pulmonary function and reduce the incidence of postoperative pulmonary complications when compared with the full median sternotomy (FS) approach.

**Methods:** A comprehensive systematic literature research was performed for studies comparing MIVS and FS up to February 2021. Randomized controlled trials (RCTs) and propensity score-matching (PSM) studies comparing early respiratory function and pulmonary complications after MIVS and FS were extracted and analyzed. Secondary outcomes included intra- and postoperative outcomes.

**Results:** A total of 10,194 patients from 30 studies (6 RCTs and 24 PSM studies) were analyzed. Early mortality differed significantly between the groups (MIVS 1.2 vs. FS 1.9%; $p = 0.005$). Compared with FS, MIVS significantly lowered the incidence of postoperative pulmonary complications (odds ratio 0.79, 95% confidence interval [0.67, 0.93]; $p = 0.004$) and improved early postoperative respiratory function status (mean difference $-24.83$ [$-29.90$, $-19.76$]; $p < 0.00001$). Blood transfusion amount was significantly lower after MIVS ($p < 0.02$), whereas cardiopulmonary bypass time and aortic cross-clamp time were significantly longer after MIVS ($p < 0.00001$).

**Conclusions:** Our study showed that minimally invasive valve surgery decreases the incidence of postoperative pulmonary complications and improves postoperative respiratory function status.

**Keywords: cardiac surgery, minimally invasive, valve repair/replacement, meta-analysis (as topic), full sternotomy**

## INTRODUCTION

Full median sternotomy (FS) has long been the standard incision for cardiac surgery due to it is excellent exposure of the heart and great vessels. However, to reduce the size of the sternotomy, cardiac surgeons have long pursued less extensive incisions to improve outcomes and thus have used minimally invasive approaches that have undergone rapid development in the last

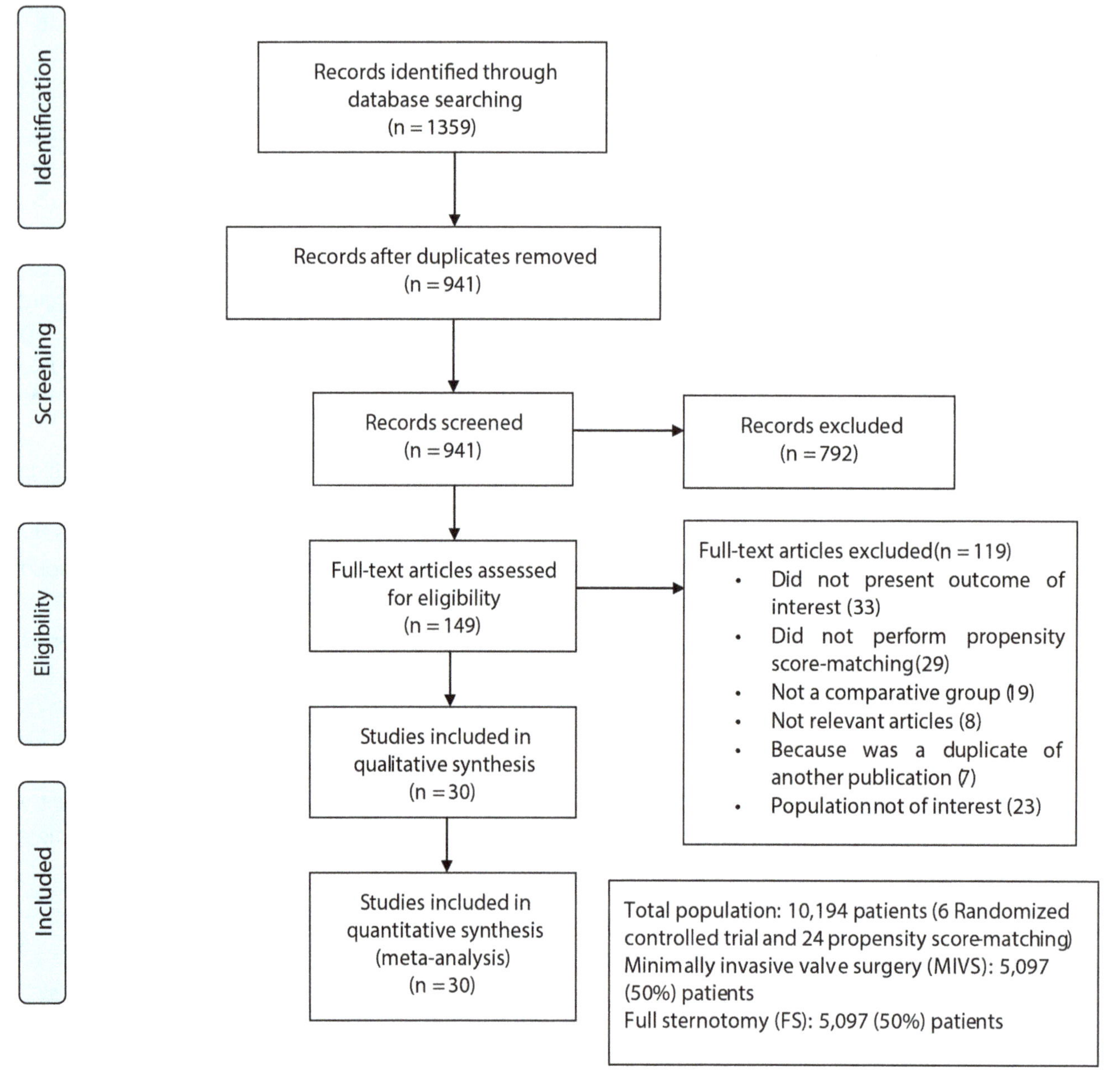


**FIGURE 1** | Flowchart for studies included in data search in accordance with PRISMA guidelines.

few decades (1–3). These approaches have multiple benefits over an FS because of a smaller surgical incision, reduced pain, earlier discharge, and quicker postoperative recovery (4, 5). On the other hand, some potential technical disadvantages tend to have prolonged cardiopulmonary bypass (CPB) and aortic cross-clamp time (6, 7).

Given such developments in surgical management and patients' treatment over the years, postoperative pulmonary complications remain a leading cause of mortality and morbidity following cardiac surgery (8, 9). These complications contribute to longer hospital stays and more readmissions into the ICU, significantly affecting health care and increasing healthcare systems' financial burden (8, 10). Atelectasis and pleural effusions, pneumonia, pneumothorax, diaphragm paralysis because of phrenic nerve damage, and pulmonary infection are the most common pulmonary complications (11).

Although considerable benefits were associated with the MIVS over FS, there is still ongoing debate about the advantage of MIVS on postoperative pulmonary complications (PPCs), and the associations remain unclear. To our knowledge, there is still limited evidence on PPCs and respiratory system function analysis of patients after MIVS compared with the FS approach has not been analyzed. Therefore, based on the existing clinical literature, we conducted this systematic review and meta-analysis of high-quality randomized controlled trials (RCTs) and propensity score-matched (PSM) studies to analyze the incidence of PPCs and respiratory function of patients who underwent a minimally invasive approach for mitral or aortic valve vs. FS.

**TABLE 1** | Characteristics of included studies.

| References | Country | Study interval | Study type | No. of patients MIVS/FS | Surgical approach | Quality assessment | LOE† | Median follow-up |
|---|---|---|---|---|---|---|---|---|
| Aris et al. (6) | Spain | NS | RCT | 20/20 | A φ | 3/5 | 2b | 6 days |
| Machler et al. (28) | Austria | 1996–1997 | RCT | 30/30 | A φ | 3/5 | 2b | 294 days$^{M}$ |
| Bonacchi et al. (14) | Italy | 1999–2001 | RCT | 40/40 | A φ | 4/5 | 1b | 9.7 ± 5.7 months$^{M}$ |
| Dogan et al. (16) | Germany | 2003–2004 | RCT | 20/20 | M § | 2/5 | 3b | NS |
| Moustafa et al. (5) | Egypt | NS | RCT | 30/30 | A φ | 2/5 | 3b | NS |
| Calderon et al. (15) | France | 2003–2007 | RCT | 39/39 | A φ | 5/5 | 2b | NS |
| Albacker et al. (12) | US | 1995–2010 | PSM | 223/223 | A § | 7 | 4 | 2 years |
| Masiello et al. (29) | Italy | 1997–1999 | PSM | 100/100 | A φ | 6 | 3b | 1 month |
| Farhat et al. (17) | France | 2000–2001 | PSM | 50/50 | A φ | 7 | 3b | 1 month |
| Tabata et al. (37) | US | 1996–2005 | PSM | 41/41 | A φ | 7 | 3b | NS |
| Iribarne et al. (25) | US | 2000–2008 | PSM | 382/382 | M § | 8 | 3b | 4.2 ± 2.4 yrs$^{M}$ |
| Holzhey et al. (24) | Germany | 1999–2009 | PSM | 143/143 | M § | 8 | 1b | 2.4 ± 2.1 yrs$^{M}$ |
| Bang et al. (13) | Korea | 1997–2010 | PSM | 73/73 | A ϕ | 7 | 3b | NS |
| Murzi et al. (31) | Italy | 2006–2010 | PSM | 100/100 | A θ | 6 | 2b | 3 years |
| Sansone et al. (32) | Italy | 2008–2010 | PSM | 50/50 | A θ | 7 | 3b | NS |
| Johnston et al. (26) | US | 1995–2004 | PSM | 832/832 | A φ | 8 | 3a | 6.5 ± 3.0 years$^{M}$ |
| Gilmanov et al. (20) | Italy | 2004–2011 | PSM | 182/182 | A θ | 7 | 3b | Until patient discharge |
| Hiraoka et al. (23) | Japan | 2007–2012 | PSM | 36/36 | A ϕ | 7 | 4 | NS |
| Ghanta et al. (19) | US | 2011–2013 | PSM | 289/289 | A ϕ | 6 | 4 | NS |
| Gilmanov et al. (21) | Italy | 2001–2013 | PSM | 100/100 | A θ | 8 | 3a | 33.7 months$^{M}$ |
| Merk et al. (30) | Germany | 2003–2012 | PSM | 477/477 | A φ | 6 | 3a | 3.1 ± 2.7 years$^{M}$ |
| Shehada et al. (34) | Germany | 2002–2012 | PSM | 585/585 | A φ | 7 | 3b | NS |
| Stoliński et al. (36) | Canada | 2010–2013 | PSM | 211/211 | A θ | 8 | 3b | NS |
| Gasparovic et al. (18) | Slovakia | 2010–2013 | PSM | 34/34 | A φ | 7 | 3a | 5 years |
| Levack et al. (27) | US | 1995–2014 | PSM | 483/483 | A φ | 8 | 3b | NS |
| Stolinski et al. (35) | Poland | 2011–2014 | PSM | 212/212 | A θ | 8 | 3a | 3 months |
| Seitz et al. (33) | Australia | 2013–2016 | PSM | 53/53 | A θ | 7 | 3b | NS |
| Hawkins et al. (22) | US | 2011–2016 | PSM | 74/74 | M § | 7 | 3b | NS |
| Wang et al. (38) | China | 2012–2015 | PSM | 67/67 | M § | 6 | 3a | 2.8 years |
| Zhao et al. (39) | China | 2013–2016 | PSM | 91/91 | C δ | 8 | 3a | 1 year |

*A, Aortic valve; C, indicated both mitral and aorta valve; FS, full sternotomy; LOE, level of evidence; MIVS, minimally invasive valve surgery; M, mitral valve; $^{M}$, mean; NS, not specified; PSM, propensity score-matching; RCT, randomized control trial; θ, indicates aortic valve surgery right mini-thoracotomy; φ, indicates aortic valve surgery upper mini-sternotomy; ϕ, indicated aortic valve surgery right mini-thoracotomy and upper mini-sternotomy; δ, indicated both mitral and aorta valve surgery right mini-thoracotomy; §, indicated mitral valve surgery right mini-thoracotomy; †Based on US Preventive Services Task Force grading system.*

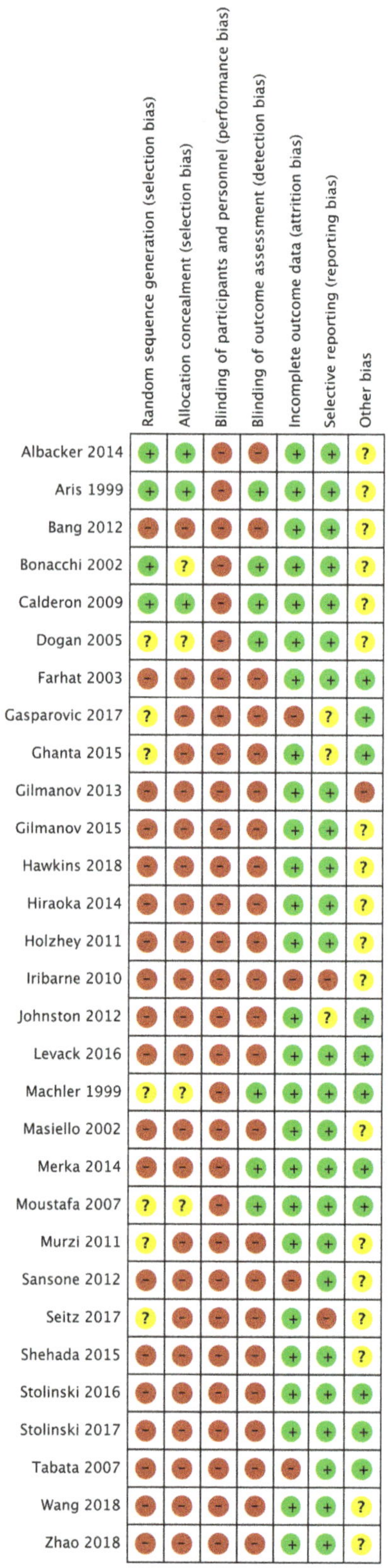


**FIGURE 2** | Risk of bias assessment summary.

# METHODS

## Selection Criteria

We included all articles reporting clinical outcomes for MIVS (repair or replacement of the mitral valve, aortic valve, or both valves) via right/lateral mini-thoracotomy or mini-sternotomy, with either a camera or direct visualization, vs. traditional FS. Studies were considered using a PICOS (Population, Intervention, Comparison, Outcome, and Study) strategy if (1) articles were published in English, (2) articles reported RCTs or PSM studies, (3) articles compared the outcomes of MIVS and FS for either mitral or aortic valve disease, and (4) outcomes included postoperative pulmonary complications and early postoperative respiratory function.

Articles without a full report available, review studies, studies with previous cardiac surgery and concomitant surgical procedures (coronary artery bypass grafting, and procedure involving ascending aortic) other than isolated mitral and aortic or both valve surgery were excluded and studies with no comparison group were also excluded.

## Information Sources

The following databases were used: PubMed, MEDLINE, Web of Science, Cochrane Central Register of Controlled Trials, Scopus, and Google Scholar. The reference lists of identified articles were also included in manual searches.

## Search Strategy

We searched articles and studies comparing FS vs. MIVS using the following medical subject headings: aortic valve, aortic valve surgery, mitral valve or mitral valve surgery, minimally/partial invasive, full/conventional/partial sternotomy or mini-sternotomy, anterolateral/right mini-thoracotomy, partial upper Hemi-sternotomy or upper mini-sternotomy.

## Study Selection

Search strategies, inclusion with exclusion criteria, statistical analysis, and outcomes were predefined. Thirty publications fulfilled our eligibility criteria (5, 6, 12–39). Two independent investigators (MA, SZ) reviewed all abstracts that fulfilled the search criteria. When there were differences of opinion between these investigators, other authors were included to resolve disagreements. **Figure 1** summarizes the search strategy.

## Data Extraction

Two reviewers independently extracted data from each included study and performed the quality assessment. Data extracted included the first author's name, year of publication, country, study interval, study type, the number of subjects who underwent MIVS or FS, and outcomes of interest. The following clinical outcomes of interest from each study were extracted to compare MIVS with FS: postoperative pulmonary complications (overall complications, pneumonia, pleural effusion, pneumothorax, pulmonary infection, and respiratory insufficiency), early postoperative pulmonary function variables after 1 week (forced expiratory volume in 1 second [FEV1], forced total lung capacity (TLC), and forced vital capacity [FVC%]). Secondary outcomes of interest included early mortality, blood transfusion and, cardiopulmonary bypass (CPB) time, aortic cross-clamp time, and operative time.

## Risk-of-Bias and Study Quality Assessment

Two independent reviewers (SZAS and NID) assessed the risk-of-bias using the Cochrane risk-of-bias (RoB2) tool. The risk-of-bias was categorized as low, high, or unclear risk-of-bias. The RoB2 Excel tool was applied to individual studies, and results were entered into Cochrane's Review Manager 5.3 (40). The Newcastle–Ottawa Scale (NOS) was used to assess the methodological quality of all observational studies. The NOS assesses the following characteristics of a study: selection of the general population, comparability, and adequate assessment of outcomes, to evaluate the methodological quality of studies (41). Based on the NOS, a maximum of 9 points can be given to each study. In this review, the modified NOS scores $\geq 7$ were considered to indicate high-quality publications. Furthermore, the methodological quality of RCTs was assessed using the Jadad scale, which evaluates RCT quality using a maximum score of 5. A Jadad score $\geq 3$ was considered to indicate high-quality RCTs (42).

## Definitions of Outcomes

MIVS was defined as any procedure not performed with an FS. A full sternotomy was performed from the sternal notch to the xiphoid process. The definitions of the postoperative outcomes mainly depend on the descriptions mentioned in the original articles (8, 18, 39, 43–45). Besides postoperative pulmonary complications were defined as complications occurring in the postoperative period and producing clinical diseases, such as pneumonia, pleural effusion, pneumothorax, pulmonary infection, and respiratory insufficiency (defined as the need for reintubation or tracheostomy after initial extubation), and prolonged ventilation time, which was defined as mechanical ventilatory support requirement for more than 24 h. Pulmonary function tests, represented by FEV1, TLC, and FVC, were assessed based on a spirometry test 1 week after surgery. The incidence of early mortality was defined as death in the hospital or within 30 days post-surgery.

## Statistical Analysis

As per Cochrane Collaboration guidelines, all statistical meta-analyses were performed using Review Manager 5.3 software (Cochrane Collaboration, Copenhagen, Denmark). We calculated pooled odds ratios (ORs) with their 95% confidence intervals (CIs) for dichotomous data, which are presented as numbers and percentages. Weighted mean differences (WMDs) were used to assess continuous data, which are presented as means $\pm$ standard deviation or medians with interquartile ranges. We assessed the heterogeneity of studies by means of $I^2$ and chi-square test. As a sensitivity analysis, FS and MIVS from RCTs and from PSM studies were compared separately. The reported results all are two-sided, and a $p < 0.05$ was considered to indicate statistical significance.

**TABLE 2** | Overall and subgroup analysis of postoperative respiratory function and complications comparing MIVS and FS.

| Outcome of interest | n/N | No. patients MIVS/FS | Overall effect | P | Study heterogeneity | | | |
|---|---|---|---|---|---|---|---|---|
| | | | WMD/OR (95% CI)† | | chi²-test | df | $I^2$ (%) | P-value |
| **Postoperative respiratory function status after 1 week** | | | | | | | | |
| **Overall spirometry** | 6 (1,928) | 964/964 | MD −24.83 [−29.90,-19.76]† | <0.00001 | 11770.40 | 13 | 100 | <0.00001 |
| **Subgroup analysis** | | | | | | | | |
| FEV1% | 6 (722) | 361/361 | −74.06 [−89.14, −58.99]† | <0.00001 | 1089.82 | 5 | 100 | <0.00001 |
| FVC% | 5 (642) | 321/321 | 4.99 [1.23, 8.75]† | 0.009 | 287.63 | 4 | 99 | <0.00001 |
| TLC | 3 (564) | 282/2,282 | 8.39 [2.00, 14.78]† | 0.01 | 72.03 | 2 | 97 | <0.00001 |
| **Overall PPCs** | 30 (10,194) | 5,097/5,097 | 0.79 [0.67, 0.93] | 0.004 | 28.51 | 27 | 5 | 0.39 |
| RCT | 6 (418) | 209/209 | OR 0.32 [0.12, 0.90] | 0.03 | 4.29 | 4 | 7 | 0.37 |
| PSM | 24 (9,776) | 4,888/4,888 | OR 0.80 [0.69, 0.94] | 0.005 | 20.98 | 22 | 0 | 0.52 |
| **Subgroup analysis** | | | | | | | | |
| Pneumonia | 5 (916) | 458/458 | 1.42 [0.44, 4.55] | 0.56 | 2.81 | 4 | 0 | 0.59 |
| Pleural Effusion | 8 (1,454) | 727/727 | 0.81 [0.45, 1.45] | 0.47 | 10.28 | 7 | 32 | 0.17 |
| Pneumothorax | 4 (420) | 210/210 | 1.55 [0.30, 8.12] | 0.60 | 4.50 | 3 | 33 | 0.21 |
| Respiratory insufficient | 12 (5,848) | 2,924/2,924 | 0.75 [0.62, 0.91] | 0.004 | 9.30 | 11 | 0 | 0.59 |
| Pulmonary infection | 2 (246) | 123/123 | 1.35 [0.16, 11.30] | 0.78 | 1.24 | 1 | 19 | 0.27 |
| Prolonged ventilation time | 10 (3,564) | 1,782/1,782 | 0.72 [0.51, 1.01] | 0.06 | 6.92 | 9 | 0 | 0.65 |

*n, number of studies; N, number of participants; MIVS, minimally invasive valve surgery; FS, full sternotomy; PPC, postoperative pulmonary complications; WMD, weighted mean difference; OR, odds ratio; CI, confidence interval; $I^2$, test of heterogeneity; FEV1, forced expiratory volume in 1 s; FVC, Forced vital capacity; TLC, total lung capacity; †Values of WMD.*

# RESULTS

## Characteristics of Eligible Studies

Our literature search revealed 30 studies that met our selection criteria (5, 6, 12–39). The total number of patients in these studies was 10,194; 5,097 (50%) patients underwent MIVS, and 5,097 (50%) patients underwent FS. Six studies were RCTs ($n$ = 418 patients) (5, 6, 14–16, 28) and 24 were PSM studies ($n$ = 9,776 patients) (12, 13, 17–27, 29–39). The characteristics of these studies are shown in **Table 1**. **Figure 1** shows the PRISMA flowchart of the search and selection strategy (46).

The RCTs scored at least 3 out of 5 on the Jadad scale, and most of the PSM studies scored at least 7 out of 9, based on a modified version of the NOS scale (**Table 1** and **Figure 2**). Therefore, overall, the studies were considered to be of high quality.

## Postoperative Pulmonary Complications Outcomes

We analyzed data on postoperative pulmonary complications from 27 studies (6, 12–14, 16–34, 36–39). The overall complications were less in MIVS patients than in FS patients (OR

| Study or Subgroup | MIVS Events | MIVS Total | FS Events | FS Total | Weight | Odds Ratio M-H, Random, 95% CI |
|---|---|---|---|---|---|---|
| **1.3.1 Randomized controlled trials (RCT)** | | | | | | |
| Aris 1999 | 1 | 20 | 0 | 20 | 0.2% | 3.15 [0.12, 82.16] |
| Bonacchi 2002 | 3 | 40 | 7 | 40 | 1.3% | 0.38 [0.09, 1.60] |
| Calderon 2009 | 0 | 39 | 0 | 39 | | Not estimable |
| Dogan 2005 | 1 | 20 | 2 | 20 | 0.4% | 0.47 [0.04, 5.69] |
| Machler 1999 | 1 | 60 | 12 | 60 | 0.6% | 0.07 [0.01, 0.54] |
| Moustafa 2007 | 0 | 30 | 1 | 30 | 0.2% | 0.32 [0.01, 8.24] |
| **Subtotal (95% CI)** | | **209** | | **209** | **2.8%** | **0.32 [0.12, 0.90]** |
| Total events | 6 | | 22 | | | |
| Heterogeneity: $Tau^2$ = 0.10; $Chi^2$ = 4.29, df = 4 (P = 0.37); $I^2$ = 7% | | | | | | |
| Test for overall effect: Z = 2.17 (P = 0.03) | | | | | | |
| **1.3.2 Propensity-matched observational studies (POS)** | | | | | | |
| Albacker 2014 | 9 | 223 | 18 | 223 | 3.7% | 0.48 [0.21, 1.09] |
| Bang 2012 | 3 | 73 | 1 | 73 | 0.5% | 3.09 [0.31, 30.38] |
| Farhat 2003 | 0 | 50 | 1 | 50 | 0.3% | 0.33 [0.01, 8.21] |
| Gasparovic 2017 | 3 | 34 | 4 | 34 | 1.0% | 0.73 [0.15, 3.52] |
| Ghanta 2015 | 26 | 289 | 25 | 289 | 7.1% | 1.04 [0.59, 1.86] |
| Gilmanov 2013 | 24 | 182 | 22 | 182 | 6.2% | 1.10 [0.59, 2.05] |
| Gilmanov 2015 | 24 | 100 | 22 | 100 | 5.6% | 1.12 [0.58, 2.16] |
| Hawkins 2018 | 5 | 74 | 8 | 74 | 1.9% | 0.60 [0.19, 1.92] |
| Hiraoka 2014 | 1 | 36 | 0 | 36 | 0.3% | 3.08 [0.12, 78.27] |
| Holzhey 2011 | 22 | 143 | 22 | 143 | 5.8% | 1.00 [0.53, 1.90] |
| Iribarne 2010 | 17 | 382 | 29 | 382 | 6.3% | 0.57 [0.31, 1.05] |
| Johnston 2012 | 24 | 832 | 45 | 832 | 9.0% | 0.52 [0.31, 0.86] |
| Levack 2016 | 10 | 483 | 12 | 483 | 3.5% | 0.83 [0.36, 1.94] |
| Masiello 2002 | 7 | 100 | 5 | 100 | 1.8% | 1.43 [0.44, 4.67] |
| Merka 2014 | 52 | 477 | 67 | 477 | 14.0% | 0.75 [0.51, 1.10] |
| Murzi 2011 | 3 | 100 | 4 | 100 | 1.1% | 0.74 [0.16, 3.41] |
| Sansone 2012 | 6 | 50 | 0 | 50 | 0.3% | 14.75 [0.81, 269.34] |
| Seitz 2017 | 3 | 53 | 3 | 53 | 1.0% | 1.00 [0.19, 5.19] |
| Shehada 2015 | 50 | 585 | 69 | 585 | 14.2% | 0.70 [0.48, 1.03] |
| Stolinski 2016 | 28 | 211 | 36 | 211 | 8.1% | 0.74 [0.44, 1.27] |
| Stolinski 2017 | 0 | 212 | 0 | 212 | | Not estimable |
| Tabata 2007 | 1 | 41 | 3 | 41 | 0.5% | 0.32 [0.03, 3.18] |
| Wang 2018 | 5 | 67 | 3 | 67 | 1.2% | 1.72 [0.39, 7.51] |
| Zhao 2018 | 18 | 91 | 13 | 91 | 4.0% | 1.48 [0.68, 3.23] |
| **Subtotal (95% CI)** | | **4888** | | **4888** | **97.2%** | **0.80 [0.69, 0.94]** |
| Total events | 341 | | 412 | | | |
| Heterogeneity: $Tau^2$ = 0.00; $Chi^2$ = 20.98, df = 22 (P = 0.52); $I^2$ = 0% | | | | | | |
| Test for overall effect: Z = 2.82 (P = 0.005) | | | | | | |
| **Total (95% CI)** | | **5097** | | **5097** | **100.0%** | **0.79 [0.67, 0.93]** |
| Total events | 347 | | 434 | | | |
| Heterogeneity: $Tau^2$ = 0.01; $Chi^2$ = 28.51, df = 27 (P = 0.39); $I^2$ = 5% | | | | | | |
| Test for overall effect: Z = 2.88 (P = 0.004) | | | | | | |
| Test for subgroup differences: $Chi^2$ = 2.97, df = 1 (P = 0.08), $I^2$ = 66.3% | | | | | | |

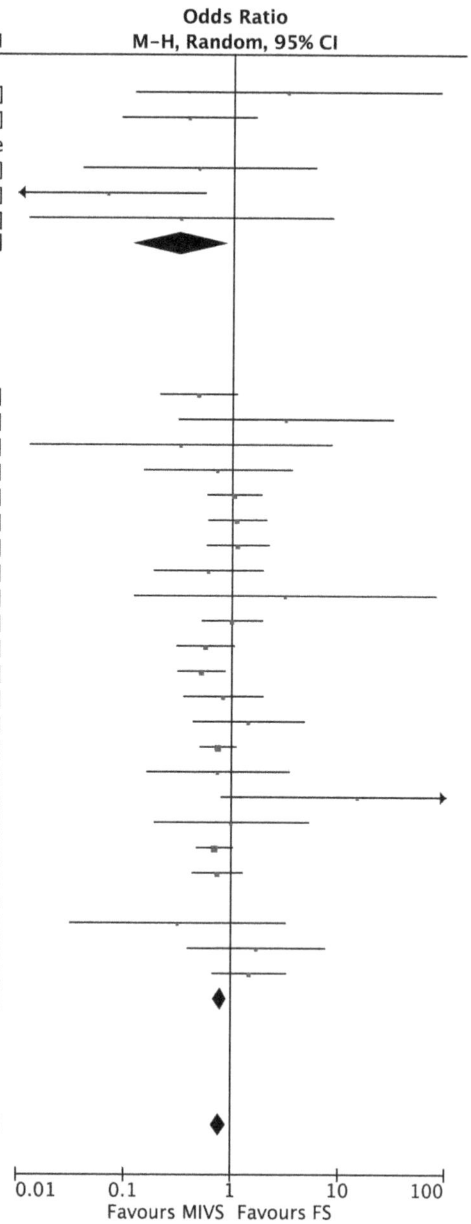


**FIGURE 3** | Forest plot demonstrating the overall study incidence of postoperative pulmonary complications between MIVS and FS.

| Study or Subgroup | MIVS Events | MIVS Total | FS Events | FS Total | Weight | Odds Ratio M-H, Random, 95% CI |
|---|---|---|---|---|---|---|
| **1.2.1 Pneumonia** | | | | | | |
| Dogan 2005 | 1 | 20 | 0 | 20 | 0.2% | 3.15 [0.12, 82.16] |
| Gilmanov 2015 | 2 | 100 | 0 | 100 | 0.2% | 5.10 [0.24, 107.62] |
| Hawkins 2018 | 1 | 74 | 2 | 74 | 0.4% | 0.49 [0.04, 5.56] |
| Seitz 2017 | 1 | 53 | 2 | 53 | 0.4% | 0.49 [0.04, 5.58] |
| Stolinski 2016 | 3 | 211 | 1 | 211 | 0.4% | 3.03 [0.31, 29.35] |
| **Subtotal (95% CI)** | | **458** | | **458** | **1.7%** | **1.42 [0.44, 4.55]** |
| Total events | 8 | | 5 | | | |
| Heterogeneity: Tau² = 0.00; Chi² = 2.81, df = 4 (P = 0.59); I² = 0% | | | | | | |
| Test for overall effect: Z = 0.59 (P = 0.56) | | | | | | |
| **1.2.2 Pleural effusion** | | | | | | |
| Aris 1999 | 1 | 20 | 0 | 20 | 0.2% | 3.15 [0.12, 82.16] |
| Dogan 2005 | 0 | 20 | 1 | 20 | 0.2% | 0.32 [0.01, 8.26] |
| Gasparovic 2017 | 3 | 34 | 4 | 34 | 0.9% | 0.73 [0.15, 3.52] |
| Gilmanov 2013 | 10 | 182 | 5 | 182 | 1.9% | 2.06 [0.69, 6.14] |
| Gilmanov 2015 | 4 | 100 | 5 | 100 | 1.3% | 0.79 [0.21, 3.04] |
| Machler 1999 | 1 | 60 | 12 | 60 | 0.5% | 0.07 [0.01, 0.54] |
| Masiello 2002 | 6 | 100 | 5 | 100 | 1.5% | 1.21 [0.36, 4.11] |
| Stolinski 2016 | 25 | 211 | 35 | 211 | 7.5% | 0.68 [0.39, 1.18] |
| **Subtotal (95% CI)** | | **727** | | **727** | **14.2%** | **0.81 [0.45, 1.45]** |
| Total events | 50 | | 67 | | | |
| Heterogeneity: Tau² = 0.21; Chi² = 10.28, df = 7 (P = 0.17); I² = 32% | | | | | | |
| Test for overall effect: Z = 0.72 (P = 0.47) | | | | | | |
| **1.2.3 Pneumothorax** | | | | | | |
| Bonacchi 2002 | 2 | 40 | 3 | 40 | 0.7% | 0.65 [0.10, 4.11] |
| Dogan 2005 | 0 | 20 | 1 | 20 | 0.2% | 0.32 [0.01, 8.26] |
| Masiello 2002 | 1 | 100 | 0 | 100 | 0.2% | 3.03 [0.12, 75.28] |
| Sansone 2012 | 6 | 50 | 0 | 50 | 0.3% | 14.75 [0.81, 269.34] |
| **Subtotal (95% CI)** | | **210** | | **210** | **1.4%** | **1.55 [0.30, 8.12]** |
| Total events | 9 | | 4 | | | |
| Heterogeneity: Tau² = 0.96; Chi² = 4.50, df = 3 (P = 0.21); I² = 33% | | | | | | |
| Test for overall effect: Z = 0.52 (P = 0.60) | | | | | | |
| **1.2.4 Respiratory insufficient** | | | | | | |
| Albacker 2014 | 9 | 223 | 18 | 223 | 3.4% | 0.48 [0.21, 1.09] |
| Bonacchi 2002 | 1 | 40 | 2 | 40 | 0.4% | 0.49 [0.04, 5.60] |
| Ghanta 2015 | 26 | 289 | 25 | 289 | 7.0% | 1.04 [0.59, 1.86] |
| Gilmanov 2015 | 14 | 100 | 10 | 100 | 3.1% | 1.47 [0.62, 3.47] |
| Hiraoka 2014 | 1 | 24 | 0 | 24 | 0.2% | 3.13 [0.12, 80.68] |
| Holzhey 2011 | 22 | 143 | 22 | 143 | 5.6% | 1.00 [0.53, 1.90] |
| Johnston 2012 | 24 | 832 | 45 | 832 | 9.0% | 0.52 [0.31, 0.86] |
| Merka 2014 | 52 | 477 | 67 | 477 | 15.4% | 0.75 [0.51, 1.10] |
| Seitz 2017 | 2 | 53 | 1 | 53 | 0.4% | 2.04 [0.18, 23.19] |
| Shehada 2015 | 50 | 585 | 69 | 585 | 15.7% | 0.70 [0.48, 1.03] |
| Wang 2018 | 3 | 67 | 5 | 67 | 1.1% | 0.58 [0.13, 2.54] |
| Zhao 2018 | 2 | 91 | 3 | 91 | 0.7% | 0.66 [0.11, 4.04] |
| **Subtotal (95% CI)** | | **2924** | | **2924** | **61.9%** | **0.75 [0.62, 0.91]** |
| Total events | 206 | | 267 | | | |
| Heterogeneity: Tau² = 0.00; Chi² = 9.30, df = 11 (P = 0.59); I² = 0% | | | | | | |
| Test for overall effect: Z = 2.89 (P = 0.004) | | | | | | |
| **1.2.5 Pulmonary infection** | | | | | | |
| Bang 2012 | 3 | 73 | 1 | 73 | 0.4% | 3.09 [0.31, 30.38] |
| Farhat 2003 | 0 | 50 | 1 | 50 | 0.2% | 0.33 [0.01, 8.21] |
| **Subtotal (95% CI)** | | **123** | | **123** | **0.7%** | **1.35 [0.16, 11.30]** |
| Total events | 3 | | 2 | | | |
| Heterogeneity: Tau² = 0.49; Chi² = 1.24, df = 1 (P = 0.27); I² = 19% | | | | | | |
| Test for overall effect: Z = 0.28 (P = 0.78) | | | | | | |
| **1.2.7 Prolonged ventilation time** | | | | | | |
| Bonacchi 2002 | 0 | 40 | 2 | 40 | 0.2% | 0.19 [0.01, 4.09] |
| Ghanta 2015 | 5 | 289 | 6 | 289 | 1.6% | 0.83 [0.25, 2.75] |
| Gilmanov 2013 | 4 | 182 | 9 | 182 | 1.6% | 0.43 [0.13, 1.43] |
| Gilmanov 2015 | 4 | 100 | 7 | 100 | 1.4% | 0.55 [0.16, 1.95] |
| Hawkins 2018 | 4 | 74 | 6 | 74 | 1.3% | 0.65 [0.18, 2.40] |
| Iribarne 2010 | 17 | 382 | 29 | 382 | 6.1% | 0.57 [0.31, 1.05] |
| Levack 2016 | 10 | 483 | 12 | 483 | 3.2% | 0.83 [0.36, 1.94] |
| Murzi 2011 | 3 | 100 | 4 | 100 | 1.0% | 0.74 [0.16, 3.41] |
| Tabata 2007 | 1 | 41 | 3 | 41 | 0.4% | 0.32 [0.03, 3.18] |
| Zhao 2018 | 16 | 91 | 10 | 91 | 3.2% | 1.73 [0.74, 4.04] |
| **Subtotal (95% CI)** | | **1782** | | **1782** | **20.1%** | **0.72 [0.51, 1.01]** |
| Total events | 64 | | 88 | | | |
| Heterogeneity: Tau² = 0.00; Chi² = 6.92, df = 9 (P = 0.65); I² = 0% | | | | | | |
| Test for overall effect: Z = 1.90 (P = 0.06) | | | | | | |
| **Total (95% CI)** | | **6224** | | **6224** | **100.0%** | **0.77 [0.66, 0.90]** |
| Total events | 340 | | 433 | | | |
| Heterogeneity: Tau² = 0.00; Chi² = 37.07, df = 40 (P = 0.60); I² = 0% | | | | | | |
| Test for overall effect: Z = 3.39 (P = 0.0007) | | | | | | |
| Test for subgroup differences: Chi² = 2.24, df = 5 (P = 0.82), I² = 0% | | | | | | |

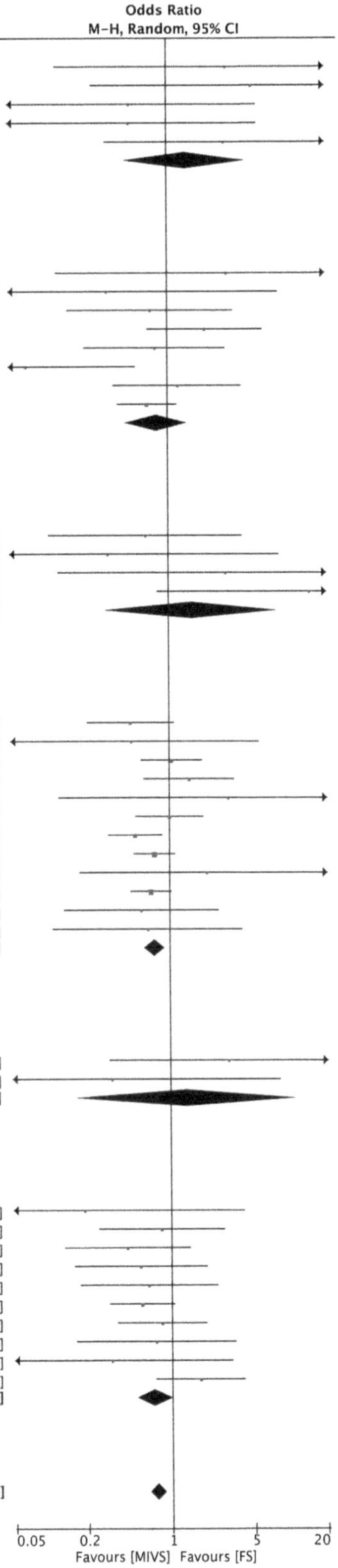


**FIGURE 4 |** Forest plot demonstrating the subgroup study of the incidence of postoperative pulmonary between MIVS and FS.

| Study or Subgroup | MIVS Mean | MIVS SD | MIVS Total | FS Mean | FS SD | FS Total | Weight | Mean Difference IV, Random, 95% CI |
|---|---|---|---|---|---|---|---|---|
| **1.1.1 FEV1% after 1 week** | | | | | | | | |
| Aris 1999 | 62 | 16 | 20 | 526 | 12 | 20 | 6.2% | -464.00 [-472.77, -455.23] |
| Bonacchi 2002 | 80.8 | 18.6 | 40 | 81.7 | 21.5 | 40 | 6.2% | -0.90 [-9.71, 7.91] |
| Calderon 2009 | 53.4 | 15.6 | 39 | 55 | 16 | 39 | 6.7% | -1.60 [-8.61, 5.41] |
| Dogan 2005 | 1.9 | 0.8 | 20 | 1.7 | 0.6 | 20 | 7.6% | 0.20 [-0.24, 0.64] |
| Moustafa 2007 | 80.47 | 0.51 | 30 | 78.47 | 0.51 | 30 | 7.6% | 2.00 [1.74, 2.26] |
| Stolinski 2017 | 79.5 | 10.1 | 212 | 74 | 11.3 | 212 | 7.5% | 5.50 [3.46, 7.54] |
| **Subtotal (95% CI)** | | | **361** | | | **361** | **41.9%** | **-74.06 [-89.14, -58.99]** |
| Heterogeneity: Tau² = 346.15; Chi² = 10894.82, df = 5 (P < 0.00001); I² = 100% | | | | | | | | |
| Test for overall effect: Z = 9.63 (P < 0.00001) | | | | | | | | |
| **1.1.2 FVC% after 1 week** | | | | | | | | |
| Aris 1999 | 60 | 17 | 20 | 53 | 12 | 20 | 6.1% | 7.00 [-2.12, 16.12] |
| Calderon 2009 | 55.9 | 14.1 | 39 | 57.9 | 15.2 | 39 | 6.8% | -2.00 [-8.51, 4.51] |
| Dogan 2005 | 2.5 | 0.9 | 20 | 2.1 | 0.8 | 20 | 7.6% | 0.40 [-0.13, 0.93] |
| Moustafa 2007 | 91.5 | 0.51 | 30 | 86.6 | 0.95 | 30 | 7.6% | 4.90 [4.51, 5.29] |
| Stolinski 2017 | 64.8 | 8.8 | 212 | 51.5 | 11.1 | 212 | 7.5% | 13.30 [11.39, 15.21] |
| **Subtotal (95% CI)** | | | **321** | | | **321** | **35.7%** | **4.99 [1.23, 8.75]** |
| Heterogeneity: Tau² = 14.34; Chi² = 287.63, df = 4 (P < 0.00001); I² = 99% | | | | | | | | |
| Test for overall effect: Z = 2.60 (P = 0.009) | | | | | | | | |
| **1.1.3 TLC after 1 week** | | | | | | | | |
| Bonacchi 2002 | 65.9 | 10 | 40 | 59.6 | 8.3 | 40 | 7.3% | 6.30 [2.27, 10.33] |
| Moustafa 2007 | 65.5 | 0.51 | 30 | 60.5 | 0.51 | 30 | 7.6% | 5.00 [4.74, 5.26] |
| Stolinski 2017 | 67.1 | 7.5 | 212 | 53.3 | 13 | 212 | 7.5% | 13.80 [11.78, 15.82] |
| **Subtotal (95% CI)** | | | **282** | | | **282** | **22.4%** | **8.39 [2.00, 14.78]** |
| Heterogeneity: Tau² = 30.23; Chi² = 72.03, df = 2 (P < 0.00001); I² = 97% | | | | | | | | |
| Test for overall effect: Z = 2.57 (P = 0.01) | | | | | | | | |
| **Total (95% CI)** | | | **964** | | | **964** | **100.0%** | **-24.83 [-29.90, -19.76]** |
| Heterogeneity: Tau² = 87.70; Chi² = 11770.40, df = 13 (P < 0.00001); I² = 100% | | | | | | | | |
| Test for overall effect: Z = 9.60 (P < 0.00001) | | | | | | | | |
| Test for subgroup differences: Chi² = 104.02, df = 2 (P < 0.00001), I² = 98.1% | | | | | | | | |

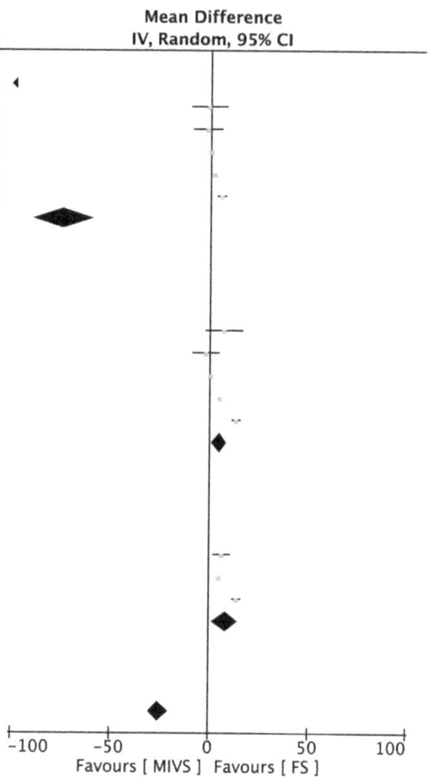


**FIGURE 5** | Forest plot demonstrating the incidence of postoperative respiratory function between the MIVS and FS.

0.79; 95% CI [0.67, 0.93]; $p = 0.004$). The results of our meta-analysis are summarized in **Table 2**, and forest plots are shown in **Figure 3**.

In subgroup analysis, postoperative pulmonary complications differed significantly between the two groups ($p = 0.0007$) in terms of the incidence of postoperative respiratory insufficiency, reported by 12 studies (12, 14, 19, 21, 23, 24, 26, 30, 33, 34, 38, 39) (OR 0.75; 95% CI [0.62, 0.91]; $p = 0.004$). Two studies reported on pulmonary infection: MIVS was associated with a lower chance of infection, but this difference was not significant (OR 1.35; 95% CI [0.16, 11.30]; $p = 0.78$) (13, 17). The incidence of postoperative pleural effusion was reported in 8 studies; this was not significantly different between the groups (OR 0.81; 95% CI [0.45, 1.45]; $p = 0.47$) (6, 16, 18, 20, 21, 28, 29, 36). We also compared the incidence of prolonged ventilation time based on data pooled from 10 studies; there was no significant difference between the groups (OR 0.72; 95% CI [0.51, 1.01]; $p = 0.06$) (14, 19–22, 25, 27, 31, 37, 39). Although the observed proportions of patients with pneumonia (OR 1.42; 95% CI [0.44, 4.55]; $p = 0.56$) and pneumothorax (OR 1.55 95% CI; [0.30, 8.12]; $p = 0.60$) were less among MIVS patients, these were not significantly different between the groups. Subgroup analysis are summarized in **Table 2** and forest plots are shown in **Figure 4**.

Six studies (5, 6, 14–16, 35) reported on postoperative respiratory function tests based on spirometry, revealing that the overall complications were significantly reduced with MIVS compared to FS (964 vs. 964, WMD −24.83 95% CI [−29.90, −19.76]; $p = < 0.00001$). Most pulmonary function tests showed that the MIVS group had better respiratory function than the FS group 1 week after surgery. There was significant heterogeneity among the studies ($p < 0.00001$).

A subgroup analysis of postoperative respiratory function identified that FEV1% (WMD: −78.06; 95% CI [−89.14, −58.99]; $p < 0.00001$), FVC% (WMD: 4.99; 95% CI [1.23, 8.75]; $p = 0.009$), and TLC (WMD: 8.39; 95% CI [2.00, 14.78]; $p = 0.01$) were all significantly better in the MIVS group. There was significant heterogeneity among the studies overall, as well as in the RCT and PSM subgroup ($p < 0.00001$) (**Table 2** and **Figure 5**).

## Early Mortality Outcomes

Early mortality was reported as an outcome in 30 studies (5, 6, 12–39), including 5 RCTs (6, 14–16, 28) and 25 PSM studies (12, 13, 17–27, 29–39). The incidence of early death was 1.2 and 1.9% with MIVS, and FS approaches, respectively. Thus, the early mortality rate after MIVS was significantly lower than that after FS (OR 1.58 95% CI: 1.15, 2.16; $p = 0.005$). There was no significant heterogeneity between the groups ($p = 0.97$) (**Figures 6A,B**).

## Intraoperative Variable Outcomes

MIVS was associated with a significantly prolonged CPB time (WMD: 11.06; 95% CI: 4.29, 17.84 min; $p = 0.001$) (**Figure 7**)

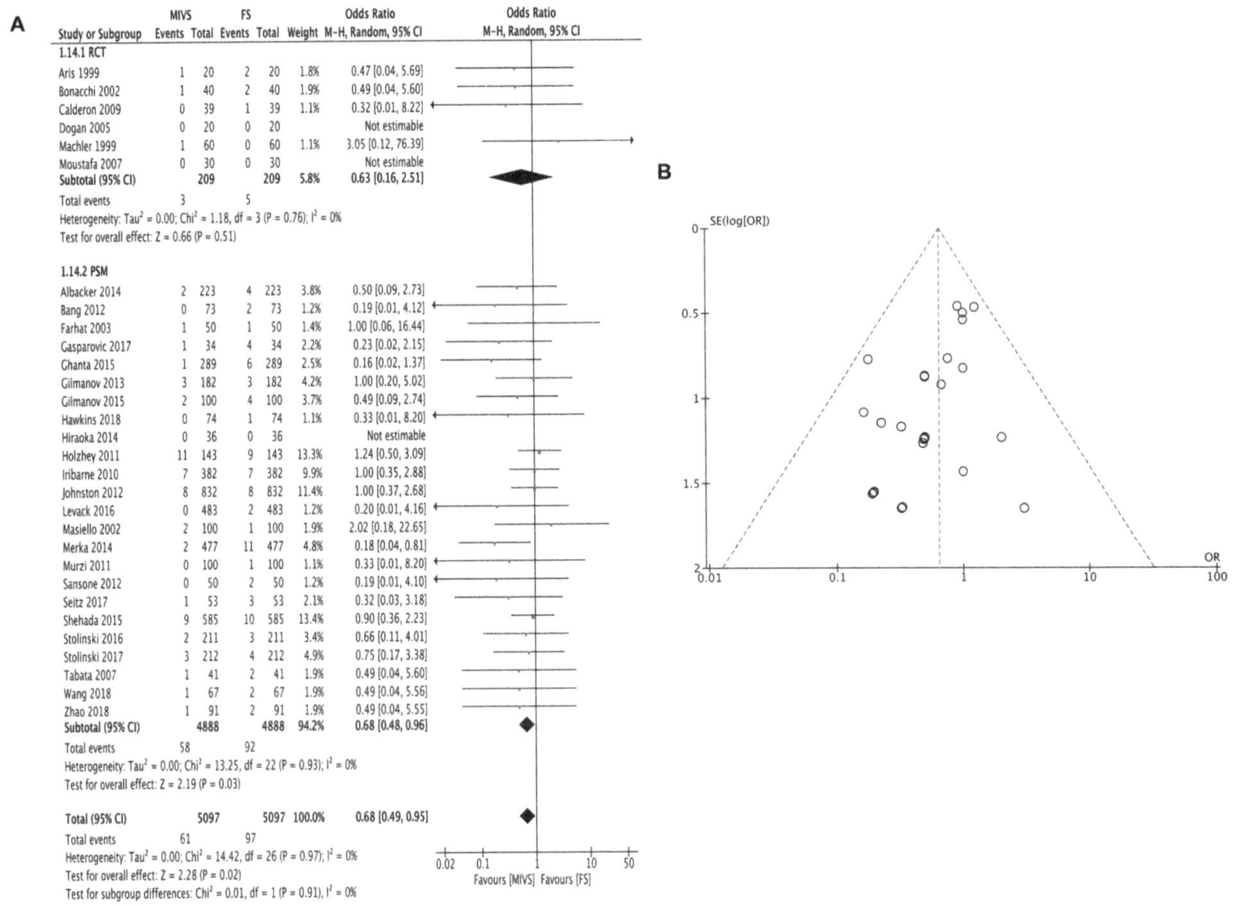

FIGURE 6 | **(A)** Forest plot MIVS vs. FS (Overall early mortality) and **(B)** Funnel plot MIVS vs. FS (overall early mortality).

and aortic cross-clamping time (WMD: 23.28; 95% CI: 5.65, 40.87 min; $p = 0.009$) (**Figure 8**). Thus, the MIVS approach took longer than the FS surgery, although there was no significant difference in the operative time (WMD: 0.39; 95% CI: −0.39, 1.77 h; $p = 0.32$) between the groups (**Figure 9**). However, the overall heterogeneity between the two approaches was significantly different ($p < 0.00001$). **Table 3** provides a summary of these studies.

## Need for Blood Transfusion Outcomes

Fourteen studies [2 RCTs (15, 16) and 12 PSM studies (19, 20, 22, 23, 26, 27, 30, 32, 33, 36, 37, 39)] reported on the need for blood transfusion in patients. Twenty-two percent of patients required red blood cell (RBC) transfusion after MIVS, compared to 28% after FS (OR 0.69, 95% CI 0.51, 0.93; $p = 0.02$) (**Figure 10**).

Ten studies [3 RCTs (5, 13, 14) and 7 PSM studies (16–18, 24, 31, 36, 38)] reported the units of RBC transfused after MIVS and FS. Those who underwent MIVS used significantly fewer units of RBCs for transfusion than those who underwent FS (WMD −0.59, 95%CI [−2.08, 0.90 U]; $p = 0.44$). There was significant heterogeneity among the studies overall as well for the RCTs and PSM studies ($p < 0.00001$) (**Figure 11**).

## DISCUSSION

Over the past decades, a steady evolution has taken place in the practice of MIVS, with excellent postoperative outcomes, according to the literature. The minimally invasive approach used for the aorta or mitral valve has advantages over the FS method in terms of decreased surgical trauma, postoperative blood loss, and length of ICU and hospital stay (4, 47). Nevertheless, postoperative pulmonary complications remain a common cause of postcardiac surgical morbidity, poor outcomes, increased cost, and hospital stays (48). Therefore, in the context of postoperative pulmonary complications and recovery of early respiratory system function, we considered it necessary to compare MIVS with FS.

In this meta-analysis, we analyzed data of 10,194 patients (5,097 [50%] vs. 5,097 [50%] patients in MIVS vs. FS groups, respectively), from 30 studies (6 RCTs and 24 PSM studies) to evaluate postoperative pulmonary functions status and pulmonary complications after MIVS vs. FS. We also assessed early mortality, CPB time, aortic cross-clamp time, procedure time, and need for blood transfusion between the MIVS and FS. Using the best available level of evidence based

| Study or Subgroup | MIVS Mean | MIVS SD | MIVS Total | FS Mean | FS SD | FS Total | Weight | Mean Difference IV, Random, 95% CI |
|---|---|---|---|---|---|---|---|---|
| **1.5.1 RCT** | | | | | | | | |
| Aris 1999 | 95 | 20 | 20 | 83 | 19 | 20 | 3.6% | 12.00 [−0.09, 24.09] |
| Calderon 2009 | 77.1 | 32.4 | 39 | 71.3 | 30.4 | 39 | 3.5% | 5.80 [−8.14, 19.74] |
| Dogan 2005 | 141.7 | 32.1 | 20 | 132.6 | 35.6 | 20 | 3.0% | 9.10 [−11.91, 30.11] |
| Machler 1999 | 84 | 32.1 | 60 | 82 | 61.25 | 60 | 3.2% | 2.00 [−15.50, 19.50] |
| Moustafa 2007 | 85.67 | 6.79 | 30 | 90 | 8.3 | 30 | 4.1% | −4.33 [−8.17, −0.49] |
| **Subtotal (95% CI)** | | | **169** | | | **169** | **17.4%** | **3.26 [−4.83, 11.34]** |
| Heterogeneity: Tau² = 43.08; Chi² = 9.03, df = 4 (P = 0.06); I² = 56% | | | | | | | | |
| Test for overall effect: Z = 0.79 (P = 0.43) | | | | | | | | |
| **1.5.2 PSM** | | | | | | | | |
| Bang 2012 | 106.3 | 45.3 | 73 | 101.9 | 39.6 | 73 | 3.5% | 4.40 [−9.40, 18.20] |
| Farhat 2003 | 89 | 18 | 50 | 70 | 11 | 50 | 4.0% | 19.00 [13.15, 24.85] |
| Gasparovic 2017 | 79.9 | 14.9 | 34 | 61.9 | 13.7 | 34 | 4.0% | 18.00 [11.20, 24.80] |
| Gilmanov 2013 | 117.5 | 41.9 | 100 | 104.1 | 34.6 | 100 | 3.7% | 13.40 [2.75, 24.05] |
| Gilmanov 2015 | 92 | 7.17 | 74 | 94 | 6.17 | 74 | 4.1% | −2.00 [−4.16, 0.16] |
| Hawkins 2018 | 155 | 35 | 36 | 108 | 65 | 36 | 2.7% | 47.00 [22.88, 71.12] |
| Hiraoka 2014 | 129 | 28 | 36 | 125 | 47 | 36 | 3.2% | 4.00 [−13.87, 21.87] |
| Holzhey 2011 | 142 | 54 | 143 | 102 | 45 | 143 | 3.7% | 40.00 [28.48, 51.52] |
| Iribarne 2010 | 139.7 | 2.6 | 382 | 117.1 | 2 | 382 | 4.1% | 22.60 [22.27, 22.93] |
| Johnston 2012 | 73 | 32 | 832 | 95 | 37 | 832 | 4.1% | −22.00 [−25.32, −18.68] |
| Levack 2016 | 70 | 26 | 483 | 87 | 36 | 483 | 4.1% | −17.00 [−20.96, −13.04] |
| Masiello 2002 | 82.4 | 22 | 100 | 66.8 | 16 | 100 | 4.0% | 15.60 [10.27, 20.93] |
| Merka 2014 | 82.2 | 217 | 477 | 81 | 19.9 | 477 | 3.1% | 1.20 [−18.36, 20.76] |
| Murzi 2011 | 119 | 30 | 100 | 106 | 32 | 100 | 3.9% | 13.00 [4.40, 21.60] |
| Sansone 2012 | 101.4 | 35.2 | 50 | 62.8 | 18.3 | 50 | 3.7% | 38.60 [27.60, 49.60] |
| Seitz 2017 | 112 | 44 | 53 | 98 | 25 | 53 | 3.5% | 14.00 [0.38, 27.62] |
| Shehada 2015 | 93.5 | 25 | 585 | 88 | 28 | 585 | 4.1% | 5.50 [2.46, 8.54] |
| Stolinski 2016 | 111 | 25 | 211 | 97.6 | 19.4 | 211 | 4.1% | 13.40 [9.13, 17.67] |
| Stolinski 2017 | 109.3 | 26.5 | 212 | 97.6 | 19.6 | 212 | 4.1% | 11.70 [7.26, 16.14] |
| Tabata 2007 | 122.2 | 48.5 | 41 | 112.1 | 39.8 | 41 | 3.1% | 10.10 [−9.10, 29.30] |
| Wang 2018 | 138.4 | 34.6 | 67 | 112.4 | 28.8 | 67 | 3.7% | 26.00 [15.22, 36.78] |
| Zhao 2018 | 112.5 | 12.9 | 91 | 103.5 | 12.2 | 91 | 4.1% | 9.00 [5.35, 12.65] |
| **Subtotal (95% CI)** | | | **4230** | | | **4230** | **82.6%** | **12.43 [4.97, 19.89]** |
| Heterogeneity: Tau² = 289.78; Chi² = 1746.47, df = 21 (P < 0.00001); I² = 99% | | | | | | | | |
| Test for overall effect: Z = 3.27 (P = 0.001) | | | | | | | | |
| **Total (95% CI)** | | | **4399** | | | **4399** | **100.0%** | **11.06 [4.29, 17.84]** |
| Heterogeneity: Tau² = 289.56; Chi² = 1924.40, df = 26 (P < 0.00001); I² = 99% | | | | | | | | |
| Test for overall effect: Z = 3.20 (P = 0.001) | | | | | | | | |
| Test for subgroup differences: Chi² = 2.67, df = 1 (P = 0.10), I² = 62.6% | | | | | | | | |

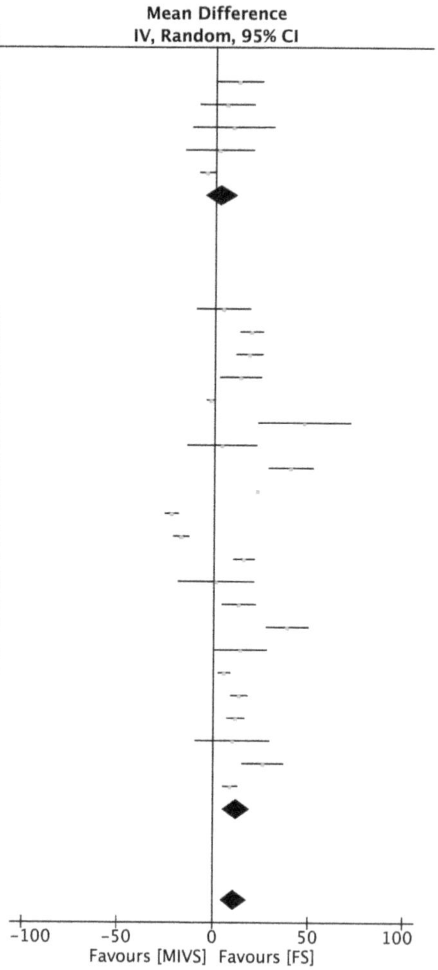


**FIGURE 7** | Forest plot of cardiopulmonary bypass time (minutes) between MIVS vs. FS.

on RCTs and PSM studies, our meta-analysis added to the literature that the MIVS is safe and had a significantly reduced overall incidence of postoperative pulmonary complications and respiratory insufficiency and decreased mechanical ventilation time compared with FS.

Moreover, the overall findings for the secondary outcomes suggested that MIVS, both aortic and mitral, significantly reduced early mortality and blood transfusion requirements. To the best of our knowledge, no previous meta-analyses have indicated whether the incidence of pulmonary complications is lower after MIVS compared with FS. Most studies that describe the effect of cardiac surgery on pulmonary complications were related to patients who underwent a coronary bypass operation through full median sternotomy (49).

It has been reported that the MIVS showed better preserved early postoperative respiratory function status and reduced the time needed to make a full recovery of pulmonary status compared with FS (50). However, there has not been explained this improved respiratory function in the MIVS group so far. This study found that patients undergoing MIVS had a reduced incidence of postoperative pulmonary complications and better postoperative respiratory function outcomes than patients undergoing valve surgery via full median sternotomy. Therefore, we believe that our finding of a reduced incidence of pulmonary complications after the MIVS group may explain the improved lung function than patients with a full median sternotomy. As a result, we believe these phenomena are more likely caused by preserving the chest wall's integrity and reduced surgical trauma. Because of their improved respiratory condition, patients could begin mobilization quicker and perform pulmonary bronchial tree ventilation and cleaning more adequately.

Several risk factors may influence the impairment of spirometry and change in pulmonary gas exchange after cardiac surgery performed via a sternotomy; these include surgical trauma, prolonged operative and CPB time (6, 12, 14, 51). CPB causes an inflammatory cascade of compounds associated with the systemic inflammatory syndrome due to blood interaction with the CPB circuit and decreased pulmonary regeneration,

| Study or Subgroup | MIVS Mean | MIVS SD | MIVS Total | FS Mean | FS SD | FS Total | Weight | Mean Difference IV, Random, 95% CI |
|---|---|---|---|---|---|---|---|---|
| **1.7.1 RCT** | | | | | | | | |
| Aris 1999 | 70 | 19 | 20 | 51 | 13 | 20 | 3.6% | 19.00 [8.91, 29.09] |
| Bonacchi 2002 | 517 | 12.2 | 40 | 52.4 | 9.8 | 40 | 3.6% | 464.60 [459.75, 469.45] |
| Calderon 2009 | 55 | 9.3 | 39 | 50.6 | 11.9 | 39 | 3.6% | 4.40 [-0.34, 9.14] |
| Dogan 2005 | 84.8 | 24.4 | 20 | 88 | 19 | 20 | 3.5% | -3.20 [-16.75, 10.35] |
| Machler 1999 | 60 | 20.25 | 60 | 60 | 19 | 60 | 3.6% | 0.00 [-7.03, 7.03] |
| Moustafa 2007 | 85.67 | 6.79 | 30 | 90 | 8.3 | 30 | 3.6% | -4.33 [-8.17, -0.49] |
| **Subtotal (95% CI)** | | | **209** | | | **209** | **21.4%** | **80.10 [-98.13, 258.32]** |
| Heterogeneity: Tau² = 49595.70; Chi² = 27352.47, df = 5 (P < 0.00001); I² = 100% | | | | | | | | |
| Test for overall effect: Z = 0.88 (P = 0.38) | | | | | | | | |
| **1.7.2 PSM** | | | | | | | | |
| Bang 2012 | 106.3 | 45.3 | 73 | 101.9 | 39.6 | 73 | 3.5% | 4.40 [-9.40, 18.20] |
| Farhat 2003 | 66 | 15 | 50 | 49 | 10 | 50 | 3.6% | 17.00 [12.00, 22.00] |
| Gasparovic 2017 | 63.4 | 12.7 | 34 | 50.3 | 11.6 | 34 | 3.6% | 13.10 [7.32, 18.88] |
| Gilmanov 2013 | 83.8 | 28.5 | 182 | 71.3 | 27.5 | 182 | 3.6% | 12.50 [6.75, 18.25] |
| Gilmanov 2015 | 59 | 4.667 | 100 | 63 | 4.333 | 100 | 3.6% | -4.00 [-5.25, -2.75] |
| Hawkins 2018 | 101 | 24 | 74 | 77 | 44 | 74 | 3.5% | 24.00 [12.58, 35.42] |
| Hiraoka 2014 | 91 | 22 | 36 | 90 | 30 | 36 | 3.5% | 1.00 [-11.15, 13.15] |
| Holzhey 2011 | 74 | 44 | 143 | 64 | 28 | 143 | 3.6% | 10.00 [1.45, 18.55] |
| Iribarne 2010 | 83.7 | 1.9 | 382 | 79.6 | 1.5 | 382 | 3.6% | 4.10 [3.86, 4.34] |
| Johnston 2012 | 58 | 25 | 832 | 71 | 28 | 832 | 3.6% | -13.00 [-15.55, -10.45] |
| Levack 2016 | 55 | 21 | 483 | 70 | 30 | 483 | 3.6% | -15.00 [-18.27, -11.73] |
| Masiello 2002 | 63.8 | 17.2 | 100 | 50.2 | 13 | 100 | 3.6% | 13.60 [9.37, 17.83] |
| Merka 2014 | 59.4 | 16 | 477 | 56.9 | 14.6 | 477 | 3.6% | 2.50 [0.56, 4.44] |
| Murzi 2011 | 83 | 20 | 100 | 74 | 28 | 100 | 3.6% | 9.00 [2.26, 15.74] |
| Sansone 2012 | 74.6 | 26.7 | 50 | 44.8 | 13.4 | 50 | 3.6% | 29.80 [21.52, 38.08] |
| Seitz 2017 | 76 | 35 | 53 | 76 | 17 | 53 | 3.5% | 0.00 [-10.48, 10.48] |
| Shehada 2015 | 65.6 | 18.4 | 585 | 64.3 | 19.8 | 585 | 3.6% | 1.30 [-0.89, 3.49] |
| Stolinski 2016 | 78.2 | 13.6 | 211 | 63.4 | 12.9 | 211 | 3.6% | 14.80 [12.27, 17.33] |
| Stolinski 2017 | 77.7 | 14.9 | 212 | 62.6 | 13.1 | 212 | 3.6% | 15.10 [12.43, 17.77] |
| Tabata 2007 | 81.9 | 31.8 | 41 | 71.6 | 30 | 41 | 3.5% | 10.30 [-3.08, 23.68] |
| Wang 2018 | 80.4 | 19.6 | 67 | 67.5 | 18.2 | 67 | 3.6% | 12.90 [6.50, 19.30] |
| Zhao 2018 | 79.5 | 12.5 | 91 | 72.9 | 11.8 | 91 | 3.6% | 6.60 [3.07, 10.13] |
| **Subtotal (95% CI)** | | | **4376** | | | **4376** | **78.6%** | **7.21 [3.98, 10.43]** |
| Heterogeneity: Tau² = 49.03; Chi² = 729.99, df = 21 (P < 0.00001); I² = 97% | | | | | | | | |
| Test for overall effect: Z = 4.38 (P < 0.0001) | | | | | | | | |
| **Total (95% CI)** | | | **4585** | | | **4585** | **100.0%** | **23.28 [5.69, 40.87]** |
| Heterogeneity: Tau² = 2240.41; Chi² = 35361.85, df = 27 (P < 0.00001); I² = 100% | | | | | | | | |
| Test for overall effect: Z = 2.59 (P = 0.009) | | | | | | | | |
| Test for subgroup differences: Chi² = 0.64, df = 1 (P = 0.42), I² = 0% | | | | | | | | |

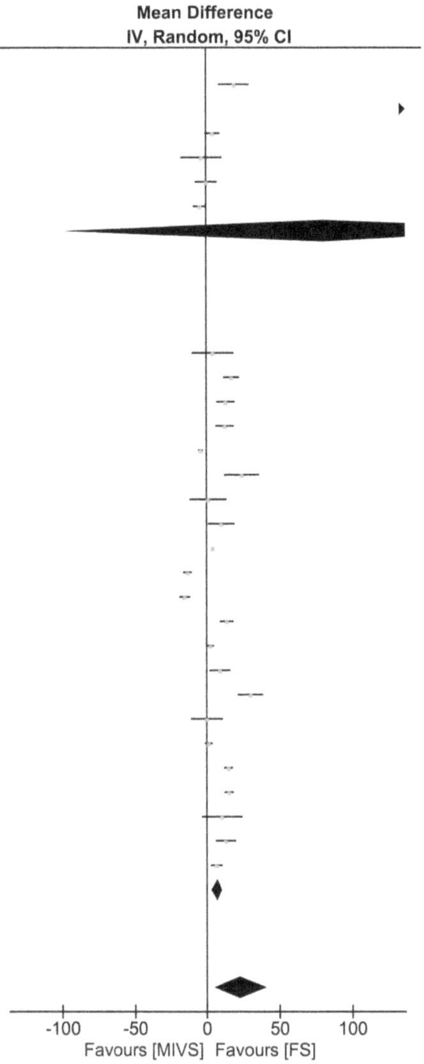


**FIGURE 8 |** The forests plot demonstrates aortic cross-clamp time (minutes) between MIVS and FS.

mostly because of insufficient surfactant release triggered by poor perfusion of the alveolar epithelium during CPB (49). Because of the more technical problem, patients in the MIVS group had a longer mean CPB duration than those in the FS group. However, we believe that this variation has no influence impact on postoperative pulmonary complications.

However, if CPB duration were the underlying cause, we would predict the MIVS group to have more significant postoperative pulmonary complications. This study found that patients who underwent MIVS had significantly longer cardiopulmonary bypass time, which may have contributed to the lower number of pulmonary complications observed in this group. A randomized clinical trial would be the only approach to analyze the influence of these independent factors on the incidence of postoperative pulmonary problems. MIVS did not result in an adverse postoperative pulmonary complication. It is likely that patients in whom the MIVS approach was used tended to have better early recovery and more favorable improvement of postoperative pulmonary function because of the shorter mechanical ventilation time, preservation of the chest wall integrity, and reduced postoperative pain, as compared with FS (50, 52, 53). Previous studies drew a similar conclusion to ours: there is less impaired respiratory function among patients who underwent surgery using the MIVS approach (11).

However, other investigators found no significant differences between the MIVS and FS regarding postoperative respiratory function system improvement (14, 15, 36, 54).

Moreover, we found that patients who underwent MIVS had a significant reduction in the incidence of early mortality (1.2%) compared with FS (1.9%). This finding was in line with that of previously published studies. A study by Mark et al. (30), who analyzed 477 PSM patients who underwent MIVS or FS, showed

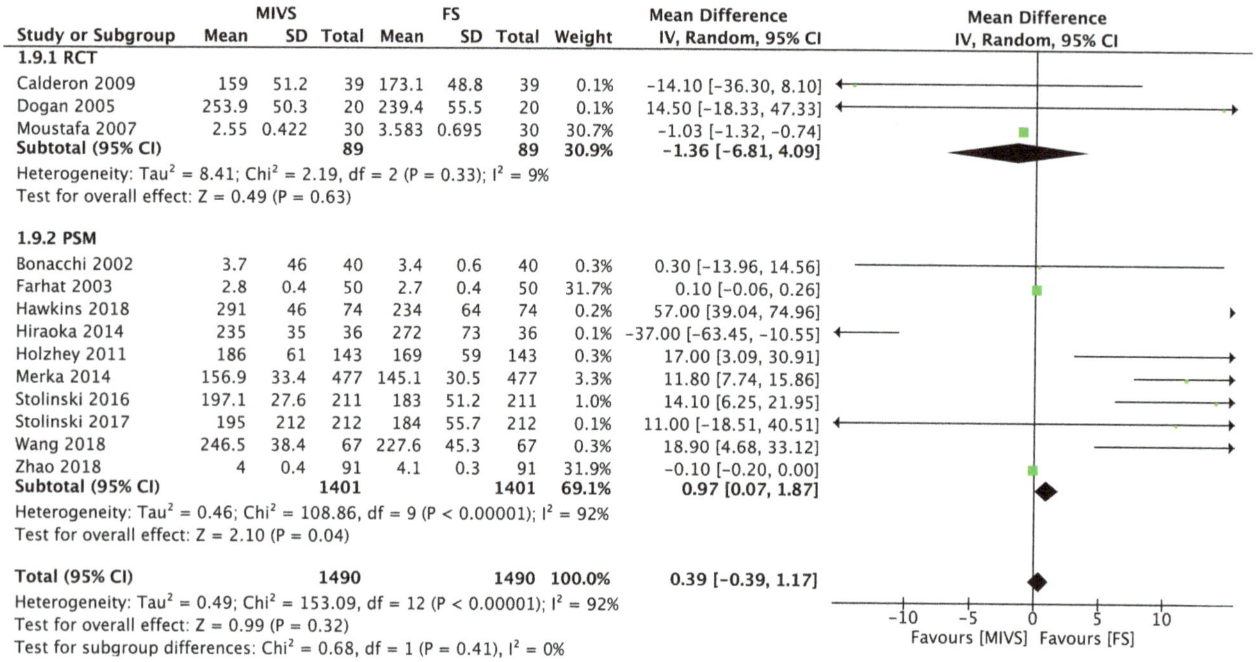


**FIGURE 9 |** The forests plot demonstrates operative time (hours) between MIVS and FS.

**TABLE 3 |** Overall analysis of demographic, intraoperative, and postoperative outcomes comparing MIVS and FS.

| Variables | n(N) | No. patients MIVS/FS | Overall effect WMD/OR (95% CI)† | *P* | Study heterogeneity | | | |
|---|---|---|---|---|---|---|---|---|
| | | | | | chi²-test | df | $I^2$(%) | *p* |
| Age, y ± SD | 30 (10,194) | 5,097/5,097 | −0.43 [−1.05, −0.18]† | 0.17 | 91.87 | 29 | 68 | <0.00001 |
| Male, % | 27 (9,628) | 4,814/4,814 | 1.01 [0.95, 1.12] | 0.48 | 9.61 | 26 | 0 | 1.00 |
| LVEF %, ± SD | 23 (2,910) | 3,455/3,455 | 0.65 [−0.09, 1.39]† | 0.09 | 1288.37 | 22 | 98 | <0.00001 |
| COPD, % | 17 (8,132) | 4,066/4,066 | 0.87 [0.74, 1.03] | 0.11 | 4.51 | 15 | 0 | 1.00 |
| Early mortality, % | 30 (10,194) | 5,097/5,097 | 0.68 [0.49, 0.95] | 0.02 | 14.42 | 26 | 0 | 0.97 |
| Blood transfusion (unit) ± SD | 10 (1,536) | 768/768 | −0.59 [−2.08, 0.90]† | 0.44 | 166.69 | 9 | 95 | <0.00001 |
| Blood transfusion (patient), % | 14 (5,756) | 2,878/2,878 | 0.69 [0.51, 0.93] | 0.02 | 48.53 | 13 | 73 | <0.00001 |
| CBP time ± SD | 27 (8,798) | 4,399/4,399 | 11.06 [4.29, 17.84]† | 0.001 | 1924.40 | 26 | 99 | <0.00001 |
| Cross clamping time, minutes ± SD | 28 (9,170) | 4,585/4,585 | 23.28 [5.69, 40.87]† | 0.009 | 35361.85 | 27 | 100 | <0.00001 |
| Operative time, minutes ± SD | 13 (2980) | 1,490/1,490 | 0.39 [−0.39, 1.17]† | 0.32 | 153.09 | 12 | 92 | <0.00001 |

*COPD, chronic obstructive pulmonary disease; CBP, cardiopulmonary bypass; CI, confidence interval; FS, Full sternotomy; $I^2$, test of heterogeneity; LVEF, left ventricular ejection fraction; MIVS, minimally invasive valve surgery; n, number of studies; N, number of participants; OR, odds ratio; SD, standard deviation; WMD, weighted mean difference;* †*Values of WMD.*

that MIVS was associated with lower hospital mortality (0.4 vs. 2.3%, respectively). This result was also in line with the results of Paparella et al. (55), who reported on 5,801 patients from different centers who underwent mini-aortic valve replacement vs. conventional aortic valve replacement.

Shehada et al. and Johnston et al. (26, 34) reported on 2,103 and 2,689 patients, respectively, in PSM analyses that compared minimally invasive to conventional aortic valve surgery. They reported a significantly lower incidence of the need for blood transfusion, as well as respiratory insufficiency in MIVS patients. Similarly, we found that the number of patients who required blood transfusion and the number of units of RBC required for transfusion were significantly reduced in MIVS than in FS.

Our observations provide evidence for the value of MIVS as an acceptable alternative option to traditional FS for patients at higher risk of developing pulmonary complications and for patients with chronic lung

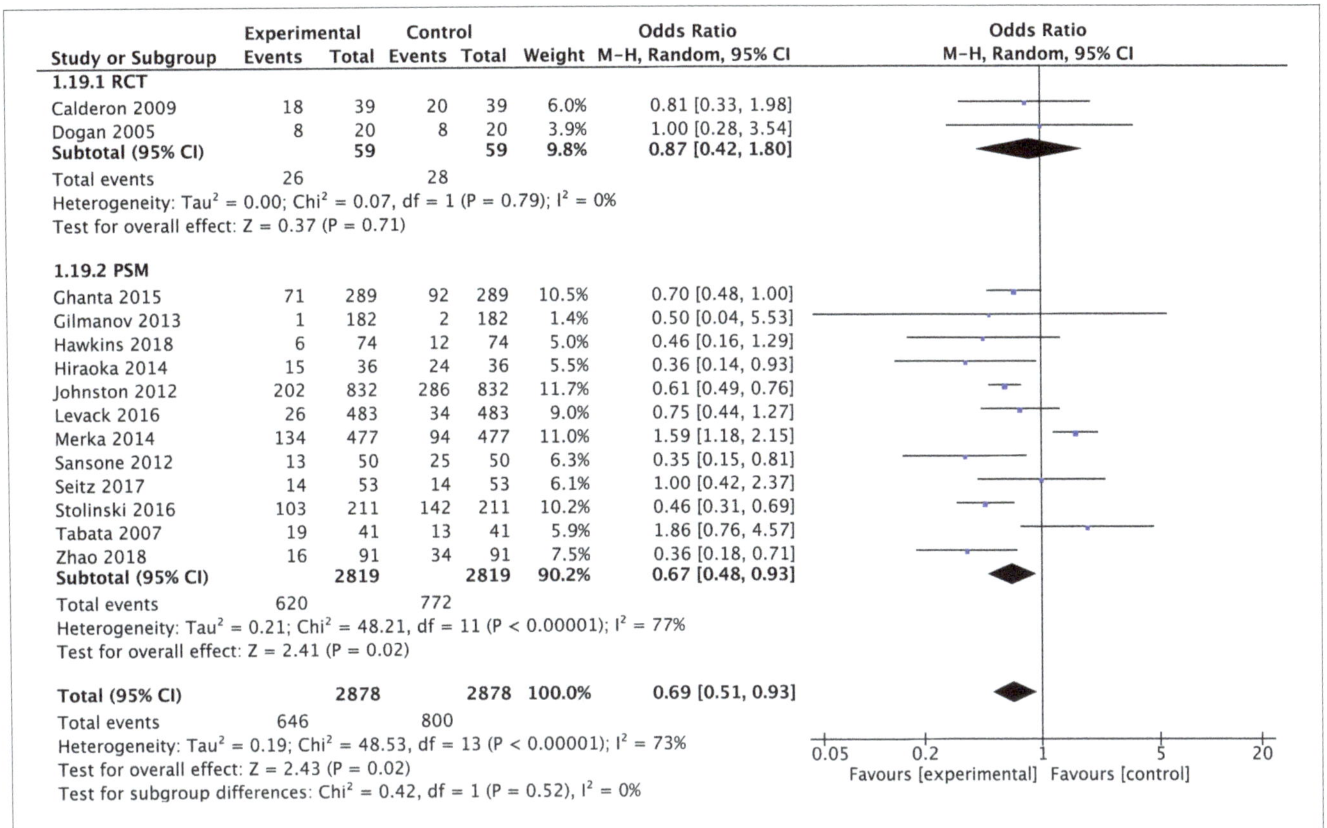


**FIGURE 10** | Forest plot of patients transfused red blood cells between MIVS and FS.

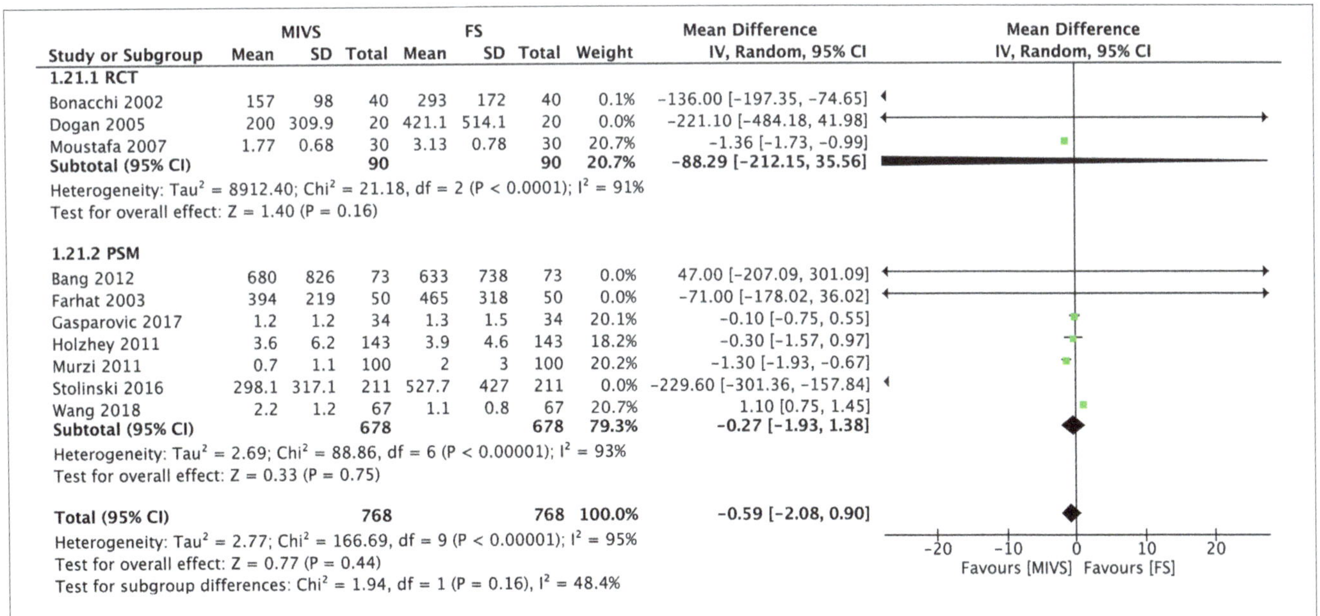


**FIGURE 11** | Forest plot of units of red blood transfused between MIVS and FS.

disease and chronic obstructive pulmonary disease undergoing mitral or/and aortic valve operations (12, 56).

Nevertheless, our study has certain limitations. Most studies did not report similar outcomes, and there was limited information about the pulmonary effects of MIVS. Follow-up for most studies was limited; hence, we were unable to compare long-term results.

## CONCLUSIONS

Based on the above findings in our meta-analysis, MIVS, both mitral and aortic, seem to provide better clinical and surgical outcomes than FS, particularly the benefits of early recovery of postoperative respiratory system functions and reduced incidence of postoperative pulmonary complications. Moreover, MIVS was not associated with an increased incidence of early mortality or a greater need for blood transfusion than FS. We believe that our findings might help surgeons in patient selection, particularly when dealing with patients with a high risk of pulmonary disease undergoing cardiac valve surgical repair or replacement. Finally, further studies comparing MIVS and FS are recommended to validate our findings.

## AUTHOR CONTRIBUTIONS

MM and SA: data analysis/writing. MM and SD: data collection/writing. RL, ND, CC, and XW: reviewers/editing. All authors contributed to the article and approved the submitted version.

## REFERENCES

1. Doll N, Borger MA, Hain J, Bucerius J, Walther T, Gummert JF, et al. Minimal access aortic valve replacement: effects on morbidity and resource utilization. *Ann Thorac Surg.* (2002) 74:S1318–22. doi: 10.1016/s0003-4975(02)03911-5
2. Chitwood WR, Wixon CL, Elbeery JR, Moran JF, Chapman WHH, Lust RM. Video-assisted minimally invasive mitral valve surgery. *J Thorac Cardiov Sur.* (1997) 114:773–80. doi: 10.1016/S0022-5223(97)70081-3
3. Boix-Garibo R, Uzzaman MM, Bapat VN. Review of minimally invasive aortic valve surgery. *Interv Cardiol.* (2015) 10:144–48. doi: 10.15420/icr.2015.10.03.144
4. Bouhout I, Morgant MC, Bouchard D. Minimally invasive heart valve surgery. *Can J Cardiol.* (2017) 33:1129–37. doi: 10.1016/j.cjca.2017.05.014
5. Moustafa MA, Abdelsamad AA, Zakaria G, Omarah MM. Minimal vs median sternotomy for aortic valve replacement. *Asian Cardiovasc Thorac Ann.* (2007) 15:472–5. doi: 10.1177/021849230701500605
6. Aris A, Camara ML, Montiel J, Delgado LJ, Galan J, Litvan H. Ministernotomy versus median sternotomy for aortic valve replacement: a prospective, randomized study. *Ann Thorac Surg.* (1999) 67:1583–7. doi: 10.1016/s0003-4975(99)00362-8
7. Cheng DC, Martin J, Lal A, Diegeler A, Folliguet TA, Nifong LW, et al. Minimally invasive versus conventional open mitral valve surgery: a meta-analysis and systematic review. *Innovations.* (2011) 6:84–103. doi: 10.1097/IMI.0b013e3182167feb
8. Miskovic A, Lumb AB. Postoperative pulmonary complications. *Br J Anaesth.* (2017) 118:317–34. doi: 10.1093/bja/aex002
9. Weissman C. Pulmonary complications after cardiac surgery. *Semin Cardiothorac Vasc Anesth.* (2004) 8:185–211. doi: 10.1177/108925320400800303
10. Canet J, Gallart L, Gomar C, Paluzie G, Valles J, Castillo J, et al. Prediction of postoperative pulmonary complications in a population-based surgical cohort. *Anesthesiology.* (2010) 113:1338–50. doi: 10.1097/ALN.0b013e3181fc6e0a
11. Weissman C. Pulmonary function after cardiac and thoracic surgery. *Curr Opin Anaesthesiol.* (2000) 13:47–51. doi: 10.1097/00000539-199906000-00014
12. Albacker TB, Blackstone EH, Williams SJ, Gillinov AM, Navia JL, Roselli EE, et al. Should less-invasive aortic valve replacement be avoided in patients with pulmonary dysfunction? *J Thorac Cardiovasc Surg.* (2014) 147:355–61. doi: 10.1016/j.jtcvs.2012.12.014
13. Bang JH, Kim JW, Lee JW, Kim JB, Jung SH, Choo SJ, et al. Minimally invasive approaches versus conventional sternotomy for aortic valve replacement: a propensity score matching study. *Korean J Thorac Cardiovasc Surg.* (2012) 45:80–4. doi: 10.5090/kjtcs.2012.45.2.80
14. Bonacchi M, Prifti E, Giunti G, Frati G, Sani G. Does ministernotomy improve postoperative outcome in aortic valve operation? A prospective randomized study. *Ann Thorac Surg.* (2002) 73:460–5. doi: 10.1016/s0003-4975(01)03402-6
15. Calderon J, Richebe P, Guibaud JP, Coiffic A, Branchard O, Asselineau J, et al. Prospective randomized study of early pulmonary evaluation of patients scheduled for aortic valve surgery performed by ministernotomy or total median sternotomy. *J Cardiothorac Vasc Anesth.* (2009) 23:795–801. doi: 10.1053/j.jvca.2009.03.011
16. Dogan S, Aybek T, Risteski PS, Detho F, Rapp A, Wimmer-Greinecker G, et al. Minimally invasive port access versus conventional mitral valve surgery: prospective randomized study. *Ann Thorac Surg.* (2005) 79:492–8. doi: 10.1016/j.athoracsur.2004.08.066
17. Farhat F, Lu Z, Lefevre M, Montagna P, Mikaeloff P, Jegaden O. Prospective comparison between total sternotomy and ministernotomy for aortic valve replacement. *J Card Surg.* (2003) 18:396–401. doi: 10.1046/j.1540-8191.2003.02047.x
18. Gasparovic I, Artemiou P, Hudec V, Hulman M. Long-term outcomes following minimal invasive versus conventional aortic valve replacement: a propensity match analysis. *Bratisl Lek Listy.* (2017) 118:479–84. doi: 10.4149/BLL_2017_092
19. Ghanta RK, Lapar DJ, Kern JA, Kron IL, Speir AM, Fonner E, et al. Minimally invasive aortic valve replacement provides equivalent outcomes at reduced cost compared with conventional aortic valve replacement: A real-world multi-institutional analysis. *J Thorac Cardiovasc Surg.* (2015) 149:1060–5. doi: 10.1016/j.jtcvs.2015.01.014
20. Gilmanov D, Bevilacqua S, Murzi M, Cerillo AG, Gasbarri T, Kallushi E, et al. Minimally invasive and conventional aortic valve replacement: a propensity score analysis. *Ann Thorac Surg.* (2013) 96:837–43. doi: 10.1016/j.athoracsur.2013.04.102
21. Gilmanov D, Farneti PA, Ferrarini M, Santarelli F, Murzi M, Miceli A, et al. Full sternotomy versus right anterior minithoracotomy for isolated aortic valve replacement in octogenarians: a propensity-matched study dagger. *Interact Cardiovasc Thorac Surg.* (2015) 20:732–41. doi: 10.1093/icvts/ivv030
22. Hawkins RB, Mehaffey JH, Kessel SM, Dahl JJ, Kron IL, Kern JA, et al. Minimally invasive mitral valve surgery is associated with excellent resource utilization, cost, and outcomes. *J Thorac Cardiovasc Surg.* (2018) 156:611–16. doi: 10.1016/j.jtcvs.2018.03.108
23. Hiraoka A, Totsugawa T, Kuinose M, Nakajima K, Chikazawa G, Tamura K, et al. Propensity score-matched analysis of minimally invasive aortic valve replacement. *Circ J.* (2014) 78:2876–81. doi: 10.1253/circj.CJ-14-0861
24. Holzhey DM, Shi W, Borger MA, Seeburger J, Garbade J, Pfannmuller B, et al. Minimally invasive versus sternotomy approach for mitral valve surgery in patients greater than 70 years old: a propensity-matched comparison. *Ann Thorac Surg.* (2011) 91:401–5. doi: 10.1016/j.athoracsur.2010.08.006
25. Iribarne A, Russo MJ, Easterwood R, Hong KN, Yang J, Cheema FH, et al. Minimally invasive versus sternotomy approach for mitral valve surgery: a propensity analysis. *Ann Thorac Surg.* (2010) 90:1471–7. doi: 10.1016/j.athoracsur.2010.06.034
26. Johnston DR, Atik FA, Rajeswaran J, Blackstone EH, Nowicki ER, Sabik JF, et al. Outcomes of less invasive J-incision approach to aortic valve surgery. *J Thorac Cardiovasc Surg.* (2012) 144:852–58. doi: 10.1016/j.jtcvs.2011.12.008
27. Levack MM, Aftab M, Roselli EE, Johnston DR, Soltesz EG, Gillinov AM, et al. Outcomes of a less-invasive approach for proximal aortic operations. *Ann Thorac Surg.* (2017) 103:533–40. doi: 10.1016/j.athoracsur.2016.06.008
28. Machler HE, Bergmann P, Anelli-Monti M, Dacar D, Rehak P, Knez I, et al. Minimally invasive versus conventional aortic valve operations: a prospective study in 120 patients. *Ann Thorac Surg.* (1999) 67:1001–5. doi: 10.1016/s0003-4975(99)00072-7

29. Masiello P, Coscioni E, Panza A, Triumbari F, Preziosi G, Di Benedetto G. Surgical results of aortic valve replacement via partial upper sternotomy: comparison with median sternotomy. *Cardiovasc Surg.* (2002) 10:333–8. doi: 10.1016/s0967-2109(02)00026-1
30. Merk DR, Lehmann S, Holzhey DM, Dohmen P, Candolfi P, Misfeld M, et al. Minimal invasive aortic valve replacement surgery is associated with improved survival: a propensity-matched comparison. *Eur J Cardiothorac Surg.* (2015) 47:11–7. doi: 10.1093/ejcts/ezu068
31. Murzi M, Cerillo AG, Bevilacqua S, Gilmanov D, Farneti P, Glauber M. Traversing the learning curve in minimally invasive heart valve surgery: a cumulative analysis of an individual surgeon's experience with a right minithoracotomy approach for aortic valve replacement. *Eur J Cardiothorac Surg.* (2012) 41:1242–6. doi: 10.1093/ejcts/ezr230
32. Sansone F, Punta G, Parisi F, Dato GM, Zingarelli E, Flocco R, et al. Right minithoracotomy versus full sternotomy for the aortic valve replacement: preliminary results. *Heart Lung Circ.* (2012) 21:169–73. doi: 10.1016/j.hlc.2011.10.004
33. Seitz M, Goldblatt J, Paul E, Marcus T, Larobina M, Yap CH. Minimally invasive aortic valve replacement via right anterior mini-thoracotomy: propensity matched initial experience. *Heart Lung Circ.* (2019) 28:320–26. doi: 10.1016/j.hlc.2017.11.012
34. Shehada SE, Ozturk O, Wottke M, Lange R. Propensity score analysis of outcomes following minimal access versus conventional aortic valve replacement. *Eur J Cardiothorac Surg.* (2016) 49:464–9. doi: 10.1093/ejcts/ezv061
35. Stolinski J, Musial R, Plicner D, Fijorek K, Medrzycki M, Andres J, et al. Respiratory functional status after conventional and minimally invasive aortic valve replacement surgery - a propensity score analysis. *Kardiochir Torakochirurgia Pol.* (2017) 14:5–9. doi: 10.5114/kitp.2017.66922
36. Stolinski J, Plicner D, Grudzien G, Wasowicz M, Musial R, Andres J, et al. A comparison of minimally invasive and standard aortic valve replacement. *J Thorac Cardiovasc Surg.* (2016) 152:1030–9. doi: 10.1016/j.jtcvs.2016.06.012
37. Tabata M, Umakanthan R, Cohn LH, Bolman RM, 3rd, Shekar PS, Chen FY, et al. Early and late outcomes of 1000 minimally invasive aortic valve operations. *Eur J Cardiothorac Surg.* (2008) 33:537–41. doi: 10.1016/j.ejcts.2007.12.037
38. Wang Q, Xi W, Gao Y, Shen H, Min J, Yang J, et al. Short-term outcomes of minimally invasive mitral valve repair: a propensity-matched comparison. *Interact Cardiovasc Thorac Surg.* (2018) 26:805–12. doi: 10.1093/icvts/ivx402
39. Zhao D, Wei L, Zhu SJ, Zhang Z, Liu H, Yang Y, et al. Combined mitral and aortic valve procedure via right mini-thoracotomy versus full median sternotomy insights from a single-center study of propensity-matched data. *Int Heart J.* (2019) 60:336–44. doi: 10.1536/ihj.18-186
40. Higgins JPT, Altman DG. Assessing risk of bias in included studies. In: Higgins JPT, Green S, editors. *Cochrane Handbook for Systematic Reviews of Interventions.* Chichester: Wiley (2008). p. 187–241.
41. Ottawa Hospital Research Institu. *The Newcastle-Ottawa Scale (nos) for Assessing the Quality of Nonrandomised Studies in Meta-Analyses.* (2019). Available online at: http://www.ohri.ca/programs/clinical_epidemiology/oxford.asp (accessed August 14, 2019).
42. Jadad AR, Carroll D, Glynn CJ, Moore RA, McQuay HJ. Morphine responsiveness of chronic pain: double-blind randomised crossover study with patient-controlled analgesia. *Lancet.* (1992) 339:1367–71. doi: 10.1016/0140-6736(92)91194-d
43. Gallart L, Canet J. Post-operative pulmonary complications: understanding definitions and risk assessment. *Best Pract Res Clin Anaesthesiol.* (2015) 29:315–30. doi: 10.1016/j.bpa.2015.10.004
44. Szelkowski LA, Puri NK, Singh R, Massimiano PS. Current trends in preoperative, intraoperative, and postoperative care of the adult cardiac surgery patient. *Curr Problems Surg.* (2014) 52:531–69. doi: 10.1067/j.cpsurg.2014.10.001
45. Tanner TG, Colvin MO. Pulmonary complications of cardiac surgery. *Lung.* (2020) 198:889–96. doi: 10.1007/s00408-020-00405-7
46. Moher D, Liberati A, Tetzlaff J, Altman DG, Group P. Preferred reporting items for systematic reviews and meta-analyses: the PRISMA statement. *PLoS Med.* (2009) 6:e1000097. doi: 10.1371/journal.pmed.1000097
47. Cosgrove DM, 3rd, Sabik JF. Minimally invasive approach for aortic valve operations. *Ann Thorac Surg.* (1996) 62:596–7.
48. Badenes R, Lozano A, Belda FJ. Postoperative pulmonary dysfunction and mechanical ventilation in cardiac surgery. *Crit Care Res Pract.* (2015) 2015:420513. doi: 10.1155/2015/420513
49. Chetta A, Bobbio A, Aiello M, Del Donno M, Castagnaro A, Comel A, et al. Changes in lung function and respiratory muscle strength after sternotomy vs. laparotomy in patients without ventilatory limitation. *Eur Surg Res.* (2006) 38:489–93. doi: 10.1159/000096008
50. e Silva AM, Saad R, Stirbulov R, Rivetti LA. Off-pump versus on-pump coronary artery revascularization: effects on pulmonary function. *Interact Cardiovasc Thorac Surg.* (2010) 11:42–5. doi: 10.1510/icvts.2009.229617
51. Ragnarsdottir M, KristjAnsdottir A, Ingvarsdottir I, Hannesson P, Torfason B, Cahalin L. Short-term changes in pulmonary function and respiratory movements after cardiac surgery via median sternotomy. *Scand Cardiovasc J.* (2004) 38:46–52. doi: 10.1080/14017430310016658
52. Shenkman Z, Shir Y, Weiss YG, Bleiberg B, Gross D. The effects of cardiac surgery on early and late pulmonary functions. *Acta Anaesthesiol Scand.* (1997) 41:1193–9.
53. Khoshbin E, Prayaga S, Kinsella J, Sutherland FW. Mini-sternotomy for aortic valve replacement reduces the length of stay in the cardiac intensive care unit: meta-analysis of randomised controlled trials. *BMJ Open.* (2011) 1:e000266. doi: 10.1136/bmjopen-2011-000266
54. Lim JY, Deo SV, Altarabsheh SE, Jung SH, Erwin PJ, Markowitz AH, et al. Conventional versus minimally invasive aortic valve replacement: pooled analysis of propensity-matched data. *J Card Surg.* (2015) 30:125–34. doi: 10.1111/jocs.12493
55. Paparella D, Malvindi PG, Santarpino G, Moscarelli M, Guida P, Fattouch K, et al. Full sternotomy and minimal access approaches for surgical aortic valve replacement: a multicentre propensity-matched study. *Eur J Cardiothorac Surg.* (2020) 57:709–16. doi: 10.1093/ejcts/ezz286
56. Santana O, Reyna J, Benjo AM, Lamas GA, Lamelas J. Outcomes of minimally invasive valve surgery in patients with chronic obstructive pulmonary disease. *Eur J Cardiothorac Surg.* (2012) 42:648–52. doi: 10.1093/ejcts/ezs098

# Permissions

All chapters in this book were first published by Frontiers; hereby published with permission under the Creative Commons Attribution License or equivalent. Every chapter published in this book has been scrutinized by our experts. Their significance has been extensively debated. The topics covered herein carry significant findings which will fuel the growth of the discipline. They may even be implemented as practical applications or may be referred to as a beginning point for another development.

The contributors of this book come from diverse backgrounds, making this book a truly international effort. This book will bring forth new frontiers with its revolutionizing research information and detailed analysis of the nascent developments around the world.

We would like to thank all the contributing authors for lending their expertise to make the book truly unique. They have played a crucial role in the development of this book. Without their invaluable contributions this book wouldn't have been possible. They have made vital efforts to compile up to date information on the varied aspects of this subject to make this book a valuable addition to the collection of many professionals and students.

This book was conceptualized with the vision of imparting up-to-date information and advanced data in this field. To ensure the same, a matchless editorial board was set up. Every individual on the board went through rigorous rounds of assessment to prove their worth. After which they invested a large part of their time researching and compiling the most relevant data for our readers.

The editorial board has been involved in producing this book since its inception. They have spent rigorous hours researching and exploring the diverse topics which have resulted in the successful publishing of this book. They have passed on their knowledge of decades through this book. To expedite this challenging task, the publisher supported the team at every step. A small team of assistant editors was also appointed to further simplify the editing procedure and attain best results for the readers.

Apart from the editorial board, the designing team has also invested a significant amount of their time in understanding the subject and creating the most relevant covers. They scrutinized every image to scout for the most suitable representation of the subject and create an appropriate cover for the book.

The publishing team has been an ardent support to the editorial, designing and production team. Their endless efforts to recruit the best for this project, has resulted in the accomplishment of this book. They are a veteran in the field of academics and their pool of knowledge is as vast as their experience in printing. Their expertise and guidance has proved useful at every step. Their uncompromising quality standards have made this book an exceptional effort. Their encouragement from time to time has been an inspiration for everyone.

The publisher and the editorial board hope that this book will prove to be a valuable piece of knowledge for researchers, students, practitioners and scholars across the globe.

# List of Contributors

**Guangxian Chen, Lin Huang, Zhuoming Zhou, Jiantao Chen, Guangguo Fu, Jian Hou, Sida Chen, Suiqing Huang, Yuan Yue, Liqun Shang, Linhua Lv, Mengya Liang and Zhongkai Wu**
Department of Cardiac Surgery, The First Affiliated Hospital of Sun Yat-Sen University, Guangzhou, China
NHC Key Laboratory of Assisted Circulation, Sun Yat-Sen University, Guangzhou, China

**Divyatha Arun**
Department of Endocrinology, Columbia Asia Referral Hospital, A Unit of Manipal Hospital, Yeshwanthpur, Bengaluru, India

**Wahaj Munir, Lara Victoria Schmitt, Rohan Vyas and Jeuela Iris Ravindran**
Barts and the London School of Medicine and Dentistry, Queen Mary University of London, London, United Kingdom

**Mohamad Bashir, Bashi Velayudhan and Mohammed Idhrees**
Institue of Cardiac and Aortic Disorders, SRM Institutes for Medical Science (SIMS Hospitals), Chennai, India

**Ian Michael Williams**
Vascular Surgery, University Hospital of Wales, Cardiff, United Kingdom

**Dongjie Li, Yulin Guo, Yingdi Gao, Xiangguang An, Yan Liu, Song Gu, Xitao Zhang, Jie Gao and Pixiong Su**
Department of Cardiac Surgery, Heart Center and Beijing Key Laboratory of Hypertension, Beijing Chaoyang Hospital, Capital Medical University, Beijing, China

**Jiuchang Zhong**
Heart Center and Beijing Key Laboratory of Hypertension, Beijing Chaoyang Hospital, Capital Medical University, Beijing, China

**Gabby Elbaz-Greener, Merav Yarkoni, Ronny Alcalai and David Planer**
Department of Cardiology, Hadassah Medical Center, Jerusalem, Israel
Faculty of Medicine, Hebrew University of Jerusalem, Jerusalem, Israel

**Guy Rozen**
Cardiology Division, Hillel Yaffe Medical Center, Hadera, Israel
The Ruth and Bruce Rappaport Faculty of Medicine, Technion, Haifa, Israel
Cardiology Division, Harvard Medical School, Massachusetts General Hospital, Boston, MA, United States

**Offer Amir**
Department of Cardiology, Hadassah Medical Center, Jerusalem, Israel
Faculty of Medicine, Hebrew University of Jerusalem, Jerusalem, Israel
Division of Cardiovascular Medicine, Baruch Padeh Medical Center, Poriya, Israel
The Azrieli Faculty of Medicine in the Galilee, Bar-Ilan University, Safed, Israel

**Shemy Carasso, Fabio Kusniec and Ibrahim Marai**
Division of Cardiovascular Medicine, Baruch Padeh Medical Center, Poriya, Israel
The Azrieli Faculty of Medicine in the Galilee, Bar-Ilan University, Safed, Israel

**Bradley Strauss and Harindra C. Wijeysundera**
Division of Cardiology, Schulich Heart Centre, Sunnybrook Health Sciences Centre, University of Toronto, Toronto, ON, Canada

**Frank W. Smart**
Louisiana State University School of Medicine, New Orleans, LA, United States

**Eldad Erez**
Department of Cardio Surgery, Hadassah Medical Center, Hebrew University of Jerusalem, Jerusalem, Israel

**Yige Huyan, Yuan Chang and Jiangping Song**
The Cardiomyopathy Research Group at Fuwai Hospital, State Key Laboratory of Cardiovascular Disease, Chinese Academy of Medical Sciences and Peking Union Medical College, Beijing, China

**Jiehui Li, Shuiyun Wang, Hansong Sun, Jianping Xu, Chao Dong, Min Song and Qibin Yu**
State Key Laboratory of Cardiovascular Disease, Department of Cardiac Surgery, National Center for Cardiovascular Diseases, Peking Union Medical College, Fuwai Hospital, Chinese Academy of Medical Sciences, Beijing, China

**Ming-Chon Hsiung, Kuan-Chih Huang and Wei-Hsuan Chiang**
Heart Center, Cheng Hsin General Hospital, Taipei, Taiwan

**Wei-Hsian Yin**
Heart Center, Cheng Hsin General Hospital, Taipei, Taiwan
Faculty of Medicine, National Yang Ming University, Taipei, Taiwan

**Yung-Tsai Lee**
Heart Center, Cheng Hsin General Hospital, Taipei, Taiwan
School of Medicine, Institute of Microbiology and Immunology, National Yang Ming University, Taipei, Taiwan

**Tien-Ping Tsao, Kuo-Chen Lee and Jeng Wei**
Heart Center, Cheng Hsin General Hospital, Taipei, Taiwan
Faculty of Medicine, National Defense Medical Center, Taipei, Taiwan

**Pei-En Chen**
Institute of Health Policy and Management, National Taiwan University, Taipei, Taiwan
Taiwan Association of Health Industry Management and Development, Taipei, Taiwan

**Tao-Hsin Tung**
Department of Medical Research and Education, Cheng Hsin General Hospital, Taipei, Taiwan
Evidence-Based Medicine Center, Taizhou Hospital of Zhejiang Province, Wenzhou Medical University, Linhai, China

**Aleksander Dokollari**
St. Michael's Hospital, Toronto, ON, Canada

**Basel Ramlawi, Gianluca Torregrossa, Michel Pompeu Sá and Serge Sicouri**
Department of Cardiac Surgery, Lankenau Heart Institute, Wynnewood, PA, United States
Department of Cardiac Surgery Research, Lankenau Institute for Medical Research, Wynnewood, PA, United States

**Edvin Prifti**
Mother Teresa Hospital, University of Tirana, Tirana, Albania

**Sandro Gelsomino**
Department of Cardiac Surgery, Maastricht University Medical Center, Maastricht, Netherlands
Department of Cardiothoracic Surgery, Cardiovascular Research Institute Maastricht—CARIM, Maastricht, Netherlands

**Massimo Bonacchi**
Cardiac Surgery Unit, Department of Experimental and Clinical Medicine, University of Florence, Florence, Italy

**Thaïs Pittet**
Cardiology Department, University Fribourg, Fribourg, Switzerland

**Stéphane Cook, Gregory Khatchatourov and Nicolas Theumann**
Hirslanden Clinics Lausanne, Lausanne, Switzerland

**Cristina Barbero, Erik Cura Stura, Claudia Calia, Viviana Sebastiano, Giovanni Marchetto and**

**Massimo Boffini**
Department of Cardiovascular Surgery, Città della Salute e della Scienza, University of Turin, Turin, Italy
Mauro Rinaldi and Marco Pocar Department of Cardiovascular Surgery, Città della Salute e della Scienza, University of Turin, Turin, Italy
Department of Clinical Sciences and Community Health, University of Milan, Milan, Italy

**Claudia Filippini**
Department of Anesthesia and Critical Care,University of Turin, Turin, Italy

**Davide Ricci**
Cardiac Surgery Unit, Scientific Institute for Research, Hospitalization and Healthcare Policlinic Hospital San Martino, Genova, Italy
Department of Integrated Surgical and Diagnostic Sciences, University of Genova, Genova, Italy

**Xiaogao Pan, Yang Zhou, Guifang Yang, Zhibiao He, Hongliang Zhang, Zhenyu Peng, Wen Peng, Tuo Guo, Mengping Zeng and Xiangping Chai**
Department of Emergency Medicine, Second Xiangya Hospital, Central South University, Changsha, China
Emergency Medicine and Difficult Diseases Institute, Second Xiangya Hospital, Central South University, Changsha, China

**Ning Ding**
Emergency Department, Changsha Central Hospital, University of South China, Changsha, China

**Tomonori Shirasaka, Shingo Kunioka, Yuta Kikuchi, Natsuya Isikawa and Hiroyuki Kamiya**
Department of Cardiac Surgery, Asahikawa Medical University, Asahikawa, Japan

**Hirotsugu Kanda**
Department of Anesthesiology and Critical Care Medicine, Asahikawa Medical University, Asahikawa, Japan

**David Levy, Driss Laghlam, Philippe Estagnasie, Alain Brusset, Pierre Squara and Lee S. Nguyen**
Intensive Care Medicine Department, CMC Ambroise Paré, Neuilly-sur-Seine, France

**Xuelian Chen, Jia Yang and Siwen Wang**
Division of Nephrology, Department of Medicine, West China Hospital of Sichuan University, Chengdu, China

**Jiaojiao Zhou**
Division of Ultrasound, West China Hospital, Sichuan University, Chengdu, China

**Miao Fang**
Department of Orthopedics, Second People's Hospital of Chengdu, Chengdu, China

**Xin Wang**
Department of Pediatric Nephrology, West China Second University Hospital, Sichuan University, Chengdu, China

**Linji Li and Tao Zhu**
Department of Anesthesiology, West China Hospital, Sichuan University, The Research Units of West China (2018RU012), Chinese Academy of Medical Sciences, Chengdu, China

**Ling Ji and Lichuan Yang**
Division of Nephrology, West China Hospital of Sichuan University, Chengdu, China

**Weina Li and Rong Cao**
Department of Anesthesiology, Chengdu Women's and Children's Central Hospital, Chengdu, China

**Fei Xu and Cheng Zhang**
Department of Anesthesiology, The Affiliated Hospital, School of Medicine, Chengdu Women's & Children's Central Hospital, UESTC, Chengdu, China
Department of Anesthesiology, Chengdu Women's and Children's Central Hospital, Chengdu, China

**Lunchang Wang, Junwei Wang, Feng Gu, Quanming Li, Hao He, Xin Li, Jian Qiu, Tun Wang, Chenzi Yang, Mo Wang, Jiehua Li, Hui Wang and Likun Sun**
Department of Vascular Surgery, The Second Xiangya Hospital of Central South University, Changsha, China
Vascular Disease Institute of Central South University, Changsha, China

**Chang Shu**
Department of Vascular Surgery, The Second Xiangya Hospital of Central South University, Changsha, China
Vascular Disease Institute of Central South University, Changsha, China
Department of Vascular Surgery, Fuwai Hospital, Chinese Academy of Medical Sciences & Peking Union Medical College, Beijing, China

**Yin Shi**
Department of Vascular Surgery, Fuwai Yunnan Cardiovascular Hospital, Kunming, China

**Ming Li**
Department of Vascular Surgery, Second Xiangya Hospital, Central South University, Changsha, China
Department of Vascular Surgery, The First Affiliated Hospital of Medical School of Zhejiang University, Hangzhou, China
Vascular Disease Institute of Central South University, Changsha, China

**Sheng Zhang, Dan Zheng, Xiao-Qiong Chu, Yong-Po Jiang, Qiao-Min Zhang, Lin-Zhu Qian, Wei-Ying Yang, Wen-Yuan Zhang and Rong-Hai Lin**
Department of Critical Care Medicine, Taizhou Hospital of Zhejiang Province, Wenzhou Medical University, Linhai, China

**Chun-Guo Wang**
Department of Cardiothoracic Surgery, Taizhou Hospital of Zhejiang Province, Wenzhou Medical University, Linhai, China

**Alina-Adriana Mistirian, Martin T. Yates and Wael I. Awad**
Department of Cardiothoracic Surgery, St Bartholomew's Hospital, London, United Kingdom

**Xiaodong Zhuang**
NHC Key Laboratory of Assisted Circulation, Sun Yat-Sen University, Guangzhou, China
Department of Cardiology, The First Affiliated Hospital of Sun Yat-Sen University, Guangzhou, China
Center for Information Technology & Statistics, The First Affiliated Hospital of Sun Yat-Sen University, Guangzhou, China

**Keke Wang**
Department of Emergency, The First Affiliated Hospital of Sun Yat-Sen University, Guangzhou, China

**Daniele Linardi, Romel Mani, Angela Murari, Maddalena Tessari, Sara Martinazzi, Giovanni B. Luciani, Giuseppe Faggian and Alessio Rungatscher**
Division of Cardiac Surgery, Department of Surgery, University of Verona, Verona, Italy

**Sissi Dolci, Loris Mannino and Ilaria Decimo**
Department of Pharmacology, University of Verona, Verona, Italy

**Leonardo Gottin**
Division of Cardio-Thoracic Anesthesiology and Intensive Care, Department of Surgery, University of Verona, Verona, Italy

**Yi Chang, Hongyuan Lin, Xiangyang Qian, Hongwei Guo, Cuntao Yu, Xiaogang Sun, Bo Wei, Qiong Ma, Yizhen Wei and Yi Shi**
Department of Vascular Surgery, National Center for Cardiovascular Diseases, Fuwai Hospital, Cardiovascular Institute, Chinese Academy of Medical Science & Peking Union Medical College, Beijing, China

**Jung-Chi Hsu**
Division of Cardiology, Department of Internal Medicine, Camillian Saint Mary's Hospital Luodong, Yilan, Taiwan
Division of Cardiology, Department of Internal Medicine, National Taiwan University Hospital, Taipei, Taiwan

**Chen-Yu Huang**
Division of Cardiology, Department of Internal Medicine, National Taiwan University Hospital, Taipei, Taiwan
Division of Cardiology, Department of Internal Medicine, Taoyuan General Hospital, Ministry of Health and Welfare, Taoyuan, Taiwan

**Shu-Lin Chuang**
Department of Medical Research, National Taiwan University Hospital, Taipei, Taiwan
Graduate Institute of Epidemiology and Preventive Medicine, College of Public Health, National Taiwan University, Taipei, Taiwan

**Hsu-Yu Yu, Yih-Sharng Chen and Chih-Hsien Wang**
Division of Cardiovascular Surgery, Department of Surgery, National Taiwan University Hospital and College of Medicine, National Taiwan University, Taipei, Taiwan

**Lian-Yu Lin**
Division of Cardiology, Department of Internal Medicine, National Taiwan University Hospital, Taipei, Taiwan
Department of Internal Medicine, College of Medicine, National Taiwan University, Taipei, Taiwan
Division of Electrophysiology, Cardiovascular Center, National Taiwan University Hospital, Taipei, Taiwan

**Chao Liu**
Department of Anesthesiology, The Affiliated Hospital, School of Medicine, Chengdu Women's & Children's Central Hospital, UESTC, Chengdu, China

**Siwei Bi**
West China of Medical School, Sichuan University, Chengdu, China

**Jun Gu**
Department of Cardiovascular Surgery, West China Hospital, Sichuan University, Chengdu, China

**Weiguo Fu**
Department of Vascular Surgery, Institute of Vascular Surgery, Zhongshan Hospital, Fudan University, Shanghai, China

**Erping Xi**
Department of Vascular Surgery, Wuhan General Hospital of Guangzhou Military Region, Wuhan, China

**Shuguang Guo**
Department of Vascular Surgery General Hospital of Chengdu Military Region, Kunming, China

**Xueming Chen**
Department of Vascular Surgery, Beijing Friendship Hospital, Capital Medical University, Beijing, China

**Zhanxiang Xiao**
Department of Vascular Surgery, Hainan Provincial People's Hospital, Haikou, China

**Shiqiang Yu**
Department of Vascular Surgery, The First Affiliated Hospital of the Fourth Military Medical University, Xi'an, China

**Jianhua Huang**
Department of Vascular Surgery, Xiangya Hospital, Central South University, Changsha, China

**Xiangchen Dai**
Department of Vascular Surgery, General Hospital of Tianjin Medical University, Tianjin, China

**Zhiwei Wang**
Department of Vascular Surgery, Wuhan University People's Hospital, Wuhan, China

**Wei Li**
Medical Research and Statistics Center, Fuwai Hospital, Chinese Academy of Medical Sciences, Beijing, China

**Qingshan Zheng**
Drug Clinical Research Center, Shanghai University of Traditional Chinese Medicine, Shanghai, China

**Mohamed Abdulkadir Mohamed, Shuai Ding, Cai Cheng and Xiang Wei**
Division of Cardiothoracic and Vascular Surgery, Tongji Hospital, Tongji Medical College, Huazhong University of Science and Technology, Wuhan, China

**Sayed Zulfiqar Ali Shah and Rui Li**
Department of Rehabilitation Medicine, Tongji Hospital, Tongji Medical College, Huazhong University of Science and Technology, Wuhan, China

**Najib Isse Dirie**
Division of Urology, Tongji Hospital, Tongji Medical College, Huazhong University of Science and Technology, Wuhan, China

# Index

www.ingramcontent.com/pod-product-compliance
Lightning Source LLC
LaVergne TN
LVHW082140200926
848484LV00008B/2085